Recent Advances in Renal Transplantation

Recent Advances in Renal Transplantation

Editor: Joe Taylor

FOSTER
ACADEMICS
www.fosteracademics.com

www.fosteracademics.com

FOSTER ACADEMICS

Cataloging-in-Publication Data

Recent advances in renal transplantation / edited by Joe Taylor.
p. cm.
Includes bibliographical references and index.
ISBN 978-1-63242-811-0
1. Kidneys--Transplantation. 2. Kidneys--Transplantation--Technique. 3. Kidneys--Surgery.
4. Kidneys--Diseases. 5. Transplantation of organs, tissues, etc. I. Taylor, Joe.
RD575 .R43 2019
617.461 059 2--dc23

Foster Academics,
118-35 Queens Blvd., Suite 400,
Forest Hills, NY 11375, USA

ISBN 978-1-63242-811-0 (Hardback)

Printed and bound in China.

Contents

Preface

The organ transplant of a kidney into a patient having end-stage renal disease is known as renal or kidney transplantation. Diabetes mellitus, malignant hypertension, infections, focal segmental glomerulosclerosis and polycystic kidney disease are some of the common disorders which often lead to end-stage renal disease. In case of renal transplantation, the donor and the recipient should be ABO blood group and crossmatch (human leukocyte antigen – HLA) compatible. The renal transplantation surgery usually takes around three hours. The transplanted donor kidney is placed in the lower abdomen and its blood vessels are then connected to the arteries and veins in the recipient's body. Renal transplantation is an upcoming field of medicine that has undergone rapid development over the past few decades. It strives to provide a fair idea about this discipline and to help develop a better understanding of the latest advances within this field. The book is appropriate for students seeking detailed information in this area as well as for doctors and experts.

All of the data presented henceforth, was collaborated in the wake of recent advancements in the field. The aim of this book is to present the diversified developments from across the globe in a comprehensible manner. The opinions expressed in each chapter belong solely to the contributing authors. Their interpretations of the topics are the integral part of this book, which I have carefully compiled for a better understanding of the readers.

At the end, I would like to thank all those who dedicated their time and efforts for the successful completion of this book. I also wish to convey my gratitude towards my friends and family who supported me at every step.

Editor

Beneficial Effect of Conversion to Belatacept in Kidney-Transplant Patients with a Low Glomerular-Filtration Rate

Julie Belliere,[1] Céline Guilbeau-Frugier,[2,3] Arnaud Del Bello,[1] Laure Esposito,[1] Caroline Capuani,[2,3] Isabelle Cardeau-Desangles,[1] Lionel Rostaing,[1,2,4] and Nassim Kamar[1,2,4]

[1] *Department of Nephrology and Organ Transplantation, CHU Rangueil, TSA 50032, 31059 Toulouse Cedex 9, France*
[2] *Université Paul Sabatier, 31062 Toulouse, France*
[3] *Department of Pathology, CHU Rangueil, 31059 Toulouse, France*
[4] *INSERM U1043, IFR-BMT, CHU Purpan, 31059 Toulouse, France*

Correspondence should be addressed to Nassim Kamar; kamar.n@chu-toulouse.fr

Academic Editor: Mariano Ferraresso

Belatacept has been found to be efficient at preserving good kidney function in maintenance kidney-transplant patients. Herein, we report on the use of belatacept as a rescue therapy for two kidney-transplant patients presenting with severe adverse events after treatment with calcineurin inhibitors (CNIs) and mammalian target-of-rapamycin (mTOR) inhibitors. Two kidney-transplant patients developed severely impaired kidney function after receiving CNIs. The use of everolimus was associated with severe angioedema. Belatacept was then successfully used to improve kidney function in both cases, even though estimated glomerular-filtration rate before conversion was <20 mL/min. These case reports show that belatacept can be used as a rescue therapy, even if kidney function is very low in kidney-transplant patients who cannot tolerate CNIs and/or mTOR inhibitors.

1. Introduction

Interstitial fibrosis and tubular atrophy (IFTA) are two of the major causes of graft loss after kidney transplantation. Calcineurin inhibitors (CNIs) are well known to have nephrotoxic effects on the kidney allograft, leading to IFTA and graft loss [1]. Mammalian target-of-rapamycin (mTOR) inhibitors, such as sirolimus and everolimus, have been used in CNI-free regimens or in association with low-dose CNIs to reduce CNI dosage and, thus, nephrotoxicity [2]. However, although mTOR-based immunosuppression regimens can improve kidney function and reduce IFTA, their safety profile remains worrisome [2]. Indeed, their side effects are often unpredictable and lead to interruption of treatment in 40% of cases [3]. Hence, in some situations, patients can be intolerant and/or contraindicated to the large majority of immunosuppressive drugs. Consequently, preserving graft function and avoiding acute rejection then become a medical challenge.

Recently, belatacept (CTLA4-Ig) has been developed to block CD80/86 and thereby inhibit T-cell costimulation [4, 5]. Two phase-III trials have compared the efficacy and safety of belatacept to that of cyclosporine A in association with mycophenolate mofetil (MMF) and steroids in *de novo* kidney-transplant patients who had received a kidney allograft from standard- and extended-criteria donors. In belatacept-treated patients, although the incidence of acute rejection was slightly higher, long-term kidney function was significantly improved [6–9]. In addition, tolerance to belatacept was excellent.

Another phase-III study has assessed the effect of converting from CNIs (cyclosporine A or tacrolimus) to belatacept. Kidney-transplant patients, who had an estimated glomerular-filtration rate (using the MDRD equation) of between 35 and 75 mL/min, were randomized to be either maintained on CNIs or were converted to belatacept [10, 11]. The data collected over 3 years showed significantly better

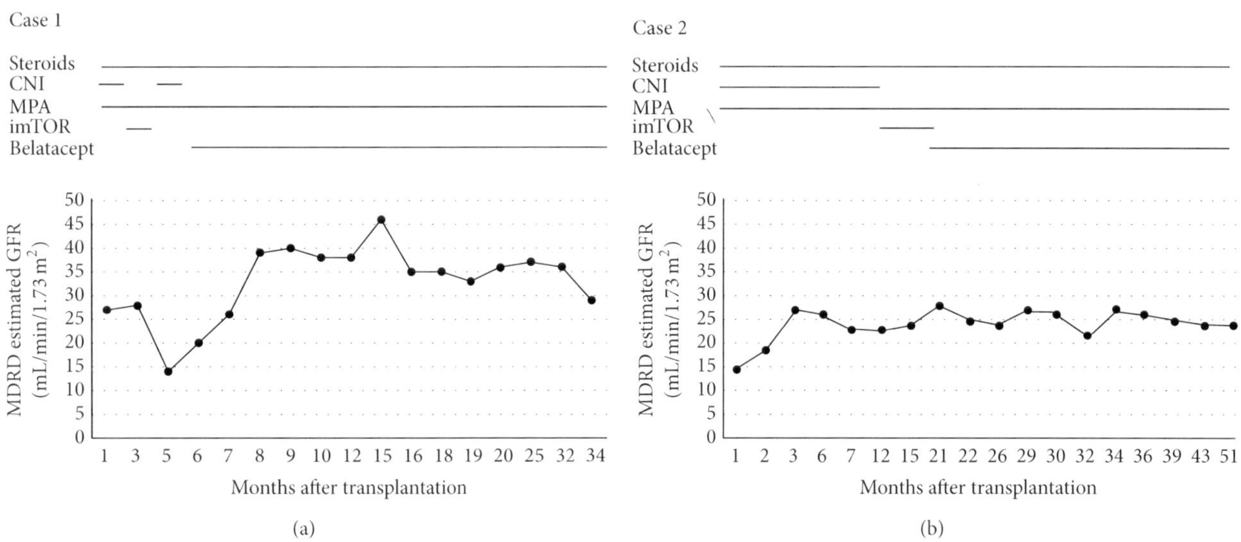

FIGURE 1: Kidney function. Glomerular-filtration rate (GFR) values were estimated with MDRD and reported for each case according to the time after transplantation. CNI: calcineurin inhibitors; MPA: mycophenolic acid; imTOR: mTOR (mammalian target of rapamycin) inhibitors.

kidney function in patients converted to belatacept compared to those receiving CNIs (either tacrolimus or cyclosporine A) [12]. The effect of conversion from CNIs to belatacept, as a rescue therapy for kidney-transplant patients with a glomerular-filtration rate (GFR) of <35 mL/min, is unknown.

Herein, we describe two kidney-transplant recipients with severe intolerance to CNIs and mTOR inhibitors who were successfully converted to belatacept. Glomerular-filtration rate (GFR) values are reported for each case in Figure 1.

2. Cases Reports

The patients' and donors' characteristics are presented in Table 1.

Case 1. A 52-year-old woman received a second kidney allograft for lupus nephritis and antiphospholipid antibody syndrome. The initial immunosuppressive therapy included basiliximab, tacrolimus, mycophenolic acid (MPA), and steroids. At one month after transplantation, because of persisting impaired kidney function (creatinine level 171 μmol/L, eGFR of 27 mL/min/1.73 m^2), a kidney biopsy was performed and showed ischemic tubular necrosis and signs of severe nephroangiosclerosis (t0 i0 g0 v0 ptc0 ah0 cg0 ci0 ct0 cv2 mm0, according to the Banff classification [13]), which was attributed to the donor, that is, a 77-year-old woman with a history of hypertension and who had died from a stroke. At that time, in order to avoid tacrolimus-induced nephrotoxicity, tacrolimus was replaced by everolimus. Kidney function remained unchanged. However, a switch back from everolimus to tacrolimus (target trough level 3–5 ng/mL) was done 2 months later because of severe angioedema. By five months after transplantation, the patient presented with heart failure, which was related to severe mitral-valve disease; thus, heart surgery was performed. After surgery, she developed acute kidney failure, which required dialysis for 6 days. Thereafter, her kidney function slightly improved but remained at ~400 μmol/L (eGFR of 10 mL/min/1.73 m^2). Hence, in order to avoid CNI-induced nephrotoxicity, tacrolimus was replaced by belatacept (5 mg/kg/month) at 6 months after transplantation, plus MPA (2 g/d) and steroids (5 mg/day). By 12 months after the switch, serum-creatinine level was 138 μmol/L and eGFR was 35 mL/min/1.73 m^2.

At the last follow-up, that is, 29 months after the switch, serum-creatinine level and eGFR were, respectively, 162 μmol/L and 29 mL/min/1.73 m^2. Proteinuria, which was 80 mg/g of creatinine before the switch, had decreased to 18 mg/g of creatinine at the last follow-up. Tolerance to the immunosuppressive treatment was excellent. No acute-rejection episode occurred and no donor-specific anti-HLA antibodies (DSAs) were detected using the Luminex single-antigen assay before or after the switch to belatacept.

Case 2. A 69-year-old man received a first kidney allograft for vascular nephropathy from an extended-criteria donor. The donor was a 74-year-old man with a history of diabetes and hypertension. The initial immunosuppressive therapy was based on basiliximab, tacrolimus, MPA, and steroids. After transplantation, his kidney function remained very poor. eGFR was 15, 26, and 23 mL/min/1.73 m^2 at 1, 6, and 12 months, respectively. A kidney biopsy, performed at 3 months posttransplantation, revealed signs of diabetic nephropathy and mild tubulopathy, but no rejection (t0 i0 g0 v0 ptc0 ah3 cg0 ci1 ct1 cv1 mm1, according to the Banff classification). At one year, tacrolimus was replaced by everolimus. Consequently, he presented with severe dyslipidemia and anemia, which required large doses of erythropoietin. In addition, steroid dose had to be reduced because of bilateral femoral osteonecrosis.

Another kidney biopsy was performed 6 months later, which showed grade-2 IFTA and severe vascular lesions (cv3,

Table 1: Donors' and recipients' characteristics.

	Case 1	Case 2
Donor		
Age (years)	77	60
Gender	W	W
Body mass index (kg/m^2)	25.4	29
Cause of death	Hemorrhagic stroke	Ischemic stroke
Cardiac arrest	no	no
Serum creatinine level (μmol/L)	52	71
Proteinuria (g/L)	0.12	0.17
Estimated MDRD GFR (mL/min/1.73 m^2)	100	74
Recipient		
Age (years)	52	69
Gender	W	M
Body mass index (kg/m^2)	26.4	24.4
Cause of kidney disease	Lupus	Vascular nephropathy
Cold ischemia time (min)	765	690
Warm ischemia time (min)	45	60

W: woman; M: male; GFR: glomerular-filtration rate.

according to the Banff classification). Kidney function was altered; serum-creatinine level was 256 μmol/L, eGFR was 22 mL/min/1.73 m^2, and proteinuria was 1.5 mg/g of creatinine. At that time, that is, 19 months after transplantation, everolimus was replaced by belatacept (5 mg/kg/month). MPA (2 g/d) and low-dose steroids (5 mg/d) were continued. At the last follow-up, that is, 33 months after the switch, serum-creatinine level was 224 μmol/L, eGFR was 24 mL/min/1.73 m^2, and proteinuria had decreased to 0.7 mg/g. Metabolic and hematological parameters were both improved. No DSAs were detected before or after the switch to belatacept.

3. Discussion

Within the last decade, the number of extended-criteria donors has increased. Consequently, for a large number of kidney-allograft recipients, the use of CNIs, which are known to have nephrotoxic effects, can be problematic. In *de novo* kidney-transplant patients who receive a kidney from an extended-criteria donor, the use of belatacept has been associated with significantly better kidney function at 5 years compared to patients that received cyclosporine A [6]. In maintenance kidney-transplant patients with preserved kidney function (eGFR between 35 and 75 mL/min), conversion from CNIs to belatacept significantly improved kidney function compared to those maintained on CNIs [10–12]. However, the effect of belatacept on kidney function in patients with impaired kidney function, that is, eGFR <35 mL/min, is unknown.

mTOR inhibitors have been used in conversion protocols to avoid CNI-induced nephrotoxicity [2]. However, late conversion from CNIs to mTOR inhibitors, when eGFR is <30 mL/min and/or when proteinuria is >0.5 mg/g of creatinine, does not prevent a decline in kidney function [14, 15]. In addition, mTOR inhibitors have several side effects that result in a high rate of treatment withdrawal, that is, 40% [3].

Herein, we have described two kidney-transplant recipients who were intolerant to both CNIs and mTOR inhibitors. The two kidney-transplant patients had severe impaired kidney function because of severe histological lesions related to the donor. The use of CNIs led to very low eGFR (<20 mL/min). The use of everolimus was associated with severe angioedema, requiring its withdrawal. Hence, belatacept was successfully used and led to improved kidney function in both cases, even though eGFR before conversion was <20 mL/min. Neither of the patients developed a serious adverse event, donor-specific antibodies, or posttransplant lymphoma disease.

In conclusion, these case reports highlight the fact that belatacept can be used as a rescue therapy, even if kidney function is very low, in kidney-transplant patients who cannot tolerate CNIs and/or mTOR inhibitors.

Authors' Contribution

Julie Belliere collected the data and wrote the paper. Céline Guilbeau-Frugier and Caroline Capuani did the pathological work-up. Arnaud Del Bello, Laure Esposito, and Isabelle Cardeau-Desangles did the follow-up to patients. Lionel Rostaing designed the study, participated in the patients' follow-up, and reviewed the paper. Nassim Kamar designed the study, participated in the patients' follow-up, and wrote the paper.

References

[1] M. Pascual, T. Theruvath, T. Kawai, N. Tolkoff-Rubin, and A. Benedict Cosimi, "Strategies to improve long-term outcomes after renal transplantation," *The New England Journal of Medicine*, vol. 346, no. 8, pp. 580–590, 2002.

[2] L. Rostaing and N. Kamar, "mTOR inhibitor/proliferation signal inhibitors: entering or leaving the field?" *Journal of Nephrology*, vol. 23, no. 2, pp. 133–142, 2010.

[3] N. Pallet and C. Legendre, "Adverse events associated with mTOR inhibitors," *Expert Opinion on Drug Safety*, vol. 12, pp. 177–186, 2013.

[4] C. P. Larsen, T. C. Pearson, A. B. Adams et al., "Rational development of LEA29Y (belatacept), a high-affinity variant of CTLA4-Ig with potent immunosuppressive properties," *The American Journal of Transplantation*, vol. 5, no. 3, pp. 443–453, 2005.

[5] F. Vincenti, C. Larsen, A. Durrbach et al., "Costimulation blockade with belatacept in renal transplantation," *New England Journal of Medicine*, vol. 353, no. 8, pp. 770–781, 2005.

[6] B. Charpentier, J. O. Medina Pestana, C. R. M. Del et al., "Long-term exposure to belatacept in recipients of extended criteria donor kidneys," *The American Journal of Transplantation*, vol. 13, pp. 2884–2891, 2013.

[7] A. Durrbach, J. M. Pestana, T. Pearson et al., "A phase III study of belatacept versus cyclosporine in kidney transplants from extended criteria donors (BENEFIT-EXT Study)," *The American Journal of Transplantation*, vol. 10, no. 3, pp. 547–557, 2010.

[8] L. Rostaing, F. Vincenti, J. Grinyo et al., "Long-term belatacept exposure maintains efficacy and safety at 5 years: results from the long-term extension of the BENEFIT study," *The American Journal of Transplantation*, vol. 13, pp. 2875–2883, 2013.

[9] F. Vincenti, B. Charpentier, Y. Vanrenterghem et al., "A phase III study of belatacept-based immunosuppression regimens versus cyclosporine in renal transplant recipients (BENEFIT Study)," *The American Journal of Transplantation*, vol. 10, no. 3, pp. 535–546, 2010.

[10] J. Grinyó, B. Charpentier, J. M. Pestana et al., "An integrated safety profile analysis of belatacept in kidney transplant recipients," *Transplantation*, vol. 90, no. 12, pp. 1521–1527, 2010.

[11] L. Rostaing, P. Massari, V. D. Garcia et al., "Switching from calcineurin inhibitor-based regimens to a belatacept-based regimen in renal transplant recipients: a randomized phase II study," *Clinical Journal of the American Society of Nephrology*, vol. 6, no. 2, pp. 430–439, 2011.

[12] N. Kamar, J. Alberu, S. Steinberg et al., "3-year outcomes after switching to belatacept from a CNI in stable kidney transplant recipients," in *Proceedings of the 16th Conference of the European Society for Organ Transplantation*, Vienna, Austria, September.

[13] B. Sis, M. Mengel, M. Haas et al., "Banff'09 meeting report: antibody mediated graft deterioration and implementation of Banff working groups," *The American Journal of Transplantation*, vol. 10, no. 3, pp. 464–471, 2010.

[14] F. Diekmann, K. Budde, F. Oppenheimer, L. Pritsche, H. H. Neumayer, and J. M. Campistol, "Predictors of success in conversion from calcineurin inhibitor to sirolimus in chronic allograft dysfunction," *The American Journal of Transplantation*, vol. 4, no. 11, pp. 1869–1875, 2004.

[15] A. I. Sánchez-Fructuoso, J. C. Ruiz, N. Calvo et al., "Everolimus as primary immunosuppression in kidney transplantation: experience in conversion from calcineurin inhibitors," *Transplantation*, vol. 93, no. 4, pp. 398–405, 2012.

2

Absence of mTOR Inhibitor Effect on Hepatic Cyst Growth: A Case Report of a Kidney Transplant Recipient with Autosomal Dominant Polycystic Kidney Disease

L. Friedrich, F. Barbey, M. Pascual, and J.-P. Venetz

Centre de Transplantation d'Organes, Centre Hospitalier Universitaire Vaudois, Avenue du Bugnon 46, 1011 Lausanne, Switzerland

Correspondence should be addressed to L. Friedrich, lauriane.friedrich@chuv.ch

Academic Editors: C. F. Classen, C. Costa, and C. Sommerer

Some experimental studies have suggested a beneficial effect of the mammalian target of rapamycin (mTOR) inhibitor use on hepatic and renal cyst growth in patients with autosomal dominant polycystic kidney disease (ADPKD). However, the results of clinical studies are conflicting and the role of mTOR inhibitors is still uncertain. We report the case of a patient with ADPKD who underwent deceased kidney transplantation because of an end-stage renal disease. The evolution was uneventful with an excellent graft function under cyclosporine (CsA) monotherapy. Some years later, the patient developed a symptomatic hepatomegaly due to growth of cysts. CsA was replaced by sirolimus, an mTOR inhibitor, in order to reduce or control the increase in the cyst and liver volume. Despite the switch, the hepatic volume increased by 25% in two years. Finally sirolimus was stopped because of the lack of effect on hepatic cyst growth and the presence of sirolimus side effects. The interest of our case resides in the followup by MRI imaging during the mTOR inhibitor treatment and 15 months after the restart of the initial immunosuppressive therapy. This observation indicates that mTOR inhibitors did not have significant effect on cyst-associated hepatic growth in our patient, which is consistent with some results of recent large clinical studies.

1. Introduction

The autosomal dominant polycystic kidney disease (ADPKD) is the most common hereditary kidney disease and is the fourth leading cause of end-stage renal disease in adults [1]. Studies outlined the role of mammalian target of rapamycin (mTOR) in the pathogenesis of renal and hepatic cyst formation. mTOR activity is upregulated in renal cyst lining epithelial cells in patient with ADPKD, suggesting a potential benefit of mTOR inhibitor treatment in reducing renal and hepatic cyst growth. However, no randomized study has been performed yet to evaluate the effect of mTOR inhibitors in reducing hepatic cyst growth in ADPKD patients. A slowing effect of mTOR inhibitors (or absence of slowing effect of mTOR inhibitors) on hepatic cysts growth still needs to be determined. A long followup is needed, because many cyst complications could change total kidney or hepatic volume. The adequate dose of mTOR inhibitor to inhibit the mTOR pathway with a minimum side effect as well as the adequate moment to initiate the treatment is also unknown and needs to be investigated.

We report the case of an ADPKD patient who underwent a kidney transplantation and developed a progressive voluminous symptomatic hepatomegaly. Sirolimus, an mTOR inhibitors, was started because of preliminary data suggesting a potential benefit of mammalian target of rapamycin (mTOR) inhibitor therapy on hepatic cysts growth. But after two years of treatment, we did not observe any improvement in his condition and sirolimus was stopped.

2. Case Report

A 50-year-old man with autosomal dominant polycystic kidney disease (ADPKD) evolved to end-stage renal failure and hemodialysis was started in 1992. Because of voluminous kidneys, a right nephrectomy was performed in 1992, followed by the left one in 1994. In April 1998, a deceased donor kidney transplantation was performed in the right iliac fossa. Induction therapy consisted in seven days of polyclonal anti-T-cell globulin (thymoglobulin), because of delayed graft function. Maintenance immunosuppression consisted of cyclosporine (CsA) and prednisone. Steroids were withdrawn in December 1998. No acute rejection was observed. At one month, the serum creatinine was 130 μmol/L and the glomerular filtration rate was estimated at 61 mL/min/1.73 m^2 by MDRD. The serum creatinine remained stable during the followup and was of 113 μmol/L in March 2011.

During the followup in our outpatient clinic, the patient suffered from recurrent episodes of hepatic cyst infections, treated by antibiotics. In April 2007, bloating and abdominal discomfort developed. An abdominal MRI was performed showing a marked hepatomegaly with incomplete chronic Budd-Chiari syndrome, due to extrinsic venous compression by voluminous liver cysts. Because of worsening symptoms and many hepatic cyst infections, a new MRI was performed in June 2008, showing an increasing liver volume without progression of the Budd-Chiari syndrome. The liver volume was 3517 mL at this time. Because of preliminary data suggesting a potential benefit of mammalian target of rapamycin (mTOR) inhibitors therapy on hepatic cyst growth, CsA was stopped and sirolimus started at 0.5 mg/d to achieve serum levels between 4 and 6 ug/L (Table 1). MRIs were performed during the mTOR therapy because of worsening symptoms, and a followup was made with volumetric hepatic MRI. Only total hepatic volume was measured. Six months later, a new MRI showed a continuing increase in liver volume, which was estimated at 3883 mL. In November 2009, the liver volume was 4240 mL and in June 2010, 4400 mL (Figure 1). The chronic partial Budd-Chiari syndrome did not change.

Under sirolimus therapy, our patient did not report adverse events like cutaneous rash, diarrhea, and aphthous stomatitis, but he developed important legs edema. Hyperlipidemia was controlled with pravastatin and there was no significant proteinuria. Because of the continuing increase in liver volume (i.e., no significant effect of sirolimus) and the important discomfort due to bilateral legs edema, sirolimus was stopped and CsA restarted in June 2010. The differential diagnosis of leg edema was venous compression due to hepatomegaly. After restarting CsA therapy, the leg edema resolved, which was consistent with a sirolimus side effect. Fifteen months after sirolimus was stopped, a new MRI was done. The liver volume was at 4700 mL (Figure 1). The average hepatic growth over the two years of sirolimus therapy was of 37.5 mL per month versus 20 mL per month with cyclosporine.

Table 1: Serum level of sirolimus during treatment.

Date of dosage (year/month/day)	Dose (mg/d)	Sirolimus level (ug/L)
08.10.15	0.5	5.6
08.12.03	0.5	4
09.01.21	0.5	6.2
09.02.27	0.5	5.1
09.07.08	0.5	5.6
09.09.16	0.5	4.2
09.09.30	0.5	3.7
09.09.10	0.5	2.8
09.11.04	1	10.5
09.11.18	0.5	4.3
10.01.22	0.5	3
10.05.12	0.5	5.3
10.06.02	0.5	3.1
10.06.23	0.5	3.8

3. Discussion

ADPKD is the most common hereditary kidney disease, affecting 1 in 400 to 1 in 10 000 births worldwide, and the fourth leading cause of end-stage renal disease in adults [1].

ADPKD is a genetically heterogeneous disease characterized by the development of cysts in the kidneys, liver, pancreas, seminal vesicles, and arachnoid membrane [1, 2]. Approximately 85% of cases are due to mutation in the polycystic kidney disease 1 gene (PKD1) in chromosome 16 and 15% to polycystic kidney disease 2 gene (PKD2) in chromosome 4 [3]. The glomerular filtration rate decline is associated with the increase in kidney volume [4]. Patients with PKD2 mutation have a later onset of disease and develop end-stage renal failure later than those with PKD1 mutation [1].

75–90% of cases develop a polycystic hepatic disease. It consists of proliferation and dilatation of biliary ductules and peribiliary glands [1]. Estrogens stimulate hepatic cyst cell proliferation, which explain why hepatic involvement is more prevalent and more severe in a young woman than in men. Polycystic hepatic disease is usually asymptomatic but symptoms can occur by mass effect or complications as cyst hemorrhage, infection, torsion, or rupture [1].

Studies outlined the role of the mammalian target of rapamycin (mTOR) in the pathogenesis of renal and hepatic cyst formation and growing, and experimental studies suggest mTOR inhibitors efficacy as treatment in ADPKD. mTOR is a kinase which integrates signals from cytokines, hormones, and growth factors. It coordinates cell growth, cell cycle progression, and proliferation. Human studies show that mTOR activity is upregulated in renal cyst lining epithelial cells in a patient with ADPKD. Recent studies have shown that somatostatin and mTOR inhibitors may have benefit hepatic cyst. Sirolimus, an mTOR inhibitor, is used as an immunosuppressive drug mainly in transplantation. Studies in rodent models show that mTOR inhibition retarded hepatic cyst expansion. A study in ADPKD patients after kidney transplantation suggested a reduction in kidney and hepatic cyst volume in patients treated with sirolimus compared to those treated with a calcineurin inhibitor [5]. However, Sirolimus blood levels to inhibit the mTOR pathway and avoid toxicity are not known [6]. Based on those findings, a randomized, crossover study compared a 6-month treatment with sirolimus

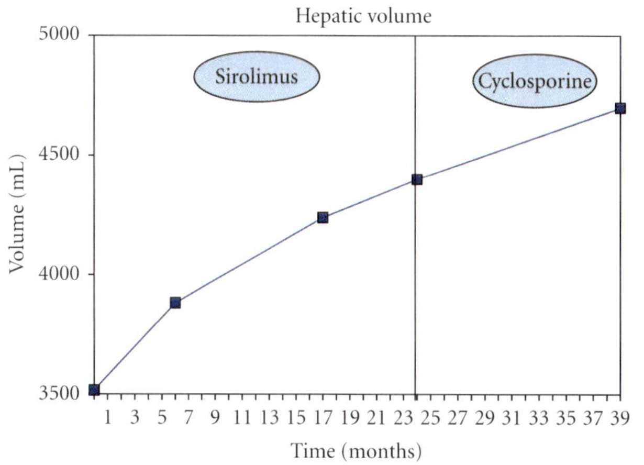

FIGURE 1: Hepatic volume since the initiation of mTOR inhibition therapy. Two-year followup by MRI. Month 0 = switch CsA to sirolimus. Month 24 = stop sirolimus because of absence of reduction growth of the hepatic volume and edema attributed to sirolimus.

or conventional therapy alone on the growth of kidney volume measured in 21 patients with ADPKD and GFR equal or more than 40 mL/min [7]. 15 patients completed the study, 7 with sirolimus. Compared with the pre-treatment values, the posttreatment mean kidney volume increased less on sirolimus than on conventional therapy, but without significant differences. However, because of the small size and the short followup of the SIRENA study, no firm conclusions about the effect of mTOR inhibition could be reached. Recently, Serra et al. [8] randomized 100 patients with a GFR of at least 70 mL/min between sirolimus and conventional therapy and followed them during 18 months by MRI imaging. The conclusion was that in patients with ADPKD and an early stage of kidney disease, sirolimus did not stop the increase in kidney volume. Similary, Walz et al. [9] randomized 433 patients followed during two years to placebo versus everolimus, another mTOR inhibitor therapy. This study showed that everolimus did not significantly slow the increase of kidney volume during the first year, but the benefit was not maintained after the second year. Moreover, Canaud et al. compared two patients who received renal transplant from a donor with a known PKD1 mutation. One patient received steroids, tacrolimus, and mycophenolate mofetil as immunosuppression therapy and the other steroids, tacrolimus, and sirolimus. A five-year follow up showed no difference in cyst growth between the two patients [6]. No difference was noticed about the GFR between the two groups. Therefore, based on the current knowledge, the effect of the mTOR inhibition on progression of ADPKD remains uncertain.

The mTOR inhibition effect on hepatic cyst progression is unknown. Qian et al. [5] retrospectively examined 16 renal transplant patients with ADPKD disease who were randomized between sirolimus-mycophenolate mofetil-prednisone therapy and tacrolimus-mycophenolate mofetil-prednisone therapy in another trial. After an average of 19.4 months of treatment, the sirolimus regimen showed a reduction in polycystic hepatic volume compared with tacrolimus, but because of the small size, the retrospective form, and the short followup of the study, no conclusion could be made about the mTOR effect on hepatic volume progression in an ADPKD patient. Recently, He et al. [10] published a meta-analysis of randomized controlled trials about the efficacy and safety of the mTOR inhibitor therapy in patients with early ADPKD. Four studies were included, and analysis of total kidney volume, cyst volume, parenchymal volume, glomerular filtration rate, and adverse events was made. They concluded that short-term mTOR inhibitor therapy may slow down the increase in kidney volume and is relatively safe but that the impact on the GFR was limited. Long-term efficacity and safety are still unknown. The adequate moment to initiate the mTOR inhibitors therapy as well as the dose of the medication needs to be investigated. Novali et al. [11] used animal models of polycystic kidney disease (PKD) to evaluate the efficacy of low-dose levels versus high-dose levels of sirolimus on renal cyst growth. They also compared early and late initiation of the treatment. They concluded that high dose of sirolimus given in an early stage of the disease reduced significantly cyst formation in ADPKD mouse models, where low-dose levels do not. When initiated at a more advanced stage, low- and high-dose levels of sirolimus have not significant effects on cyst formation. The high doses used in mouse models are 10 to 20 times higher than those used for immunosuppressive therapy after transplantation, beyond the levels tolerated by humans.

Side effects were reported in the different studies. Most of them were controlled with medical treatment. Classical adverse events are aphtous stomatitis, rash, peripheral edema, diarrhea, hyperlipidemia, proteinuria, and infection.

We reported the case of a patient in which we introduced sirolimus to achieve serum levels between 4 and 6 ug/L late in the disease progression. Our case raises several questions concerning the use of mTOR inhibitors: when should the treatment be introduced, which serum should be targeted, and is it effective and safe? In our patient, mTOR inhibitor did not improve his abdominal condition and induce important legs edema. Hepatic cysts epithelia express a high level of mTOR suggesting that mTOR inhibitors may have an effect in downregulating hepatic cyst growth [5], but no randomized study has been performed yet to evaluate the effect of this therapy. Randomized studies are needed to determine the efficacy of mTOR inhibitors on hepatic cyst growing. A long followup is needed, because many cyst complications could change the total kidney or hepatic volume. The adequate dose of sirolimus to inhibit the mTOR pathway with a minimum of side effect [6] as well as the adequate moment to initiate the therapy is still unknown and needed to be investigated. The mTOR inhibitor effect on hepatic cysts growth still needs to be determined.

References

[1] V. E. Torres, P. C. Harris, and Y. Pirson, "Autosomal dominant polycystic kidney disease," *The Lancet*, vol. 369, no. 9569, pp. 1287–1301, 2007.

[2] A. B. Chapman, "Autosomal dominant polycystic kidney disease: time for a change?" *Journal of the American Society of Nephrology*, vol. 18, no. 5, pp. 1399–1407, 2007.

[3] J. Lespinasse, J. Fourcade, and F. Schir, "La génétique des polykystoses rénales: mise au point et conseil génétique," *Néphrologie & Thérapeutique*, vol. 2, no. 3, pp. 120–126, 2006.

[4] J. J. Grantham, V. E. Torres, A. B. Chapman et al., "Volume progression in polycystic kidney disease," *The New England Journal of Medicine*, vol. 354, no. 20, pp. 2122–2130, 2006.

[5] Q. Qian, H. Du, B. F. King et al., "Sirolimus reduces polycystic liver volume in ADPKD patients," *Journal of the American Society of Nephrology*, vol. 19, no. 3, pp. 631–638, 2008.

[6] G. Canaud, B. Knebelmann, P. C. Harris et al., "Therapeutic mTOR inhibition in autosomal dominant polycystic kidney disease: what is the appropriate serum level?" *American Journal of Transplantation*, vol. 10, no. 7, pp. 1701–1706, 2010.

[7] N. Perico, L. Antiga, A. Caroli et al., "Sirolimus therapy to halt the progression of ADPKD," *Journal of the American Society of Nephrology*, vol. 21, no. 6, pp. 1031–1040, 2010.

[8] A. L. Serra, D. Poster, R. P. Wuthrich et al., "Sirolimus and kidney growth in autosomal dominant polycystic kidney disease," *The New England Journal of Medicine*, 2010.

[9] G. Walz, K. Budde, M. Mannaa et al., "Everolimus in patients with autosomal dominant polycystic kidney disease," *The New England Journal of Medicine*, vol. 363, no. 9, pp. 830–840, 2010.

[10] Q. He, C. Lin, J. Chen et al., "Efficacy and safety of mTOR inhibitor therapy in patients with early-stage autosomal dominant polycystic kidney disease: a meta-analysis of randomized controlled trials," *The American Journal of the Medical Sciences*, vol. 344, no. 6, pp. 491–497, 2012.

[11] Z. Novali, A. M. Van der Wal, D. J. M. Peters et al., "Dose-dependent effects of sirolimus on mTOR signaling and polycystic kidney disease," *Journal of the American Society of Nephrology*, vol. 23, no. 5, pp. 842–853, 2012.

3

Renal Transplantation in Secondary Amyloidosis Associated with Tuberculosis

Vivek B. Kute,[1] Aruna V. Vanikar,[2] Himanshu V. Patel,[1] Manoj R. Gumber,[1] Pankaj R. Shah,[1] Pranjal R. Modi,[3] and Hargovind L. Trivedi[1]

[1] *Department of Nephrology and Clinical Transplantation, Institute of Kidney Diseases & Research Center, Dr. H. L. Trivedi Institute of Transplantation Sciences (IKDRC-ITS), Civil Hospital Campus, Asarwa, Ahmedabad, Gujarat 380016, India*
[2] *Department of Pathology, Laboratory Medicine, Transfusion Services and Immunohematology, IKDRC-ITS, Ahmedabad, India*
[3] *Department of Urology and Transplantation, IKDRC-ITS, Ahmedabad, India*

Correspondence should be addressed to Vivek B. Kute; drvivekkute@rediffmail.com

Academic Editors: R. L. Heilman and G. Orlando

Although end-stage renal disease (ESRD) related to AA amyloidosis nephropathy secondary to tuberculosis is most common in our country, there are limited data concerning patient and graft outcome after renal transplantation (RTx). To the best of our knowledge, this is the first report of RTx in ESRD patient with secondary amyloidosis due to tuberculosis from India. A 30-year-old female with past history of pulmonary tuberculosis 3 years back was admitted with complaint of gradually progressive pedal oedema and nausea for 3 months. Renal biopsy was suggestive of secondary renal amyloidosis with vascular involvement and chronic tubulointerstitial involvement. She was transplanted with kidney from her 28-year-old brother with 3/6 human leukocyte antigen match. She had immediate good graft function without any perioperative complications (cardiovascular, infections, rejection and delayed graft function). She was discharged with serum creatinine of 0.8 mg/dL. Her last serum creatinine level was 0.9 mg/dL with cyclosporine level of 100 mg/dL at 9-month followup without any medical or surgical complication. The quality of life also improved after transplantation. With careful selection, ESRD patients with secondary amyloidosis due to tuberculosis are eligible for RTx with favorable outcome and improved quality of life.

1. Introduction

The most frequent and life-threatening complication of secondary amyloidosis (AA) is renal disease characterized by nephrotic syndrome and a progressive decline of renal function leading to end-stage renal disease (ESRD). Kidney involvement constitutes a major prognostic factor in patients with secondary amyloidosis. Chronic inflammatory diseases (rheumatoid arthritis (RA)) and infections (tuberculosis (TB)) were the most common causes of renal amyloidosis in the developed countries and developing countries [1, 2]. Estimated frequency of AA amyloidosis in Western Europe is about 1/100,000. It comprises 2-3% of total amyloidosis. Overall incidence is about 0.5–1.3/100,000 annually. A total of 2401 renal biopsies were analyzed retrospectively from 1990 to 2008 in an Indian single centre, out of which 8% showed amyloidosis [3]. ESRD patients with AA amyloidosis are considered less suitable for renal transplantation (RTx) due to fear of cardiovascular, infectious complications, risk of graft loss from recurrent amyloid/progressive disease, and high risk of mortality [4]. Although ESRD related to AA amyloidosis nephropathy secondary to TB is most common in our country, there are limited data concerning patient and graft outcome after RTx. To the best of our knowledge, this is the first report of RTx in a patient with amyloidosis due to TB from India.

2. Case Presentation

A 30-year-old female was admitted with complaint of gradually progressive pedal oedema and nausea for 3 months. There was no history of skin rash, joint pain, hair loss, or decreased urine output. She had completed the treatment for

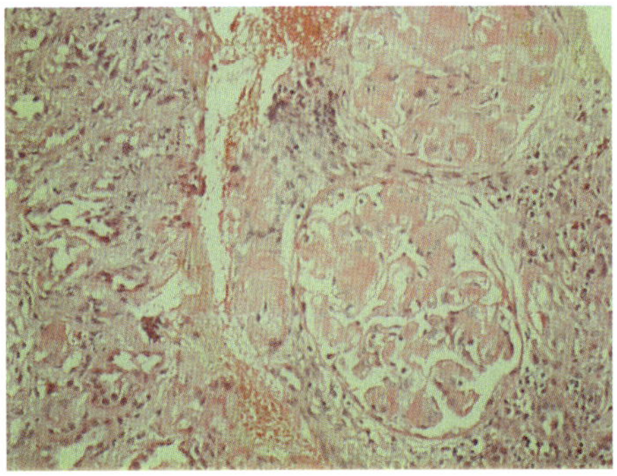

(a)

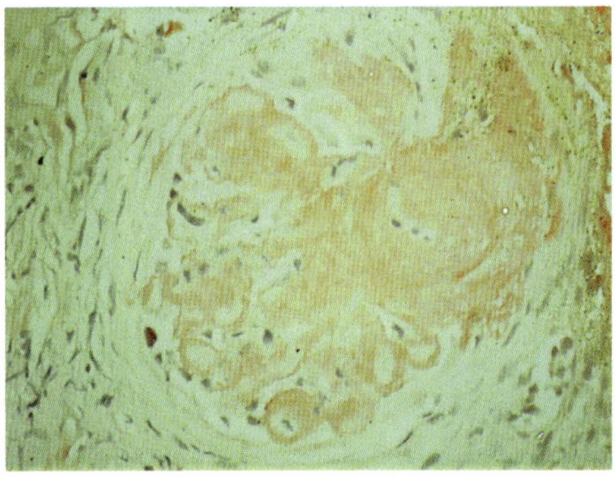

(b)

FIGURE 1: (a) Renal biopsy showing amyloid deposit, pink acellular hyaline material (hematoxylin and eosin stain ×400). (b) Renal biopsy showing congo red positive amyloid deposit, pink acellular hyaline material (congo red stain ×400).

pulmonary tuberculosis (PTB) in 2009 and responded well. She had no history of any other major illness like diabetes and hypertension. There was no other history of any other major illness in past or family. On examination she had pitting pedal oedema with blood pressure of 110/70 mmHg, temperature of 39°C, respiratory rate of 18 breaths per minute, and heart rate of 90 breaths per minute.

3. Investigations

Laboratory investigations revealed the following: hemoglobin, 6.9 gm/L; total white cell count, 11.07 × 103/μL (differential count: 67% neutrophils, 29% lymphocytes, 2% monocytes, and 3% eosinophils); platelet count, 374 × 103/μL; reticulocyte count, 1%; peripheral blood smear was negative for hemolysis; sodium, 145 mmol/L; potassium, 3.8 mEq/L; chloride, 105 mmol/L; urea, 121; creatinine was 7.2 mg/dL; calcium, 7.8 md/dL; phosphate, 8.7; serum protein 5.3 gm/dL. Serum albumin/globulin was 4.3/1.7 gm/dL. Urine examination showed proteinuria (albumin +3) with no hematuria, and pus cells. 24-hour urine protein was 5.3 gm. Enzyme-linked immunosorbent assays for human immunodeficiency virus, hepatitis B surface antigen, and hepatitis C virus were negative with antinuclear antibodies and antibodies to double-stranded DNA negative and normal C3 and C4 levels. Ultrasonography of the abdomen showed kidney size of 12.8 × 4 centimeter on the right side and 11.5 × 4.7 centimeter on the left side. Abdominal fat biopsy was suggestive of amyloidosis. Renal biopsy (Figures 1(a) and 1(b)) was done, suggestive of renal amyloidosis (secondary) with vascular involvement and chronic tubulointerstitial involvement. Blood, urine, and sputum culture did not show any organisms. Electrocardiography was normal. Sputum for acid-fast bacillus was negative. Echocardiogram was normal with ejection fraction of 60%. High resolution computed tomography of chest showed traction bronchiectasis in both lung fields with multiple enlarged lymph nodes in pretracheal, prevascular, and subcarinal and both hilar regions along with hypodense area within nodes suggesting tuberculosis. Erythrocyte sedimentation rate was 30 and 62 mm/hour at end of 1 and 2 hours. Tuberculin test was negative.

4. Treatment

Antituberculosis treatment was restarted in July 2012 with isoniazid, rifampicin, pyrazinamide, moxifloxacin, and ethambutol. Pneumococcal polyvalent vaccine was given to prevent infection. She was on maintenance hemodialysis for 4 months through left jugular dual lumen catheter initially for 3 weeks and later through arteriovenous fistula. She was transplanted with kidney from her 28-year-old brother with 3/6 human leukocyte antigen match on the 5th of November 2012. Warm ischaemia time, cold ischaemia time, and anastomosis time were 1 minute and 57 seconds, 52 minutes and 28 minutes and 32 seconds, respectively.

5. Immunosuppressive Regimen

Induction immunosuppression consisted of methylprednisolone 500 mg for 3 days. Maintenance immunosuppression consisted of prednisolone 10 mg, cyclosporine 3 mg/kg, and mycophenolate mofetil 500 mg TID. The recipient was covered with perioperative antibiotic. She was initiated on prophylaxis against cytomegalovirus infection (gancyclovir × 3 months), fungal infections (fluconazole × 3 months), and *Pneumocystis carinii* pneumonia (trimethoprim/sulfamethoxazole × 9 months) as per standard protocol.

6. Transplantation Outcome and Followup

She had immediate good graft function without any perioperative surgical or medical complications (cardiovascular, infections, rejection, and delayed graft function). She was discharged with serum creatinine of 0.8 mg/dL. Her last serum creatinine level was 0.9 mg/dL with cyclosporine level of 100 mg/dL at 9-month followup without any complication. Antituberculosis treatment was completed after RTx and continued with isoniazid for TB prophylaxis. The quality of life before and after transplant patients was evaluated using WHOQOL-BREF scale. Physical health, psychological, social relationship, and environment scores before RTx were higher (24; 23; 12; 32) than pretransplant scores (20; 17; 9; 24).

7. Discussion

Patients with renal amyloidosis who progress to ESRD can be treated with either dialysis or RTx. Hemodialysis and continuous ambulatory peritoneal dialysis (CAPD) appear to be equally effective, the limiting factors being the degree of extrarenal amyloid deposition, hypotension with hemodialysis, and peritonitis with CAPD. 14% of deaths on dialysis resulted from amyloidosis complications, emphasizing that thorough evaluation of systemic complications remains important even after patients with renal amyloidosis progress to ESRD. Underlying etiology should be corrected or controlled. Successful treatment of the underlying inflammatory process included surgical resection of the focus of infection, cytotoxic agents/biological agents in RA, and antibiotics with chronic infection. RTx should be performed, at earliest time possible after onset of maintenance dialysis prior to development of severe cardiac disease. The outcome appears to be best in patients without cardiac involvement on echocardiography [5, 6].

Fitness of transplant candidates is a major concern due to cardiovascular instability, infections, and uncontrolled underlying inflammatory process. It is important to evaluate the presence, and severity of coronary disease, heart failure, valvular disease, and arrhythmias prior to transplantation. Goals of cardiac testing are to assist in determining transplant candidacy and to identify patients who might benefit from preoperative cardiac intervention and aggressive risk factor modification to decrease perioperative and posttransplant cardiac events [7, 8].

Limited data suggest that graft survival is similar but patient survival is lower in patients with AA amyloidosis compared to other forms of renal disease [9–14]. Recurrence of amyloid nephropathy is of concern because recurrent amyloid deposition in the transplant occurs in 20 to 72% of cases due to continued activity of the underlying disease, but graft loss due to recurrence is uncommon.

Outcomes were sought among all patients attending the UK National Amyloidosis Centre [9] who received RTx between 1978 and 2011. A total of 111 RTx operations were performed in 104 patients. Outcomes following RTx were generally excellent in these diseases, reflecting their slow natural history; median graft survival was 13.1 years [9].

The Australia and New Zealand Dialysis and Transplant Registry reported long-term renal replacement therapy (RRT) outcomes of amyloidosis. The survival of amyloidosis patients receiving peritoneal dialysis was comparable with that of those receiving haemodialysis. Forty-six patients underwent RTx with first graft survival rates of 45% at 5 years and 26% at 10 years. Nine (16.4%) patients experienced amyloidosis recurrence in their allografts, which led to graft failure in six patients. Amyloidosis was associated with poor patient survival following dialysis and/or RTx, poor renal allograft survival, and a significant incidence of disease recurrence in the allograft. An appreciable proportion of amyloid ESRD patients died of amyloidosis-related complications [10].

The French multicenter study [11] reported long-term outcome of RTx in patients with amyloidosis ($n = 59$) compared to the general transplant population ($n = 177$). The overall 5- and 10-year patient survival was significantly lower for the AA amyloidosis patients, but they had similar graft survival. AA amyloidosis transplanted patients exhibited a high proportion of infectious complications after transplantation (73.2%). This study reported that patients with AA amyloidosis nephropathy are eligible for RTx but require careful management of both cardiovascular and infectious complications to reduce the high risk of mortality (73.2%).

Sherif et al. reported similar long-term (5 to 10 years) outcome of live related donor RTx in patients with amyloidosis ($n = 23$) compared to the general transplant population [12]. Emiroglu et al. reported, 5-year outcome of RTx in patients with amyloidosis ($n = 32$) similar to that in those patients who receive transplantations for other reasons [13]. Better survival was noted for ESRD patients amyloidosis who had RTx despite recurrences due to systemic. These results encourage transplantation in amyloid ESRD [14]. The recurrence of amyloid in the graft within one year after transplantation in a patient with systemic AA amyloidosis secondary to tuberculosis has been reported [15].

It is reasonable to suspect renal amyloidosis in any patient with known history of PTB presenting with pedal edema and proteinuria. The interval between the onset of tuberculosis and first evidence of amyloidosis is variable (months to years). Renal amyloidosis in children within 2 years of the onset of juvenile rheumatoid arthritis at the age of 7 years has been reported. Once amyloidosis has extensively involved the kidneys, anti-TB treatment will not cause any regression in the course of renal amyloidosis. Adequately treated patients may present with renal amyloidosis despite having effective anti-TB therapy. It could be attributed to posttubercular bronchiectasis or an irreversible process of amyloid deposition that had initiated earlier.

In the near future stem cell therapy may have a role in reducing requirement of immunosuppressants leading to less infections and better graft survival.

8. Conclusion

With careful selection, patients with secondary amyloidosis due to tuberculosis are eligible for renal transplantation with favorable outcome and improved quality of life.

Authors' Contribution

All authors made equal contribution to the study. All authors read and approved the final paper.

References

[1] D. Bunker and P. Gorevic, "AA amyloidosis: mount Sinai experience, 1997–2012," *The Mount Sinai Journal of Medicine*, vol. 79, no. 6, pp. 749–756, 2012.

[2] J. Prakash, T. Brojen, S. S. Rathore, T. A. Choudhury, and T. Gupta, "The changing pattern of renal amyloidosis in Indian subcontinent: two decades of experience from a single center," *Renal Failure*, vol. 34, no. 10, pp. 1212–1216, 2012.

[3] U. Das, K. V. Dakshinamurty, and A. Prayaga, "Pattern of biopsy-proven renal disease in a single center of south India: 19 years experience," *Indian Journal of Nephrology*, vol. 21, no. 4, pp. 250–257, 2011.

[4] T. Kofman, P. Grimbert, F. Canoüi-Poitrine et al., "Renal transplantation in patients with aa amyloidosis nephropathy: results from a french multicenter study," *American Journal of Transplantation*, vol. 11, no. 11, pp. 2423–2431, 2011.

[5] G. Moroni, G. Banfi, A. Montoli et al., "Chronic dialysis in patients with systemic amyloidosis: the experience in Northern Italy," *Clinical Nephrology*, vol. 38, no. 2, pp. 81–85, 1992.

[6] K. Sakai, M. Okamoto, K. Koshino et al., "A case of living-donor renal transplantation for chronic renal failure caused by secondary amyloidosis," *Transplantation Proceedings*, vol. 43, no. 6, pp. 2418–2420, 2011.

[7] A. Haq, S. Hussain, B. Meskat, P. Mohan, P. Conlon, and D. P. Hickey, "Complications of renal transplantation in patients with amyloidosis," *Transplantation Proceedings*, vol. 39, no. 1, pp. 120–124, 2007.

[8] A. Çelik, F. Saglam, D. Dolek et al., "Outcome of kidney transplantation for renal amyloidosis: a single-center experience," *Transplantation Proceedings*, vol. 38, no. 2, pp. 435–439, 2006.

[9] J. H. Pinney, H. J. Lachmann, P. T. Sattianayagam et al., "Renal transplantation in systemic amyloidosis-importance of amyloid fibril type and precursor protein abundance," *American Journal of Transplantation*, vol. 13, no. 2, pp. 433–441, 2013.

[10] W. Tang, S. P. McDonald, C. M. Hawley et al., "End-stage renal failure due to amyloidosis: outcomes in 490 ANZDATA registry cases," *Nephrology Dialysis Transplantation*, vol. 28, no. 2, pp. 455–461, 2013.

[11] T. Kofman, P. Grimbert, F. Canoüi-Poitrine et al., "Renal transplantation in patients with aa amyloidosis nephropathy: results from a french multicenter study," *American Journal of Transplantation*, vol. 11, no. 11, pp. 2423–2431, 2011.

[12] A. M. Sherif, A. F. Refaie, M. A.-K. Sobh, N. A.-H. Mohamed, H. A. Sheashaa, and M. A. Ghoneim, "Long-term outcome of live donor kidney transplantation for renal amyloidosis," *American Journal of Kidney Diseases*, vol. 42, no. 2, pp. 370–375, 2003.

[13] R. Emiroglu, Ö. Başaran, S. Pehlivan et al., "Effect of amyloidosis on long-term survival in kidney transplantation," *Transplantation Proceedings*, vol. 37, no. 7, pp. 2967–2968, 2005.

[14] B. H. Özdemir, F. N. Özdemir, S. Sezer, A. Şar, and M. Haberal, "Among therapy modalities of end-stage renal disease, renal transplantation improves survival in patients with amyloidosis," *Transplantation Proceedings*, vol. 38, no. 2, pp. 432–434, 2006.

[15] V. Jha, V. Sakhuja, K. Vaiphei, K. Sud, H. S. Kohli, and K. L. Gupta, "An unusual case of recurrence of AA amyloidosis in the renal allograft," *Renal Failure*, vol. 26, no. 1, pp. 89–92, 2004.

Transplantation of Horseshoe Kidney from Living, Genetically Unrelated Donor

Kazuro Kikkawa, Takahito Wakamiya, Hiroki Kusumoto, Nagahide Matsumura, Yasuo Kohjimoto, and Isao Hara

Department of Urology, Wakayama Medical University, 811-1 Kimiidera, Wakayama 641-0012, Japan

Correspondence should be addressed to Kazuro Kikkawa; kzro@wakayama-med.ac.jp

Academic Editor: Frieder Keller

We report a case of renal transplantation using a horseshoe kidney from a living, genetically unrelated donor. The recipient was a 60-year-old man with diabetic nephropathy, and the donor was the 63-year-old wife of the recipient with a horseshoe kidney free of complications. Computed tomography showed two renal arteries and one renal vein on the left side, and the isthmus was perfused by several accessory arteries and veins. To demarcate the boundary of the isthmus, the left renal artery was ligated and cannulated for in situ perfusion. Furthermore, the isthmus was clamped, and the boundary of the isthmus was confirmed. The kidney was divided at the left margin of the perfused boundary. The cut ends of the isthmus were closed by sutures. The left kidney was transplanted into the right iliac fossa of the recipient. Asymptomatic fluid collection occurred on the cut surface at the isthmus of the donor, and this fluid decreased in due course. On the other hand, the recipient experienced no surgical complication or rejection, while maintaining serum creatinine levels of 2.00–2.20 mg/dL over a 22-month follow-up period. Horseshoe kidneys may be used for transplantation in selected cases after a detailed preoperative evaluation.

1. Introduction

The number of patients with chronic kidney disease who are awaiting a transplant is increasing. The continuing donor organ shortage has led to an expansion of the criteria for acceptability of deceased-donor organs, including the use of marginal kidneys with congenital abnormalities.

The horseshoe kidney is one of the most common congenital anomalies. The incidence has been reported to range from 1 per 600–800 [1]. The vascular anatomy in the horseshoe kidney is complex, and ureteral abnormalities also may be present. Therefore, urinary tract infection, vesicoureteral reflux, nephrolithiasis, and hydronephrosis are frequent complications in patients with horseshoe kidneys.

Although several deceased-donor kidney transplantations have been performed to date, use of divided horseshoe kidneys from living donors is rare. We present our experience with a horseshoe kidney used as a renal transplant from a living, genetically unrelated donor.

2. Case Report

The recipient was a 60-year-old man with end-stage renal disease related to diabetic nephropathy. The donor was the 63-year-old wife of the recipient. Preoperative computed tomography (CT) revealed a horseshoe kidney with no hydronephrosis or calculi in the donor (Figure 1(a)). Dynamic CT showed one renal artery and one renal vein on the right side, two renal arteries and one renal vein on the left side, and several accessory arteries and veins distributed to the lower fused parenchyma (Figure 1(b)). Intravenous urography showed no communicating calyceal system (Figure 2). Because the renal function of the left kidney was slightly lower than that of the right kidney according to renal scintigraphy, the left kidney was chosen for use as a transplant.

The surgery was performed in March 2013. A donor exploration was performed through an abdominal midline incision. The accessory arteries were ligated. The left kidney was procured by clamping and ligation of the left renal artery.

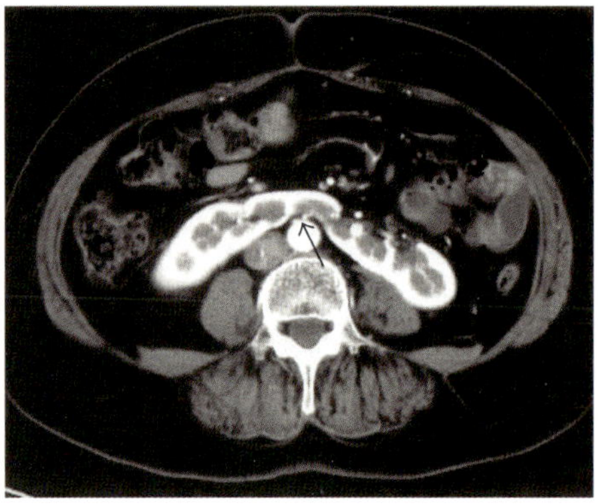

(a)

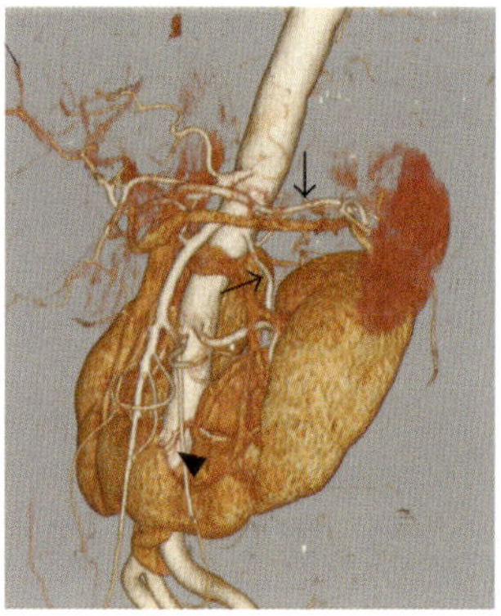

(b)

Figure 1: (a) Preoperative donor CT images with contrast enhancement showed the isthmus of the horseshoe kidney and an artery from the aorta supplying the isthmus (arrow). (b) Three-dimensional reconstruction of the CT scan of the donor revealed various blood vessels supplying the horseshoe kidney. Two left renal arteries (arrows) supplied the upper and middle poles of the left kidney and two aortic branches (arrowheads) supplied the isthmus.

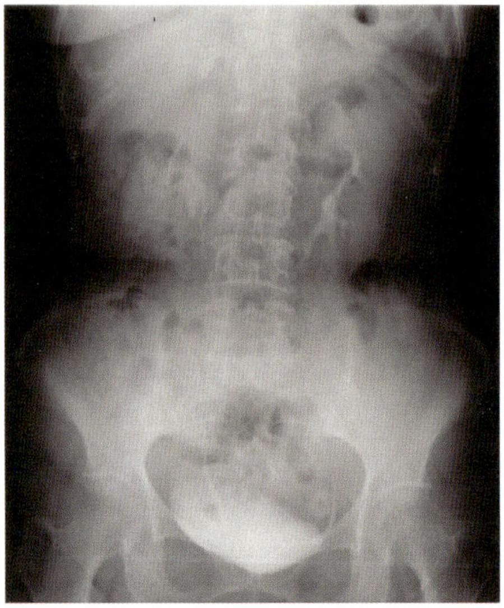

Figure 2: Intravenous urography of the donor revealed a medially rotated pelvis. Bilateral collecting systems were not connecting, and hydronephrosis was not seen.

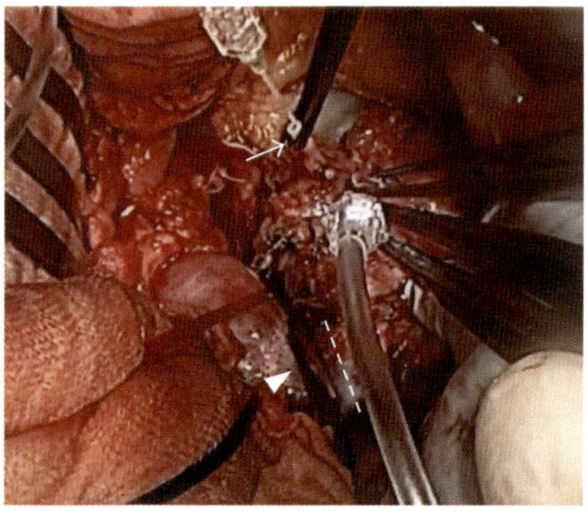

Figure 3: The left renal artery of the donor was cannulated for in situ perfusion (arrow). The isthmus was clamped during perfusion (arrowhead), and a divided fusion site of the isthmus was confirmed (dotted line).

To demarcate the boundary, the left renal artery was cannulated for in situ perfusion with perfusion solution. Because the lower vein drained the left and right kidneys, the perfused boundary of the isthmus was unclear. Furthermore, the isthmus was clamped during perfusion, and the boundary of the isthmus was confirmed (Figure 3). The kidney was divided at the left margin of the perfused boundary, and the left renal vein was ligated. The cut ends were sealed with polyglactin sutures, and the parenchyma approximated. After unclamping the isthmus in the donor, no bleeding and no urine leakage were detected from transacted surfaces.

At the back table, the superior pole renal artery was anastomosed side-to-side with the inferior renal artery. To detect injury of the vessels, indigo carmine was administered through the renal artery. Moreover, to detect injury of the collecting system and prevent urine leakage, indigo carmine was administered through the ureter. Detected injuries of vessels and collecting systems were closed with poliglecaprone sutures. The cut ends were sealed with polyglactin sutures, and the parenchyma was approximated.

The transplant was performed in the right iliac fossa of the recipient. The renal artery was anastomosed to the external iliac artery, and the renal vein was anastomosed to the external iliac vein (Figure 4). The ureter was connected to the bladder using a Lich-Gregoir technique with a ureteral stent placed in situ. After perfusion of the graft, no bleeding and no urine leakage were detected from the transacted surfaces. After 191 min of renal ischemia, including 6 min of warm ischemia, the graft began producing urine. No complications were observed after surgery. Induction therapy consisted of 20 mg basiliximab administered on days 0 and 4, and cyclosporine, mycophenolate mofetil, and methylprednisolone were initiated for maintenance immunosuppression. The patient required control of hypertension by oral medication and hyperglycemia by insulin preparation after transplantation. Subsequently, he had no indications of surgical

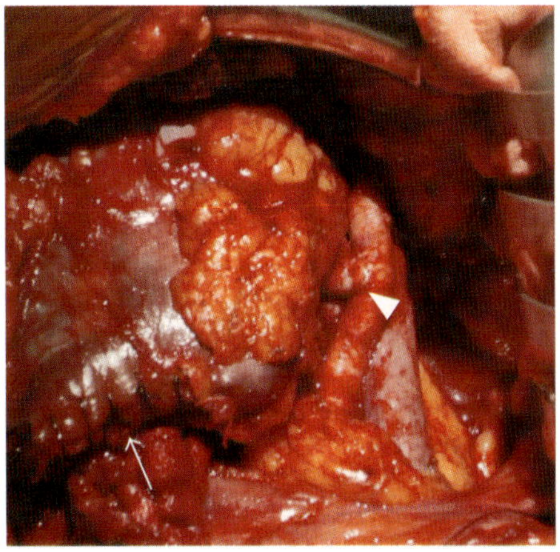

FIGURE 4: The horseshoe kidney after transplantation into the recipient. The edge of the isthmus was sutured (arrows). The renal artery was anastomosed to the external iliac artery (arrowhead), and the renal vein was anastomosed to the external iliac vein.

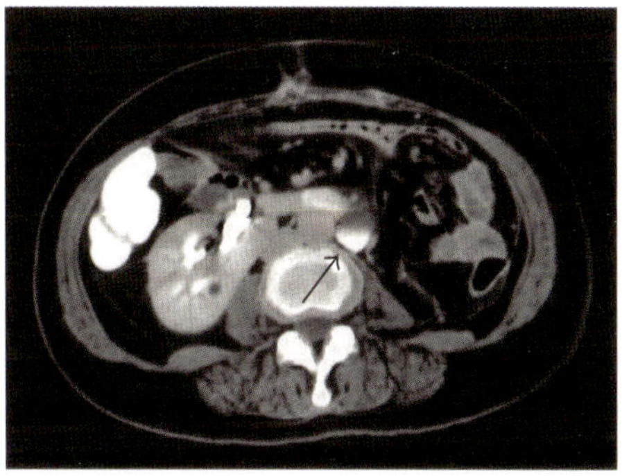

FIGURE 5: Postoperative donor CT images with contrast enhancement showed a site of fluid collection on the cut edge of the isthmus (arrow).

complications or rejection and was discharged 28 days after surgery with a serum creatinine level of 2.04 mg/dL. At 22 months' follow-up, the patient maintained serum creatinine levels between 2.00 and 2.20 mg/dL.

After donor nephrectomy, asymptomatic fluid collection, which was thought to be derived from the collecting system, occurred on the cut surface at the residual isthmus for a while (Figure 5) and decreased following a natural course 1 month after surgery. The donor's renal function has not worsened with serum creatinine levels between 0.53 and 0.66 mg/dL.

3. Discussion

A horseshoe kidney is the most common anatomic variation of the kidney, with an incidence of 1 in 600–800 adults [1]. Most horseshoe kidneys are fused at the lower poles, causing an incomplete rotation. Hence, the renal pelvises are situated in a ventral position, and the course of the ureter follows in front of the lower pole. In two-thirds of cases with horseshoe kidneys, complications occur based on ureteropelvic junction obstruction, such as hydronephrosis, renal calculi, and urinary tract infection. The vascular anatomy of horseshoe kidneys is usually complex, with only 30% of all horseshoe kidneys having a single renal artery to each side. The positions as well as the numbers of renal arteries and veins vary greatly, while the renal isthmus often has a separate blood supply. The renal isthmus connecting the pole of a horseshoe kidney is mostly composed of functional parenchyma.

Transplantation of a horseshoe kidney was first reported by Nelson and Palmer in 1975 [2]. Following their report, a few reviews of horseshoe kidney transplantation have been published [3, 4]. The horseshoe kidney from a deceased donor can be transplanted en bloc or split for 1 or 2 recipients after division. There is no consensus regarding the outcome associated with using a transplanted horseshoe kidney. Some authors claim that results from horseshoe kidney transplantation appear to be similar to those of normal kidney transplantation [3]. On the other hand, some authors have reported that horseshoe kidney transplantation is associated with a higher percentage of primary nonfunction [4], and the results of transplants using horseshoe kidneys are worse than those for normal kidneys [5].

A literature review revealed that six horseshoe kidneys were transplanted from living donors [5–9]. Among these, urine leakage occurred during the postoperative period in three cases. All transplanted kidney allografts demonstrated good function at a median follow-up of 14 months (range, 6–30 months). In living donors, the decision regarding where to divide the kidney is best made after the vascular anatomy and the anatomy of the collecting systems has been meticulously evaluated preoperatively using urography and CT. When the urinary collecting systems of the two sides are not connected and do not overextend into the contralateral part of the horseshoe kidney, the isthmus can be safely divided. If the urinary collecting system of a horseshoe kidney crosses the midline and the isthmus is divided, one or more calices are severed. This condition can be complicated by a urinary fistula, which is intractable. In the split technique, most surgeons transect the parenchyma according to the demarcation line made via methylene blue administration into the arterial system. Although the urinary collection system is frequently injured during separation of a renal isthmus, intraoperative perfusion of the graft with methylene blue into the renal artery was not sufficient to detect leakage of the urinary system in the literature. Therefore, we used a different technique for the split procedure. First, we ligated the inferior accessory artery and perfused the left renal artery in situ. After clamping the isthmus along the demarcation line, the parenchyma was transected (Figure 6). Furthermore, we administered indigo carmine through the renal artery and ureter to detect injury to the vessels and collecting system at the back table. In addition, to prevent complications such as urine leakage or hemorrhage after dividing the parenchyma in a living donor, the renal isthmus was divided at the left margin of the perfused boundary. In our case, there were no vascular complications due to multiple vascular abnormalities. Although slight urine leakage occurred from the cut end of the isthmus after donor nephrectomy, this fluid leakage was asymptomatic and decreased immediately.

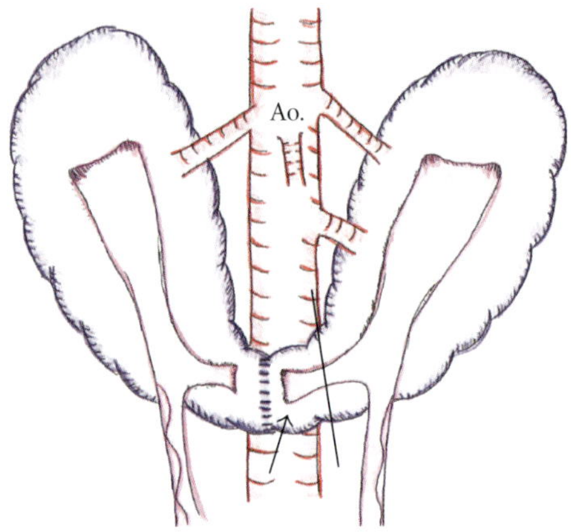

FIGURE 6: Illustration shows the horseshoe kidney with blood supplied from the aorta (Ao.) and collecting systems. The isthmus was divided on the left side position from the center (full line). A part of the left collecting system was preserved on the isthmus of the donor side (arrow).

Our case revealed that the horseshoe kidney can be an appropriate organ for transplantation. Because the number of patients awaiting a kidney transplant increases while the donor pool remains limited, we believe that using a horseshoe kidney as a renal allograft after a detailed preoperative evaluation may contribute to an expanded donor pool.

References

[1] S. B. Bauer, "Anomalies of the upper urinary tract," in *Campbell-Walsh Urology*, pp. 3269–3304, Saunders, Philadelphia, Pa, USA, 9th edition, 2007.

[2] R. P. Nelson and J. M. Palmer, "Use of horseshoe kidney in renal transplantation Technical aspects," *Urology*, vol. 6, no. 3, pp. 357–359, 1975.

[3] O. B. Stroosma, G. W. H. Schurink, J. M. A. Smits, and G. Kootstra, "Transplanting horseshoe kidneys: a worldwide survey," *The Journal of Urology*, vol. 166, no. 6, pp. 2039–2042, 2001.

[4] T. Pontinen, K. Khanmoradi, A. Kumar et al., "Horseshoe kidneys: an underutilized resource in kidney transplant," *Experimental and Clinical Transplantation*, vol. 8, no. 1, pp. 74–78, 2010.

[5] A. Dinckan, A. Tekin, S. Turkyilmaz et al., "Horseshoe kidney for transplant: report of 3 cases," *Experimental and Clinical Transplantation*, vol. 5, no. 2, pp. 716–719, 2007.

[6] S. Inoue, K. Imai, K. Kuzuhara, O. Ootubo, and A. Yamada, "Use of horseshoe kidney as renal transplant from living donor: its surgical feasibility and pitfalls," *Transplantation Proceedings*, vol. 32, no. 7, pp. 1586–1588, 2000.

[7] A. Goyal, K. Gaitonde, S. N. Sagade, B. V. Shah, and M. H. Kamat, "Transplantation of horseshoe kidney from living-related donors: report of two cases," *Transplantation Proceedings*, vol. 35, no. 1, pp. 32–34, 2003.

[8] N. Hüser, K. E. Gerauer, A. R. Novotny, V. Assfalg, and M. J. Stangl, "Successful living donor transplantation of a kidney with horseshoe malformation: extending the donor pool," *Transplant International*, vol. 18, no. 6, pp. 761–762, 2005.

[9] T. O. Sezer, I. Solak, M. Sozbilen et al., "A horseshoe kidney from a live donor as a renal transplant: case report," *Experimental and Clinical Transplantation*, vol. 11, no. 5, pp. 454–457, 2013.

5

Invasive Aspergillosis in a Renal Transplant Recipient Successfully Treated with Interferon-Gamma

C. Estrada,[1] A. G. Desai,[2] L. M. Chirch,[3] H. Suh,[1] R. Seidman,[4] F. Darras,[5] and E. P. Nord[1]

[1] *Division of Nephrology, Department of Medicine, School of Medicine, State University of New York at Stony Brook, HSC T-16 Rm 080, Stony Brook, NY 11794, USA*
[2] *Division of Pulmonology, Department of Medicine, School of Medicine, State University of New York at Stony Brook, Stony Brook, NY 11794, USA*
[3] *Division of Infectious Diseases, Department of Medicine, School of Medicine, State University of New York at Stony Brook, Stony Brook, NY 11794, USA*
[4] *Department of Pathology, School of Medicine, State University of New York at Stony Brook, Stony Brook, NY 11794, USA*
[5] *Transplantation Services, School of Medicine, State University of New York at Stony Brook, Stony Brook, NY 11794, USA*

Correspondence should be addressed to C. Estrada, chelsea.estrada@stonybrookmedicine.edu

Academic Editors: D. Capone and N. Leveque

Invasive aspergillosis is a serious complication of solid organ transplantation. An early diagnosis is hampered by the lack of reliable serum markers and, even if appropriately diagnosed and treated with current antifungal agents, has a high mortality rate. We report a case of invasive pulmonary and cerebral aspergillosis in a renal transplant patient treated with IFN-γ in conjunction with combination anti-fungal therapy for six weeks in whom complete resolution of the fungal infection was achieved. Renal function remained intact throughout the treatment period. Surveillance CT scans of the chest and head showed resolution of prior disease but revealed a new left upper lobe mass four months after completion of treatment with IFN-γ. Biopsy of the lesion was positive for primary lung adenocarcinoma, for which she underwent left upper lobe resection. The pathology report confirmed clear surgical margins and lymph nodes and no evidence of fungal hyphae. IFN-γ should be considered early in the management of invasive aspergillosis in renal transplant patients. To date, allograft rejection has not been encountered.

1. Introduction

Invasive aspergillosis (IA) is a serious complication of solid organ transplantation. Early diagnosis improves mortality but can be challenging [1]. The introduction of voriconazole has played a role in decreasing morbidity and mortality, when compared to amphotericin B [2], but concern exists regarding mounting azole resistance [3], and mortality remains as high as 70% [4, 5].

The use of interferon-gamma (IFN-γ) to treat invasive fungal infections is derived from animal models that showed resistance to disease correlated with an intact Th1 response [6] and protection was associated with high levels of tumor necrosis factor alpha (TNF-α), interleukin-2 (IL-2), interleukin-12 (IL-12), and IFN-γ [7]. Current immunosuppressive therapy blunts cell-mediated immunity, thereby predisposing organ transplant recipients to invasive fungal infections. IFN-γ has the potential to augment this defect in immunity, eradicate invasive fungal disease, and thus far has not been associated with allograft rejection [8]. We report a case of invasive pulmonary and cerebral aspergillosis, coinfected with cytomegalovirus (CMV) pneumonitis, in a renal transplant recipient, successfully treated with adjunctive IFN-γ, after combination antifungal therapy failed to eradicate the infection.

2. Case Report

A 54-year-old woman recently diagnosed with non-small-cell lung cancer was admitted for a left upper lobe resection. Her past medical history was significant for chronic bronchitis, hepatitis C treated with interferon-alpha in 1992, and hypertension. She also had chronic kidney disease secondary to glomerulonephritis (not biopsy proven), for which she

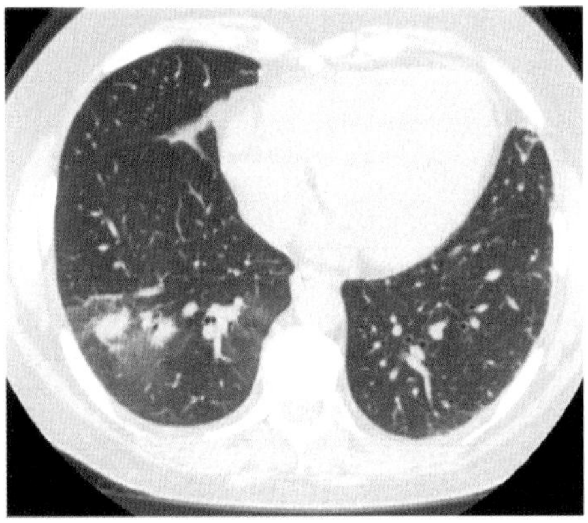

FIGURE 1: Chest CT scan without intravenous contrast on initial admission showing patchy infiltrates and a "halo sign" surrounding a right lower lobe lesion.

had a preemptive living-unrelated kidney transplant in November 2009. She was an active smoker.

Nine months posttransplant, she presented to the emergency department with a cough and dyspnea for one month. On physical examination, she was afebrile with a blood pressure of 121/56 mmHg, a heart rate of 68 beats per minute and regular, and an oxygen saturation of 97% on room air. Chest examination was significant for diffuse expiratory wheezes with scattered crackles. Heart, abdomen, and neurologic examinations were normal. Her medications included tacrolimus and mycophenolate mofetil. On laboratory evaluation, she had a white blood cell count of $9.5 \times 10^3/\text{mL}^3$ with 93.8% neutrophils, blood urea nitrogen of 25 mg/dL, and a serum creatinine of 1.1 mg/dL. Serum tacrolimus level was elevated at 14.5 mcg/mL. Computed tomography (CT) scan of her chest (Figure 1) showed multifocal infiltrates and a halo sign. Aztreonam, vancomycin, metronidazole, and capsofungin were initiated on admission for presumed multifocal pneumonia. Serum cytomegalovirus (CMV) polymerase chain reaction (PCR) and galactomannan antigen were negative. Due to lack of clinical improvement, a CT guided lung biopsy was attempted, and complicated by hemopneumothorax and cardiac arrest, from which she recovered. The biopsy result was inconclusive but sputum culture subsequently revealed moderate *Aspergillus fumigatus*. Treatment for pulmonary aspergillosis was initiated with intravenous voriconazole (6 mg/kg twice daily) for one day and then changed to oral voriconazole (4 mg/kg twice daily), which she was discharged on. Tacrolimus and mycophenolate mofetil were suspended and prednisone was initiated in their place.

Three weeks after discharge she presented to transplant clinic complaining of left-sided weakness and headache, in addition to dyspnea and cough. CT scan of her head showed extensive edema in the right cerebral hemisphere surrounding a mass-like lesion. Magnetic resonance imaging (MRI) reported this large lesion in the right basal ganglia, extending into the frontal lobe, suspicious for a fungal abscess (Figure 2(a)). She accordingly underwent stereotactic brain biopsy which showed a chronic abscess with fragments of fungal hyphae consistent with *Aspergillus* species (Figure 2(b)). Pertinent laboratory findings included elevated serum (1, 3)-beta-D-glucan at 376 pg/mL, and negative *toxoplasma gondii* PCR and galactomannan antigen. She was started on intravenous dexamethasone, and micafungin 100 mg/day was added to voriconazole. Her weakness and headache improved during the hospitalization and she was discharged home on a steroid taper, micafungin (to complete a four week course) and voriconazole.

Eight weeks later, after completing the course of micafungin, and resuming low-dose tacrolimus, a CT chest was done for persistent dyspnea and cough. It showed worsening opacities in bilateral lower lobes. Since clinical and radiographic findings were suggestive of ongoing aspergillosis, interferon gamma (IFN-γ) 200 mcg subcutaneously, three times a week was initiated and continued for six weeks. She was subsequently admitted and bronchoscopy performed. Bronchoalveolar lavage was positive for CMV and negative for *Aspergillus* species. Serum (1, 3)-beta-D-glucan level was 88 pg/mL and CMV PCR was 9650 cpy/mL. In addition to the IFN-γ, micafungin was restarted, and ganciclovir was added for her superimposed CMV pneumonitis and continued for three weeks.

Surveillance CT scans of her head and chest were done one, three, four and seven months after beginning IFN-γ. Overall improvement was seen both clinically and radiographically and CMV PCR and (1, 3)-beta-D-glucan were negative on three separate measurements. However, CT scan of her chest at four months revealed an enlarging left upper lobe density which doubled in size at seven months. A CT-guided lung biopsy was done with cytology positive for non-small cell lung cancer. The current admission, one year after her initial presentation for pulmonary aspergillosis, was for a left upper lobectomy. The post-operative course was uneventful and her graft function remained stable with serum creatinine consistently between 1.3–1.5 mg/dL. Surgical pathology demonstrated moderately-differentiated adenocarcinoma with negative margins and lymph nodes. No fungal elements were seen on multiple sections.

3. Discussion

We present a case of proven [9] invasive pulmonary and cerebral aspergillosis (and CMV pneumonitis), in a renal transplant recipient, treated successfully with adjunctive IFN-γ after combination antifungal therapy with voriconazole and micafungin that showed little clinical and radiographic improvement. Despite withdrawal or minimization of immunosuppression, renal function remained stable throughout one year. We submit that the course of IFN-γ, as described by others [8], eradicated the invasive fungal infection and in conjunction with treatment for CMV coinfection, was responsible for her symptom resolution.

Initially recognized in patients with chronic granulomatous disease [10] or neutropenia, IA is now a well-recognized complication of solid organ transplantation (SOT), with an incidence of approximately 1% [1, 4]. Overall mortality in SOT is 41–76% and up to 90% in cerebral aspergillosis [1, 4, 11, 12]. Early diagnosis improves mortality [1], however

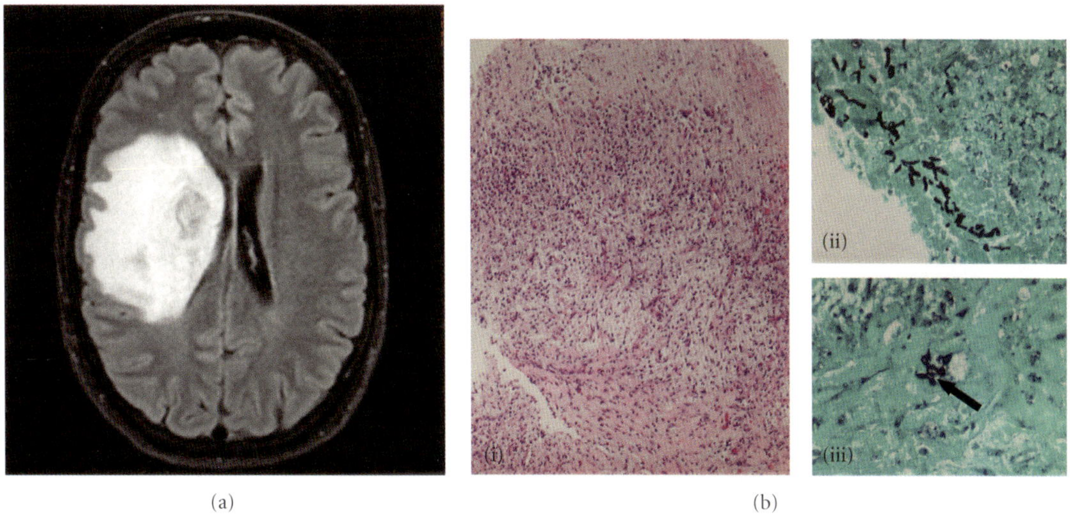

Figure 2: (a) FLAIR axial sequence of MRI of brain with gadolinium showing a large lesion in the right basal ganglia and frontal lobe with extensive edema and mass effect in keeping with a fungal abscess. (b) Brain biopsy (i). Representative area of the brain biopsy shows relatively acellular necrotic material in the top 1/5 of the image, the dense pink well-formed capsule, of a chronic abscess, occupying the bottom 1/3 of the image and a looser admixture of lymphocytes, macrophages, and new blood vessels in the center of the field. Hematoxylin and eosin, original magnification 100x (ii). The dark black structures forming a linear array running obliquely from top left to bottom center are fragments of fungi. Gomori Methenamine Silver, original magnification 400x (iii). The arrow indicates a single black fragment of a fungal structure with 45-degree branching, which is characteristic of aspergillus. Gomori Methenamine Silver, original magnification 600x.

is hampered by lack of reliable serum markers, and, at best, often only a probable diagnosis is reached, rather than proven [9]. Microbiologic evidence is rare, and sputum or bronchoalveolar lavage fluid culture cannot prove infection, as *Aspergillus* is ubiquitous. The galactomannan antigen assay has an overall sensitivity of 65–90% and a specificity of 89–98% but has primarily been studied in stem cell recipients and in hematologic malignancies [13–15] and recently was shown to be of lower yield in SOT and non-hematologic malignancies [16]. The beta-D-glucan assay appears to be more sensitive but must still be integrated with other clinical data, as it cannot differentiate between certain fungal infections, including candida and cryptococcus [13, 17]. The halo sign, a typical CT finding of IA, has been reported in 15–61% of patients; other possible radiographic findings include consolidations, cavitary lesions, and infarcts [16, 18]. Taken together, IA infection remains a lethal opportunistic infection following SOT and necessitates the integration of clinical, radiographic, microbiologic and immunologic data to effectively diagnose it.

Prior to the development of newer antifungal agents, amphotericin B was the primary therapy for invasive aspergillosis. Its use was limited by infusion reactions, nephrotoxicity and, electrolyte abnormalities and was associated with increased mortality compared with newer antifungals [1]. The introduction of voriconazole has improved survival with less toxic side effects when compared to amphotericin B [2], however mortality remains high. Since voriconazole has a strong inhibitory effect on cytochrome P450-3A4 activity, tacrolimus dosage must often be adjusted accordingly. Indeed in one case report, the potential nephrotoxic effect of this drug combination necessitated the discontinuation of tacrolimus [19]. Combination antifungal therapy has been attempted in efforts to improve outcomes; *in vitro* studies showed that for some isolates (primarily *Aspergillus fumigates*), the addition of micafungin to voriconazole raises the minimal inhibitory concentration (MIC) and enhances maximal killing effects of voriconazole against aspergillus hyphae [20]. This synergy was not seen in other species [21]. Importantly, the use of combination antifungal therapy was not associated with a mortality benefit in SOT patients with invasive aspergillosis [1]. Additionally, concern exists over increasing azole resistance; in one study of *Aspergillus fumigatus* isolates from 1997 to 2007, resistance to azoles increased from 0 to 17% over the ten-year period [3]. The relatively poor performance of current antifungals, as evident by high mortality rates, and rising azole resistance both necessitate a different approach to treatment of invasive fungal infections in immunocompromsied hosts.

Early clinical experience with IFN-γ in treating refractory invasive fungal infections has demonstrated surprisingly good outcomes. To the best of our knowledge, there are 7 reported cases of renal transplant recipients with invasive fungal infections treated with IFN-γ, in conjunction with standard antifungal therapy, of which 3 had *Aspergillus fumigatus* [8] IFN-γ was administered for six weeks, with dramatic, immediate results and no relapse. Furthermore, allograft rejection, a distinct concern when using IFN-γ in transplant patients, was not encountered. Mechanistically, protection against IA infection in mice has been associated with increased levels of TNF-α, IL-2, and IFN-γ [6], Indeed, the phagocytic cells of mice resistant to aspergillus infection were better at eradicating fungal hyphae and conida while simultaneously producing more TNF-α and IFN-γ [7]. In healthy, immunocompetent humans, exposure to *Aspergillus fumigatus* caused the release of IFN-γ, demonstrating an intact Th1 response [22]. This protective effect of IFN-γ is explained by its immunologic action of stimulating B-cells, Th1 cells, neutrophils, and phagocytes. specifically, it promotes Th1 cytokine induction of TNF-α, causing the upregulation and activation of alveolar macrophages [23]. Current immunosuppressive protocols for SOT are potent inhibitors of these cell-mediated immune responses. Tacrolimus has been shown to inhibit intragraft mRNA expression of the Th1-cytokines IFN-γ, IL-12, and TNF-α [24], and in healthy human cells treated with tacrolimus and cyclosporine, a dose-dependent reduction in natural killer cell degranulation and IFN-γ production was seen [25].

Our case adds to the literature demonstrating successful and safe use of IFN-γ in IA in renal transplant recipients. We propose that IFN-γ be considered early in the course of treatment of invasive aspergillosis either in combination with other antifungals or alone. The enhancement of the immune system with immunomodulatory agents is an attractive alternative or adjuvant to established antifungal therapy, and has potential to impact morbidity and mortality. Their role in the treatment of invasive fungal infections is evolving.

Acknowledgment

The expert secretarial assistance of Sherryl Krulik is gratefully acknowledged.

References

[1] J. W. Baddley, D. R. Andes, K. A. Marr et al., "Factors associated with mortality in transplant patients with invasive Aspergillosis," *Clinical Infectious Diseases*, vol. 50, no. 12, pp. 1559–1567, 2010.

[2] R. Herbrecht, D. W. Denning, T. F. Patterson et al., "Voriconazole versus amphotericin B for primary therapy of invasive Aspergillosis," *The New England Journal of Medicine*, vol. 347, no. 6, pp. 408–415, 2002.

[3] S. J. Howard, D. Cerar, M. J. Anderson et al., "Frequency and evolution of azole resistance in *Aspergillus* fumigatus associated with treatment failure," *Emerging Infectious Diseases*, vol. 15, no. 7, pp. 1068–1076, 2009.

[4] J. Gavalda, O. Len, R. San Juan et al., "Risk factors for invasive Aspergillosis in solid-organ transplant recipients: a case-control study," *Clinical Infectious Diseases*, vol. 41, no. 1, pp. 52–59, 2005.

[5] M. K. Ju, D. J. Joo, S. J. Kim et al., "Invasive pulmonary Aspergillosis after solid organ transplantation: diagnosis and treatment based on 28 years of transplantation experience," *Transplantation Proceedings*, vol. 41, no. 1, pp. 375–378, 2009.

[6] H. Nagai, J. Guo, H. Choi, and V. P. Kurup, "Interferon-γ and tumor necrosis factor-α protect mice from invasive Aspergillosis," *Journal of Infectious Diseases*, vol. 172, no. 6, pp. 1554–1560, 1995.

[7] E. Cenci, A. Mencacci, C. F. D'Ostiani et al., "Cytokine- and T helper-dependent lung mucosal immunity in mice with invasive pulmonary Aspergillosis," *Journal of Infectious Diseases*, vol. 178, no. 6, pp. 1750–1760, 1998.

[8] D. Armstrong-James, I. A. Teo, S. Shrivastava et al., "Exogenous interferon-γ immunotherapy for invasive fungal infections in kidney transplant patients," *American Journal of Transplantation*, vol. 10, no. 8, pp. 1796–1803, 2010.

[9] T. J. Walsh, E. J. Anaissie, D. W. Denning et al., "Treatment of Aspergillosis: clinical practice guidelines of the infectious diseases society of America," *Clinical Infectious Diseases*, vol. 46, no. 3, pp. 327–360, 2008.

[10] D. E. Morgenstern, M. A. C. Gifford, L. L. Li, C. M. Doerschuk, and M. C. Dinauer, "Absence of respiratory burst in X-linked chronic granulomatous disease mice leads to abnormalities in both host defense and inflammatory response to *Aspergillus* fumigatus," *Journal of Experimental Medicine*, vol. 185, no. 2, pp. 207–218, 1997.

[11] Y. Nivoix, M. Velten, V. Letscher-Bru et al., "Factors associated with overall and attributable mortality in invasive Aspergillosis," *Clinical Infectious Diseases*, vol. 47, no. 9, pp. 1176–1184, 2008.

[12] S. J. Lin, J. Schranz, and S. M. Teutsch, "Aspergillosis case-fatality rate: systematic review of the literature," *Clinical Infectious Diseases*, vol. 32, no. 3, pp. 358–366, 2001.

[13] G. Maschmeyer, A. Haas, and O. A. Cornely, "Invasive Aspergillosis: epidemiology, diagnosis and management in immunocompromised patients," *Drugs*, vol. 67, no. 11, pp. 1567–1601, 2007.

[14] M. D. Moragues, E. Amutio, J. C. García-Ruiz, and J. Pontón, "Usefulness of galactomannan detection in the diagnosis and follow-up of hematological patients with invasive Aspergillosis," *Revista Iberoamericana de Micologia*, vol. 20, no. 3, pp. 103–110, 2003.

[15] C. D. Pfeiffer, J. P. Fine, and N. Safdar, "Diagnosis of invasive Aspergillosis using a galactomannan assay: a meta-analysis," *Clinical Infectious Diseases*, vol. 42, no. 10, pp. 1417–1427, 2006.

[16] O. Lortholary, J. P. Gangneux, K. Sitbon et al., "Epidemiological trends in invasive Aspergillosis in France: the SAIF network (2005–2007)," *Clinical Microbiology and Infection*, vol. 17, no. 12, pp. 1882–1889, 2011.

[17] J. Acosta, M. Catalan, A. del Palacio-Pérez-Medel et al., "Prospective study in critically ill non-neutropenic patients: diagnostic potential of (1,3)-β-D-glucan assay and circulating galactomannan for the diagnosis of invasive fungal disease," *European Journal of Clinical Microbiology and Infectious Diseases*, vol. 31, no. 5, pp. 721–731, 2011.

[18] R. E. Greene, H. T. Schlamm, J. W. Oestmann et al., "Imaging findings in acute invasive pulmonary Aspergillosis: clinical significance of the halo sign," *Clinical Infectious Diseases*, vol. 44, no. 3, pp. 373–379, 2007.

[19] D. Capone, G. Tarantino, A. Gentile et al., "Effects of voriconazole on tacrolimus metabolism in a kidney transplant recipient," *Journal of Clinical Pharmacy and Therapeutics*, vol. 35, no. 1, pp. 121–124, 2010.

[20] R. E. Lewis and D. P. Kontoyiannis, "Micafungin in combination with voriconazole in *Aspergillus* species: a pharmacodynamic approach for detection of combined antifungal activity *in vitro*," *Journal of Antimicrobial Chemotherapy*, vol. 56, no. 5, pp. 887–892, 2005.

[21] K. Heyn, A. Tredup, S. Salvenmoser, and F. M. C. Müller, "Effect of voriconazole combined with micafungin against Candida, *Aspergillus*, and *Scedosporium* spp. and Fusarium solani," *Antimicrobial Agents and Chemotherapy*, vol. 49, no. 12, pp. 5157–5159, 2005.

[22] H. Hebart, C. Bollinger, P. Fisch et al., "Analysis of T-cell responses to *Aspergillus* fumigatus antigens in healthy individuals and patients with hematologic malignancies," *Blood*, vol. 100, no. 13, pp. 4521–4528, 2002.

[23] W. J. Steinbach and D. A. Stevens, "Review of newer antifungal and immunomodulatory strategies for invasive Aspergillosis,"

Clinical Infectious Diseases, vol. 37, supplement 3, pp. S157–S187, 2003.

[24] H. Krook, L. Wennberg, A. Hagberg, Z. Song, C. G. Groth, and O. Korsgren, "Immunosuppressive drugs in islet xenotransplantation: a tool for gaining further insights in the mechanisms of the rejection process," *Transplantation*, vol. 74, no. 8, pp. 1084–1089, 2002.

[25] O. Morteau, S. Blundell, A. Chakera et al., "Renal transplant immunosuppression impairs natural killer cell function *in vitro* and *in vivo*," *PLoS ONE*, vol. 5, no. 10, Article ID e13294, 2010.

6

Fatal Lactic Acidosis in a Kidney Transplant Recipient on Combination Antiretroviral Therapy after Initiation of Tacrolimus Therapy

Michael V. Holmes,[1] Ranjababu Kulasegaram,[2] Sebastian B. Lucas,[3] Terry Wong,[4] and Rachel Hilton[1]

[1] *Directorate of Nephrology, Transplantation and Urology, Guy's Hospital, Guy's and St Thomas' NHS Foundation Trust, London SE1 9RT, UK*
[2] *Department of HIV and Genitourinary Medicine, Guy's and St Thomas' NHS Foundation Trust, London SE19RT, UK*
[3] *Department of Histopathology, Guy's and St Thomas' NHS Foundation Trust, London SE19RT, UK*
[4] *Department of Gastroenterology, Guy's and St Thomas' NHS Foundation Trust, London SE19RT, UK*

Correspondence should be addressed to Rachel Hilton, rachel.hilton@gstt.nhs.uk

Academic Editors: I. Engelmann and Y. Sugawara

In general, kidney transplantation is safe and efficacious in patients receiving treatment for HIV. Although multiple drug interactions between antiviral and immunosuppressive treatments exist, few patients experience serious adverse reactions. We report a case of fatal lactic acidosis in a healthy kidney transplant recipient with stable HIV infection who had previously received treatment for and cleared hepatitis C virus infection. Death occurred less than one month following the initiation of tacrolimus therapy. Based on predicted drug interactions, appropriate tacrolimus dosing was calculated prior to its commencement, yet plasma tacrolimus levels were initially unexpectedly high. The patient subsequently developed lactic acidosis and hepatic steatosis, presumably due to mitochondrial toxicity from the antiretroviral regimen on which he had previously been stable. We suspect *CYP2C19*2* (poor metaboliser) genotype status and concomitant treatment with lansoprazole, tacrolimus, and antiretroviral (ARV) medications resulted in hepatic decompensation. This highlights the importance of careful interaction screening for all new drugs administered to patients with HIV who have complex treatment regimens as well as heightened clinical vigilance for unexpected toxicities.

1. Introduction

Since the introduction of highly active antiretroviral therapy (HAART) in 1996, mortality in patients with human immunodeficiency virus (HIV) infection has decreased markedly [1]. As a result, morbidity from other chronic conditions such as kidney, liver, and heart disease is increasing. Patients with HIV are at particular risk for development of chronic kidney disease, most notably HIV-associated nephropathy (HIVAN), which is the third most common cause of end-stage kidney disease in black individuals aged 20–64 years in the United States [2]. The presence of HIV was historically regarded as a contraindication to transplantation [3] because of the concern regarding the potential worsening of HIV disease and the increased risk of opportunistic infection by immunosuppression. However, current data suggest that transplant recipients with optimal control of HIV do as well in the short term as those without HIV, provided there is proper donor selection and recipient management [4–6]. Indeed, survival for patients with end-stage kidney disease and HIV is better after transplantation than on maintenance haemodialysis [7].

Concerns remain, however, regarding the concomitant use of antiretroviral medications and immunosuppressive agents that may be substrates for, or may induce or inhibit pharmacokinetic enzymes involved in drug handling, such as P-glycoprotein flux transporters or cytochrome P450 metabolizing enzymes found in the gut and liver. These

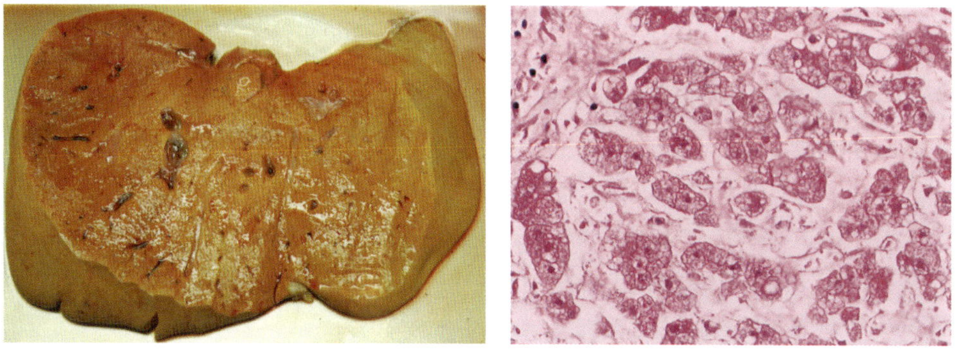

(a) (b)

Figure 1: (a) The liver showing yellow steatosis. (b) Microvesicular steatosis in hepatocytes (H&E ×400).

interactions can lead to unexpected increases or decreases in drug plasma levels leading to drug toxicity, transplant rejection, or HIV disease breakthrough. Significant drug interactions have been observed depending on the class of antiretroviral agent [8]. Clearly, predicting such interactions is mandatory to inform decisions regarding drug dosing and administration. However, because as yet relatively few patients with HIV have received organ transplants, there remains scope for emergence of presently unrecognised drug interactions due, for example, to rare genotypes encoding pharmacokinetic enzymes of high or low activity and/or idiosyncratic reactions. We report here a kidney transplant recipient who was HIV positive with cleared hepatitis C (HCV) from previous treatment who developed unpredicted mitochondrial toxicity leading to hepatic microvesicular steatosis and fatal lactic acidosis following initiation of tacrolimus immunosuppression.

2. Case Presentation

A 39-year-old Caucasian male with chronic kidney disease due to a combination of kidney stones and high blood pressure was found to have HIV infection and commenced HAART in 1995 consisting of abacavir, nevirapine, and lamivudine, on which he achieved reconstitution of CD4 count (500 cells/μL) and undetectable HIV RNA viral load (<40 copies/mL). 11 years later, he developed end-stage kidney disease and started peritoneal dialysis. Later that year, he was diagnosed with acute HCV genotype 1 infection and was treated with sustained virological response. Liver function tests at baseline were normal (Table 1). Neither liver biopsy nor transient elastography was performed. Other comorbidities included hypercholesterolaemia treated initially with bezafibrate and subsequently atorvastatin.

Eighteen months after starting dialysis, he was referred to this hospital and received a living related donor kidney transplant with a one-HLA haplotype match between donor and recipient. Immunosuppression consisted of basiliximab induction, ciclosporin microemulsion, mycophenolate mofetil, and oral prednisolone.

Six months after engraftment, there was a rise in serum creatinine above baseline, and he underwent a biopsy of his transplanted kidney which showed acute transplant rejection. This was treated with three consecutive daily doses of intravenous methylprednisolone without immediate improvement in kidney function. A decision was therefore made to switch the base immunosuppressive therapy from ciclosporin to tacrolimus. Tacrolimus is primarily metabolized in the liver by cytochrome P450 (CYP3A), and nevirapine is a slight inducer of CYP3A [9], thus by co-administering tacrolimus and nevirapine, it was predicted that plasma levels of tacrolimus would be decreased. The patient commenced tacrolimus at a standard dose (0.1 mg/kg twice daily). The initial serum tacrolimus level after 48 hours was very high (60 μg/L), and the patient complained of tremor and weakness consistent with tacrolimus toxicity. Dosing was adjusted accordingly.

Two weeks later, the patient required hospital admission with malaise, metabolic acidosis, and deranged kidney and liver function (Table 1). Bacterial septicaemia was excluded by duplicate sets of blood and urine cultures, which were negative. HCV RNA was not detected. Abdominal examination, liver ultrasonography, and abdominal CT were unremarkable. Over the course of the next 12 hours, he became drowsy, hypotensive, and peripherally vasoconstricted despite fluid resuscitation. Arterial blood gas analysis revealed severe metabolic acidosis with a serum lactate level beyond the recordable range of the blood gas analyser (>20 mmol/L). HAART and immunosuppressive agents were discontinued at this stage. He required escalating doses of inotropic and vasopressor support and in spite of 48 hours of high-volume (65 mL/kg) continuous venovenous haemofiltration (CVVHF), he remained acidotic with high serum lactate levels (16 to >20 mmol/L). He suffered a cardio-respiratory arrest from which he was resuscitated. Sedation was withdrawn to assess his neurological function, but no cortical function and limited brain stem reflexes were elicited consistent with severe brain injury. Given his poor cerebral function and clinical prognosis, active treatment was withdrawn, and he died shortly afterwards.

At autopsy, the main pathology was in the liver. Weighing 1670 gm, it was soft, bright yellow, not fibrotic, and without focal lesions (Figure 1(a)). Histopathologically, there was global microvesicular steatosis (Figure 1(b)), no hepatitis, and minimal fibrosis (Ishak stage 1-2/6; some portal fibrosis and focal spurs of connective tissue in the lobules but absence

Table 1: Haematology, biochemistry, thrombosis, and virology test results at various time points prior to and following renal transplantation.

Variable	Reference range (min, max), adults	Pretransplant	4–6 weeks prior to tacrolimus initiation	One week following tacrolimus initiation	Two weeks following tacrolimus initiation
Haematology					
Haemoglobin (g/dL)	13.0, 17.0	11.8	12.5	12.5	12.9
White cell count ($\times 10^9$)	4.0, 11.0	9.0	8.8	12.6	10.9
Platelet count ($\times 10^9$)	150, 400	268	308	255	229
CD4 Lymphocytes (per μL)	300, 1400	1188	956	235	21
Coagulation					
Activated partial thromboplastin time ratio	0.85, 1.16	0.91	1.08	1.23	1.51
International normalized ratio	0.90, 1.10	1.03	1.04	1.10	1.59
Clinical Chemistry					
Sodium (mmol/L)	135, 145	133	136	134	130
Potassium (mmol/L)	3.5, 5.0	4.3	4.3	4.6	5.1
Bicarbonate (mmol/L)	22, 30	25	26	19	15
Urea (mmol/L)	1.7, 8.3	22.0	7.8	14.4	14.1
Creatinine (μmol/L)	59, 104	1415	156	206	233
Albumin (g/L)	40, 52	46	46	37	32
Alkaline phosphatase (IU/L)	35, 129	62	205	236	383
Bilirubin (μmol/L)	0, 16	7	6	10	44
Alanine transaminase (IU/L)	4, 59	36	20	65	141
Gamma-glutamyl transferase (IU/L)	4, 72	42	61	354	1500
Creatine kinase (IU/L)	0, 229	Not measured	Not measured	Not measured	1468
Lactic acid (mmol/L)	0.4, 2.2	Not measured	Not measured	Not measured	18
Virology					
Hepatitis C RNA (IU/mL)		< 15	Not measured	Not measured	<15
HIV-1 RNA (copies/mL)		<40	<40	Not measured	<40
CMV DNA (copies/mL)		Not applicable	Not detected	Not detected	Not detected
Drug levels					
Ciclosporin level (μg/L)	100, 200	Not applicable	74	Not applicable	Not applicable
Tacrolimus level (μg/L)	8, 12	Not applicable	Not applicable	26	13
Antiviral medications		6 weeks prior to transplantation	15 weeks following transplant: on ciclosporin	NR	2 weeks after switching to tacrolimus
Abacavir (mean steady state §C_{min}, C_{max}; ng/mL)	10, 3000	1551	1611	NR	538
Lamivudine (mean steady state †C_{min}, C_{max}; ng/mL)	90, 1200	794	1615	NR	717
Nevirapine (therapeutic range min, max; ng/mL)	3000, 8000‡	5227	Not measured	NR	5488

Estimated from therapeutic doses of §300 mg abacavir twice daily and †150 mg lamivudine twice daily (values derived from Delphic Laboratories (Liverpool) ltd.).

of portal-portal bridging or diffuse perisinusoidal fibrosis). The other organs showed nonspecific changes of multi-organ failure. The steatosis was typical for toxicity associated with NRTI drugs.

Antiretroviral drug levels tested posthumously on stored serum samples lay within the therapeutic range (Table 1). Genotyping demonstrated homozygosity for variants in exon 5 of the CYP2C19 gene (*CYP2C19*2*) rendering this enzyme nonfunctional.

3. Discussion

3.1. Drug Interactions between Immunosuppressive Drugs and Antiretroviral Medication. Interactions between immunosuppressive therapy and antiretroviral medications (ARV) are common [10]. The most notable occurs as a consequence of induction or inhibition of cytochrome P450 metabolizing enzymes and P-glycoprotein flux transporters found in the liver and intestine. The CYP3A subfamily is the most highly expressed of the cytochrome P450 enzymes, and CYP3A4 is the most abundant isoform. CYP3A4 is responsible for the metabolism of calcineurin inhibitors (CNI; cyclosporin and tacrolimus), mammalian target of rapamycin (mTOR) inhibitors (sirolimus and everolimus), and HIV protease inhibitors (PI). CNIs and PIs are not only substrates but also inhibitors of CYP3A4 and tend to increase systemic blood levels of CYP3A4 substrates, whereas some nonnucleoside analogue reverse transcriptase inhibitors (NNRTIs) such as efavirenz induce CYP3A, so increasing metabolism and decreasing blood levels of CYP3A4 substrates. In addition, many of these drugs are also substrates and inhibitors of P-glycoprotein (ATP-binding cassette, PGP), a membrane-bound efflux protein involved in drug transportation across cell membranes. In the intestine, PGP limits oral bioavailability of drugs by expelling them from the interior of enterocytes into the gut lumen. Thus, coadministration of inhibitors and substrates of both P-glycoprotein and CYP3A4, such as CNIs with PIs, would be expected to increase both CNI and PI uptake and systemic blood levels. Although the extent of these drug interactions is not fully characterized for all available therapeutic combinations, careful anticipation of appropriate drug dosing is essential prior to organ transplantation to minimize the risk of treatment failure or drug toxicity. In the case reported here, the patient was not receiving a PI. The only significant predicted drug interaction was an anticipated decrease in tacrolimus plasma concentration due to coadministration of nevirapine.

3.2. Tacrolimus and Proton Pump Inhibition. Proton pump inhibitors such as lansoprazole are metabolized by both CYP2C19 and CYP3A4 isoforms of cytochrome P450. This leads to potential drug interactions with other substrates of CYP3A4 (such as tacrolimus), particularly when CYP2C19 activity is impaired [11]. Possession of the G → A allelic variation at the single nucleotide polymorphism rs4244285 is a marker of *CYP2C19*2* status. This mutation alters the mRNA reading frame, resulting in a premature stop codon, yielding a truncated nonfunctioning protein (and consequent low phenotypic CYP2C19 enzymatic activity). In Caucasians, homozygosity for the risk allele (A/A) is rare (5%). Posthumous genotyping revealed that our patient was homozygous for *CYP2C19*2*, rendering this enzyme nonfunctional. This resulted in competition between lansoprazole and tacrolimus for CYP3A4-mediated metabolism and accounted for the unexpectedly high tacrolimus levels.

3.3. Lactic Acidosis and ARV. Lactic acidosis is a rare but potentially life-threatening condition associated with exposure to nucleoside/tide reverse transcriptase inhibitors (NRTIs), particularly stavudine and didanosine, although reported with all NRTIs. Other reported risk factors include female gender, pregnancy, obesity, prolonged ARV duration, and use of ribavirin with didanosine in patients with hepatitis C coinfection [12]. The cause is inhibition of human mitochondrial polymerase-γ resulting in impaired synthesis of mitochondrial enzymes that generate adenosine triphosphate (ATP) by oxidative phosphorylation. Although 20–60% of patients on NRTI therapy have elevated lactate levels, only 0.1% to 0.4% develop lactic acidosis [13], which may be difficult to diagnose because the presenting symptoms (e.g., lethargy, nausea, vomiting, and abdominal pain) may be nonspecific. The liver is consistently involved, and pathological examination usually reveals steatosis, which may be macrovesicular, microvesicular, or mixed [14]. Treatment consists of prompt recognition and discontinuation of the offending NRTIs. Several adjunctive therapies have been tried, with limited success, including essential vitamin coenzymes (thiamine and riboflavin), ubiquinone, biotin, zinc picolinate, *n*-acetylcysteine, uridine, and l-carnitine [15]. The mortality rate is almost 60% [16]. Other than prolonged use of ARV and the presence of HCV (discussed below), in the patient we report here, there were no obvious predictors of a heightened risk of lactic acidosis.

3.4. HCV and HIV Coinfection in Transplant Recipients. Due to similar routes of transmission, coinfection of HIV with other sexual and blood-borne viruses such as hepatitis B virus (HBV) and HCV is relatively common. Of the 35 million people living with HIV worldwide, around 20% have chronic HCV infection. The mechanism of interaction between the two viruses and their impact on liver injury is not completely understood, but patients with HIV are less likely to achieve spontaneous HCV clearance and progress more rapidly to liver fibrosis and end-stage liver disease than HIV-negative individuals. Furthermore, HIV/HCV coinfected patients are more susceptible to liver toxicity and steatosis from ARV, more so with the use of NRTIs, and in such patients, hepatic steatosis is associated with more advanced hepatic fibrosis [17]. Risk factors for hepatic steatosis in HIV-HCV coinfected patients include white race, increasing age, higher body mass index, insulin resistance, lower levels of high-density lipoprotein cholesterol, presence of lipodystrophy, HCV genotype 3, higher HCV plasma viral load, stavudine or didanosine use, and raised serum ferritin [18]. Among liver transplant recipients, poorer outcomes have been observed in patients coinfected with HIV and HCV in comparison with HIV or HCV monoinfected patients [6, 19], principally due to recurrent HCV infection. HCV-positive kidney transplant recipients have equivalent patient but decreased graft survival in comparison with HCV-negative recipients, poorer graft outcome being partly explained by mesangioproliferative glomerulonephritis in the allograft [20].

In the case we report here, although the patient had cleared HCV and remained HCV RNA negative with normal liver function tests, he had not had assessment of liver fibrosis by biopsy or transient elastography prior to kidney transplantation. Features which argue against a causal role of HCV in this case are sustained virological response to HCV eradication therapy; presence of Ishak stage 1-2 hepatic fibrosis on autopsy (a sign of early fibrosis often present in the general population); microvesicular steatosis, which is unrelated to HCV and consistent with a drug-induced lactic acidosis (typically NRTI); an AST-to-platelet ratio index (APRI) of 0.08, measured when the patient was stable, indicating haematological and biochemical absence of fibrosis.

3.5. In Search of Occam's Razor. The close temporal association between the initiation of tacrolimus and the onset of progressive liver dysfunction suggests a causal relationship, but the mechanism for this remains unexplained. The unexpectedly high tacrolimus levels probably resulted from *CYP2C19*2* status and concomitant lansoprazole, both of which affected tacrolimus metabolism by CYP3A4. However, this does not explain the mitochondrial uncoupling with lactic acidosis and steatosis that occurred shortly after tacrolimus initiation; there are no previous reports of tacrolimus-induced lactic acidosis. It is possible that a steatosis diathesis was created by existing treatment with NRTI, which, coupled with the presence of elevated tacrolimus levels, resulted in hepatic decompensation. Yet, serum levels of HAART were normal (although this may not accurately reflect intrahepatic levels, nor is it indicative of increased risk of mitochondrial oxidative uncoupling). An alternative hypothesis is that the unique combination of genetic variation and polypharmacy precipitated hepatic decompensation through unknown pathways.

Organ transplantation for patients with HIV remains a novel therapy [21] and carries a risk of unanticipated drug interactions that may cause increased drug toxicity or diminished therapeutic effect. While these may shed new light on mechanisms of drug metabolism and disposition, our case highlights the need for careful interaction screening of all new treatment regimens in such patients as well as heightened clinical vigilance for unexpected toxicities.

Acknowledgments

For their kind help, the auhors thank Dr. Peter Green (Genomics Laboratory, Department of Medical and Molecular Genetics, King's College London), Helen Dunn (Virology Department, Guys' and St Thomas' NHS Foundation Trust), and Lesley Robinson (Delphic Diagnostics ltd.). The authors acknowledge financial support from the Department of Health via the National Institute for Health Research (NIHR) and comprehensive Biomedical Research Centre award to Guy's and St Thomas' NHS Foundation Trust in partnership with King's College London and King's College Hospital NHS Foundation Trust.

References

[1] E. J. Schwartz, L. A. Szczech, M. J. Ross, M. E. Klotman, J. A. Winston, and P. E. Klotman, "Highly active antiretroviral therapy and the epidemic of HIV+ end-stage renal disease," *Journal of the American Society of Nephrology*, vol. 16, no. 8, pp. 2412–2420, 2005.

[2] M. Monahan, N. Tanji, and P. E. Klotman, "HIV-associated nephropathy: an urban epidemic," *Seminars in Nephrology*, vol. 21, no. 4, pp. 394–402, 2001.

[3] "European best practice guidelines for renal transplantation (part 1)," *Nephrology Dialysis Transplantation*, vol. 15, supplement 7, pp. 1–85, 2000.

[4] J. E. Locke, R. A. Montgomery, D. S. Warren, A. Subramanian, and D. L. Segev, "Renal transplant in HIV-positive patients: long-term outcomes and risk factors for graft loss," *Archives of Surgery*, vol. 144, no. 1, pp. 83–86, 2009.

[5] J. Qiu, P. I. Terasaki, K. Waki, J. Cai, and D. W. Gjertson, "HIV-positive renal recipients can achieve survival rates similar to those of HIV-negative patients," *Transplantation*, vol. 81, no. 12, pp. 1658–1661, 2006.

[6] M. E. Roland, B. Barin, L. Carlson et al., "HIV-infected liver and kidney transplant recipients: 1- and 3-year outcomes," *American Journal of Transplantation*, vol. 8, no. 2, pp. 355–365, 2008.

[7] M. S. Kumar, D. R. Sierka, A. M. Damask et al., "Safety and success of kidney transplantation and concomitant immunosuppression in HIV-positive patients," *Kidney International*, vol. 67, no. 4, pp. 1622–1629, 2005.

[8] L. A. Frassetto, M. Browne, A. Cheng et al., "Immunosuppressant pharmacokinetics and dosing modifications in HIV-1 infected liver and kidney transplant recipients," *American Journal of Transplantation*, vol. 7, no. 12, pp. 2816–2820, 2007.

[9] H. Izzedine, V. Launay-Vacher, A. Baumelou, and G. Deray, "Antiretroviral and immunosuppressive drug-drug interactions: an update," *Kidney International*, vol. 66, no. 2, pp. 532–541, 2004.

[10] K. Seden, D. Back, and S. Khoo, "Antiretroviral drug interactions: often unrecognized, frequently unavoidable, sometimes unmanageable," *Journal of Antimicrobial Chemotherapy*, vol. 64, no. 1, pp. 5–8, 2009.

[11] F. Itagaki, M. Homma, K. Yuzawa, K. Fukao, and Y. Kohda, "Drug interaction of tacrolimus and proton pump inhibitors in renal transplant recipients with CYP2C19 gene mutation," *Transplantation Proceedings*, vol. 34, no. 7, pp. 2777–2778, 2002.

[12] C. J. Fichtenbaum, "Metabolic abnormalities associated with HIV infection and antiretroviral therapy," *Current Infectious Disease Reports*, vol. 11, no. 1, pp. 84–92, 2009.

[13] A. Carr and D. A. Cooper, "Adverse effects of antiretroviral therapy," *The Lancet*, vol. 356, no. 9239, pp. 1423–1430, 2000.

[14] Y. E. Claessens, J. D. Chiche, J. P. Mira, and A. Cariou, "Bench-to-bedside review: severe lactic acidosis in HIV patients treated with nucleoside analogue reverse transcriptase inhibitors," *Critical Care*, vol. 7, no. 3, pp. 226–232, 2003.

[15] K. Brinkman, S. Vrouenraets, R. Kauffmann, H. Weigel, and J. Frissen, "Treatment of nucleoside reverse transcriptase inhibitor-induced lactic acidosis," *AIDS*, vol. 14, no. 17, pp. 2801–2802, 2000.

[16] V. Falco, D. Rodriguez, E. Ribera et al., "Severe nucleoside-associated lactic acidosis in human immunodeficiency virus-infected patients: report of 12 cases and review of the literature," *Clinical Infectious Diseases*, vol. 34, no. 6, pp. 838–846, 2002.

[17] M. Nunez, R. Lana, J. L. Mendoza, L. Martín-Carbonero, and V. Soriano, "Risk factors for severe hepatic injury after introduction of highly active antiretroviral therapy," *Journal of Acquired Immune Deficiency Syndromes*, vol. 27, no. 5, pp. 426–431, 2001.

[18] F. Bani-Sadr, F. Carrat, P. Bedossa et al., "Hepatic steatosis in HIV-HCV coinfected patients: analysis of risk factors," *AIDS*, vol. 20, no. 4, pp. 525–531, 2006.

[19] S. Norris, C. Taylor, P. Muiesan et al., "Outcomes of liver transplantation in HIV-infected individuals: the impact of HCV

and HBV infection," *Liver Transplantation*, vol. 10, no. 10, pp. 1271–1278, 2004.
[20] K. L. Brown, J. M. El-Amm, M. D. Doshi et al., "Intermediate-term outcomes of hepatitis C-positive compared with hepatitis C-negative deceased-donor renal allograft recipients," *American Journal of Surgery*, vol. 195, no. 3, pp. 298–303, 2008.
[21] S. Bhagani, P. Sweny, and G. Brook, "Guidelines for kidney transplantation in patients with HIV disease," *HIV medicine*, vol. 7, no. 3, pp. 133–139, 2006.

Utility of Iron Staining in Identifying the Cause of Renal Allograft Dysfunction in Patients with Sickle Cell Disease

Yingchun Wang,[1] Mona Doshi,[2] Salman Khan,[3] Wei Li,[1] and Ping L. Zhang[1]

[1]*Department of Anatomic and Clinical Pathology, Beaumont Health System, Royal Oak, MI 48073, USA*
[2]*Division of Nephrology, Wayne State University School of Medicine, Detroit, MI 48201, USA*
[3]*Dallas Nephrology Associates, Dallas, TX 75204, USA*

Correspondence should be addressed to Ping L. Zhang; ping.zhang@beaumont.edu

Academic Editor: Frieder Keller

Sickle cell nephropathy (SCN) is associated with iron/heme deposition in proximal renal tubules and related acute tubular injury (ATI). Here we report the utility of iron staining in differentiating causes of renal allograft dysfunction in patients with a history of sickle cell disease. Case 1: the patient developed acute allograft dysfunction two years after renal transplant. Her renal biopsy showed ATI, supported by patchy loss of brush border and positive staining of kidney injury molecule-1 in proximal tubular epithelial cells, where diffuse increase in iron staining (2+) was present. This indicated that ATI likely resulted from iron/heme toxicity to proximal tubules. Electron microscope confirmed aggregated sickle RBCs in glomeruli, indicating a recurrent SCN. Case 2: four years after renal transplant, the patient developed acute allograft dysfunction and became positive for serum donor-specific antibody. His renal biopsy revealed thrombotic microangiopathy (TMA) and diffuse positive C4d stain in peritubular capillaries. Iron staining was negative in the renal tubules, implying that TMA was likely associated with acute antibody-mediated rejection (AAMR, type 2) rather than recurrent SCN. These case reports imply that iron staining is an inexpensive but effective method in distinguishing SCN-associated renal injury in allograft kidney from other etiologies.

1. Introduction

In native renal biopsies from patients with sickle cell disease (SCD), sickle cell nephropathy (SCN) may include dominant glomerular disorders, renal tubular injury, or both. SCN has been considered predominantly a vascular disorder with sickle shaped red blood cells (RBCs) clogging the peritubular capillaries leading to papillary necrosis and scarring. Membranoproliferative changes similar to chronic thrombotic microangiopathy (TMA) are the common findings [1–3], as clustered sickle cells result in thrombotic injury. In addition to nonspecific tubular atrophy, due to hemolysis of the vulnerable sickled RBCs, iron/heme deposition in the renal tubules has been described as a tubular injury pattern causing renal failure in native kidneys [4–6]. However, not all renal disease in patients with SCD is due to SCN. Further, there is no pathognomonic lesion that defines SCN. Currently, there is no reliable test to distinguish SCN-associated renal tubular injury from other injury etiologies.

Acute tubular injury (ATI) is also a common finding in renal transplant biopsies, up to 28% of all renal transplant biopsies in our institution (unpublished observation). The most common cause of ATI results from ischemic-reperfusion injury occurring shortly after deceased renal grafts. Calcineurin toxicity, volume depletion, and acute antibody-mediated rejection are other possible causes.

Here we present how to use iron staining to differentiate SCN-associated tubular injury from other etiologies in two renal transplant biopsies from patients with known SCD.

2. Cases Presentation

2.1. Case 1. A 46-year-old woman with a medical history of SCD and end stage renal disease (ESRD) underwent renal transplantation two years before this biopsy. She was found to have elevated serum creatinine up to 1.4 mg/dL from baseline of 0.9 mg/dL, and her renal graft was biopsied to rule out rejection.

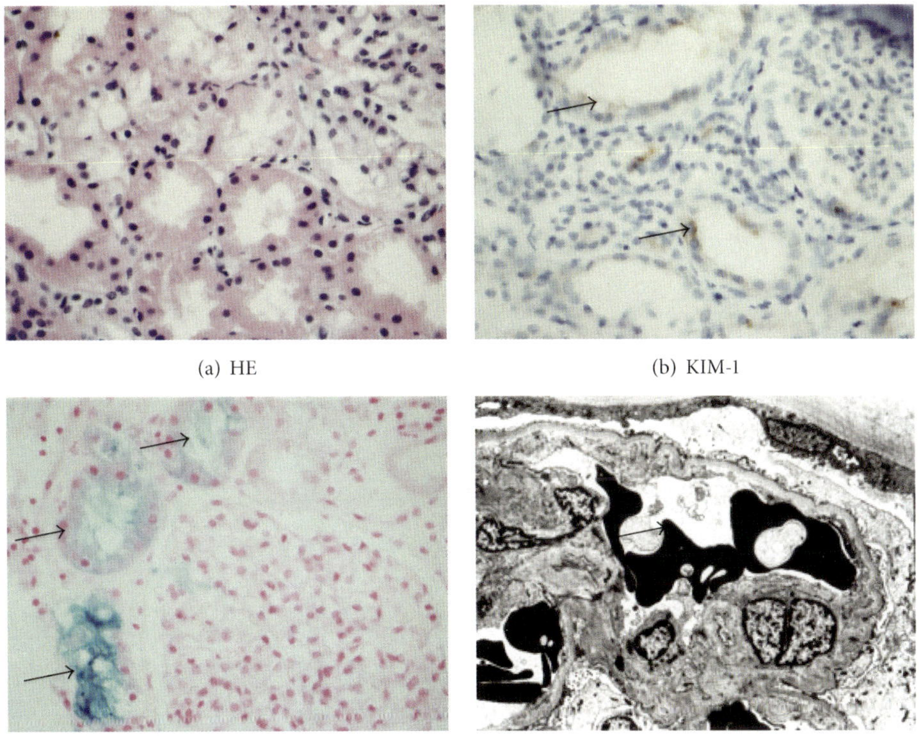

(a) HE (b) KIM-1

(c) Iron (d) EM

FIGURE 1: Iron deposition associated with acute tubular injury in the allograft kidney. (a) Dilated proximal tubules with focal disruption of brush border. No inflammatory infiltration is seen (hematoxylin and eosin, original magnification ×400). (b) Acute tubular injury was confirmed by positive kidney injury molecule-1 staining (arrow) along the luminal surface of proximal tubules (original magnification ×400). (c) Iron staining was moderately (2+) positive in the injured proximal tubules (arrow) (original magnification ×400). (d) Electron photomicrograph depicting sickle shaped red blood cells (arrow) clustered in the glomerular capillary loops (original magnification ×4000).

The hematoxylin and eosin (HE) sections revealed three biopsy cores with 10 glomeruli. None of the glomeruli was either segmentally or globally sclerosed. There was no glomerulitis or double contours of glomerular basement membranes noted. Except for focal tubular atrophy, the majority of renal tubules were back-to-back without significant interstitial fibrosis (Figure 1(a)). The proximal tubules were mildly dilated with focal disruption of the brush borders. There was no significant inflammatory infiltration in the renal parenchyma, tubulitis, or vasculitis. BK virus staining was negative with a good positive control. C4d staining by immunofluorescent method was negative in peritubular capillaries. There was no specific glomerular staining for IgA, IgG, IgM, C1q, C3, kappa, or lambda light chain. An immunohistochemical stain for kidney injury molecule-1 (KIM-1) was positive along the luminal surface of some proximal tubules (Figure 1(b)), consistent with acute tubular injury. Approximately 20% of proximal tubules stained 1+ to 2+ positive for iron (Figure 1(c)), implying that the ATI was associated with iron/heme deposition from hemolyzed sickled RBCs into the renal tubules. Two glomeruli were present on Methylene Blue Azure II stained sections. Ultrastructurally, there was good preservation of foot processes. Focal thickening of glomerular basement membranes was noted. Some irregular shaped RBCs were identified in the glomerular capillary loops, consistent with sickled RBCs (Figure 1(d)). No immune complex deposits were present in the mesangial areas, subendothelial or subepithelial spaces. In summary, the mild ATI was most likely associated with iron nephrotoxicity secondary to recurrent SCN.

2.2. Case 2. The 35-year-old man underwent a renal transplantation four years before due to SCN-associated ESRD. His recent serum test was positive for donor-specific antibody, and his current serum creatinine was elevated to 3.8 mg/dL before the renal allograft biopsy.

Sections of light microscopy revealed two biopsy cores of renal cortex containing totally ten glomeruli (Figure 2(a)). One glomerulus was globally sclerosed and the remaining glomeruli showed membranoproliferative pattern with thrombi in one glomerulus. There was lymphocytic infiltration involving more than 20% of the renal cortex with mild tubulitis. No vasculitis was identified. Trichrome-stained section showed mild to moderate interstitial fibrosis and tubular atrophy. BK virus staining was negative with a good positive control. C4d staining by immunohistochemical method was strongly and diffusely positive in glomeruli and peritubular capillaries (Figure 2(b)). Iron staining was essentially negative in the renal tubules (Figure 2(c)). Three glomeruli were present for immunofluorescence studies. At least two glomeruli showed segmentally positive staining for fibrinogen (2+) and IgM (1+). The remaining staining including IgG,

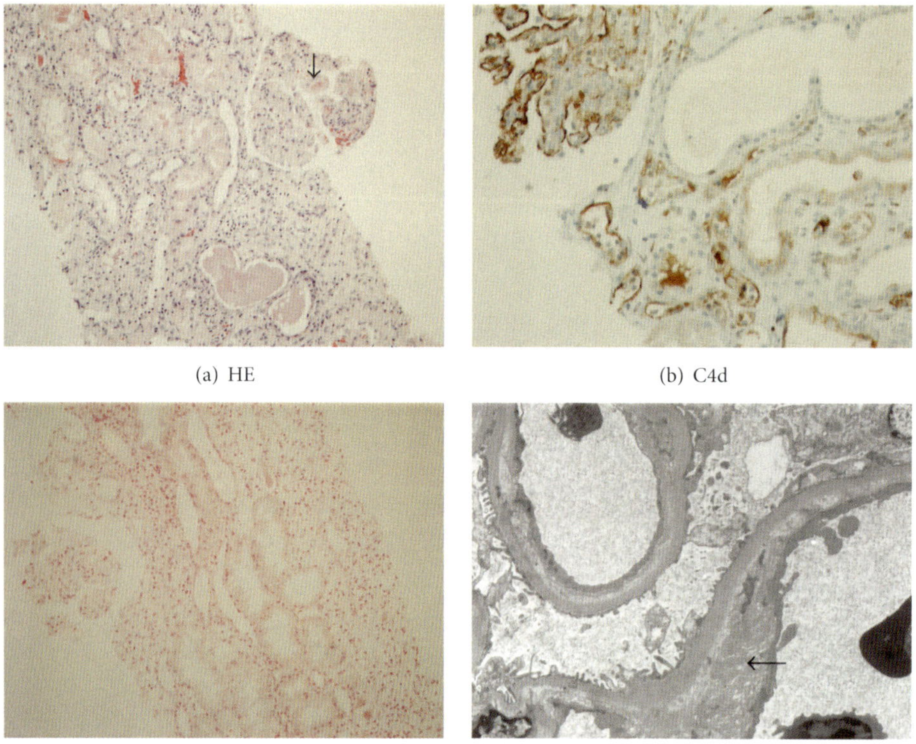

(a) HE

(b) C4d

(c) Iron

(d) EM

Figure 2: Acute tubular injury caused by type 2 antibody-mediated rejection in the allograft kidney. (a) Light microscopy showed a glomerulus with lobular configuration and focal fibrin thrombi (arrow). Renal tubules are mildly dilated with mild tubulitis. Interstitial mononuclear infiltrate is also seen (hematoxylin and eosin, original magnification ×100). (b) C4d diffusely positive in peritubular capillaries and glomerular capillary loops (original magnification ×200). (c) Iron staining is essentially negative (original magnification ×100). (d) Electron photomicrograph showed double contoured glomerular capillary loops with lucency and subendothelial deposit of fibrin (arrow), consistent with thrombotic microangiopathy (original magnification ×4000).

IgA, C3, C1q, kappa, and lambda was negative. C4d stained sections showed strong positive staining in 80% of the peritubular capillaries, consistent with antibody-mediated rejection. Four glomeruli were identified on Methylene Blue Azure II stained sections for electron microscopy. Ultrastructurally, there was segmental fusion of foot processes. The glomerular basement membrane showed prominent double contour with lucent appearance and scattered foci of subendothelial fibrin deposits (Figure 2(d)). Occasional irregular shaped RBCs were present, but they do not form thrombus. No immune complex deposits were identified in the mesangial areas, subendothelial or subepithelial spaces. We commented that the TMA can be either secondary to the antibody-mediated rejection or SCN. However, the negative iron stain in the renal tubules implied that SCN was not the major cause for this current TMA. Instead, the TMA was most likely associated with the antibody-mediated rejection and thus classified as type II acute antibody-mediated rejection.

2.3. Prussian Blue Iron Staining. The intensity for Prussian blue iron staining within the luminal surface of proximal tubular epithelial cells was graded from 0 to 3+ (0, no staining; 1+, weak fine granular staining along the luminal surface; 2+, moderate granular staining; and 3+, strong large granular staining).

2.4. Immunohistochemistry. Immunohistochemistry on renal biopsy was performed as previously described [7]. KIM-1, AKG7 monoclonal antibody, was kindly provided by Dr. Joseph V. Bonventre, Renal Division, Brigham and Women's Hospital, Boston. C4d, rabbit polyclonal antibody, was from Cell Marque, Rocklin, California.

3. Discussion

SCD in native kidneys can be associated with iron/heme deposition in renal tubules and its related acute tubular injury (Figure 3), as reported previously [4–6]. In order to evaluate the utility of iron staining in renal tubules to identify SCN-associated tubular injury from other causes, we also performed Prussian blue iron staining in 29 renal biopsies without a history of SCD. These included 25 biopsies from native kidneys, 13 TMA and 12 IgA nephropathy, and four ATI, one acute cellular rejection and one acute antibody-mediated rejection from allograft kidneys. Among the 13 TMA cases, three had 1+ weak iron staining in less than 10% of renal tubules, whereas the remaining ten cases stained negative for iron. Among the 12 cases of IgA nephropathy, three cases showed 1+ iron staining in less than 1% of the renal tubules, while the other nine cases were negatively stained for tubular iron. In allograft kidneys, four cases with ATI and one case

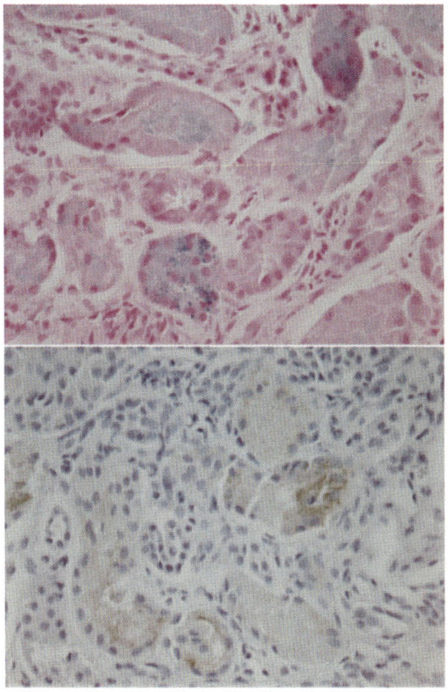

Figure 3: Native renal biopsy with sickle cell nephropathy associated iron deposition and acute tubular injury. A 17-year-old male, with a medical history of SCD, developed acute renal failure. Findings of his renal biopsy were consistent with SCN. Top panel: the proximal tubules were deposited with large amount of iron broken from sickle red blood cells (positive Prussian blue iron staining). Bottom panel: the iron-associated nephrotoxicity in the proximal tubules was confirmed by positive KIM-1 staining. *(Top and bottom panels, original magnification ×400.)*

with acute cellular rejection stained negatively for the tubular iron, and one case with antibody-mediated rejection was found to have 1+ iron stain in less than 1% of renal tubules. In the IgA nephropathy and TMA, normal shaped RBCs that went through nephrons are unlikely to be damaged, and thus, there was minimal iron spill into renal tubules. However, renal deposits of iron, hemosiderosis, have been observed in a number of diseases featuring intravascular hemolysis [8], including SCD. Mechanical trauma to erythrocytes liberates hemoglobin into plasma, where hemoglobin is bound by haptoglobin and degraded or filtered and incorporated into proximal tubules through the megalin-cubilin receptor system present on the apical surface of these cells. Heme proteins can cause acute kidney injury through three main mechanisms: decreased renal perfusion, direct cytotoxicity, and intratubular casts formed from the interaction of heme proteins with Tamm-Horsfall protein. Cytotoxic effects of large amounts of heme result from its lipophilic, oxidant, proinflammatory, and apoptotic effects [9, 10].

In our current transplant Case 1, the strong iron staining was found in allograft renal tubules, most likely being the cause of ATI, which was confirmed by positive staining for kidney injury molecule-1, a specific injury marker of proximal tubules [11, 12]. In the second renal transplant case, iron staining was essentially negative in renal tubules, while a type 2 acute antibody-mediated rejection was identified in the allograft biopsy, which is known to cause ischemia type of insult to renal glomeruli and tubules [13, 14]. The different iron staining results from these renal allograft biopsies indicate that the inexpensive iron staining could help differentiate allograft dysfunction secondary to recurrent SCN from other etiologies in patients with known SCD.

References

[1] C. Vogler, E. Wood, P. Lane, E. Ellis, B. Cole, and C. Thorpe, "Microangiopathic glomerulopathy in children with sickle cell anemia," *Pediatric Pathology & Laboratory Medicine*, vol. 16, no. 2, pp. 275–284, 1996.

[2] A. G. Morgan, D. J. Shah, and W. Williams, "Renal pathology in adults over 40 with sickle-cell disease," *West Indian Medical Journal*, vol. 36, no. 4, pp. 241–250, 1987.

[3] I. B. Elfenbein, A. Patchefsky, W. Schwartz, and A. G. Weinstein, "Pathology of the glomerulus in sickle cell anemia with and without nephrotic syndrome," *The American Journal of Pathology*, vol. 77, no. 3, pp. 357–374, 1974.

[4] D. B. Bhathena and J. H. Sondheimer, "The glomerulopathy of homozygous sickle hemoglobin (SS) disease: morphology and pathogenesis," *Journal of the American Society of Nephrology*, vol. 1, no. 11, pp. 1241–1252, 1991.

[5] J. A. Pitcock, E. E. Muirhead, F. E. Hatch, J. G. Johnson, and B. J. Kelly, "Early renal changes in sickle cell anemia," *Archives of Pathology*, vol. 90, no. 5, pp. 403–410, 1970.

[6] R. J. Falk, J. Scheinman, G. Phillips, E. Orringer, A. Johnson, and J. C. Jennette, "Prevalence and pathologic features of sickle cell nephropathy and response to inhibition of angiotensin-converting enzyme," *The New England Journal of Medicine*, vol. 326, no. 14, pp. 910–915, 1992.

[7] D. Cosner, X. Zeng, and P. L. Zhang, "Proximal tubular injury in medullary rays is an early sign of acute tacrolimus nephrotoxicity," *Journal of Transplantation*, vol. 2015, Article ID 142521, 6 pages, 2015.

[8] P. Leonardi and A. Ruol, "Renal hemosiderosis in the hemolytic anemias: diagnosis by means of needle biopsy," *Blood*, vol. 16, pp. 1029–1038, 1960.

[9] Q. Qian, K. A. Nath, Y. Wu, T. M. Daoud, and S. Sethi, "Hemolysis and acute kidney failure," *American Journal of Kidney Diseases*, vol. 56, no. 4, pp. 780–784, 2010.

[10] M. J. Tracz, J. Alam, and K. A. Nath, "Physiology and pathophysiology of heme: implications for kidney disease," *Journal of the American Society of Nephrology*, vol. 18, no. 2, pp. 414–420, 2007.

[11] P. L. Zhang, L. I. Rothblum, W. K. Han, T. M. Blasick, S. Potdar, and J. V. Bonventre, "Kidney injury molecule-1 expression in transplant biopsies is a sensitive measure of cell injury," *Kidney International*, vol. 73, no. 5, pp. 608–614, 2008.

[12] W. K. Han, V. Bailly, R. Abichandani, R. Thadhani, and J. V. Bonventre, "Kidney Injury Molecule-1 (KIM-1): a novel biomarker for human renal proximal tubule injury," *Kidney International*, vol. 62, no. 1, pp. 237–244, 2002.

[13] R. K. Johnson, D. Sarmarapungavan, R. K. Parasuraman et al., "Acute tubular injury is an important component in type I acute antibody-mediated rejection," *Transplantation Proceedings*, vol. 45, no. 9, pp. 3262–3268, 2013.

[14] R. Nair, M. Fraer, N. Agrawal, and M. Suneja, "Acute Transplant glomerulopathy is associated with antibody-mediated rejection and poor graft outcome," *Transplantation Proceedings*, vol. 42, no. 9, pp. 3507–3512, 2010.

8

Inferior Epigastric Artery Pseudoaneurysm in a Kidney Transplant Recipient

M. Tozzi,[1] B. Molteni,[2] M. Franchin,[2] G. Ietto,[2] G. Soldini,[2] V. Bertocchi,[2] and G. Carcano[2]

[1] *Vascular Surgery, Insubria University, Circolo University Teaching Hospital, Via Guicciardini 9, 21100 Varese, Italy*
[2] *Department of Organ Transplant, Insubria University, Circolo University Teaching Hospital, Via Guicciardini 9, 21100 Varese, Italy*

Correspondence should be addressed to M. Tozzi; matteo.tozzi@uninsubria.it

Academic Editors: A. Beiras-Fernandez and M. Klinger

Pseudoaneurysm of inferior epigastric artery (IEA) is a very rare clinical entity. We reported a case of combined kidney transplant and pseudoaneurysmectomy in a young HBV-HCV-HIV recipient. This case emphasizes the possibility of planning a safe and correct surgical treatment and the best timing to treat IEA pseudoaneurysm. An exhaustive preoperative radiological study in all patients candidate to kidney transplant could identify the possible aortoiliac disease both stenotic or dilatative even if it is rare and helps to define the best treatment options.

1. Introduction

Pseudoaneurysm of inferior epigastric artery (IEA) is a very rare clinical entity, with just a few cases reported in the literature. It is described as a complication of surgery, trauma, arterial puncture, paracentesis, and removal of Tenckhoff catheters and sometimes is idiopathic.

IEA pseudoaneurysm can be diagnosed by a contrast enhanced computer tomography (CT) scan or by a color Doppler ultrasound (US).

The treatment options include surgery with excision and ligation of IEA, percutaneous embolization with placement of metallic coils or with N-butyl cyanoacrylate (NCBA), percutaneous thrombin injection, sonographic-guided compression, and conservative treatment [1–25].

2. Case Report

A 51-year-old male marble cutter, with chronic hepatopathy HBV-HCV related, HIV infection, hypertension, and chronic obstructive pulmonary disease, developed end-stage HIV nephropathy. The patient had no prior surgical treatment. The patient started dialysis in 2009. In 2010, he was considered for kidney transplant. In consideration of comorbidities, angiographic-CT scan was performed and detected a 8 mm pseudoaneurysm of left IEA close to the vassel origin (Figure 1). The patient did not refer to pain or discomfort; no tender mass was detected at palpatory examination. Kidney transplant was performed approximately 20 months after trough a "hockey stick" incision; renal graft was anastomized to common-iliac vessels. Contemporary IEA ligation at vassel origin and pseudoaneurymectomy were performed (Figure 2). Postoperative course was regular. During hospitalization, a renal tract US was performed in 4th and 10th postoperative days and no perigraft or pericystic fluid collection was detected. Hospitalization time was 12 days and at the discharge creatinine serical level was 1,4 mg/dL, haemoglobin 13,6 g/dL. At 1 month, creatinine level was 1.2 mg/dL.

3. Discussion

The IEA arises as a branch of the external iliac artery just above the inguinal ligament. From its origin, it courses upward and medially to enter the rectus sheath. Within the rectus sheath, it lies just at anterior to posterior wall of the sheath [1]. Pseudoaneurysm of the IEA is a recognised but very rare clinical entity with just a few cases reported in the literature as complication of surgery, trauma, and arterial puncture [2–4]. Other very unusual causes are sutures, drain-tube or Tenckoff catheters insertion, therapeutic paracentesis, manipulation of

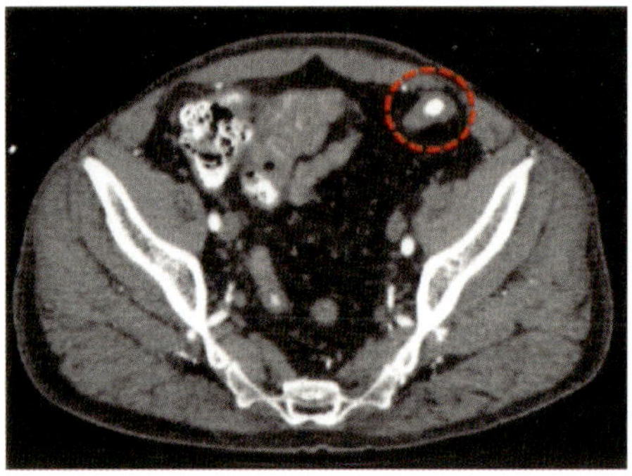

Figure 1

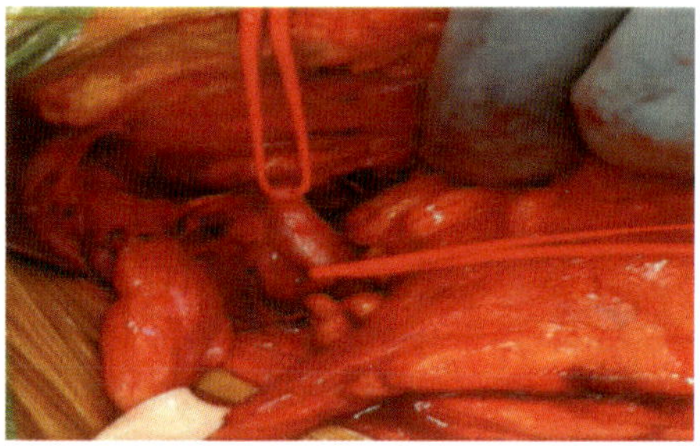

Figure 2

laparoscopic instruments [26], and abdominal wall surgery [19]; only 3 cases of idiopathic IEA pseudoaneurysm were described in the literature [11]. An IEA pseudoaneurysm and arteriovenous fistula as a complication of IEA surgical injury are reported [13].

IEA pseudoaneurysm could be treated by feeding vessel surgical ligation and aneurysmectomy [2, 4–7, 9, 10, 12, 25], by percutaneous coil embolisation [3, 8, 13–15, 17–19, 22, 24], by ultrasound guided thrombin injection, by ultrasound guided compression, or by conservative treatment with a spontaneous regression [16, 20, 23]. Surgery is the most invasive treatment and includes the necessity of general anaesthesia and postoperative pain treatment, but the advantage is the quick resolution of the symptoms with the removal of the mass effect caused by the pseudoaneurysm [18]. Ferrer et al. recommended surgery for large pseudoaneurysm [5]. Percutaneous embolization is generally used, but the disadvantages of percutaneous transcatheter approach for the management of IEA pseudoaneurysms include the necessity of arterial access, sheath placement, and increased potential for femoral pseudoaneurysm (0,8–2,2%) [27]. Lam et al. suggested that percutaneous transcatheter techniques may be preferable in patients with portal hypertension caused by chronic liver disease, who often have a coagulopathy and increased venous collateral in their abdominal wall [8]. Embolization with metallic coils or microcoils is successful, but it depends on the anatomy, the size of the arterial lesion, and the technical ability to place selectivity or superselectivity catheters or microcatheters [1]; also NBCA has been successfully used to treat IEA pseudoaneurysm [24]. US-guided probe compression may be useful for initial management of the pseudoaneurysms, but it may not be adequate if the pseudoaneurysm is deep seated either secondary to a large haematoma or it has a wide neck [15]; pain and discomfort at the compression site, the longtime compression (30–50 min), and incomplete occlusion constitute drawbacks [3, 4]. Ultrasonographic-guided thrombin injection is simple, safe, and quick to perform, painless and extremely effective, but the risk of thrombosis of patent artery because of the leakage of thrombin into the supply artery should be considered [1]. Spontaneous thrombosis has been reported after conservative management; the authors believe that the rise of intracompartimental pressure caused by hematoma was enough to achieve thrombosis [23].

Clinically, IEA pseudoaneurysms are difficult to diagnose because they usually present as diffuse tender masses that are not pulsatile. They are therefore difficult to differentiate from simple haematomas, which can also present as tender masses [1]. Epigastric vassels are usually located in the area between 4 and 8 cm from the midline [28]; clinical suspicions for an IEA pseudoaneurysm should be raised when any patient presents with a painful abdominal wall mass <8 cm from either side of midline whether or not is found to be pulsatile [18]. Because of the communication with the injured artery, an audible bruit may sometimes be present over the pseudoaneurysm [2, 6, 26], which excludes a hematoma.

Diagnosis of IEA pseudoaneurysms is usually by a contrast-enhanced CT scan or a color Doppler US with the latter being the imaging modality of choice [9, 11–13, 15]. Dopple US has a sensitivity and specificity of 100% in the differentiation of pseudoaneurysms from periarterial hematoma [29] and shows the classic "to-and-fro" sign of a pseudoaneurysm, which is caused by flow change within the pseudoaneurysm during the systole and diastole [1].

4. Conclusion

IEA pseudoaneurysm surgical treatment is a good choice if it can be performed contextually with another surgical laparotomy as in kidney transplant. That implies that the disadvantages of surgery, as general anesthesia and postoperative pain, are reduced from 2 times to just 1 time. In addition, during kidney transplantation, ligation of IEA is usually performed; therefore in our patient surgical treatment contextually with the kidney transplant was the best choice even if pseudoaneurysm size was small. In our patient an exhaustive radiological imaging study was important in order to detect possible vascular abnormalities in kidney recipient prior to transplantation, that give us the opportunity to detect IEA pseudoaneurysm. The literature largely demonstrates how physical examination alone cannot be always sufficient to detect aortoiliac district damage either in stenotic or dilatative way. In our experience, abdominal contrast-enhanced CT or Doppler study is mandatory for all patients waiting a kidney transplant with two or more risk factors for vasculopathies or elder than 55 years in order to plan and timing the correct surgical treatment of vascular lesions. Preoperative studies can also help to detect rare vascular lesions and give the opportunity to plan the correct treatment and timing, as in this case report during the kidney transplant laparotomy.

Abbreviations and Acronyms

CT: Computer tomography
IEA: Inferior epigastric artery
NBCA: n-Butyl cyanoacrylate
US: Ultrasound.

References

[1] S. K. Venkatesh, V. B. Reynolds, H. R. Sidhu, and P. K. Maran, "Spontaneous inferior epigastric artery pseudoaneurysm," *Journal of Clinical Ultrasound*, vol. 38, no. 5, pp. 259–262, 2010.

[2] F. V. Ello and D. B. Nunn, "False aneurysm of the inferior epigastric artery as a complication of abdominal retention sutures," *Surgery*, vol. 74, no. 3, pp. 460–461, 1973.

[3] T. S. Gage, S. K. Sussman, F. U. Conard III, D. Hull, and S. A. Bartus, "Pseudoaneurysm of the inferior epigastric artery: diagnosis and percutaneous treatment," *American Journal of Roentgenology*, vol. 155, no. 3, pp. 529–530, 1990.

[4] Y. Segev, D. Orron, R. Alon, and M. Graif, "Pseudoaneurysm of the inferior epigastric artery mimicking abdominal wall hematoma," *Journal of Ultrasound in Medicine*, vol. 13, no. 6, pp. 483–484, 1994.

[5] J. V. Ferrer, P. Soriano, C. Zazpe, F. Vicente, J. Herrera, and J. M. Lera, "Pseudoaneurysm of the inferior epigastric artery: pathogenesis, diagnosis, and treatment," *Archives of Surgery*, vol. 131, no. 1, pp. 102–103, 1996.

[6] J. Verbist, F. Stillaert, P. Dujardin, and G. Dewaele, "Pseudoaneurysm of the inferior epigastric artery," *Acta Chirurgica Belgica*, no. 4, pp. 196–198, 1997.

[7] D. Weishaupt and N. Goebel, "Rectus sheath hematoma—detection of a still active bleeding from an aneurysm of the epigastric artery by CT," *Vasa*, vol. 26, no. 1, pp. 55–57, 1997.

[8] E. Y. Lam, R. B. McLafferty, J. Taylor L.M. et al., "Inferior epigastric artery pseudoaneurysm: a complication of paracentesis," *Journal of Vascular Surgery*, vol. 28, no. 3, pp. 566–569, 1998.

[9] M. Werner, J. Bernheim, M. Witz, Y. Gritton, H. Savin, and Z. Korzets, "Pseudoaneurysm of the inferior epigastric artery—a rare complication of Tenckhoff catheter removal," *Nephrology Dialysis Transplantation*, vol. 14, no. 5, pp. 1297–1299, 1999.

[10] R. Wutke, T. Reck, and W. Bantz, "Pseudoaneurysm of the A. epigastrica inferior after laparoscopic cholecystectomy," *RoFo*, vol. 171, no. 6, pp. 494–496, 1999.

[11] A. G. S. Shabani and G. M. Baxter, "Inferior epigastric artery pseudoaneurysm: ultrasound diagnosis and treatment with percutaneous thrombin," *British Journal of Radiology*, vol. 75, no. 896, pp. 689–691, 2002.

[12] S. V. R. C. Murthy, S. T. Hussain, S. Gupta, S. Thulkar, and V. Seenu, "Pseudoaneurysm of inferior epigastric artery following abdominal paracentesis," *Indian Journal of Gastroenterology*, vol. 21, no. 5, pp. 197–198, 2002.

[13] A. Piñero, M. Reus, B. Agea, A. Capel, J. Riquelme, and P. Parrilla, "Conservative management of an arteriovenous fistula of the inferior epigastric artery," *British Journal of Radiology*, vol. 76, no. 902, pp. 135–136, 2003.

[14] J. D. Bennett and C. Coblentz, "Continuing professional development evidence-based radiology problems inferior epigastric artery pseudoaneurysm: computed tomographic diagnosis and transcatheter therapy February 2004—January 2005," *Canadian Association of Radiologists Journal*, vol. 55, no. 1, pp. 8–11, 2004.

[15] K. Takase, T. Kazama, K. Abe, Y. Chiba, H. Saito, and S. Takahashi, "Pseudoaneurysm of the inferior epigastric artery successfully treated by ultrasound-guided compression," *CardioVascular and Interventional Radiology*, vol. 27, no. 5, pp. 520–522, 2004.

[16] J. S. Williamson, R. L. Harries, G. Davies, and A. Woodward, "Spontaneous resolution of an inferior epigastric artery pseudoaneurysm secondary to surgical drain placement," *Annals of The Royal College of Surgeons of England*, vol. 94, no. 6, pp. e193–e194, 2012.

[17] K. L. Splinter and C. L. Cook, "Inferior epigastric artery pseudoaneurysm following trocar injury," *Journal of Minimally Invasive Gynecology*, vol. 19, no. 3, pp. 393–395, 2012.

[18] K. Nichols-Totten, T. Pollema, and M. Moncure, "Pseudoaneurysm of the inferior epigastric artery: a rare complication of laparoscopic ventral hernia repair," *Surgical Laparoscopy, Endoscopy and Percutaneous Techniques*, vol. 22, no. 1, pp. e25–e27, 2012.

[19] C. N. Parnaby, D. Nicholls, and J. G. Docherty, "Inferior epigastric artery false aneurysm following incisional hernia repair," *International Journal of Surgery Case Reports*, vol. 2, no. 7, pp. 178–180, 2011.

[20] J.-M. Kim, N.-H. Jun, H.-K. Kim, and K. T. Min, "Pseudoaneurysm in the inferior epigastric artery and scrotal hematoma following removal of a femoral vein catheter," *Korean Journal of Anesthesiology*, vol. 59, supplement, pp. S3–S5, 2010.

[21] N. A. Bildzukewicz, B. Durkan, P. J. Maxwell IV, and G. A. Isenberg, "A pseudoaneurysm of the inferior epigastric artery after laparoscopic right hemicolectomy," *American Surgeon*, vol. 75, no. 12, pp. 1266–1268, 2009.

[22] M. Krokidis, A. Hatzidakis, J. Petrakis, T. Lagoudis, and D. Tsetis, "Coil embolization of inferior epigastric artery pseudoaneurysm after percutaneous thrombin injection failure: a case report," *Cases Journal*, vol. 2, no. 8, article 6562, 2009.

[23] J. Ruiz-Tovar, M. Rubio, S. Conde, V. Morales, and E. Martinez-Molina, "Inferior epigastric artery pseudoaneurysm: complication of surgical drain insertion," *ANZ Journal of Surgery*, vol. 78, no. 12, article 1139, 2008.

[24] S. W. Park, W. H. Choe, C. H. Lee et al., "Transcatheter embolization of a pseudoaneurysm of the inferior epigastric artery with N-butyl cyanoacrylate," *The British Journal of Radiology*, vol. 81, no. 963, pp. e64–e67, 2008.

[25] F. Karimian, K. Darbanian, and A. Paydar, "Pseudoaneurysm of inferior epigastric artery complicating ileostomy construction," *Singapore Medical Journal*, vol. 47, no. 10, pp. 910–912, 2006.

[26] G. S. Georgiadis, V. D. Souftas, T. T. Papas, M. K. Lazarides, and P. Prassopoulos, "Inferior epigastric artery false aneurysms: review of the literature and case report," *European Journal of Vascular and Endovascular Surgery*, vol. 33, no. 2, pp. 182–186, 2007.

[27] M. Lenartova and T. Tak, "Iatrogenic pseudoaneurysm of femoral artery: case report and literature review," *Clinical Medicine & Research*, vol. 1, no. 3, pp. 243–247, 2003.

Drug Interaction between Sirolimus and Ranolazine in a Kidney Transplant Patient

Joanna C. Masters,[1] Mita M. Shah,[2,3] and Ashley A. Feist[2]

[1] *Skaggs School of Pharmacy and Pharmaceutical Sciences, University of California, San Diego, La Jolla, CA 92093, USA*
[2] *University of California, San Diego Medical Center, Center for Transplantation, La Jolla, CA 92037, USA*
[3] *University of California, San Diego Medical Center, Department of Medicine, Division of Nephrology and Hypertension, San Diego, CA 92103, USA*

Correspondence should be addressed to Ashley A. Feist; aafeist@ucsd.edu

Academic Editors: P. A. Andrews, D. Capone, R. Grenda, and H. P. Tan

Purpose. The case of a kidney transplant recipient who experienced a probable drug interaction between sirolimus and ranolazine is reported. *Summary.* The narrow therapeutic window of immunosuppressive therapy in transplant recipients requires close monitoring for potential drug-drug interactions. The patient, a 57-year-old Caucasian male kidney transplant recipient, was stable for years on sirolimus as his primary immunosuppressive agent and had a history of chronic angina, for which he was prescribed ranolazine. Upon addition and dose escalation of ranolazine, whole blood sirolimus levels more than tripled, rising to immeasurably high concentrations. After holding sirolimus on multiple occasions and reducing dosage more than 50%, blood levels returned to therapeutic range, while continuing ranolazine. *Conclusion.* Since ranolazine is a documented P-GP and CYP3A inhibitor, and sirolimus a known substrate for both pathways, it is proposed that ranolazine inhibition of P-GP and CYP3A4 contributed to the significant elevation in sirolimus exposure. No alternative causes for the rise in sirolimus exposure were found, and assessment with the Drug Interaction Probability Scale finds this interaction to be probable. Clinicians should be aware of the potential for this interaction to cause elevated sirolimus exposure and subsequent increase in clinical effect or toxicity, in this case overimmunosuppression.

1. Introduction

Immunosuppressive agents used in solid organ transplant have narrow therapeutic windows, making drug-drug interactions a major concern. As new drugs are brought to market, clinically significant drug interactions may be identified that have not been previously reported in the literature. This case report describes a possible drug interaction between sirolimus and ranolazine in a kidney transplant patient, leading to supratherapeutic blood concentrations of sirolimus.

Ranolazine is a piperazine derivative approved for treatment of refractory angina; however, its exact mechanism of action is unclear. Ranolazine is metabolized primarily by intestinal and liver enzymes CYP3A (cytochrome P450, family 3A), and to a lesser extent CYP2D6, resulting in active metabolites, with less than 5% of compounds excreted in the urine. It is reported to be a mild inhibitor of CYP3A. Ranolazine is also a substrate and moderate inhibitor of p-glycoprotein (P-GP), an active transporter that serves as an intestinal efflux pump [1, 2].

The immunosuppressant sirolimus is a mammalian target of rapamycin (mTOR) inhibitor, which is used in transplant patients in place of, or along with, calcineurin inhibitors such as cyclosporine and tacrolimus. Sirolimus is metabolized primarily by CYP3A4 and about 2% is excreted in urine. Sirolimus is also a substrate and mild inhibitor of the P-GP efflux pump [3]. Due to the narrow therapeutic window, drug interactions through CYP or P-GP mechanisms are of concern, and increased knowledge about such interactions can prevent unnecessary toxic accumulation of sirolimus and significant adverse events.

The purpose of this paper is to report a probable drug interaction between sirolimus and ranolazine, leading to elevations in sirolimus blood levels. To further assess this interaction, an advanced literature search of the PubMed database was performed, using the search terms ranolazine and sirolimus. No results were reported. This lack of published information regarding concomitant use of these two agents highlights the importance of presenting this case report.

2. Case Report

A 57-year-old Caucasian male presented to the long-term kidney transplant clinic for routine follow-up. The patient's medical history was significant for type 1 diabetes mellitus since the age of ten leading to complications of coronary artery disease with chronic angina and end-stage renal disease. Four years prior to presentation, the patient received a simultaneous pancreas and kidney transplant. The patient underwent pancreatectomy shortly after transplantation due to graft thrombosis, but the kidney allograft continued to function. Additionally, he underwent a redo coronary artery bypass graft (CABG) one year after transplant. Due to an intolerance of mycophenolate mofetil and tremor on therapeutic-dose tacrolimus, he has been maintained on an immunosuppressive regimen of sirolimus, low-dose tacrolimus, and prednisone since shortly after transplantation. His renal function has been stable with a serum creatinine ranging from 1.3 to 1.7 mg/dL.

The patient had remained adherent and stable on sirolimus for several years with whole blood levels of 8–12 ng/mL on doses of 5 to 7 mg by mouth daily. Approximately seven months prior to presentation to our transplant clinic, the sirolimus dose was increased from 6 mg to 7 mg daily. One week later, the patient presented to his cardiologist with worsening angina and was started on ranolazine 500 mg by mouth twice daily (Figure 1). Four months after the addition of ranolazine, sirolimus trough concentration was measured to be 19.1 ng/mL, higher than previous values, but still within the target therapeutic range. No changes were made to his immunosuppressive regimen at this time. Due to ongoing angina, shortly thereafter the ranolazine dose was increased twofold to 1 gram twice daily. No other significant changes in his medication profile were made throughout this time period.

One month following this ranolazine dose increase, the patient presented to the emergency department for pain, dehydration, and malaise following a recent oral surgery. In the emergency department, the sirolimus level was found to be greater than 60 ng/mL, which is beyond the upper limit of detection of the assay. A repeat level confirmed this value. After consultation with the transplant nephrology service, the sirolimus was held for four days, until concentrations reached 15.5 ng/mL. All other laboratory values were within normal limits, including renal and hepatic function tests. Sirolimus was then restarted at a decreased dose of 6 mg daily; however, repeat levels were once again above the therapeutic target, and therefore the dose was further reduced one week later to 5 mg daily (see Figure 1 for detailed timeline). At this time, the etiology of the elevated sirolimus levels was unclear and had not been associated with a possible drug-drug interaction.

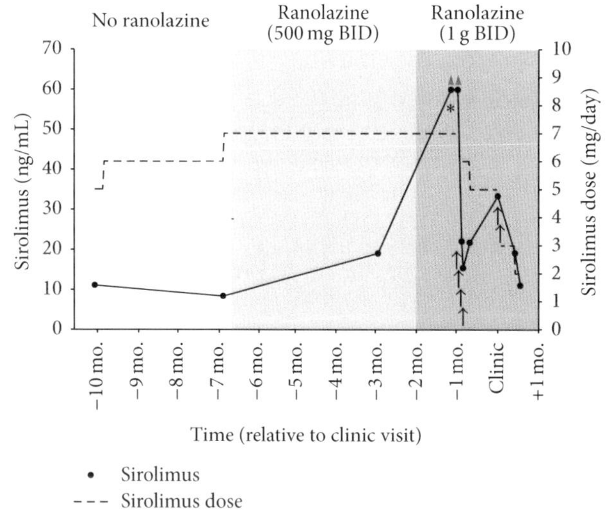

Figure 1: Timeline of sirolimus dosing and whole blood concentrations with ranolazine titration. ▲: level above limit of detection; ↑: sirolimus held for 1 day; ∗: patient presents to emergency department.

In following month the patient presented for follow-up to our kidney transplant clinic. His medication list at presentation included sirolimus 5 mg daily with a target trough concentration of 10–20 ng/mL, low-dose tacrolimus 1 mg daily, prednisone 5 mg daily, clopidogrel 75 mg daily, aspirin 325 mg daily, ranolazine 1 gram twice daily, amlodipine besylate 10 mg daily, lisinopril 10 mg daily, metoprolol tartrate 100 mg twice daily, furosemide 20 mg twice daily, nitroglycerin sublingual spray 0.4 mg as needed for chest pain, hydromorphone hydrochloride 4 mg every 4 hours as needed for pain, vitamin D 5,000 IU daily, and insulin lispro administered via insulin pump. The patient reported taking all medications as prescribed, and the only major medication changes in the recent past were titration of ranolazine and sirolimus as described previously. At this visit his steady-state sirolimus trough level was elevated to 33.4 ng/mL. Close review of his recent sirolimus levels and dosing history was made by the clinical pharmacist and transplant nephrologist, and an association between the addition of ranolazine and the highly elevated sirolimus levels was identified. A drug interaction was suspected between ranolazine and sirolimus, based on ranolazine's moderate P-GP inhibition and mild CYP3A inhibition. The patient was instructed to hold two doses of sirolimus, and reduce his daily dose to 3 mg thereafter with close monitoring of his sirolimus levels. He would continue on ranolazine 1 gram twice daily as instructed by his cardiologist and was advised to notify the transplant clinic of any future changes in ranolazine therapy.

The patient returned for labs in two weeks, at which time his sirolimus level was 19.2 ng/mL. He was then instructed to completely discontinue his low-dose tacrolimus due to the risk of potential overimmunosuppression. Six months later his sirolimus levels have remained within the target range on 2-3 mg daily, and he has continued on the same dose of ranolazine 1 gram twice daily.

3. Discussion

Ranolazine is reported to be a moderate inhibitor of P-GP, and the manufacturer includes a caution that dose reduction may be needed in agents transported by P-GP when used in combination with ranolazine. Ranolazine is also a CYP3A inhibitor, and package information contains a generic caution for use with drugs with narrow therapeutic windows, including sirolimus, tacrolimus, and cyclosporine. However, no published reports were found on the specific drug interaction or magnitude of interaction between sirolimus and ranolazine. Two published case reports describe an interaction between tacrolimus and ranolazine in transplant recipients, proposing that both the weak CYP3A inhibition and the moderate P-GP inhibition were responsible for observed elevated tacrolimus levels, which in one case required a 70% decrease in tacrolimus dose [4, 5]. Another case report suggests that the same dual P-GP and CYP3A inhibition was responsible for increased simvastatin exposure upon addition of ranolazine, which resulted in toxicity of rhabdomyolysis [6]. Ranolazine concentrations were not measured for this patient during the reported time period, and therefore systemic ranolazine levels cannot be assessed in this case.

Of note, this patient was also concurrently on tacrolimus. However, he was on a low dose given once daily with levels below the limit of detection of the assay and had no changes in tacrolimus dose during the time period detailed in this report. After the addition of ranolazine, tacrolimus levels increased to the detectable range but still remained subtherapeutic, therefore requiring no dose adjustment. For this reason, the drug interaction between ranolazine and tacrolimus, which has been reported previously [4, 5], was not a primary focus of this case report.

Drugs such as ranolazine that have both CYP and P-GP inhibition have the potential to create large increases in systemic concentrations of agents that are substrates of both, such as sirolimus. An increase in bioavailability through inhibited P-GP efflux, in addition to a decrease in first-pass metabolism and systemic clearance through inhibition of CYP enzymes, may result in sirolimus blood levels several-fold above the target systemic concentration. Such an event was described in a patient whose sirolimus levels increased more than eightfold upon addition of clarithromycin, a potent inhibitor of both P-GP and CYP3A [7]. Sirolimus blood levels far above the therapeutic window can have dire consequences for the patient, including complications of overimmunosuppression leading to serious infections. Patients on immunosuppressants such as sirolimus and concomitant dual CYP and P-GP inhibitors require closer monitoring of systemic drug levels, particularly after any relevant medication and/or dose changes. Patients should be clearly instructed to report any changes instituted by other providers to the transplant clinic team for appropriate follow-up, including up-to-date drug levels and increased monitoring, if necessary.

Alternative explanations do exist for the phenomenon described here; however, upon review we have determined none to be highly probable in this patient case. Of course, we assume that the patient was adherent to the prescribed sirolimus regimen, as this is what he reported during discussion with providers and there was no evidence of changes in prescription refill patterns that would suggest overdosing. The presence of other concomitant medications resulting in a drug interaction with sirolimus and/or ranolazine would also contribute to supratherapeutic sirolimus exposure. We could identify no other alterations in medication regimen with the potential to significantly impact ranolazine or sirolimus exposure. The patient's hepatic function remained normal throughout this time, making acute hepatic impairment an unlikely explanation for impaired sirolimus clearance. High fat meals have been shown to increase the mean total exposure (AUC) of sirolimus by 23 to 35% [3]; however, an unreported change in dosing time with regard to meals or any dietary changes is also not likely to explain the magnitude and the duration of change in sirolimus level seen in this case.

There is also a possibility that the degree of the P-GP interaction between ranolazine and sirolimus and subsequent increase in sirolimus bioavailability is impacted by dosing times. Simultaneous administration of sirolimus and modified cyclosporine, a known CYP3A4 and P-GP inhibitor, has been shown to increase the mean maximum concentration (C_{max}) of sirolimus by 512% and AUC by 148% compared with administration of sirolimus alone. However, administering sirolimus four hours after modified cyclosporine, as directed by the package insert, results in only a 33% increase in both C_{max} and AUC [3]. Perhaps a similar phenomenon could be observed with ranolazine and sirolimus, and thus minimizing the amount of ranolazine present in the gut to inhibit P-GP efflux could reduce the extent of increase in sirolimus exposure.

4. Conclusion

In this case we observed that upon the addition of ranolazine 1 gram twice daily, sirolimus dosing had to eventually be reduced by greater than fifty percent. Based on the sequence of events and known mechanisms listed above, we believe that the doubling of the daily ranolazine dose was the precipitating factor in the significant elevation of sirolimus trough levels. The phenomenon observed here did not represent an acute event, but a sustained interaction that persisted while the patient continued on ranolazine. No reasonable alternative causes for the magnitude of increase in sirolimus exposure could be found. The combination of inhibition of P-GP efflux and CYP3A4 enzymatic clearance by ranolazine explains the mechanism that may have caused the great increase in sirolimus concentration that occurred shortly thereafter.

This is the first published report of a drug interaction between ranolazine and sirolimus resulting in elevated sirolimus exposure. The patient was able to continue treatment on both sirolimus and ranolazine once doses were appropriately adjusted based on frequent blood level measurements. We determined the patient experienced a probable drug interaction through evaluation with the Drug Interaction Probability Scale (DIPS). This scale is a tool which aids in objective assessment of causation in patient cases involving suspected drug interactions [8]. Further study is needed to improve understanding of the mechanism and extent of the drug interaction, as well as methods to reduce the severity, such as dose separation. Transplant recipients taking sirolimus should be instructed to report any medication changes to the providers managing their transplant medications and take care to monitor for any signs of infection or other new adverse effects. Furthermore, other providers should be encouraged to check for any potential interactions with narrow therapeutic range immunosuppressants before adding or removing medications for comorbid conditions.

References

[1] *Ranexa (Ranolazine) Package Insert*, Gilead Sciences, Foster City, Calif, USA, 2011.

[2] M. Jerling, "Clinical pharmacokinetics of ranolazine," *Clinical Pharmacokinetics*, vol. 45, no. 5, pp. 469–491, 2006.

[3] *Rapamune (Sirolimus) Package Insert*, Wyeth Pharmaceuticals, Philadelphia, Pa, USA, 2011.

[4] D. A. Pierce and A. M. Reeves-Daniel, "Ranolazine-tacrolimus interaction," *Annals of Pharmacotherapy*, vol. 44, no. 11, pp. 1844–1849, 2010.

[5] H. Patni, M. Gitman, A. Hazzan, and K. D. Jhaveri, "Ranolazine, tacrolimus, and diltiazem might be a hazardous combination in a transplant patient," *Renal Failure*, vol. 34, no. 2, pp. 251–253, 2012.

[6] A. C. Hylton and T. O. Ezekiel, "Rhabdomyolysis in a patient receiving ranolazine and simvastatin," *American Journal of Health-System Pharmacy*, vol. 67, no. 21, pp. 1829–1831, 2010.

[7] D. Capone, G. Palmiero, A. Gentile et al., "A pharmacokinetic interactions between clarithromycin and sirolimus in kidney transplant recipient," *Current Drug Metabolism*, vol. 8, no. 4, pp. 379–381, 2007.

[8] J. R. Horn, P. D. Hansten, and L. Chan, "Proposal for a new tool to evaluate drug interaction cases," *Annals of Pharmacotherapy*, vol. 41, no. 4, pp. 674–680, 2007.

10

Pediatric Renal Transplantation in a Highly Sensitised Child—8 Years On

Catherine Quinlan,[1] Atif Awan,[1] Denis Gill,[1] Mary Waldron,[2] Dilly Little,[3] David Hickey,[3] Peter Conlon,[3] and Mary Keogan[4]

[1] *Paediatric Renal Transplant Centre, The Children's University Hospital, Temple Street, Dublin 1, Ireland*
[2] *Our Lady's Children's Hospital, Crumlin, Dublin 12, Ireland*
[3] *Renal Transplant Unit, Beaumont Hospital, Dublin 9, Ireland*
[4] *National Histocompatibility and Immunogenetics Services for Solid Organ Transplantation, Beaumont Hospital, Dublin 9, Ireland*

Correspondence should be addressed to Catherine Quinlan, catherine.quinlan@gosh.nhs.uk

Academic Editors: J. A. Kari and M. Sadeghi

Highly sensitised children have markedly reduced chances of receiving a successful deceased donor renal transplant, increased risk of rejection, and decreased graft survival. There is limited experience with the long-term followup of children who have undergone desensitization. Following 2 failed transplants, our patient was highly sensitised. She had some immunological response to intravenous immunoglobulin (IVIg) but this was not sustained. We developed a protocol involving sequential therapies with rituximab, IVIg, and plasma exchange. Immunosuppressant therapy at transplantation consisted of basiliximab, tacrolimus, mycophenolate mofetil, and steroids. At the time of transplantation, historical crossmatch was ignored. Current CDC crossmatch was negative, but T and B cell flow crossmatch was positive, due to donor-specific HLA Class I antibodies. Further plasma exchange and immunoglobulin therapy were given pre- and postoperatively. Our patient received a deceased donor-kidney-bearing HLA antigens to which she originally had antibodies, which would have precluded transplant. The graft kidney continues to function well 8 years posttransplant.

1. Introduction

Kidney transplantation remains the optimal treatment for end-stage renal failure (ESRF). However, highly sensitised children continue to have markedly reduced chances of receiving a successful kidney transplant and, if transplanted, they have a greater number of rejection episodes with decreased graft survival [1]. Over the last 10–15 years, there has been increased interest in transplanting sensitised children, due to increased rates of living-donor transplants, better immunosuppressive regimes, improved methods of detecting anti-HLA antibodies, and a greater understanding of antibody-mediated rejection (AMR) [2].

Several protocols have been suggested for desensitization of patients who have a positive cross-match against a potential donor, utilizing a combination of IVIg [3–5], plasmapheresis [6], MMF [7], sirolimus [8], and rituximab [9–15]. There is limited data on desensitization facilitating deceased donor transplantation and little long-term followup data. We describe a patient who underwent successful deceased donor transplantation 7 years ago using a hybrid of the John Hopkins [6] and Cedars Sinai [5] desensitization protocols.

2. Patient

Our patient was a 12-year-old Caucasian girl with ESRF secondary to congenital nephrotic syndrome of the Finnish variety [16]. She had renal transplants at age 3 and 5 years. The first was lost to chronic allograft nephropathy at 18 months. The second was lost to acute rejection necessitating nephrectomy, within 2 weeks of transplantation. During the transplant nephrectomy, blood loss necessitated resuscitation with 7 units of red cells. Her first allograft remained in situ.

She was then maintained on hemodialysis for 8 years without a suitable kidney becoming available. Her antibody levels remained high with a panel reactive antibody (PRA) determined by Complement Dependent Lymphocytotoxic (CDC) of 95% against peripheral blood lymphocytes and 100% against chronic lymphocytic leukaemia (CLL) cells. No suitable living donor was available. After 60 months on the waiting list for a deceased donor transplant, the decision was made to attempt desensitization. After failure of IVIg on its own to desensitize her, a novel regime was developed as outlined below.

3. Desensitization Regime

3.1. Pretransplant

(i) Rituximab (375 mg/m^2), four infusions administered weekly.

(ii) Single volume plasma exchange with fresh frozen plasma (FFP) replacement monthly for 3 months.

(iii) Infusion of IVIg (flebogamma 2 g/kg over 2 days) monthly for 3 months after each plasma exchange.

3.2. Immediately Pretransplant

(i) Plasma exchange with FFP replacement.

(ii) Infusion of IVIg (flebogamma 500 mg/kg).

3.3. Immediately Posttransplant (Week 1)

(i) Plasma exchange with 4.5% human albumin replacement.

(ii) Infusion of IVIg (500 mg/kg) daily for 4 days on day 3, 4, 5, and 6.

(iii) Infusion of rituximab (375 mg/m^2).

4. Immunosuppression Regime

4.1. Pretransplant

(i) Basiliximab 10 mg IV 2 hours pretransplant.

(ii) Prednisolone 600 mg/m^2 IV.

(iii) Tacrolimus 0.15 mg/kg IV.

4.2. Posttransplant

(i) Mycophenolate mofitil 250 mg twice daily (14 mg/kg/day).

(ii) Prednisolone tapered to 10 mg/day by day 7 posttransplant.

(iii) Basiliximab 10 mg IV day 4 posttransplant.

(iv) Tacrolimus 0.3 mg/kg/day post transplant adjusted with serum drug levels (aim 12–15 in first 3 months).

Our patient received a blood group identical, HLA 1,1,2 mismatch kidney from an unrelated, standard criteria, deceased donor. CDC crossmatch was negative, but flow cytometry crossmatch was significantly positive against both T and B cells. Subsequent investigation of the day of transplant serum showed donor-specific antibodies against A31 and borderline reactivity to DQ2. The A31 and DQ2 antibodies were presumed to be due to transfusion, while the historic reactivity to DR53 was related to previous mismatches.

Donor-specific antibodies were monitored by flow cytometry using donor cells or ELISA thrice weekly for 3 weeks, weekly for 6 weeks, and monthly thereafter. Donor-specific antibodies were noted to be mildly raised, day 3 posttransplant, and this was treated with plasma exchange and further doses of IVIg (total dose 2 g/kg) on day 3, 4, 5, and 6 as outlined above. Donor-specific antibodies were no longer detectable by ELISA. Retrospective reanalysis of stored sera using Luminex single antigen technology has shown persisting donor-specific weak positivity against HLA A31 and DQ2, however, this has remained stable over the last 6.5 years.

She is now 8 years post transplant and has had no episodes of rejection. Her most recent estimated glomerular filtration rate (eGFR) is 71 mL/minute/1.73 m^2 with a serum creatinine of 104 μmol/L.

5. Discussion

Sensitizing events include previous transplantation, blood transfusions, and pregnancy [17]. As many HLA antigens are closely related, exposure to a small number of HLA antigens can give rise to broad sensitization in individuals who generate antibodies to "public," or cross-reactive, epitopes. Desensitization is an attempt to firstly remove anti-HLA immunoglobulin (IgG), transplant when crossmatch is negative or acceptable, and finally to prevent formation of further donor-specific anti-HLA IgG after transplantation.

At the time of transplantation, 10% of patients on the renal transplant deceased donor waiting list have >60% panel reactive antibody (PRA) levels to HLA [18]. A high PRA limits the number of negative crossmatches with potential donors, thus the waiting time for a suitable kidney is increased. In the past, the presence of these preformed anti-HLA donor specific antibodies (DSA) in the recipient's serum at the time of transplantation was a contraindication to proceeding [2, 19–22]. However, in the last 15 years, there has been increased research in the area of desensitization and a number of approaches have emerged [6, 23, 24].

The cautious and cost-effective approach is to firstly maximise the chance of their receiving negative crossmatch grafts. This can be achieved through acceptable mismatch programs [25] and living donor kidney exchange programs [7]. Results from the Eurotransplant Acceptable Mismatch Program [26] are encouraging, no additional immunosuppression is necessary and graft survival in the sensitised group is identical to that of nonsensitised recipients. The Dutch National Living Donor Kidney Exchange Program [27], The New England Program for Kidney Exchange, the

Mid-Atlantic Paired Exchange Program [7], and computer match programs for paired kidney exchanges [28, 29] also offer effective strategies to expand the donor pool. Much work is needed to fund and build such programs at national, European, and international levels.

IVIg is known to have immunomodulatory effects [3, 4], when used as part of a desensitization protocol, it results in decreased anti-HLA antibody levels, decreased ischemia reperfusion injuries, decreased episodes of acute rejection, and improved long-term survival of the graft [8, 30, 31]. It is the only element of the desensitization protocol that has been evaluated in a placebo-controlled, multicentre, double-blinded trial [32]. The NIH IG02 trial enrolled 101 highly sensitised patients with ESRF over 3 years. Patients in the treatment group were given high-dose IVIg (2 g/kg) monthly for 4 months and had significantly lower anti-HLA antibody levels and greater transplantation rates when compared to the placebo group (35% versus 17% $P = 0.02$). 3-year graft survival rate was not significantly affected.

Plasmapheresis has been used with success in an *ex vivo* model of xenograft hyperacute rejection [33], in patients transplanted across ABO blood groups [34, 35], in heart transplant patients with acute rejection [36], and as part of the pretransplantation management of adult sensitised patients [37–40]. It is used along with cytomegalovirus immunoglobulin as part of the John Hopkins desensitization protocol [6].

The increased understanding of the role played by B-cells in rejection led to the use of agents which specifically target this facet of the immune response [9]. One such agent is rituximab, a genetically engineered chimeric mouse/human monoclonal antibody [10, 11] directed against the CD20 antigen found on the surface of B-lymphocytes. Rituximab eliminates B cells by a combination of antibody-dependent cell-mediated cytotoxicity [12], complement-dependent cytotoxicity [13], and activation of apoptotic pathways [14]. Phase 1 trials of rituximab in nine highly sensitised adults on dialysis showed prolonged depletion of B cells and reductions in PRA [15]. However, rituximab has no effect on plasma cells and no immediate effect on circulating antibody levels, thus it is better used in combination therapy (i.e., with IVIG $\pm$ plasma exchange).

We developed a regime which involved sequential therapies with rituximab, IVIg, and plasma exchange. This resulted in a marked sustained reduction in antibody levels, allowing transplantation. Our patient remains well, 102 months posttransplant. She has been successfully transitioned to adult services. Immunosuppression is maintained on MMF and tacrolimus. Her most recent estimated glomerular filtration rate (eGFR) is 71 mL/minute/1.73 m^2 with a serum creatinine of 104 μmol/L.

References

[1] R. Patel and P. I. Terasaki, "Significance of the positive crossmatch test in kidney transplantation," *The New England Journal of Medicine*, vol. 280, pp. 735–739, 1969.

[2] S. K. Takemoto, A. Zeevi, S. Feng et al., "National conference to assess antibody-mediated rejection in solid organ transplantation," *American Journal of Transplantation*, vol. 4, pp. 1033–1041, 2004.

[3] S. C. Jordan, A. A. Vo, D. Tyan, C. C. Nast, and M. Toyoda, "Current approaches to treatment of antibody-mediated rejection," *Pediatric Transplantation*, vol. 9, no. 3, pp. 408–415, 2005.

[4] M. D. Kazatchkine and S. V. Kaveri, "Immunomodulation of autoimmune and inflammatory diseases with intravenous immune globulin," *The New England Journal of Medicine*, vol. 345, no. 10, pp. 747–755, 2001.

[5] S. C. Jordan, A. A. Vo, C. C. Nast, and D. Tyan, "Use of high-dose human intravenous immunoglobulin therapy in sensitized patients awaiting transplantation: the Cedars-Sinai experience," *Clinical Transplants*, pp. 193–198, 2003.

[6] R. A. Montgomery and A. A. Zachary, "Transplanting patients with a positive donor-specific crossmatch: a single center's perspective," *Pediatric Transplantation*, vol. 8, no. 6, pp. 535–542, 2004.

[7] R. L. Hanto, W. Reitsma, and F. L. Delmonico, "The development of a successful multiregional kidney paired donation program," *Transplantation*, vol. 86, no. 12, pp. 1744–1748, 2008.

[8] S. C. Jordan, A. Vo, S. Bunnapradist et al., "Intravenous immune globulin treatment inhibits crossmatch positivity and allows for successful transplantation of incompatible organs in living-donor and cadaver recipients," *Transplantation*, vol. 76, no. 4, pp. 631–636, 2003.

[9] M. D. Pescovitz, "The use of rituximab, anti-CD20 monoclonal antibody, in pediatric transplantation," *Pediatric Transplantation*, vol. 8, no. 1, pp. 9–21, 2004.

[10] V. D. Garcia, J. L. Bonamigo Filho, J. Neumann et al., "Rituximab in association with rapamycin for post-transplant lymphoproliferative disease treatment," *Transplant International*, vol. 16, no. 3, pp. 202–206, 2003.

[11] K. Nozu, K. Iijima, M. Fujisawa, A. Nakagawa, N. Yoshikawa, and M. Matsuo, "Rituximab treatment for posttransplant lymphoproliferative disorder (PTLD) induces complete remission of recurrent nephrotic syndrome," *Pediatric Nephrology*, vol. 20, no. 11, pp. 1660–1663, 2005.

[12] D. G. Maloney, T. M. Liles, D. K. Czerwinski et al., "Phase I clinical trial using escalating single-dose infusion of chimeric anti-CD20 monoclonal antibody (IDEC-C2B8) in patients with recurrent B-cell lymphoma," *Blood*, vol. 84, no. 8, pp. 2457–2466, 1994.

[13] M. E. Reff, K. Carner, K. S. Chambers et al., "Depletion of B cells in vivo by a chimeric mouse human monoclonal antibody to CD20," *Blood*, vol. 83, no. 2, pp. 435–445, 1994.

[14] J. Rodriguez and A. Gutierrez, "Pharmacokinetic properties of rituximab," *Reviews on Recent Clinical Trials*, vol. 3, no. 1, pp. 22–30, 2008.

[15] C. A. Vieira, A. Agarwal, B. K. Book et al., "Rituximab for reduction of anti-HLA antibodies in patients awaiting renal transplantation: 1. Safety, pharmacodynamics, and pharmacokinetics," *Transplantation*, vol. 77, no. 4, pp. 542–548, 2004.

[16] K. E. Papez and W. E. Smoyer, "Recent advances in congenital nephrotic syndrome," *Current Opinion in Pediatrics*, vol. 16, no. 2, pp. 165–170, 2004.

[17] P. Gailiunas Jr., M Suthanthiran, G. J. Busch, C. B. Carpenter, and M. R. Garovoy, "Role of humoral presenitization in human renal transplant rejection," *Kidney International*, vol. 17, pp. 638–646, 1980.

[18] A. Soosay, D. O'Neill, A. Counihan, D. Hickey, and M. Keogan, "Causes of sensitisation in patients awaiting renal

transplantation in Ireland," *Irish Medical Journal*, vol. 96, no. 4, pp. 109–112, 2003.

[19] H. M. Gebel, R. A. Bray, and P. Nickerson, "Pre-transplant assessment of donor-reactive, HLA-specific antibodies in renal transplantation: contraindication vs. risk," *American Journal of Transplantation*, vol. 3, no. 12, pp. 1488–1500, 2003.

[20] A. L. Girnita, S. A. Webber, and A. Zeevi, "Anti-HLA alloantibodies in pediatric solid organ transplantation," *Pediatric Transplantation*, vol. 10, no. 2, pp. 146–153, 2006.

[21] D. Glotz, C. Antoine, and A. Duboust, "Antidonor antibodies and transplantation: how to deal with them before and after transplantation," *Transplantation*, vol. 79, no. 3, pp. S30–S32, 2005.

[22] M. P. Emonds, J. Herman, J. Dendievel, M. Waer, and R. van Damme-Lombaerts, "Evaluation of anti-human leukocyte antigen allo-immunization in pediatric cadaveric kidney transplantation," *Pediatric Transplantation*, vol. 4, no. 1, pp. 6–11, 2000.

[23] R. E. Shaddy and T. C. Fuller, "The sensitized pediatric heart transplant candidate: causes, consequences, and treatment options," *Pediatric Transplantation*, vol. 9, no. 2, pp. 208–214, 2005.

[24] C. C. Magee, "Transplantation across previously incompatible immunological barriers," *Transplant International*, vol. 19, no. 2, pp. 87–97, 2006.

[25] F. H. Claas, M. D. Witvliet, R. J. Duquesnoy, G. G. Persijn, and I. I. Doxiadis, "The acceptable mismatch program as a fast tool for highly sensitized patients awaiting a cadaveric kidney transplantation: short waiting time and excellent graft outcome," *Transplantation*, vol. 78, no. 2, pp. 190–193, 2004.

[26] I. I. N. Doxiadis, J. M. A. Smits, G. G. Persijn, U. Frei, and F. H. J. Claas, "It takes six to boogie: allocating cadaver kidneys in Eurotransplant," *Transplantation*, vol. 77, no. 4, pp. 615–617, 2004.

[27] M. De Klerk, K. M. Keizer, F. H. J. Claas, M. Witvliet, B. J. J. M. Haase-Kromwijk, and W. Weimar, "The Dutch national living donor kidney exchange program," *American Journal of Transplantation*, vol. 5, no. 9, pp. 2302–2305, 2005.

[28] I. Kaplan, J. A. Houp, R. A. Montgomery, M. S. Leffell, J. M. Hart, and A. A. Zachary, "A computer match program for paired and unconventional kidney exchanges," *American Journal of Transplantation*, vol. 5, pp. 2306–2308, 2005.

[29] F. L. Delmonico, P. E. Morrissey, G. S. Lipkowitz et al., "Donor kidney exchanges," *American Journal of Transplantation*, vol. 4, no. 10, pp. 1628–1634, 2004.

[30] S. C. Jordan, A. W. Quartel, L. S. C. Czer et al., "Posttransplant therapy using high-dose human immunoglobulin (intravenous gammaglobulin) to control acute humoral reaction in renal and cardiac allograft recipients and potential mechanism of action," *Transplantation*, vol. 66, no. 6, pp. 800–808, 1998.

[31] S. C. Jordan, A. Vo, D. Tyan, and M. Toyota, "Desensitization therapy with intravenous gammaglobulin (IVIG): applications in solid organ transplantation," *Trans Am Clin Climatol Assoc*, vol. 117, pp. 199–211, 2006, discussion p. 211.

[32] S. C. Jordan, D. Tyan, D. Stablein et al., "Evaluation of intravenous immunoglobulin as an agent to lower allosensitization and improve transplantation in highly sensitized adult patients with end-stage renal disease: report of the NIH IG02 trial," *Journal of the American Society of Nephrology*, vol. 15, no. 12, pp. 3256–3262, 2004.

[33] T. J. Kroshus, A. P. Dalmasso, J. R. Leventhal, R. John, A. J. Matas, and R. M. Bolman III, "Antibody removal by column immunoabsorption prevents tissue injury in an ex vivo model of pig-to-human xenograft hyperacute rejection," *Journal of Surgical Research*, vol. 59, no. 1, pp. 43–50, 1995.

[34] T. Sawada, S. Fuchinoue, T. Kawase, K. Kubota, and S. Teraoka, "Preconditioning regimen consisting of anti-CD20 monoclonal antibody infusions, splenectomy and DFPP-enabled non-responders to undergo ABO-incompatible kidney transplantation," *Clinical Transplantation*, vol. 18, no. 3, pp. 254–260, 2004.

[35] Y. Yamazaki, H. Kawaguchi, K. Ito, K. Takahashi, H. Toma, and K. Ota, "ABO incompatible kidney transplantation in children," *Journal of Urology*, vol. 154, no. 2, pp. 914–916, 1995.

[36] E. Berglin, C. Kjellstrom, V. Mantovani, G. Stelin, C. Svalander, and L. Wiklund, "Plasmapheresis as a rescue therapy to resolve cardiac rejection with vasculitis and severe heart failure: a report of five cases," *Transplant International*, vol. 8, no. 5, pp. 382–387, 1995.

[37] P. Fauchald, T. Leivestad, D. Albrechtsen, Y. Willassen, A. Jacobsen, and A. Flatmark, "Plasma exchange and immunoadsorption prior to renal transplantation in allosensitized patients," *Transplantation Proceedings*, vol. 22, no. 1, pp. 149–150, 1990.

[38] D. L. Segev, C. E. Simpkins, D. S. Warren et al., "ABO incompatible high-titer renal transplantation without splenectomy or anti-CD20 treatment," *American Journal of Transplantation*, vol. 5, no. 10, pp. 2570–2575, 2005.

[39] R. Ben-Youssef, Y. Iwaki, P. Baron et al., "Successful living related kidney transplantation across an anti-donor HLA antibody," *Transplantation Proceedings*, vol. 38, no. 5, pp. 1280–1282, 2006.

[40] A. V. Reisaeter, T. Leivestad, D. Albrechtsen et al., "Pretransplant plasma exchange or immunoadsorption facilitates renal transplantation in immunized patients," *Transplantation*, vol. 60, no. 3, pp. 242–248, 1995.

11

Transitional Cell Carcinoma of the Kidney Graft: An Extremely Uncommon Presentation of Tumor in Renal Transplant Recipients

Vital Hevia,[1] Victoria Gómez,[1] Sara Álvarez,[1] Víctor Díez Nicolás,[1] Carmen Gómez del Cañizo,[1] Andrea Orosa,[1] Cristina Galeano Álvarez,[2] and F. J. Burgos Revilla[1]

[1] *Department of Urology, Hospital Ramón y Cajal, Ctra. Colmenar km 9,100, 28034 Madrid, Spain*
[2] *Department of Nephrology, Hospital Ramón y Cajal, Ctra. Colmenar km 9,100, 28034 Madrid, Spain*

Correspondence should be addressed to Vital Hevia; vital.hevia.uro@gmail.com

Academic Editors: M. G. H. Betjes, C. Costa, and F. Keller

Purpose. Transitional cell carcinoma (TCC) affecting the graft after renal transplantation is a very infrequent way of presentation of this tumor. Our aim is to present our single institution experience with 2 cases, as well as to perform a review of the literature about this tumor after the transplant. *Materials and Methods.* TCC of the graft developed in 2 of 1365 patients from 1977 to 2010, both cases in women. Data were analyzed for incidence, clinical presentation, treatment, and outcomes. *Results.* Both cases occurred in 2 mid-age women and resulted to be high grade and locally advanced TCCs, representing an incidence of 0,14% (2/1365). Clinical presentation was urinary obstruction for the first case and incidental ultrasound finding for the second. Preoperative staging was made with CT, cytology, pyelography, ureterorenoscopy, and biopsy. Treatment performed was nephroureterectomy of the graft with bladder cuff and regional lymphadenectomy. Pathological examination showed in both cases a locally advanced and high grade urothelial carcinoma of the pelvis allograft. After 24 and 14 months of followup, both patients are disease free. *Conclusions.* TCC of the kidney graft is an infrequent tumor that has only been reported in a few cases in the literature. It usually appears at a lower age, more often locally advanced, and with poor differentiation. A multidisciplinary approach to treatment should be required in these cases.

1. Introduction

Nowadays, it is widely known that renal transplantation (RT) is the optimal treatment for end stage renal disease. However, after solid organ transplantation, there is a significant increased risk of developing a malignant neoplasm that varies based on cancer type [1]. This condition after RT is believed to depend on the length and type of immunosuppression or is associated with some viral infections. This risk is especially high for nonmelanoma skin cancer, hematological neoplasms, renal cell carcinoma, and thyroid cancer. Instead of this, prostate, testicular, or breast cancers have a lower risk [2]. Other tumors associated to viral infections and induced by that condition—such as hepatobiliary, cervical, or vulvovaginal neoplasms—have a higher incidence on transplant recipients.

Transitional cell carcinoma (TCC) of the urinary tract is one of those tumors that appear also more commonly on transplanted population than nontransplanted, varying its incidence according to the series from 0,07% [3] to 1,9% [4]. The possible cause for the increased risk of cancer in this population is due to immunosuppression, which decreases the host ability to defend against viral infections. In contrast, an important meta-analysis by Grulich et al. [5] compared the cancer risk in patients infected by HIV against patients who have received a solid organ transplant. TCC did not show an increased incidence in HIV population, so this finding could suggest that immunodeficiency would not be the leading and solitary cause for pathogenesis in this subgroup of neoplasms. Regarding the TCC, two main viruses had been related with an increased risk developing this neoplasm: BK virus (BKV) [6] and human papillomavirus (HPV) types 16 and 18 [7].

Most of these tumors are located in the bladder, but they can also appear at any location in the urinary tract: ureter, urethra, renal calyces, or pelvis. The risk increase for renal transplant recipients (RTRs) suffering a TCC has been estimated around 3 times higher than nontransplanted population [3]. Moreover, TCC in RTRs is regarded as being more aggressive, poorly differentiated, rapidly progressive, and more often fatal than in normal population. It is not surprising to find in these patients a higher incidence of locally advanced disease or metastatic presentation, as well as a significantly lower age at diagnosis [8, 9].

There are many reports and reviews in the literature about bladder TCC, assessing many aspects such as incidence, clinical presentation, treatment, or outcomes. Nevertheless, only a few cases of TCC affecting the renal allograft have been published. Our aim is to present our experience with 2 cases of TCC in the kidney allograft, as well as to perform a review of the existing literature about this extremely infrequent kind of presentation.

2. Patients and Methods

2.1. Case 1. A 61-year-old female patient developed chronic renal failure secondary to polycystic kidney disease and began hemodialysis in 1999. One year later she received a renal transplant from a deceased donor and underwent an immunosuppressive therapy based on corticoids, tacrolimus (FK506), and mycophenolate, with a mild chronic dysfunction at the moment of the diagnosis. After 12 years of transplantation, she came to the Emergency Department complaining of fever, urinary symptoms, and pain in the allograft region. An expansive process in allograft pelvis with secondary moderate hydronephrosis was detected on ultrasound, as well as higher serum creatinine levels. A percutaneous nephrostomy was placed, so creatinine returned to its baseline. Antegrade pyelography (Figure 1) revealed a big filling defect and a stop to the contrast at ureteropelvic junction, and the CT showed a big mass at renal pelvis that could infiltrate the adjacent fat.

Selective urinary cytology and biopsy were positive for a high grade urothelial carcinoma. Inferior urinary tract was negative for tumor invasion. A nephroureterectomy of the renal allograft was performed. Histological analysis revealed a high grade urothelial carcinoma of the pelvis allograft with fat invasion and extension to proximal portion of the ureter, where it infiltrates the muscular layer. Surgical ureteral margin was free of tumor (stage pT3G4).

2.2. Case 2. A 59-year-old female patient developed chronic renal failure secondary to focal and segmental hyalinosis and began hemodialysis in 1987. In 1988 she underwent a renal transplantation but presented an acute rejection that required transplantectomy. A second RT was performed

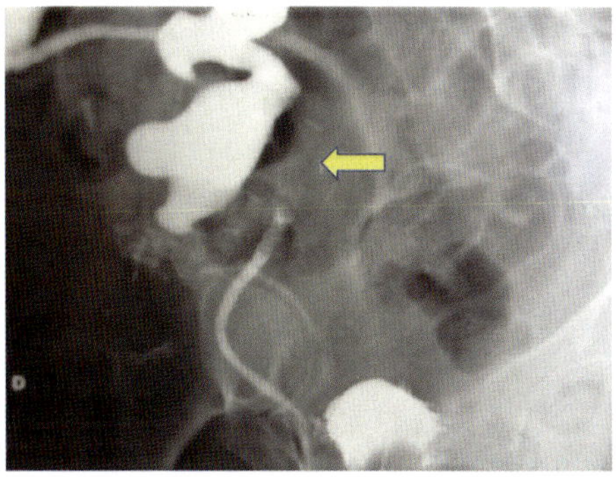

FIGURE 1: Antegrade pyelography showing a big filling defect in the kidney allograft secondary to a pelvis mass with moderate hydronephrosis.

in 1991. After years she developed a chronic allograft dysfunction that made her return to hemodialysis in 2009, as well as undergoing another transplantectomy because of graft intolerance syndrome. Third RT was performed in 2010, using a renal allograft from a deceased male donor. Immunosuppressive therapy used was thymoglobulin, corticoids, tacrolimus (FK506), and mycophenolate. Immediate renal allograft function was achieved, and her baseline creatinine serum levels were around 1,2 mg/dL. After 14 months of third RT, in a routine review, ultrasound examinations revealed a heterogeneous renal mass located on inferior pole with moderate hydronephrosis associated. CT confirms the suspect (Figure 2) and shows a big mass in the kidney graft depending on the pelvis and probably infiltrating fat.

Antegrade pyelography showed a big filling defect with amputation of medium and inferior calyxes. Selective urinary cytology was positive for a high grade urothelial carcinoma, and cystoscopy was negative for tumor invasion in the low urinary tract. Once again, a transplantectomy including ureter and bladder cuff was performed. Histological analysis revealed a high grade urothelial carcinoma of the pelvis allograft with fat invasion (Figure 3). Surgical ureteral margin was free of tumor (stage pT3(m)G3). Cytogenetic analysis of the tumor's cells (Figure 4) showed the presence of chromosomes XY, so it allowed us to establish the origin of the neoplasm in the donor cells, which was probably accelerated by high doses of immunosuppressants used.

Both patients had a successful postoperative period, returning to dialysis (first with hemodialysis and later with a peritoneal catheter) immediately. At the present moment, and after 24 and 14 months of followup with cystoscopy, urinary cytology, and CT, they are free of malignancy and no recurrence was diagnosed.

3. Discussion

The overall incidence of de novo malignancies after RT is about 4 to 5 times greater than in general population. Several malignancies do not show more risk, while others are significantly enhanced after transplantation [10]. Patients with an RT are at a higher risk of having a TCC compared to

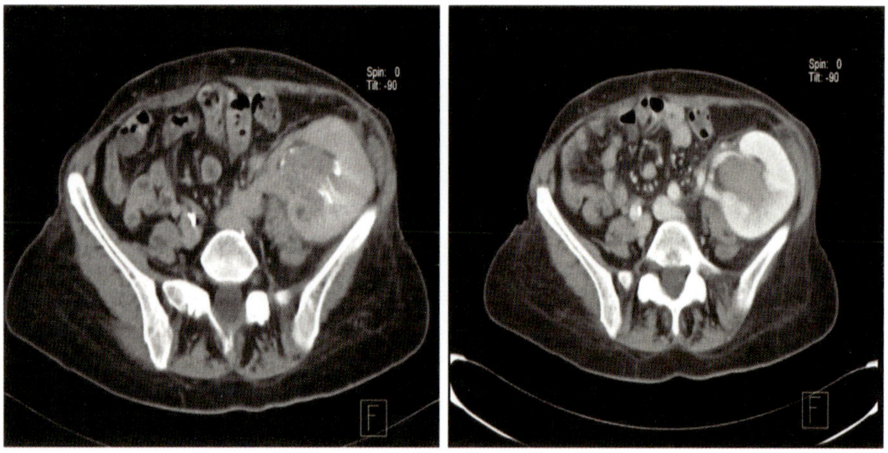

FIGURE 2: Pelvic CT demonstrating the presence of a big mass in the allograft, located in left iliac fossa, affecting renal pelvis and calyx.

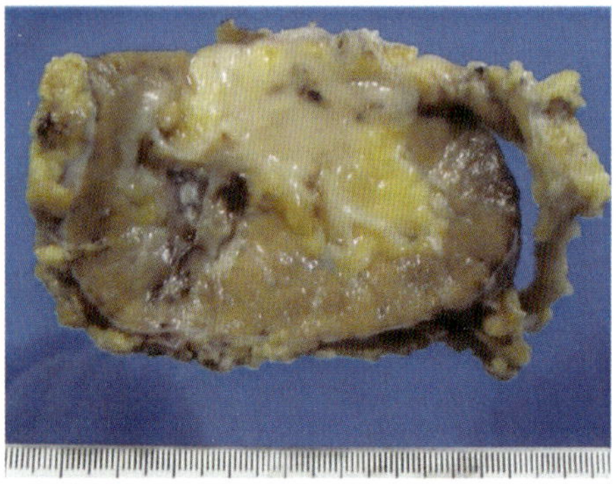

FIGURE 3: Macroscopic study after surgery that revealed a TCC of the renal pelvis with fat invasion and extension to proximal portion of the ureter, where it infiltrates the muscular layer. Surgical margin was free of tumor, and the stage was a pT3G4.

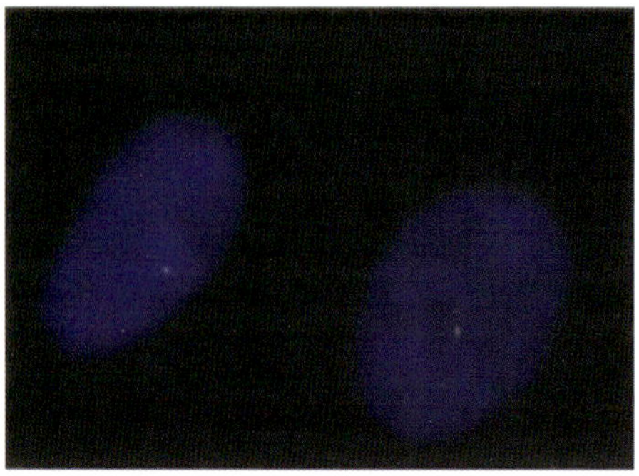

FIGURE 4: Cytogenetic analysis of the tumor's cells, demonstrating the presence of XY chromosomes.

nontransplanted recipients, and it has been estimated around 3 times greater [3]. This fact, like many others related to epidemiology, varies substantially depending on the demographic area. Thus, there are series with an incidence of TCC in RTRs from 0,07% in University of California study [3] to 1,9% in Beijing group study [4]. This significant difference between the two regions is due in part to aristolochic acid, a substance in a Chinese herb which is known as an important risk factor of urothelial carcinoma [11] and was present as a risk factor in 16/27 (59,3%) of the RTRs diagnosed of TCC.

Another important and widely known risk factor of TCC is Balkan endemic nephropathy (BEN), which is a primary renal disease that occurs in endemic regions of Croatia, Bulgaria, Bosnia, Romania, and Serbia. It produces end stage renal failure and is classically associated with 100 times greater incidence of TCC, especially in upper urinary tract [12, 13]. In fact, one of the few cases present in the literature of TCC in a renal allograft was in a Croatian 52-year-old male transplanted because of a CRF due to BEN. He first developed a low grade pTa TCC in left native kidney 3 years after RT (treated with left nephroureterectomy). Later, 6 years after RT, another low grade but pT2 TCC appeared in the allograft, limited to superior calyx. The uncommon of the case was the conservative treatment performed: a resection of the upper quarter of the allograft followed by a prophylactic right nephroureterectomy with bladder cuff resection. Cytopathological and genetic findings confirmed that the tumor arose from recipient urothelium and was not transferred by the donor. After 1-year followup, the patient maintained a normal renal function and was free of tumor recurrence [14].

Regarding clinical presentation of TCC in RTRs, it can occur in many ways. Painless gross hematuria is usually the most common symptom, as occurred in Li et al. [4] and Cox and Colli [9] studies. That is the main reason why some authors recommend a quick and thorough evaluation of gross hematuria [9, 15]. Other possibilities such as incidental finding, microhematuria, hydronephrosis, or irritative syndrome can be the first manifestation of a TCC. In the case of RTRs with the allograft affected by tumor, it is logical to think that hydronephrosis would be quite frequent, according to the high invasiveness of these tumors which can cause an obstruction of the urinary tract. Actually, the two cases presented hydronephrosis at the moment of diagnose, also with acute renal failure in case 1 due to obstructive uropathy.

High incidence of neoplasms and their aggressive course are associated with immunosuppressive therapy. Some immunosuppressant drugs such as cyclosporine (CsA) can promote cancer progression by a direct cellular effect [16]. Overimmunosuppression was also reported as one of factors related to the development of TCC [17], but it is still difficult to determine which dose of these drugs such as CsA or tacrolimus (FK506) is optimal and balanced between their side effects and their immunologic capacity. One last factor to consider is uremia. It is one of the preexisting factors that increase the risk of developing a TCC. Immunological dysfunction caused by uremia has been reported as an important factor involved in developing a TCC [2, 18].

Regarding to the location of TCC in RTRs population, bladder is the most common site in urinary tract where this tumor appears [4, 9]. It is followed by native upper urinary tract. Other locations reported in some articles are the urethra and the renal allograft, but much more infrequently. Actually, as commented previously, only a few cases of urothelial cancer in the allograft have been reported in the literature [6, 9, 14, 19, 20].

Another important fact is that maybe due to immunosuppression, the tumor stage at diagnosis is frequently more locally advanced, poorly differentiated, and with a lower age at the time of presentation [10].This is the reason why some groups recommend an exhaustive followup and evaluation of these patients in order to prevent aggressive clinical presentations of TCC, especially if they complain of gross hematuria [9].

The way of treatment of TCC in RTRs is not so different from the way in nontransplanted population. In the low urinary tract, it goes from bladder transurethral resection (TURB) for nonmuscle-invasive bladder cancer (NMIBC) to radical cystectomy (RC) and Urinary diversion for muscle-invasive bladder cancer (MIBC). TCCs of native upper urinary tract are classically treated with radical nephroureterectomy (RNU); sometimes it is performed as a prophylactic treatment in high risk cases. In those cases that the TCC appears affecting the renal allograft, the standard treatment should be the radical transplantectomy including the ureter and a bladder cuff, considering as an option for selected cases with low grade tumors the percutaneous resection. Mokos et al. [14] report a case treated with partial nephrectomy including the upper quarter of the allograft in a low grade TCC with *muscularis propria* invasion of the superior calyx, being free of recurrence after 1 year followup. It could maybe represent a less safety treatment from an oncological point of view, but the approach should consider also every medical aspect such as the return to dialysis. Because of particularities of TCC in RTRs already discussed, such as higher grade, multicentricity, more locally advanced and more metastatic presentation, radical nephroureterectomy of the allograft including ureter and bladder cuff would be the standard of treatment, even knowing that it would make the patient return to dialysis.

4. Conclusion

Transitional cell carcinoma, such as other malignancies, appears more commonly in renal transplant recipients than in nontransplanted population. Gross hematuria is the more frequent symptom of the TCC, but not the only one. The renal allograft is a very uncommon location of TCC; bladder is the most often place in the urinary tract. They usually appear at a lower age and are often more locally advanced, poorly differentiated, and with metastatic disease. Proper treatments should be tailored to each case according to a multidisciplinary approach, including urologists, nephrologists, and oncologists.

References

[1] J. H. Stewart, C. M. Vajdic, M. T. van Leeuwen et al., "The pattern of excess cancer in dialysis and transplantation," *Nephrology Dialysis Transplantation*, vol. 24, no. 10, pp. 3225–3231, 2009.

[2] C. M. Vajdic, S. P. McDonald, M. R. E. McCredie et al., "Cancer incidence before and after kidney transplantation," *The Journal of the American Medical Association*, vol. 296, no. 23, pp. 2823–2831, 2006.

[3] V. A. Master, M. V. Meng, G. D. Grossfeld, T. M. Koppie, R. Hirose, and P. R. Carroll, "Treatment and outcome of invasive bladder cancer in patients after renal transplantation," *Journal of Urology*, vol. 171, no. 3, pp. 1085–1088, 2004.

[4] X. B. Li, N. Z. Xing, Y. Wang, X. P. Hu, H. Yin, and X. D. Zhang, "Transitional cell carcinoma in renal transplant recipients: a single center experience," *International Journal of Urology*, vol. 15, no. 1, pp. 53–57, 2008.

[5] A. E. Grulich, M. T. van Leeuwen, M. O. Falster, and C. M. Vajdic, "Incidence of cancers in people with HIV/AIDS compared with immunosuppressed transplant recipients: a meta-analysis," *The Lancet*, vol. 370, no. 9581, pp. 59–67, 2007.

[6] R. Saquib, Y. M. Barri, R. Saad et al., "Transitional cell carcinoma of renal allograft associated with BK virus infection," *Dialysis and Transplantation*, vol. 38, no. 12, pp. 518–519, 2009.

[7] J. Xiao, X. Zhu, G. Y. Hao et al., "Association between urothelial carcinoma after renal transplantation and infection by human papillomavirus types 16 and 18," *Transplantation Proceedings*, vol. 43, no. 5, pp. 1638–1640, 2011.

[8] B. Ehdaie, G. J. Stukenborg, and D. Theodorescu, "Renal transplant recipients and patients with end stage renal disease present with more advanced bladder cancer," *Journal of Urology*, vol. 182, no. 4, pp. 1482–1487, 2009.

[9] J. Cox and J. L. Colli, "Urothelial cancers after renal transplantation," *International Urology and Nephrology*, vol. 43, no. 3, pp. 681–686, 2011.

[10] B. L. Kasiske, J. J. Snyder, D. T. Gilbertson, and C. Wang, "Cancer after kidney transplantation in the United States," *The American Journal of Transplantation*, vol. 4, no. 6, pp. 905–913, 2004.

[11] J. L. Nortier, M. C. M. Martinez, H. H. Schmeiser et al., "Urothelial carcinoma associated with the use of a Chinese herb (*Aristolochia fangchi*)," *The New England Journal of Medicine*, vol. 342, no. 23, pp. 1686–1692, 2000.

[12] S. D. Petkovic, "Epidemiology and treatment of renal pelvic and ureteral tumors," *Journal of Urology*, vol. 114, no. 6, pp. 856–865, 1975.

[13] S. Jankovic, J. Marinkovic, and Z. Radovanovic, "Survival of the upper-urothelial-cancer patient from the Balkan nephropathy endemic and nonendemic areas," *European Urology*, vol. 15, no. 1-2, pp. 59–61, 1988.

[14] I. Mokos, J. Pasini, R. Stern-Padovan, S. Mrsic, and S. Ries, "Conservative surgical treatment of low-grade urothelial carcinoma in the renal allograft recipient: a case report," *Transplantation Proceedings*, vol. 38, no. 5, pp. 1363–1365, 2006.

[15] M. M. Kamal, S. M. Soliman, A. A. Shokeir, H. Abol-Enein, and M. A. Ghoneim, "Bladder carcinoma among live-donor renal transplant recipients: a single-centre experience and a review of the literature," *The British Journal of Urology International*, vol. 101, no. 1, pp. 30–35, 2008.

[16] M. Hojo, T. Morimoto, M. Maluccio et al., "Cyclosporine induces cancer progression by a cell-autonomous mechanism," *Nature*, vol. 397, no. 6719, pp. 530–534, 1999.

[17] H. M. Kauffman, W. S. Cherikh, M. A. McBride, Y. Cheng, and D. W. Hanto, "Post-transplant de novo malignancies in renal transplant recipients: the past and present," *Transplant International*, vol. 19, no. 8, pp. 607–620, 2006.

[18] S. Satoh, N. Tsuchiya, T. Habuchi, T. Ishiyama, K. Seimo, and T. Kato, "Renal cell and transitional cell carcinoma in a Japanese population undergoing maintenance dialysis," *Journal of Urology*, vol. 174, no. 5, pp. 1749–1753, 2005.

[19] I. Vervloessem, R. Oyen, Y. Vanrenterghem et al., "Transitional cell carcinoma in a renal allograft," *European Radiology*, vol. 8, no. 6, pp. 936–938, 1998.

[20] P. Jensen, B. P. Ulhøi, and E. H. Nielsen, "Transitional-cell carcinoma in a 25-year-old renal allograft," *Nephrology Dialysis Transplantation*, vol. 13, no. 12, pp. 3240–3241, 1998.

12

Torsion of the Retroperitoneal Kidney: Uncommon or Underreported?

Michael Sosin,[1] Wuya Lumeh,[2] and Matthew Cooper[1]

[1] *Medstar Georgetown Transplant Institute, Georgetown University Hospital, 3800 Reservoir Road, NW, Main Hospital Building, Second Floor, Washington, DC 20007, USA*
[2] *Georgetown University School of Medicine, Medical Dental Building, 3900 Reservoir Road, NW, Washington, DC 20057, USA*

Correspondence should be addressed to Matthew Cooper; matthew.cooper@gunet.georgetown.edu

Academic Editors: D. Conti and M. Klinger

Vascular torsion in a renal allograft after placement in the retroperitoneum is rare and has only been reported twice in the literature. It is an extrinsically mediated process that occurs at the vascular pedicle resulting in graft compromise and potential loss. Rapid diagnosis and immediate surgical intervention may salvage allograft function. Herein, we present a unique case of a 42-year-old male that developed renal allograft torsion following a second kidney transplant placed in the retroperitoneum. Immediate detorsion did not resolve allograft dysfunction, and a biopsy revealed acute cellular mediated rejection. After antithymocyte globulin treatment, allograft function was salvaged. A review of the current literature shows that the incidence, morbidity, and long term allograft function of intraperitoneal and extraperitoneal torsion are different. As such, torsion of the retroperitoneal kidney demonstrates encouraging allograft salvage rates. Only the third case reported to date, this serves as a contribution to the growing body of literature in retroperitoneal renal torsion and reviews the risks, medication considerations, diagnostic tests, and treatment modalities in a unique disease process.

1. Introduction

Commonly reported short-term complications following kidney transplant include postoperative hemorrhage, thrombosis, urine leak, ureteral stricture, and acute rejection [1, 2]. Thrombosis can occur from intrinsic mediators or extrinsic factors that compromise vascular inflow or outflow [3]. Vascular torsion is an extrinsically mediated, rare, and potentially reversible complication that occurs at the vascular pedicle resulting in graft compromise and/or loss. Rapid diagnosis and immediate surgical intervention may salvage allograft function. However, a delay in diagnosis increases the risk of acute rejection or frank necrosis sometimes requiring transplant nephrectomy [4, 5]. Herein, we present a case complicated by renal torsion and subsequent acute rejection. Early recognition and treatment of both complications allowed for successful salvage of the graft. This case serves as only the third report of renal hilar torsion in retroperitoneal placement of a kidney allograft [6, 7].

2. Case Report

A 42-year-old male with hemodialysis-dependent (HD), end stage renal disease (ESRD) underwent a second deceased donor kidney transplant (DDKT). His past medical history included glomerulonephritis, the etiology of his ESRD, for which he underwent an initial DDKT at the age of 30. Following this first transplant, the patient was diagnosed with donor-derived metastatic melanoma. Immediate discontinuation of immunosuppression was followed by a donor nephrectomy that same year. The patient was disease-free without evidence of metastasis for the following 11 years. In lieu of a prior malignancy, he did not undergo center-standard induction therapy with alemtuzumab and instead received 500 mg of intravenous methylprednisolone and 40 mg of intravenous basiliximab. The standard criteria donor was a 20-year-old male that suffered from head trauma following a motor vehicle accident. Cold ischemia time was 4 hours. Incision and placement of the allograft was in the left retroperitoneal iliac fossa due to the patient's prior right sided surgeries. The donor had an accessory renal artery and a single arterial anastomosis was completed using a single aortic cuff receiving inflow from both tributary vessels. The venous anastomosis was completed in standard fashion. Operative time was 1.5 hours. Intraoperative urine output was 225 mL and postoperatively continued at a rate of 40–500 mL/hr for the following 10 hours. Urine output then began to decrease acutely from 25 mL/hr to 10 mL/hr. Renal ultrasound obtained at postoperative hour 11 demonstrated elevated velocity at the main renal artery anastomosis. A loss of tardus parvus waveform with a decreased resistive index was concerning for external compression, kink, stenosis, or impending thrombosis. No perinephric fluid collection was visible. The concern for a technical error prompted immediate return to the operating room on postoperative day (POD) 1. Intraoperatively, the allograft was torsed medially across the vascular pedicle with mild discoloration suggestive of ischemia. No evidence of frank necrosis was observed. After detorsion, intraoperative ultrasound assessment confirmed reestablishment of arterial and venous flow. A biopsy was not performed at the time of reexploration. Nephropexy of the superior pole to adjacent soft tissue and the lateral abdominal wall was then completed. The iliac fossa space was more intimately closed to decrease the potential space.

The patient remained oliguric requiring hemodialysis with ongoing elevations in serum creatinine. With a concern for rejection, on hospital day 6 the patient underwent an ultrasound-guided biopsy with final pathology revealing Banff 2B acute cellular rejection. A 5-day cycle of anti-thymocyte globulin treatment was initiated with the patient producing urine after 18 hours of treatment. The creatinine level markedly decreased from 6 at initiation of treatment to 1.35 upon discharge. Throughout his perioperative and postoperative course, the immunosuppression regimen consisted of prednisone, mycophenolate mofetil beginning on POD 2, and tacrolimus was initiated on POD 8.

3. Discussion

Torsion of the transplanted allograft is a rare complication. Only two reports of vascular torsion in a renal allograft have been reported in retroperitoneal transplants [6, 7]. The majority of vascular torsion has been reported in the intraabdominally placed kidney associated with simultaneous pancreas kidney (SPK) transplants [8]. The purported risk factors for intraperitoneal renal torsion include pediatric transplant recipients, patients with Prune Belly syndrome, and patients taking chronic corticosteroids [9–14]. Immunosuppressive medication is believed to induce an adhesion-free intraabdominal environment, acknowledging a potential role for nephropexy to adjacent structures. Although multiple authors recommend prophylactic nephropexy for SPK transplantation, there is a paucity of data to support it in retroperitoneal kidney transplantation [8, 12, 13]. Modi et al. have reported 2 of 6 patients undergoing a laparoscopic kidney transplant without nephropexy developed renal torsion and subsequently underwent nephrectomy. The following 38 cases completed by the same group utilized laparoscopic prophylactic nephropexy yielding a 0% torsion rate [15]. Despite such promising findings, a randomized control trial would better elucidate the efficacy of such practice in open SPKs or open retroperitoneal kidney transplants.

Torsion has been described to occur as early as POD 1, as evidenced in this case, to as long as 10 years postoperatively [16]. Lucewicz et al. provide a detailed description of varying mechanisms of torsion in a review of 16 intraperitoneal cases. In this case, the mechanism of twist occurred anteromedially, from left to right along the sagittal axis. Rotation along the coronal or transverse axis ranging from 120 to 360 degrees has also been described [9, 10, 12, 13, 16, 17]. We attributed our complication to a large potential space in the iliac fossa. However, other possible explanations include a long vascular pedicle, long ureter, increased laxity in the abdominal wall, or excessive fluid in the perinephric space.

Lymphocele is the most common perinephric fluid collection following extraperitoneal kidney transplants, and it has a lower incidence in intraperitoneally placed transplants because of the absorptive capacity of the peritoneum [18]. Fenestration techniques have been advocated for prevention of retroperitoneal fluid collections [19, 20]. However, Zaontz and Firlit only studied pediatric patients [19]. Syversveen et al. defined lymphocele so broadly that interpretation of other perinephric fluid collections may have been misdiagnosed as lymphoceles [20]. To date there is insufficient evidence to support prophylactic fenestration for prevention of renal torsion.

Renal allograft ultrasonography is a routine method of serially monitoring for vascular complications. Including color flow Doppler imaging is a rapid, inexpensive, and accurate method of assessing vascular patency. The overall sensitivity of this method when evaluating the renal pedicle is 95%, with specificity of 92% [6]. Computerized tomography angiography (CTA) and magnetic resonance imaging angiography (MRA) are superior methods of imaging but are costly and may delay intervention in the acute setting. In the setting of a nonacute, subclinical presentation of kidney torsion, MRA provides a reconstructed 3-dimensional image and can serve as an excellent modality in diagnosing renal torsion as an etiology of renal artery stenosis, hypertension, and chronic rejection [4].

Once recognized, treatment involves immediate detorsion in the operating room. Rates of graft salvage after detorsion are approximately 44%. Immediate nephrectomy has been reported in 38% of torsion cases, with 19% of delayed allograft loss following detorsion [8]. Exclusive to intraabdominal torsion, these rates differ from retroperitoneal torsion case reports. Including our case, now 3 retroperitoneal torsed kidneys have been reported to have a 100% salvage rate in allograft function after detorsion. We do recognize that this may be overly optimistic and is likely subject to publication bias.

Intraoperative findings confirmed torsion as the etiology of our patient's acute onset of oliguria. A biopsy was deferred as the source of allograft dysfunction seemed to be apparent and suspicion of acute rejection was low. In retrospect, a biopsy should have been obtained as the risk of acute cellular mediated rejection increases in the setting of renal ischemia [21]. This episode served as a second warm ischemic episode thereby increasing the risk of rejection. Despite rapid restoration of allograft perfusion, ensuing graft dysfunction prompted a kidney biopsy confirming Banff 2B rejection. Upon treatment with anti-thymocyte globulin, allograft function returned within 18 hours, ultimately salvaging allograft function and avoiding the loss of our patient's second and potentially final transplant.

Exceptional to this case was the patient's prior history of a donor-transmitted malignancy. Attenuated immunosuppressive regimens have been advocated for transplant recipients with prior malignancy [22, 23]. In lieu of his donor-transmitted metastatic melanoma, we avoided aggressive induction therapy. Additionally, multiple trips to the operating room and poor renal function altered our standardized immunosuppressive protocol.

This case underscores the importance of maintaining a high suspicion of renal torsion despite placement of the allograft in the retroperitoneum. Salvage rates after detorsion dramatically differ from that of intraperitoneally placed allografts suggesting that retroperitoneal torsion may result in better outcomes after detorsion and should be studied as a distinct entity. We also emphasize the importance of obtaining a biopsy upon detorsion of the graft. It is unclear whether this was an isolated technical complication as the etiology for rejection, whether an attenuated immunosuppressive regimen was a culpable source, or both issues contributed to the outcome. We describe a series of rare events occurring in one case. Circumventing a complete workup can only be pursued with caution and in retrospect may delay a diagnosis. After detorsion, if transplant nephrectomy is avoided, we recommend obtaining a biopsy in the operating room. We emphasize the fundamentals of a thorough evaluation following persistent graft dysfunction are of paramount importance in salvaging a threatened renal allograft.

References

[1] D. Dimitroulis, J. Bokos, G. Zavos et al., "Vascular complications in renal transplantation: a single-center experience in 1367 renal transplantations and review of the literature," *Transplantation Proceedings*, vol. 41, no. 5, pp. 1609–1614, 2009.

[2] H. Karakayah, O. Basaran, G. Moray, R. Emiroglu, and M. Haberal, "Major postoperative complications of renal transplantation: results from a single center in Turkey," *Transplantation Proceedings*, vol. 35, no. 7, pp. 2657–2659, 2003.

[3] T. Sutherland, F. Temple, S. Chang, O. Hennessy, and W.-K. Lee, "Sonographic evaluation of renal transplant complications," *Journal of Medical Imaging and Radiation Oncology*, vol. 54, no. 3, pp. 211–218, 2010.

[4] P. Rodrigues, F. Hering, and A. Gil, "A well-documented case of chronic renal failure due to misplacement of the transplanted kidney," *Clinics*, vol. 63, no. 1, pp. 147–148, 2008.

[5] Z. Zilinska, M. Chrastina, B. Trebaticky et al., "Vascular complications after renal transplantation," *Bratislava Medical Journal*, vol. 111, no. 11, pp. 586–589, 2010.

[6] M. M. Ozmen, I. Bilgic, I. Ziraman, and M. Koc, "Torsion of extraperitoneally transplanted kidney: an unusual complication," *Experimental and Clinical Transplantation*, vol. 11, no. 2, pp. 186–190, 2013.

[7] T. C. Winter, A. L. Clarke, and J. Campsen, "Acute torsion of a retroperitoneal renal transplant mimicking renal vein thrombosis," *Ultrasound Quarterly*, vol. 29, no. 3, pp. 203–204, 2013.

[8] A. Lucewicz, A. Isaacs, R. D. M. Allen, V. W. T. Lam, S. Angelides, and H. C. C. Pleass, "Torsion of intraperitoneal kidney transplant," *ANZ Journal of Surgery*, vol. 82, no. 5, pp. 299–302, 2012.

[9] L. Badet, P. Petruzzo, N. Lefrancois, M. Colombel, H. Fassi-Fehri, and X. Martin, "Torsion of the renal pedicle due to rotation of the kidney after simultaneous kidney-pancreas transplantation," *Progres en Urologie*, vol. 13, no. 4, pp. 675–678, 2003.

[10] R. G. Marvin, G. A. Halff, and I. Elshihabi, "Renal allograft torsion associated with prune-belly syndrome," *Pediatric Nephrology*, vol. 9, no. 1, pp. 81–82, 1995.

[11] P. L. Abbitt, R. L. Chevalier, B. M. Rodgers, and S. S. Howards, "Acute torsion of a renal transplant: cause of organ loss," *Pediatric Nephrology*, vol. 4, no. 2, pp. 174–175, 1990.

[12] A. M. Roza, C. P. Johnson, and M. Adams, "Acute torsion of the renal transplant after combined kidney-pancreas transplant," *Transplantation*, vol. 67, no. 3, pp. 486–488, 1999.

[13] M. S. West, R. B. Stevens, P. Metrakos et al., "Renal pedicle torsion after simultaneous kidney-pancreas transplantation," *Journal of the American College of Surgeons*, vol. 187, no. 1, pp. 80–87, 1998.

[14] A. M. Palestrant and W. C. DeWolf, "The pseudostricture of transplant ureteral torsion," *Radiology*, vol. 145, no. 1, pp. 49–50, 1982.

[15] P. Modi, B. Pal, J. Modi et al., "Retroperitoneoscopic living-donor nephrectomy and laparoscopic kidney transplantation: experience of initial 72 cases," *Transplantation*, vol. 95, no. 1, pp. 100–105, 2013.

[16] S. Nangia and E. R. Saad, "Torsion of renal transplant 10 years after simultaneous kidney-pancreas transplantation: imaging as a diagnostic tool," *Transplantation*, vol. 87, no. 10, p. 1590, 2009.

[17] J. J. Wong-You-Cheong, K. Grumbach, T. L. Krebs et al., "Torsion of intraperitoneal renal transplants: imaging appearances," *American Journal of Roentgenology*, vol. 171, no. 5, pp. 1355–1359, 1998.

[18] B. G. Dammeier, A. Lehnhardt, S. Glüer, G. Offner, B. Nashan, and B. M. Ure, "Laparoscopic fenestration of posttransplant lymphoceles in children," *Journal of Pediatric Surgery*, vol. 39, no. 8, pp. 1230–1232, 2004.

[19] M. R. Zaontz and C. F. Firlit, "Pelvic lymphocele after pediatric renal transplantation: a successful technique for prevention," *Journal of Urology*, vol. 139, no. 3, pp. 557–559, 1988.

[20] T. Syversveen, K. Midtvedt, K. Brabrand, O. Øyen, A. Foss, and T. Scholz, "Prophylactic peritoneal fenestration to prevent morbidity after kidney transplantation: a randomized study," *Transplantation*, vol. 92, no. 2, pp. 196–202, 2011.

[21] C. Troppmann, K. J. Gillingham, E. Benedetti et al., "Delayed graft function, acute rejection, and outcome after cadaver renal transplantation: a multivariate analysis," *Transplantation*, vol. 59, no. 7, pp. 962–968, 1995.

13

Clear Cell Papillary Renal Cell Carcinoma in the Bilateral Native Kidneys after 2 Years of Renal Transplantation

Zhanyong Bing and John E. Tomaszewski

Department of Pathology and Laboratory Medicine, Hospital of the University of Pennsylvania, 3400 Spruce Street, Philadelphia, PA 19104, USA

Correspondence should be addressed to Zhanyong Bing, bingz@uphs.upenn.edu

Academic Editors: A. Beiras-Fernandez, D. Capone, R. Grenda, and H. J. Jeong

Renal transplantation increases the probability of malignant tumors by about 2–4-fold overall with a much higher rate for renal epithelial malignancy. Renal tumors in renal transplant recipients are commonly conventional clear cell or papillary renal cell carcinoma. Clear cell papillary renal cell carcinoma is a recently described unique renal epithelial neoplasm with scant eosinophilic or moderate amount of clear cytoplasm and pyknotic small nuclei oriented commonly toward the apical surfaces. No such tumor has been reported in renal transplant recipients. In this paper, we describe a clear cell papillary renal cell carcinoma involving bilateral native kidneys in a patient who had received a renal transplant 2 years earlier. Clear cell papillary renal cell carcinoma commonly presents with low pathologic stage and lower Fuhrman grade and is clinically indolent. Additional cases are needed to evaluate the clinical behavior of this type of tumor in renal transplant recipients.

1. Introduction

Renal transplantation has greatly improved the lives of the patients with end-stage renal disease; however, their life expectancies are still not at par with general population. One of factors that contribute to such outcome is increased tendency to develop malignancy. The incidence of cancer development in renal transplants is increased 2–4-fold [1–3] overall, while there is greater increase in the incidence of kidney malignancies (15-fold) in renal transplants.

Clear cell papillary renal cell carcinoma (CCPRCC) is a recently described low-grade renal cell carcinoma [4–9]. It is usually strongly positive for cytokeratin 7 (CK7) and mostly negative for CD10. Genetically no deletion of chromosome 3p or loss of chromosome Y has been found [5]. In addition, Aydin et al. studied gain of chromosome 7 or 17 in such tumors and found only low copy number of such chromosomal changes in 1 out of 10 cases [4]. This unique type of tumor has been described in kidneys with [9] or without [5] end-stage renal diseases. Such type of tumor has not been reported in the patients with renal transplants. In this paper, we described a renal transplant recipient with multiple cystic clear cell papillary renal cell carcinomas in both native kidneys.

2. Clinical History

The patient was a 67-year-old lady with end-stage renal disease secondary to type II diabetes and hypertension. She received a cadaveric kidney from a 51-year-old man who died from an intracranial event. The patient was immunosuppressed with tacrolimus/mycophenolate/prednisone. Tacrolimus levels were monitored for toxicity. Two years later, the patient was found to have bilateral renal masses and underwent bilateral nephrectomies of the native kidneys. The patient was alive without recurrence of carcinoma 21 months status after surgery.

2.1. Pathology Findings

2.1.1. Macroscopic Findings. The left kidney measured 8.0 × 3.2 × 3.3 cm. The kidney was atrophic. The cortical thickness

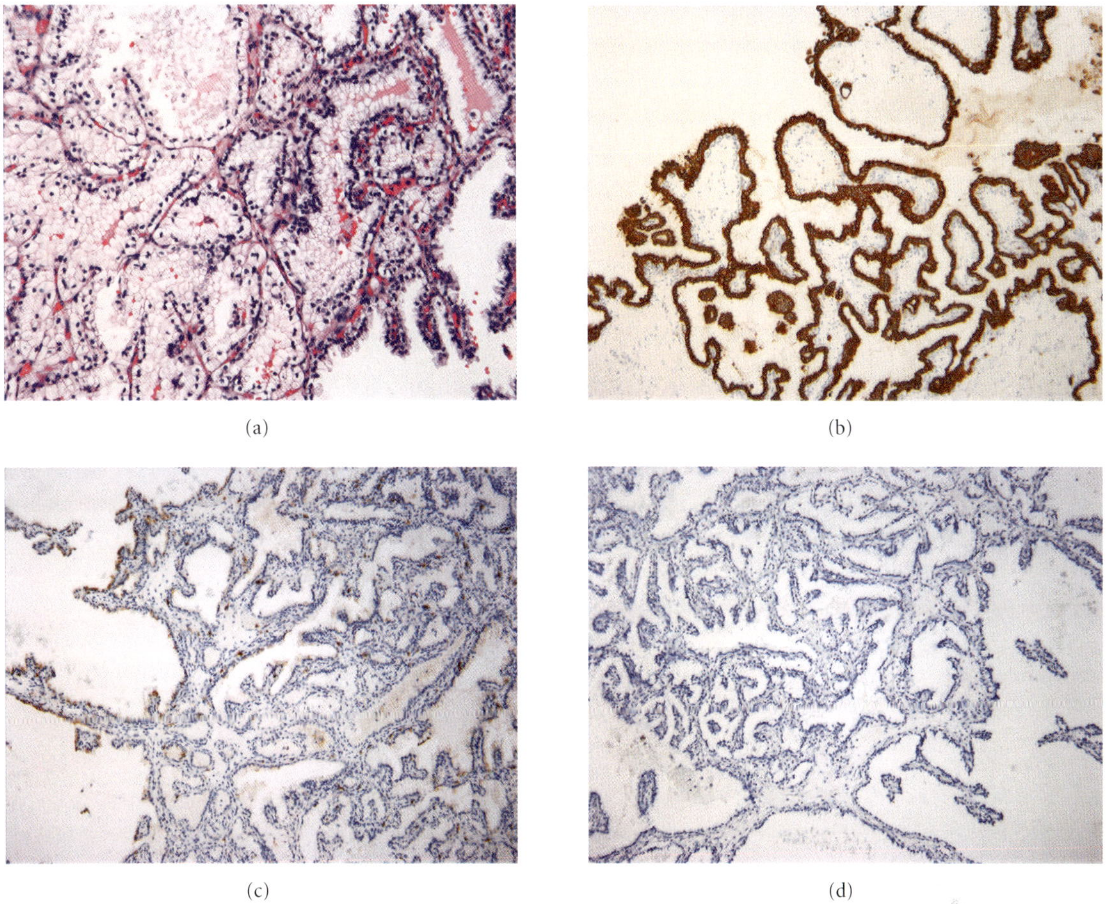

FIGURE 1: Clear cell papillary renal cell carcinoma in native kidneys of a renal transplant recipient. (a) Single layers of clear cells with moderate amount of clear cytoplasm and pyknotic nuclei oriented toward the apical surfaces, H&E 400×; (b) diffuse CK7 positivity, 100×; (c) weak CD10 stain, 100×; (d) negative RCC stain, 100×.

was 2 mm. There were 4 cystic lesions in the kidney which measured 0.6 cm, 0.5 cm, 0.4 cm, and 0.3 cm in diameter.

The right kidney measured 8.6 × 5.0 × 3.0 cm. The kidney was also atrophic. There was an exophytic polar mass which measured 2.2 × 1.3 × 1.0 cm, and the mass was partially cystic and partially gelatinous with a well-defined tan-white capsule. Adjacent to this mass, there was a cystic lesion measuring 0.9 cm in diameter. At the opposite pole, there was a cystic lesion measured 1.1 cm in diameter and multiple cysts ranging from 0.3 cm to 0.5 cm in diameter. In addition, in the middle pole, there was a gelatinous lesion measuring 0.3 cm in diameter.

2.1.2. Microscopic Findings. There were four cystic lesions in each kidney. In the left kidney, one tumor had a complete capsule. The remaining tumors did not have any capsules. In the right kidney, two tumors were completely encapsulated while one had a partial capsule and one no capsule. Some cysts contained colloid-like secretion. The tumors did not have a prominent fibrotic stroma. The tumors showed several morphologic patterns including tubules, acini, papillae, or ribbons lined with single layer of clear cells. The clear cells showed scant eosinophilic or moderate amount of clear cytoplasm. The nuclei of the clear cells were pyknotic, small, and mostly oriented toward the apical surfaces (Fuhrman grade 1). No necrosis or sarcomatoid changes were identified. No microscopic vascular invasion or perinephric or renal sinus invasion was seen. All of resection margins were negative. Immunohistochemically, the tumor cells showed diffuse positivity for CK7 and E-cadherin, weakly positive for CD10, and negative staining for renal cell carcinoma antigen (RCC). The background kidneys showed end-stage changes including extensive global glomerulosclerosis, tubular atrophy, and diffuse interstitial fibrosis (see Figure 1).

3. Discussion

Clear cell papillary renal cell carcinoma (CCPRCC) is a recently described low-grade renal cell cancer [4, 5, 7–9]. It can occur in both end-staged kidneys [9] and normal kidneys [5]. No coagulative necrosis, sarcomatoid changes, or vascular invasion has been identified [4].

The tumors are commonly cystic, with multiple growth patterns, including cysts, tubules, acini, papillae, and clear cell nests [4]. Branching tubules and clear cell ribbons are reported to be the characteristic morphologic patterns [4]. The tubules, acini, ribbons, or papillae are lined with single layer of tumor cells. The tumor cells usually show moderate clear cytoplasm with low nuclear grade. The nuclei were oriented away from the basement membranes and toward the apical surfaces.

The tumors show a characteristic immunophenotype. The tumor cells are diffusely positive for CK7 and negative for alpha-methylacyl-CoA racemase (AMACR); the majority of the tumors are also negative for CD10 [4]. The stain for carbonic anhydrase IX (CA9) is variable.

Genetically, the tumor does not show deletion of chromosome 3P. Aydin et al. showed that only 1 out of 10 tumors had low copy number gains of chromosomes 7 and 17 [4]. In addition, two tumors whose entire VHL gene sequences and promoter regions were analyzed showed no alterations [4].

CCPRCC usually presents with low pathologic stage. In 82 of reported cases, 80 were categorized as pathologic stage 1 and the remaining 2 tumors as pathologic stage 2 tumors [4, 5, 7–10]. The current case is pathologic stage 1. CCPRCC appears to be clinically indolent. Follow-up in 40 cases with a mean follow-up period of 28 months showed no evidence of disease after treatment [4]. In our case the patient is alive 21 months after the surgery.

The main differential diagnoses include clear cell renal cell carcinoma (CCRCC) and papillary renal cell carcinoma (PRCC). The primary morphological clue to CCPRCC is the recognition of papillary architecture. The tubules and cysts lined with clear cells may raise the suspicion for conventional CCRCC. However, CCPRCC lacks the delicate sinusoidal vascular networks seen in the CCRCC, while CCRCC does not have the branched tubules and complex clear cell ribbons seen in the former. In a difficult case, immunohistochemical stains can help to confirm the diagnosis. CCRCC is usually positive for RCC, CA9, and CD10 and negative for CK7 while CCPRCC is diffusely positive for CK7, commonly negative for CD10, and variably positive for CA 9. In the current case, we also stained the tumor for RCC; it was negative. Genetically, while CCRCC shows a deletion of chromosome 3p [11] and mutation in VHL gene in majority of sporadic cases [12], CCPRCC does not have such changes.

PRCC may show clear cell changes, which may be confused with CCPRCC. In addition to the characteristic morphological features, CCPRCC has unique immunohistochemical and genetic profiles. CCPRCC is diffusely positive for CK7, negative for AMACR, and also mostly negative for CD10 and variably positive for CA9, while PRCC is positive for CK7, CD10, and AMACR, usually negative for CA9. Gains of chromosome 7 and 17 are commonly seen in PRCC while such chromosomal changes were only seen in 1 out of 10 tested cases in CCRRCC [4].

Besides CCRCC and PRCC, several other renal tumors may enter in the differential diagnosis including multilocular cystic renal cell carcinoma (MLCRCC) and mixed epithelial and stromal tumor (MEST). MLCRCC is a variant of CCRCC with multilocular cystic growth pattern. The cysts are lined by clear cells with low nuclear grade [13, 14]. Genetically, MLCRCC also has chromosome 3p alteration [13]. Although CCPRCC can have abundant smooth muscle stroma, it does not, however, have the overall characteristic morphology of MEST.

Solid organ transplant recipients have higher risk for cancer development, which contributes to a far worse outcome than in the general population [1]. Renal transplant recipients have a 2–4-fold increase in overall cancer development [2, 3]. For kidney malignancy there is approximately a 15-fold increase [15]. The histologic types are approximately 2/3 conventional clear cell renal cell carcinoma and 1/3 of papillary renal cell carcinoma [16]. No clear cell papillary renal cell carcinoma has been previously reported in a renal transplant recipient. Renal cell carcinoma has been shown to be more aggressive tumors in renal transplant recipients compared to the general and dialysis population [17, 18], which may be partially attributed to the immunosuppression. The current case is the first case of CCPRCC reported in a kidney transplant recipient. The patient did not have tumor recurrence 21 months after surgery; however, the clinical behavior of this tumor in the kidney transplant recipients needs to be further evaluated with more cases and longer follow-up periods.

References

[1] J. Alber, "Clinical insights for cancer outcomes in renal transplant patients," *Transplantation Proceedings*, vol. 42, no. 9, pp. S36–S40, 2010.

[2] A. Andres, "Cancer incidence after immunosuppressive treatment following kidney transplantation," *Critical Reviews in Oncology/Hematology*, vol. 56, no. 1, pp. 71–85, 2005.

[3] J. D. Briggs, "Causes of death after renal transplantation," *Nephrology Dialysis Transplantation*, vol. 16, no. 8, pp. 1545–1549, 2001.

[4] H. Aydin, L. Chen, L. Cheng et al., "Clear cell tubulopapillary renal cell carcinoma: a study of 36 distinctive low-grade epithelial tumors of the kidney," *American Journal of Surgical Pathology*, vol. 34, no. 11, pp. 1608–1621, 2010.

[5] S. Gobbo, J. N. Eble, D. J. Grignon et al., "Clear cell papillary renal cell carcinoma: a distinct histopathologic and molecular genetic entity," *American Journal of Surgical Pathology*, vol. 32, no. 8, pp. 1239–1245, 2008.

[6] N. Kuroda, M. Michal, O. Hes et al., "Renal angiomyoadenomatous tumor: fluorescence in situ hybridization," *Pathology International*, vol. 59, no. 9, pp. 689–691, 2009.

[7] K. T. Mai, D. M. Kohler, E. C. Belanger, S. J. Robertson, and D. Wang, "Sporadic clear cell renal cell carcinoma with diffuse cytokeratin 7 immunoreactivity," *Pathology*, vol. 40, no. 5, pp. 481–486, 2008.

[8] M. Michal, O. Hes, and F. Havlicek, "Benign renal angiomyoadenomatous tumor: a previously unreported renal tumor," *Annals of Diagnostic Pathology*, vol. 4, no. 5, pp. 311–315, 2000.

[9] S. K. Tickoo, M. N. dePeralta-Venturina, L. R. Harik et al., "Spectrum of epithelial neoplasms in end-stage renal disease: an experience from 66 tumor-bearing kidneys with emphasis on histologic patterns distinct from those in sporadic adult renal neoplasia," *American Journal of Surgical Pathology*, vol. 30, no. 2, pp. 141–153, 2006.

[10] M. Michal, O. Hes, J. Nemcova et al., "Renal angiomyoadenomatous tumor: morphologic, immunohistochemical, and molecular genetic study of a distinct entity," *Virchows Archiv*, vol. 454, no. 1, pp. 89–99, 2009.

[11] L. Cheng, S. Zhang, G. T. MacLennan, A. Lopez-Beltran, and R. Montironi, "Molecular and cytogenetic insights into

the pathogenesis, classification, differential diagnosis, and prognosis of renal epithelial neoplasms," *Human Pathology*, vol. 40, no. 1, pp. 10–29, 2009.

[12] C. L. Cowey and W. K. Rathmell, "VHL gene mutations in renal cell carcinoma: role as a biomarker of disease outcome and drug efficacy," *Current Oncology Reports*, vol. 11, no. 2, pp. 94–101, 2009.

[13] S. Halat, J. N. Eble, D. J. Grignon et al., "Multilocular cystic renal cell carcinoma is a subtype of clear cell renal cell carcinoma," *Modern Pathology*, vol. 23, no. 7, pp. 931–936, 2010.

[14] S. Suzigan, A. Lopez-Beltran, R. Montironi et al., "Multilocular cystic renal cell carcinoma: a report of 45 cases of a kidney tumor of low malignant potential," *American Journal of Clinical Pathology*, vol. 125, no. 2, pp. 217–222, 2006.

[15] B. L. Kasiske, J. J. Snyder, D. T. Gilbertson, and C. Wang, "Cancer after kidney transplantation in the United States," *American Journal of Transplantation*, vol. 4, no. 6, pp. 905–913, 2004.

[16] I. Tsaur, N. Obermuller, D. Jonas et al., "De novo renal cell carcinoma of native and graft kidneys in renal transplant recipients," *BJU International*.

[17] S. M. Moudouni, A. Lakmichi, M. Tligui et al., "Renal cell carcinoma of native kidney in renal transplant recipients," *BJU International*, vol. 98, no. 2, pp. 298–302, 2006.

[18] Y. Neuzillet, F. Lay, A. Luccioni et al., "De novo renal cell carcinoma of native kidney in renal transplant recipients," *Cancer*, vol. 103, no. 2, pp. 251–257, 2005.

14

Unusual Fungal Infections in Renal Transplant Recipients

Mahesh Eswarappa,[1] P. Vijay Varma,[1] Rakesh Madhyastha,[1] Sujeeth Reddy,[1] M. S. Gireesh,[1] K. C. Gurudev,[1] Vijaya V. Mysorekar,[2] and Beena Hemanth[3]

[1]*Department of Nephrology, M. S. Ramaiah Medical College and Teaching Hospital, MSR Nagar, MSRIT Post, Bangalore, Karnataka 560054, India*
[2]*Department of Pathology, M. S. Ramaiah Medical College and Teaching Hospital, MSR Nagar, MSRIT Post, Bangalore, Karnataka 560054, India*
[3]*Department of Microbiology, M. S. Ramaiah Medical College and Teaching Hospital, MSR Nagar, MSRIT Post, Bangalore, Karnataka 560054, India*

Correspondence should be addressed to Mahesh Eswarappa; manasnephro2002@yahoo.co.in

Academic Editor: Graeme Forrest

Fungal infections are an important cause of morbidity and mortality in renal transplant recipients. The causative agent and the risk factors differ depending on the period after the kidney transplant. Also the incidence varies according to the geographical area. We are reporting three cases of fungal infections in renal transplant recipients. Two of them have etiological agents which are common among immunosuppressed patients, but with an atypical clinical presentation, while one of them is a subcutaneous infection caused by a less frequent dematiaceous fungus, *Aureobasidium pullulans*. These cases highlight how a high index of clinical suspicion and prompt diagnosis is very much essential for better outcome. The emerging fungal infections and paucity of data regarding their management pose a challenge to the transplant physicians.

1. Introduction

Fungal infections account for 5% of all infections in renal transplant recipients [1]. The incidence varies according to the geographical area. Because of environmental exposure and the effects of immunosuppressive regimens, systemic mycosis is a significant problem in transplant patients worldwide and remains the major cause of death in those individuals [2]. In an Indian study 6.1% of renal transplant recipients were affected by systemic fungal infections and resulted in a 63% mortality rate [3]. The causative agent and the risk factors differ depending on the period after the kidney transplant. *Aspergillus* species, Mucorales species, *Candida* species, and *Cryptococcus neoformans* are the opportunistic fungi that cause most infections.

Herein we report three cases of fungal infection in renal transplant recipients. Two of them have etiological agents which are common among immunosuppressed patients, but with an atypical clinical presentation, while one of them is a subcutaneous infection caused by a less frequent dematiaceous fungus, *Aureobasidium pullulans*.

2. Case 1

A 33-year-old male who underwent renal transplantation in May 2012 with his mother as donor (haplomatch) was started on antituberculous treatment (ATT) for pulmonary tuberculosis prior to transplant from December 2011 and continued up to September 2012. In view of graft dysfunction biopsy was done in November 2013 which showed evidence of interstitial fibrosis and tubular atrophy (IF/TA). This patient presented to us in April 2014 with pain in the posterior aspect of the right side of the chest. He was on tacrolimus [(TAC) 3 mg/day], mycophenolate mofetil [(MMF) 1 g/day], and prednisolone (10 mg/day) immunosuppression. Serum creatinine at the time of admission was 2.5 mg/dL.

Chest radiograph showed homogenous lobulated opacity in the right hilar region. Computed tomography (CT) of

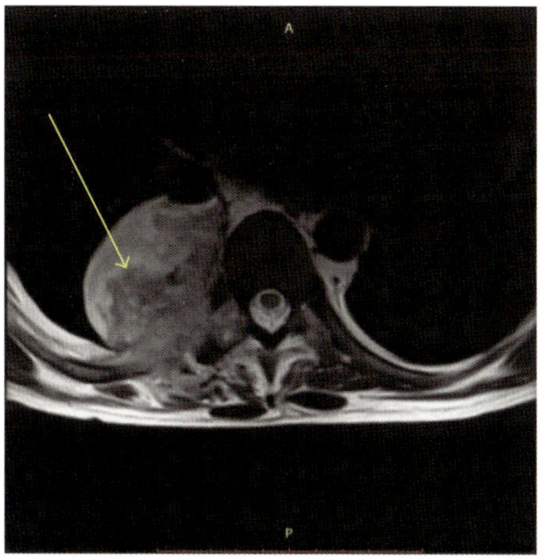

FIGURE 1: MRI spine (axial T1 and T2) showing paraspinal abscess on the right side with an air fluid level (arrow).

the chest revealed a cold abscess in the D9 vertebra-rib region. In the background of old pulmonary tuberculosis he was empirically restarted on ATT. However patient had worsening of symptoms with fever spikes. MRI spine revealed well-defined heterogeneously hyperintense signal lesion in the paravertebral region bilaterally and predominantly on the right side (Figure 1). Surgical drainage of the lesion was done and pus showed fungal elements of *Aspergillus* species. He was treated with IV liposomal amphotericin B [(LAmpB) 3 mg/kg/day] for 7 days followed by oral voriconazole (VOR) 200 mg twice a day and the dose of TAC was adjusted accordingly. Patient developed progressive worsening of renal function and severe metabolic acidosis requiring initiation of hemodialysis. He was also treated with broad spectrum antibiotics. On day 14 of admission, patient developed acute onset paraplegia and hypotension requiring inotropic support. Repeat MRI showed collapse of T8, T9 vertebrae with evidence of spinal cord indentation. However he could not be taken for surgical intervention owing to poor hemodynamic status. Patient developed refractory shock and ultimately succumbed.

3. Case 2

A 34-year-old lady underwent renal transplantation in May 2012 with her brother as donor (HLA match—NIL). She was on triple immunosuppressive regimen. In view of graft dysfunction (serum creatinine: 2.5 mg/dL), graft biopsy was done in October 2013 which showed interstitial fibrosis and tubular atrophy (IF/TA). This lady presented to us with complaints of fever and burning micturition in December 2014. *E. coli* was isolated from the urine culture and she was started on appropriate IV antibiotics. However she continued to have fever spikes in spite of antibiotic therapy. Further evaluation revealed *Cytomegalovirus* (CMV) infection and she was started on intravenous ganciclovir (GCV) 250 mg/day. On day 7 of initiation of therapy patient developed leucopenia for which MMF dose was tapered and later stopped and intravenous GCV was withheld. In the meanwhile patient had severe dyspeptic symptoms for which esophagogastroduodenal endoscopy was done which showed esophageal candidiasis. She was started on intravenous fluconazole 100 mg/day and TAC dose was adjusted accordingly. Patient developed progressive graft dysfunction (serum creatinine: 6.5 mg/dL) for which she was initiated on hemodialysis and later subjected to graft biopsy which showed intracapillary spherical fungal structures within the glomerulus that showed periodic acid-Schiff stain (PAS) positive capsules consistent with cryptococcal organisms. Also tubular epithelium showed features of CMV nephritis (Figure 2). She was restarted on intravenous GCV, once the leucopenia resolved. In view of multiple coinfections (CMV nephritis, cryptococcal infection, and esophageal candidiasis) patient was given the option of withdrawal of immunosuppression in order to prevent dissemination. However consent for the withdrawal of immunosuppression was not given and she was started on intravenous LAmpB 150 mg/day. In spite of 10-day treatment with LAmpB there was no improvement in graft function and she was dialysis-dependent. Patient ultimately succumbed to the underlying illness.

4. Case 3

A 56-year-old male, a case of end stage renal disease due to diabetic nephropathy, underwent renal transplantation in June 2011, donor being his sister (HLA match—full house match). He was on triple immunosuppressive regimen. In June 2013 he presented to us with a nonhealing wound over the sole of right foot following a trauma and multiple subcutaneous nodules over the right leg (Figure 3). He was subjected to biopsy of the ulcer edge and pus from the nodules was sent for bacterial and fungal culture sensitivity.

He was empirically started on IV antibiotics, pending further reports. Pus from the subcutaneous nodules showed fungal elements. He was started on oral itraconazole (ITR) 200 mg/day. The serum TAC levels increased to 23 ng/mL after one-week treatment with ITR and the TAC dose was reduced to a mere 0.5 mg/day. Growth was observed on Sabouraud medium on day 10 of incubation which was later reported to be due to a mould *Aureobasidium pullulans*. He was continued on oral ITR 200 mg/day and the skin lesions gradually disappeared. Two months later patient developed recurrence of lesions while still being on ITR.

Hence treatment was changed over to oral VOR 200 mg/day and the TAC dose was adjusted accordingly. Lesions gradually disappeared over a period of 1 month. Treatment with VOR was continued for another 2 months following the resolution and then stopped.

5. Discussion

Fungal infections among renal transplant recipients are an important cause of mortality. The symptoms of systemic fungal infections are nonspecific, particularly in their early stages [2]. In the first two cases described above, although the infections were caused by common fungal agents among the transplant recipients, the site of involvement was very

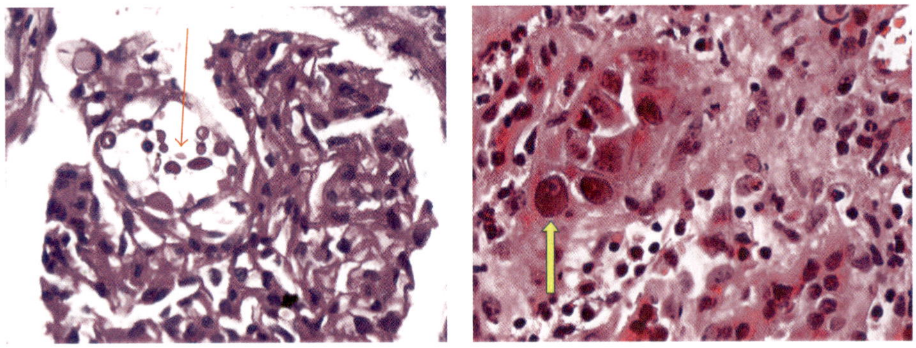

(a) (b)

Figure 2: Glomerulus exhibits intracapillary spherical fungal structures that show PAS positive capsules consistent with cryptococcal organism (red arrow). Few of the tubular epithelial cells show homogenous smudgy appearing intranuclear inclusions (yellow arrow).

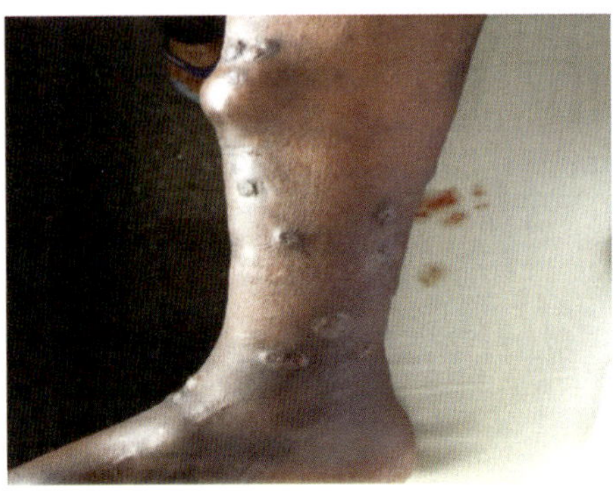

Figure 3: Photograph showing emerging subcutaneous nodule with healed lesions over the right lower limb.

unusual. The third case of subcutaneous mycosis due to *Aureobasidium pullulans* is a rare infection with only a few cases reported so far.

In the first case, the diagnosis was delayed due to initial treatment with ATT as the patient had prior pulmonary tuberculosis and also because tuberculous paraspinal abscess is a more common entity in tropical countries like India. The frequency of invasive aspergillosis (IA), the second-highest cause of invasive fungal infection in renal transplant recipients after candidiasis, ranges from 0.5% to 2.2%, with a mortality rate up to 88% [4–7]. Although pulmonary involvement is the most common presentation of IA, the spectrum of disease is broad and virtually every organ of the body has been reported to be affected [8]. Spinal cord involvement by *Aspergillus* is a rare entity and could be in the form of paraspinal abscess, epidural abscess, vertebral osteomyelitis, discitis, or spinal cord necrosis [9]. A similar case scenario of *Aspergillus* paraspinal abscess causing paraparesis and ultimately death due to fungal sepsis has been described [10]. This case highlights how misdiagnosis at an early stage of a serious infection in a transplant recipient can prove to be fatal. A high index of clinical suspicion is hence necessary.

The second case had multiple coinfections: CMV nephritis, esophageal candidiasis, and cryptococcosis of the allograft. The increased occurrence of fungal infections in the background of immunomodulatory viruses such as *Cytomegalovirus* is well known. Majority of cases (53–72%) of cryptococcal disease among solid organ transplant (SOT) recipients are disseminated or involve the CNS [11]. Overall, 61% of the SOT recipients in one report had disseminated disease, 54% had pulmonary disease, and 8.1% had skin, soft-tissue, or osteoarticular cryptococcosis [12]. The detection of cryptococcal elements in the renal allograft has been rarely described in the literature. In one French study of 11 SOT recipients, 3 had urinary tract infection [13]. The case highlights the need to save the life first and then to save the kidney when inevitable.

The third case of subcutaneous nodular fungal infection caused by *Aureobasidium pullulans* is the first case being reported from India. *Aureobasidium pullulans* is a saprophytic dematiaceous fungus widely distributed in the environment, and it can be isolated from soil, decaying plant debris, wood, rock, and household dust as well as human hair, skin, and nails [14–16].

It is the best known *Aureobasidium* species for causing emerging human diseases including peritonitis in patients on peritoneal dialysis, splenic abscess, meningitis, skin, and soft tissue infections, as well as septicemia in patients with malignancies or receiving major surgery [16].

Franco et al. described a case of chromomycosis in a renal transplant recipient caused by *A. pullulans* following penetrating trauma in the same skin area with the presentation as an ulcerative lesion resembling squamous cell carcinoma [17]. In the present case also patient had a wound over the sole of the right foot prior to the development of the skin lesions which probably could have been the source of infection.

Arranz Sánchez et al. reported similar [18] skin lesions in a renal transplant recipient caused by *A. pullulans* which subsided within 2 months of ITR therapy with no relapse at one year of follow-up. However in our case the lesions recurred after 2 months despite the patient being on antifungal agents. How long these lesions have to be treated has not been clearly defined [18, 19]. This case also highlights how crucial it is to optimize the TAC dose and monitor for nephrotoxicity when the patient is treated with antifungal drugs such as triazoles, owing to the drug interactions.

6. Conclusion

The present case series highlights the unusual fungal infections and their manifestations in the renal transplant population. A high index of clinical suspicion and prompt diagnosis is very much essential for better outcome. In certain clinical situations, the decision to withdraw the immunosuppression and forgo the graft might be the call of the hour. The emerging fungal infections and paucity of data regarding their management pose a challenge to the transplant physicians.

References

[1] R. Patel and C. V. Paya, "Infections in solid-organ transplant recipients," *Clinical Microbiology Reviews*, vol. 10, no. 1, pp. 86–124, 1997.

[2] P. Badiee and A. Alborzi, "Invasive fungal infections in renal transplant recipients," *Experimental and Clinical Transplantation*, vol. 9, no. 6, pp. 355–362, 2011.

[3] K. S. Chugh, V. Sakhuja, S. Jain et al., "Fungal infections in renal allograft recipients," *Transplantation Proceedings*, vol. 24, no. 5, pp. 1940–1942, 1992.

[4] G. J. Alangaden, R. Thyagarajan, S. A. Gruber et al., "Infectious complications after kidney transplantation: current epidemiology and associated risk factors," *Clinical Transplantation*, vol. 20, no. 4, pp. 401–409, 2006.

[5] F. Ergin, H. Arslan, A. Azap, B. Demirhan, H. Karakayali, and M. Haberal, "Invasive aspergillosis in solid-organ transplantation: report of eight cases and review of the literature," *Transplant International*, vol. 16, no. 4, pp. 280–286, 2003.

[6] J. Morgan, K. A. Wannemuehler, K. A. Marr et al., "Incidence of invasive aspergillosis following hematopoietic stem cell and solid organ transplantation: interim results of a prospective multicenter surveillance program," *Medical Mycology*, vol. 43, no. 1, pp. S49–S58, 2005.

[7] S.-J. Lin, J. Schranz, and S. M. Teutsch, "Aspergillosis case-fatality rate: systematic review of the literature," *Clinical Infectious Diseases*, vol. 32, no. 3, pp. 358–366, 2001.

[8] V. T. Andriole, "Infections with *Aspergillus* species," *Clinical Infectious Diseases*, vol. 17, supplement 2, pp. S481–S486, 1993.

[9] S. A. Lee and P. Nee, "Aspergillus epidural abscess of the spine: case and review," *Infectious Diseases in Clinical Practice*, vol. 9, no. 2, pp. 88–91, 2000.

[10] S. B. Park, M. J. Kang, E. A. Whang, S. Y. Han, and H. C. Kim, "A case of fungal sepsis due to aspergillus spondylitis followed by cytomegalovirus infection in a renal transplant recipient," *Transplantation Proceedings*, vol. 36, no. 7, pp. 2154–2155, 2004.

[11] N. Singh, F. Dromer, J. R. Perfect, and O. Lortholary, "Cryptococcosis in solid organ transplant recipients: current state of the science," *Clinical Infectious Diseases*, vol. 47, no. 10, pp. 1321–1327, 2008.

[12] N. Singh, B. D. Alexander, O. Lortholary et al., "Cryptococcus neoformans in organ transplant recipients: impact of calcineurin-inhibitor agents on mortality," *The Journal of Infectious Diseases*, vol. 195, no. 5, pp. 756–764, 2007.

[13] F. Dromer, S. Mathoulin-Pélissier, O. Launay, O. Lortholary, and the French Cryptococcosis Study Group, "Determinants of disease presentation and outcome during cryptococcosis: the cryptoA/D study," *PLoS Medicine*, vol. 4, no. 2, p. e21, 2007.

[14] R. Ibanez Perez, J. Chacon, A. Fidalgo, J. Martin, V. Paraiso, and J. L. Munoz-Bellido, "Peritonitis by *Aureobasidium pullulans* in continuous ambulatory peritoneal dialysis," *Nephrology Dialysis Transplantation*, vol. 12, no. 7, pp. 1544–1545, 1997.

[15] G. Bolignano and G. Criseo, "Disseminated nosocomial fungal infection by *Aureobasidium pullulans* var. *melanigenum*: a case report," *Journal of Clinical Microbiology*, vol. 41, no. 9, pp. 4483–4485, 2003.

[16] M. Hawkes, R. Rennie, C. Sand, and W. Vaudry, "Aureobasidium pullulans infection: fungemia in an infant and a review of human cases," *Diagnostic Microbiology and Infectious Disease*, vol. 51, no. 3, pp. 209–213, 2005.

[17] A. Franco, I. Aranda, M. J. Fernandez et al., "Chromomycosis in a European renal transplant recipient," *Nephrology Dialysis Transplantation*, vol. 11, no. 4, pp. 715–716, 1996.

[18] D. M. Arranz Sánchez, M. Corral de la Calle, M. A. Martín-Díaz et al., "Subcutaneous mycosis produced by *Aureobasidium pullulans* in a renal transplant recipient," *Journal of the European Academy of Dermatology and Venereology*, vol. 20, no. 2, pp. 229–230, 2006.

[19] P. A. Wackym, G. F. Gray Jr., R. E. Richie, and C. R. Gregg, "Cutaneous chromomycosis in renal transplant recipients. Successful management in two cases," *Archives of Internal Medicine*, vol. 145, no. 6, pp. 1036–1037, 1985.

15

Late Renal Allograft Rupture Associated with Cessation of Immunosuppression following Graft Failure

Sumayah Askandarani,[1] Noura Aloudah,[2] Hanan Al Enazi,[2] Khaled O. Alsaad,[2,3] and Abdulrahman Altamimi[4]

[1] *Division of Nephrology, Department of Medicine, King Abdulaziz Medical City, P.O. Box 22490, Riyadh 11426, Saudi Arabia*
[2] *Department of Pathology and Laboratory Medicine, King Abdulaziz Medical City, P.O. Box 22490, Riyadh 11426, Saudi Arabia*
[3] *King Abdullah International Medical Research Centre and College of Medicine, King Saud bin Abdulaziz University for Health Sciences, King Abdulaziz Medical City, P.O. Box 22490, Riyadh 11426, Saudi Arabia*
[4] *Department of Hepatobiliary Sciences and Liver Transplantation, King Abdulaziz Medical City, P.O. Box 22490, Riyadh 11426, Saudi Arabia*

Correspondence should be addressed to Abdulrahman Altamimi, altamimiab@ngha.med.sa

Academic Editors: A. Beiras-Fernandez and Y. Sugawara

A 29-year-old man developed chronic allograft nephropathy 63 months after renal transplantation. He became symptomatic with advanced chronic graft failure; his immunosuppressive medications were reduced and he was commenced on haemodialysis. Two months following the withdrawal of immunosuppression, he presented with abdominal pain, haematuria, and a marked drop in haemoglobin. The patient was taken to the operating room, where the renal allograft was found to be ruptured, and graft nephrectomy was subsequently performed. Histological examination of the graft specimen showed severe haemorrhagic acute vascular cellular rejection in a background of marked chronic allograft vasculopathy. Immunostaining for C4d showed diffuse, strong, linear circumferential staining of the peritubular capillaries, indicating a concurrent antibody-mediated rejection. We report herein an unusual case of spontaneous renal allograft rupture that occurred long time after transplantation due to severe acute rejection following cessation of immunosuppressive medications for advanced chronic allograft failure. To the best of our knowledge, the time interval between transplantation and the rupture of this allograft is the longest of those reported in the literature.

1. Introduction

Renal allograft rupture is a well-recognised but rare complication of renal transplantation, which normally occurs in the first few weeks after transplantation. It is associated with severe graft pain, hypotension, and a drop in haemoglobin. The most common cause of allograft rupture is acute rejection [1]. The incidence of allograft rupture has decreased due to the use of modern potent immunosuppressive medications [2–4]. Due to its devastating clinical course and outcome, recognition and prompt management of allograft rupture is important. Usually, nephrectomy is necessary treatment measure, but conservative surgical intervention has also been attempted to preserve the renal allograft in certain cases [2, 5–8]. We report an unusual case of late renal allograft rupture secondary to severe acute rejection, which followed cessation of the patient's immunosuppressive regimen due to advanced chronic allograft failure (CAF). To the best of our knowledge, the interval period of time between renal allograft transplantation and rupture in this case is the longest of those reported in the literature.

2. Case Report

A 29-year-old man received a living-unrelated kidney transplant abroad for end-stage kidney disease secondary to neurogenic bladder. The patient had an uneventful postoperative clinical course with good early graft function. The data of HLA matching and induction protocol are lacking. He was

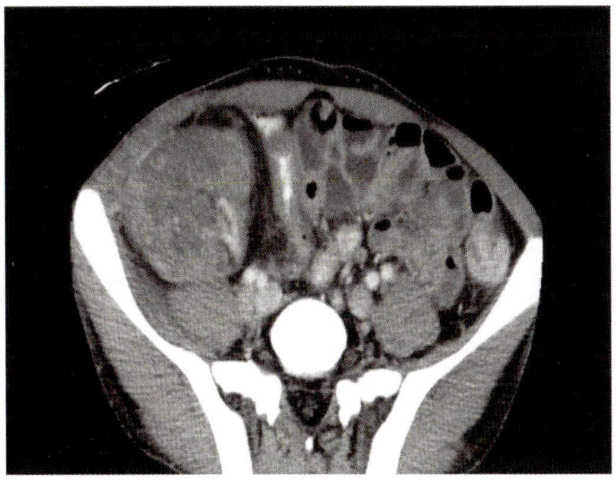

Figure 1: Computed tomography scan showing hyperdense areas in the renal allograft, in keeping with foci of parenchymal haemorrhage.

maintained on prednisone, cyclosporine, and myocophenolate mofetil. The patient was discharged on postoperative day 5, with an adequate urine output and serum creatinine 110 μmol/L. In addition, he was kept on intermittent self-catherization four times per day. Forty-eight months after transplantation, the patient was diagnosed in another institution to have chronic allograft failure based on slow rising serum creatinine. No renal allograft biopsy was obtained *as the patient refused*. His immunosuppression was modified, whereby tacrolimus was substituted for cyclosporine A, when his serum creatinine had increased to 400 μmol/L.

Sixty-three months after renal transplantation, the patient was first seen in our hospital, when he presented with hypoxic respiratory failure secondary to pneumonia, pulmonary oedema, and deteriorating kidney allograft function. His blood urea and nitrogen (BUN) was 44 mmol/L and serum creatinine 700 μmol/L. He was admitted to the intensive care unit and started on ventilatory support. Appropriate antimicrobial coverage was started for pneumonia and haemodialysis was initiated. During the hospital admission for about a month, the patient was diagnosed to have advanced graft failure based on his clinical progression. The patient refused the renal allograft biopsy. He was maintained on haemodialysis and discharged on prednisone 5 mg daily. Tacrolimus and mycophenolate mofetil were discontinued.

Two months later (65 months post renal transplant), the patient was admitted because of abdominal pain, graft tenderness, and gross haematuria. There was no history of abdominal trauma or recent renal allograft biopsy. Upon admission, the patient was pale, tachycardic, and hypotensive. His heart rate was 111 beat per minute, and the blood pressure 110/56 mmHg. Laboratory tests showed WBC of 2 × 103/μL, haemoglobin of 5.5 g/dL (dropped from 12.7 g/dL one month earlier), haematocrit of 16.6%, platelets count of 344 × 103/Ul, PT of 9.1, PTT of 33.9, BUN of 13.0 mmol/L, and serum creatinine of 809 μmol/L. The patient was resuscitated with crystalloid fluids and packed red blood cells. An enhanced abdominal computed tomography (CT) scan revealed few scattered hyperdense foci in the renal allograft, in keeping with microhaemorrhage and microperforations (Figure 1). The renal artery and vein were patent.

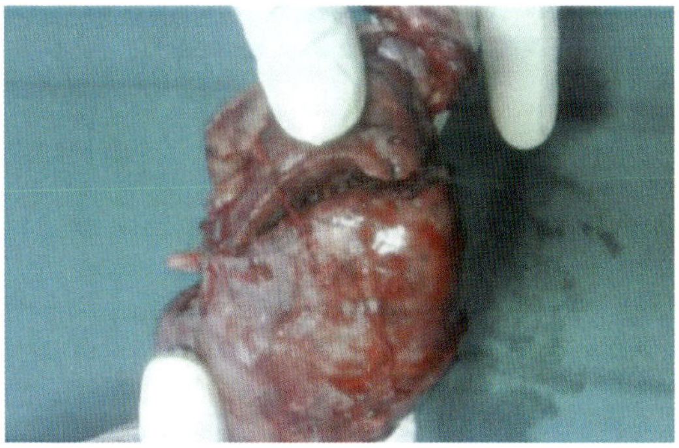

Figure 2: Oblique laceration on in the upper pole and mid portion of the kidney compatible with ruptured graft.

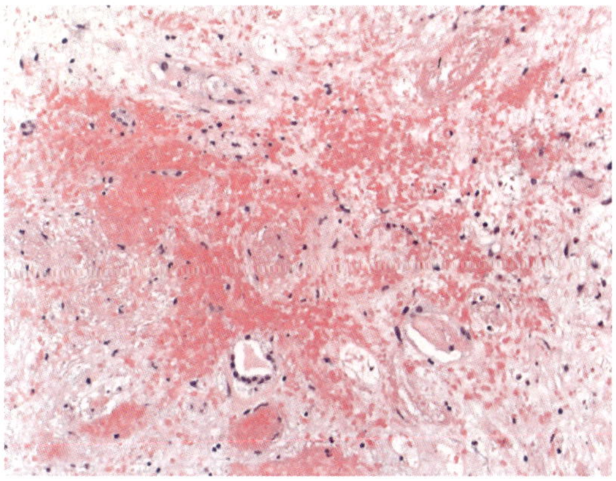

Figure 3: Marked interstitial oedema and haemorrhage (H&E × 100).

The patient was emergently taken to the operating room, where urinary bladder irrigation and washout revealed 3 litres of partially clotted blood. Exploration of the renal graft through the old transplant scar and intracapsular approach showed ruptured graft. An oblique laceration that measured 4 cm in length and involved the upper pole and the mid portion of the graft was evident (Figure 2). The renal artery and vein were dissected, clamped, and divided, along with the transplant ureter. The postoperative course was uneventful, and the patient was discharged 5 days after the graft nephrectomy.

Histological examination showed morphological features compatible with severe acute vascular T-cell mediated (cellular) rejection, in a background of marked chronic allograft arteriopathy. The interstitium was markedly oedematous and showed areas of extensive haemorrhage (Figure 3). Severe interstitial inflammation was seen and the inflammatory infiltrate consisted of lymphocytes, plasma cells, and neutrophils. Large numbers of eosinophils were also noted. This was associated with severe *lymphocytic* tubulitis, acute tubular epithelial cell degenerative and regenerative changes in the viable renal tubules, and severe endarteritis with fibrinoid necrosis (Figure 4). The vast majority of glomeruli were

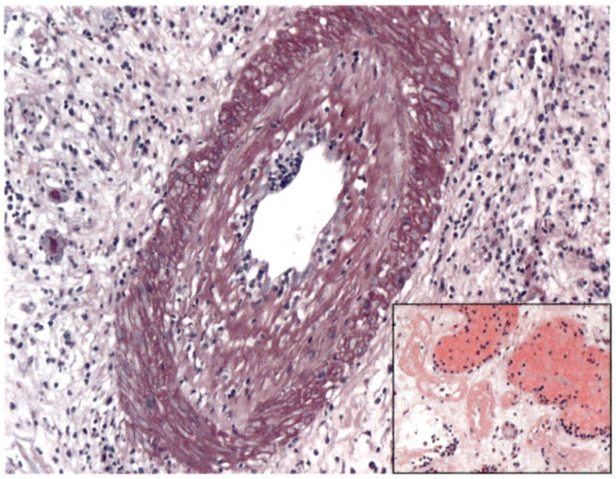

Figure 4: Severe endarteritis was readily identified in the interstitial blood vessels (PAS stain ×200), along with arterial and arteriolar fibrinoid necrosis (Inset H&E ×200).

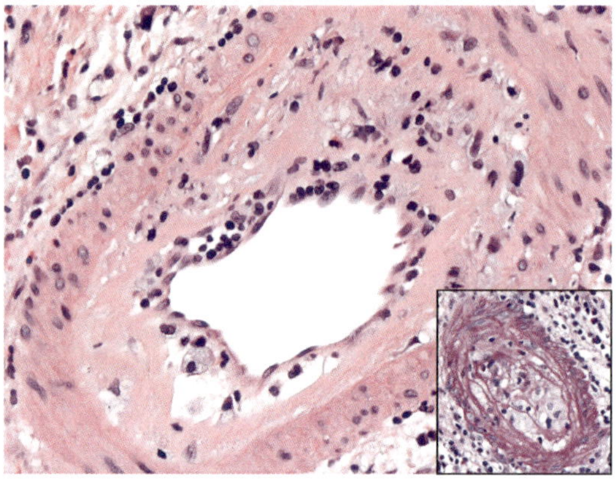

Figure 6: The morphological features of the acute rejection were found in a background of severe chronic allograft arteriopathy (H&E ×40, inset PAS ×200).

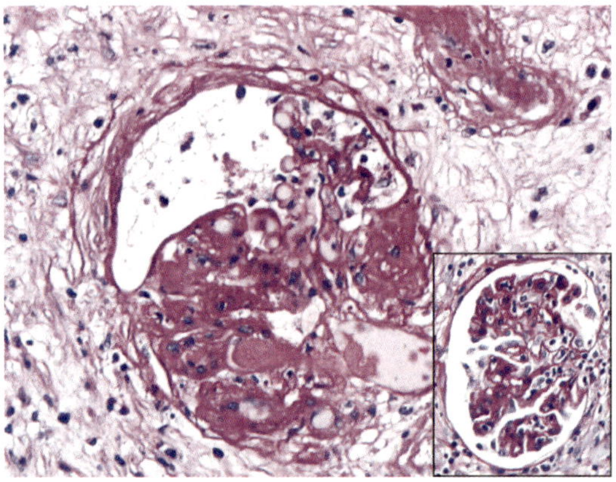

Figure 5: Fibrin microthrombi were also seen in the glomeruli (PAS ×200). Glomerulitis in the form of mononuclear inflammatory cells infiltrating the glomerular capillaries was seen (Inset PAS ×200).

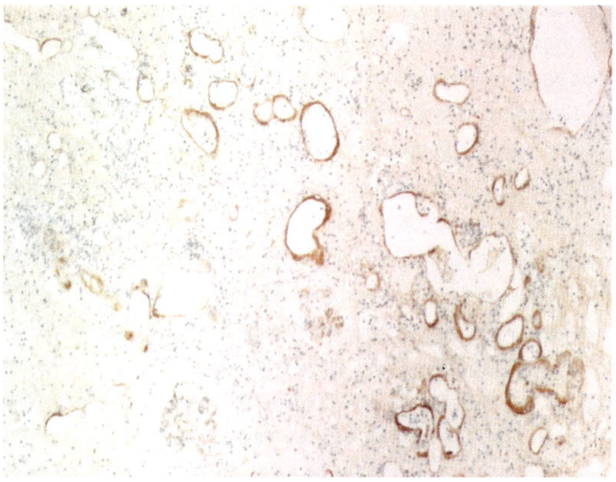

Figure 7: Immunohistochemical staining for C4d shows diffuse linear and strong circumferential staining in the peritubular capillaries, consistent with acute antibody-mediated rejection (C4d IHC ×100).

globally sclerosed, and the scattered viable glomeruli showed ischemic changes and segmental scarring. Mild glomerulitis, congestion, and fibrin microthrombi were identified in the viable glomeruli (Figure 5). Marked chronic allograft vasculopathic changes in the form of severe fibrointimal thickening and presence of intimal and subintimal foamy aggregates were readily seen in the interstitial blood vessels (Figure 6). Peritubular capillaritis was noted, of which most of the inflammatory cells were of mononuclear type. No viral cytopathic effect was identified. Immunohistochemical staining for C4d (dilution 1 : 40, polyclonal Abcam, Cambridge, UK) showed diffuse linear staining in peritubular capillaries in the renal cortex and medulla, indicating a concurrent active antibody-mediated rejection (Figure 7). Immunostaining for polyoma virus (dilution 1 : 200, clone Pab416, Abcam) was negative.

Immunologically, anti-HLA (PRA) antibody profile revealed the following specificities: Class I-A1, 24, 80, 34, 32, 68, 36, 33, 11, and 23 (A1 and A10 CREGs) and B51. Profiling for Class II PRA was negative. The donor HLA typing was not performed, since the transplantation was performed abroad.

3. Discussion

Spontaneous renal allograft rupture is one of the most serious complications of kidney transplantation [5, 9–11], which typically occurs within three weeks after transplantation [1]. The prevalence of renal allograft rupture (RAR) varies from 0.3% to 3% [5]. The pathogenesis of RAR is still not fully understood. Major precipitating factors include acute rejection, ischemic acute tubular epithelial cell damage, renal vein thrombosis, mechanically damaged hilar lymphatics, and ureteral obstruction [1, 5–7]. Rarely RAR can be triggered by graft biopsy [11]. Our case showed the typical gross and histological findings of the graft rupture.

One possible mechanism put forward for RAR is that cortical and capsular ischemia results from interstitial oedema and cellular inflammatory cell infiltration causes capsular tension and rupture. The main clinical manifestations of RAR are sudden onset of abdominal pain, graft bulging and tenderness, and haemorrhagic shock [5]. Recipients of non-heart-beating donor kidneys are at a greater risk of developing graft rupture, and this has been attributed to the higher rate of acute tubular necrosis in this type of grafts. Other risk factors are high peak PRA and younger recipient, probably due to more vigorous immunological responsiveness [6]. On the other hand, the use of ATG was found to be associated with a lower incidence of RAR, presumably due to reduced frequency and severity of rejection [6]. The diagnosis is usually made based on the typical clinical picture and conventional CT scan. In our case, the CT scan findings were helpful in the diagnosis and showed intrarenal haemorrhage and retroperitoneal bleed. There is new evidence showing superiority of multidetector computed tomography (MDCT) in the diagnosis of RAR [12]. The most common course of management in RAR is urgent graft nephrectomy; however, recent reports suggest that ruptured kidney grafts are potentially salvageable by conservative surgical repair of the rupture, with good success rates [2, 5–7, 13, 14]. This approach was not considered in our case as the patient was *clinically* labelled with advanced graft failure.

Our case has the longest time interval between the time of transplant and the graft rupture in the literature. Nevertheless, the underlying cause of rupture was still severe combined acute cellular and antibody-mediated rejection, resulted from cessation of immunosuppression. Case with the second longest interval (21 months) was also a case of RAR secondary to acute rejection that followed discontinuation of immunosuppression following chronic allograft failure [15].

In our case, the patient refused the renal allograft biopsy twice, leading to the clinical assumption of allograft failure without tissue diagnosis. Although severe chronic interstitial fibrosis and tubular atrophy (IF/TA) and chronic allograft arteriopathy were evident in the graft, severe acute cellular as well as antibody-mediated allograft rejection was severely affecting the graft. Our case indicates that RAR remains a possibility five years after transplantation, particularly when immunosuppressive agents are discontinued. This raises a question of what is the best approach for immunosuppressive drug withdrawal following graft failure; should it be abrupt or gradual? The answer for this is not clear. Abrupt cessation of immunosuppression might lead to graft rejection and subsequent RAR, as in our case. On the other hand, higher morbidity and mortality have been reported in patients continued on immunosuppressive therapy after graft failure and commencement of dialysis [16]. In our experience, the presence of advanced graft failure in the form of marked interstitial fibrosis and tubular atrophy is associated with safe abrupt cessation of immunosuppressive therapy, emphasizing the value of kidney graft biopsy before discontinuation of immunosuppression medications. Messa et al. [17] described a strategy to withdraw the immunosuppressive agents in patients with graft failure whereby, the antiproliferative agents are stopped immediately to reduce the risk of infection on patients starting the dialysis, and the calcineurin inhibitors are withdrawn over 1–3 weeks if the graft failure is slow and prolonged, and 4–8 weeks if the graft failure follows a short course of time or is immunologically mediated.

Another important point to be emphasized is the role of renal allograft biopsy before the presumption of graft failure and withdrawal of the immunosuppressive agents. Our patient might started rejecting the graft long time before his initial clinical presentation 48 months after transplantation. A graft biopsy at that time would help identifying the immunological insult to the graft, dictating appropriate management, and preventing a subsequent graft rupture. Refusing graft biopsy is not uncommon in some regions and cultures of the world, and the patients should be educated about the reasons and benefits of the graft biopsy, in attempt to deliver best clinical practice.

Although the donor HLA typing was not performed in our patient, the presence of PRA Class I specificities for CREGs A1 and A10 and B51 suggests that the antibody-mediated component in the rejection process is mediated by donor-specific antibodies. Most intriguing is what may initiate an antibody-mediated immune rejection in a sensitized patient after such a long time since transplantation. Likely possibility is that the pneumonia (as an infection) may have been the triggering stimulus in our patient.

4. Conclusion

Renal allograft rupture is a rare but a serious complication of kidney transplant, which usually occurs few weeks after transplantation. The most common cause is acute antibody-mediated allograft rejection. Discontinuation of the immunosuppressive therapy in patients with graft failure may be a significant risk factor for late RAR and renal allograft biopsy should be performed before withdrawal of immunosuppressive agents. Following cessation of immunosuppressive therapy, careful clinical follow-up should be practiced to detect the symptoms and signs of RAR, even long time after transplantation.

Authors' Contribution

Dr. S. Askandrani collected data and wrote the clinical aspects of the case report. Dr. N. Aloudah handled the pathology gross specimen, reviewed the histopathology, and wrote the pathology findings in the manuscript. Miss H. Al. Enazi performed the clinical laboratory investigations. Dr. KO. Alsaad wrote the discussion part of the manuscript, reviewed the histopathology, took images for publication, and performed the prove reading of the manuscript. Dr. A. Altamimi performed the surgery, collected clinical data, and reviewed the manuscript.

References

[1] P. Szenohradszky, G. Smehák, E. Szederkényi et al., "Renal allograft rupture: a clinicopathologic study of 37 nephrectomy cases in a series of 628 consecutive renal transplants," *Transplantation Proceedings*, vol. 31, no. 5, pp. 2107–2111, 1999.

[2] S. Guleria, R. K. Khazanchi, A. K. Dinda et al., "Spontaneous renal allograft rupture: is graft nephrectomy an option?" *Transplantation Proceedings*, vol. 35, no. 1, p. 339, 2003.

[3] J. Vallejo Herrador, J. M. Rodriguez Luna, A. Fernandez Fernandez, T. Mayayo Dehesa, R. Marcen Letosa, and S. Berenguer Sanchez, "Graft fracture in kidney transplant our clinical experience," *Actas Urologicas Espanolas*, vol. 13, no. 4, pp. 252–255, 1989.

[4] H. Oesterwitz, V. Strobelt, G. May et al., "Spontaneous kidney transplant rupture—effect of immunosuppressive therapy on incidence of rupture," *Zeitschrift für Urologie und Nephrologie*, vol. 83, pp. 157–163, 1990.

[5] H. Shahrokh, H. Rasouli, M. A. Zargar, K. Karimi, and K. Zargar, "Spontaneous kidney allograft rupture," *Transplantation Proceedings*, vol. 37, no. 7, pp. 3079–3080, 2005.

[6] M. D. Garcia Sanchez De La Nieta, A. I. Sánchez-Fructuoso, R. Alcázar et al., "Higher graft salvage rate in renal allograft rupture associated with acute tubular necular," *Transplantation Proceedings*, vol. 36, no. 10, pp. 3016–3018, 2004.

[7] N. Busi, E. Capocasale, M. P. Mazzoni et al., "Spontaneous renal allograft rupture without acute rejection," *Acta Biomedica de l'Ateneo Parmense*, vol. 75, no. 2, pp. 131–136, 2004.

[8] O. Odocha, C. O. Callender, and W. Pinn-Wiggins, "Spontaneous rupture of the renal allograft," *Journal of the National Medical Association*, vol. 83, no. 2, pp. 171–174, 1991.

[9] Y. H. Chan, K. M. Wong, K. C. Lee, and C. S. Li, "Spontaneous renal allograft rupture attributed to acute tubular necrosis," *American Journal of Kidney Diseases*, vol. 34, no. 2, pp. 355–358, 1999.

[10] J. R. Salaman, R. Y. Calne, J. Pena, R. A. Sells, H. J. White, and D. Yoffa, "Surgical aspects of clinical renal transplantation," *British Journal of Surgery*, vol. 56, no. 6, pp. 413–417, 1969.

[11] A. S. Nikonenko, S. N. Zavgorodniĭ, A. A. Kovalev, and T. N. Nikonenko, "Surgical strategies in spontaneous rupture of renal allograft," *Klinicheskaya Khirurgiya*, no. 1, pp. 37–39, 2002.

[12] C. Basaran, F. Y. Donmez, N. C. Tarhan, M. Coskun, and M. Haberal, "Multidetector computed tomography findings of spontaneous renal allograft ruptures," *Clinical Radiology*, vol. 64, no. 5, pp. 523–528, 2009.

[13] D. S. Finley and J. P. Roberts, "Frequent salvage of ruptured renal allografts: a large single center experience," *Clinical Transplantation*, vol. 17, no. 2, pp. 126–129, 2003.

[14] B. He, M. M. Rao, X. Han, X. Li, D. Guan, and J. Gao, "Surgical repair of spontaneous renal allograft rupture: a new procedure," *ANZ Journal of Surgery*, vol. 73, no. 6, pp. 381–383, 2003.

[15] A. H. Zakir, K. J. Woodside, E. C. Feliberti, S. Rajaraman, K. K. Gugliuzza, and J. A. Daller, "Late renal allograft rupture in a patient with small vessel vasculitis following discontinuation of immunosuppression," *Transplant International*, vol. 16, no. 10, pp. 761–764, 2003.

[16] P. J. Smak Gregoor, R. Zietse, J. L. C. M. Van Saase et al., "Immunosuppression should be stopped in patients with renal allograft failure," *Clinical Transplantation*, vol. 15, no. 6, pp. 397–401, 2001.

[17] P. Messa, C. Ponticelli, and L. Berardinelli, "Coming back to dialysis after kidney transplant failure," *Nephrology Dialysis Transplantation*, vol. 23, no. 9, pp. 2738–2742, 2008.

16

Transurethral Incision of the Bladder Neck in a Woman with Primary Bladder Neck Obstruction after Kidney Transplantation

Dean Markić,[1] Maksim Valenčić,[1] Anton Maričić,[1] Kristian Krpina,[1] Dražen Rahelić,[1] Juraj Ahel,[1] Nino Rubinić,[1] Lidija Orlić,[2] and Sanjin Rački[2]

[1]*Department of Urology, University Hospital Rijeka, 51000 Rijeka, Croatia*
[2]*Department of Nephrology and Dialysis, University Hospital Rijeka, 51000 Rijeka, Croatia*

Correspondence should be addressed to Dean Markić; dean.markic@ri.htnet.hr

Academic Editor: Marian Klinger

Voiding dysfunction is frequently seen in the early posttransplant period. Among other causes, this condition can arise due to bladder outlet obstruction. Primary bladder neck obstruction (PBNO) is a possible but very rare cause of bladder outlet obstruction. We present the case of a 52-year-old woman who, after kidney transplantation, presented with PBNO. The diagnosis was established based on symptoms, uroflowmetry, and multichannel urodynamics with electromyography. The transurethral incision of the bladder neck was made at the 5- and 7-o'clock position. After the operation, the maximal flow rate was significantly increased, and postvoid residual urine was decreased compared to the preoperative findings. The patient was followed for 5 years, and her voiding improvement is persistent. This is the first reported case of PBNO treated with a transurethral incision of the bladder neck in a posttransplantation female patient.

1. Introduction

Kidney transplantation (KT) is the best treatment modality for patients with end-stage renal disease (ESRD). Before transplantation, patients are placed on a renal replacement therapy, haemodialysis in most cases. During this period, the production of urine decreases with time, and the urinary bladder becomes hypotrophic (disused bladder dysfunction). Bladder capacity and compliance decreased with the longer duration of the haemodialysis [1]. After successful transplantation, urine production started again and micturition and bladder function were restored. Nevertheless, some voiding problems may become evident after years of bladder inactivity.

Bladder outlet obstruction (BOO) in women is an infrequent condition compared to men and is found among 2.7–8% of women referred for an evaluation of their lower urinary tract symptoms (LUTS) [2]. BOO in women can be generally divided, according to the cause, into functional or anatomical obstruction (pelvic organ prolapse, uterine tumour, post-anti-incontinence procedure, urethral stricture, and bladder or urethral tumour) [3]. Functional obstruction can be diagnosed only during the act of micturition, as anatomic abnormalities, which can be connected with patients' symptoms, do not exist. One of the functional causes of BOO is primary bladder neck obstruction (PBNO) [3]. PBNO may present with a variety of symptoms, such as a decreased force of the urinary stream, hesitancy, intermittent stream, incomplete emptying, frequency, urgency, urge incontinence, nocturia, and urinary retention [3]. Here, we present a case of a woman after renal transplantation with BOO caused by PBNO who was treated with a transurethral incision of the bladder neck.

2. The Case Report

Our female patient has ESRD caused by Alport syndrome. The beginning of her complaints was in childhood. Gradually her kidney function declined and she started with hemodialysis at the age of 25. At the age of 29 she received a kidney transplant from a deceased donor. The first graft lasted 14 years. The cause of graft failure was chronic graft nephropathy and she again started with hemodialysis. At that time the patient was anuric. Three years later the patient had received a kidney transplant (second transplantation) from a deceased donor. There was good match in the human leukocyte antigens (HLAs), with only three mismatches. After transplantation, immunosuppression was started with cyclosporine, mycophenolate mofetil, and prednisolone. Because of gastrointestinal side-effects, mycophenolate mofetil was replaced with azathioprine. The further postoperative clinical course was uneventful, and the function of the transplanted kidney was excellent during follow-up. Also, the patient's bladder function recovery after KT was established in just few weeks.

In the age of 52 our patient came to the urology office due to her frequency, nocturia, decreased force of urinary stream, and feeling of incomplete bladder emptying. The symptoms had started 22 months previously. Her urinary diary showed that she voided 12 times during 24 hours (nocturia 2x) with urine volume of 1500–3000 mL through 24 hours. Laboratory exams showed normal renal function with urea 4.7 mmol/L and creatinine 85 μmol/L. Physical examination and urinalysis were normal. Urinary infection was excluded by sterile culture. Pelvic ultrasound with a full bladder was performed and a possible mass compressing the urethra was excluded. The postvoidal residual urine was 60 mL. Her gynaecological exam was normal. Cystoscopy was performed using a 17 Fr rigid urethrocystoscope and revealed normal endoscopic findings in the bladder and urethra, except for the trabeculation of the urinary bladder.

In our patient, uroflowmetry and multichannel urodynamics were assessed. Uroflowmetry revealed an outflow obstruction, with a maximal flow rate of 9 mL/s (Figure 1). Multichannel urodynamics with electromyography showed normal filling and storage phase, with synchronised activity between the bladder and urinary sphincter during voiding.

The diagnosis of PBNO was established based on the symptoms, uroflowmetry, and multichannel urodynamics. After the PBNO diagnosis, therapy with tamsulosin 0.4 mg once daily for 2 months was started. However, this therapy failed, and a transurethral incision was the next therapeutic step.

The operation was performed in the standard lithotomy position. The endoscopic incision was made with a vertical diathermy electrode (Collings knife) in the bladder neck at the 5- and 7-o'clock position (Figure 2). At the end of the procedure, the Foley catheter was inserted. The catheter was removed 48 hours after the operation. No procedure-related complications occurred.

After the operation, the patient reported a better urinary stream. Her urinary diary showed that she voided 8 times over 24 hours without nocturia. The maximal flow rate was increased from 9 to 15 mL/s, and the postvoid residual urine decreased from 60 to 20 mL compared to preoperative findings (Figure 3). Now, five years after the transurethral incision of the bladder neck, her kidney function is stable, and the patient is still satisfied with voiding, with the improved urodynamics characteristics.

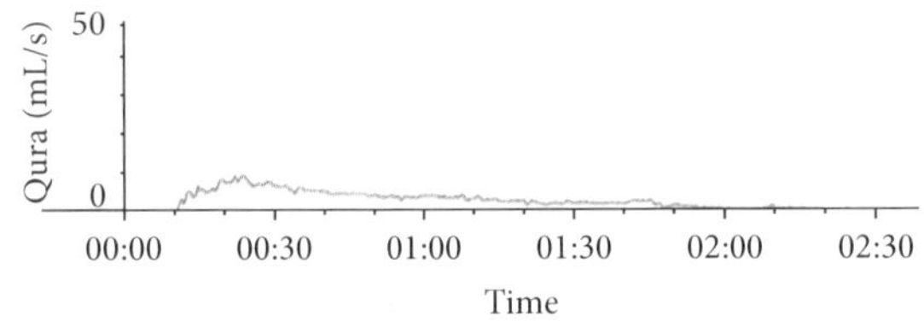

Figure 1: Uroflow before the operation revealed an obstructed flow with a maximal flow rate of 9 mL/s, voided volume of 397 mL, and voiding time of more than 2 minutes.

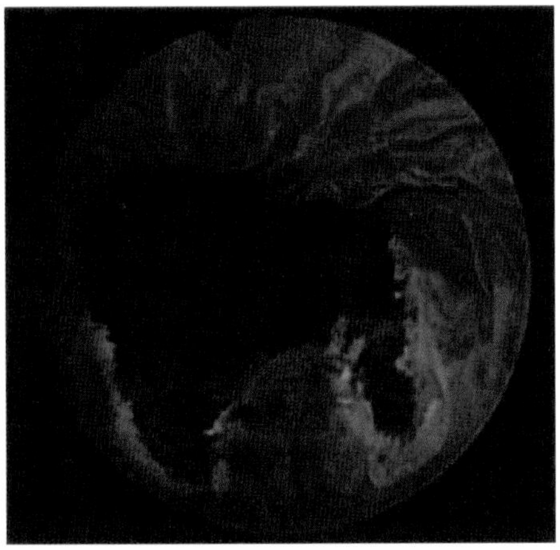

Figure 2: Transurethral incision of the bladder neck in a woman with a primary bladder neck obstruction. Final view of the transurethral incision of the bladder neck at the 5- and 7-o'clock position.

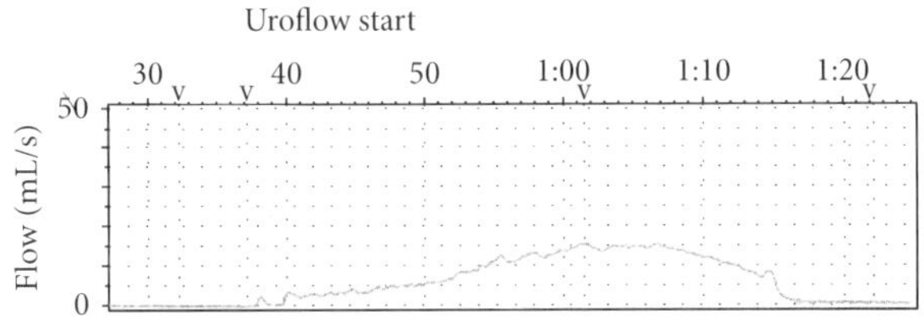

Figure 3: Uroflow after the operation revealed an increased flow with a maximal flow rate of 15 mL/s, voided volume of 351 mL, and voiding time of 45 s.

The use of her medical record was approved by the Ethics Committee of the University Hospital Rijeka, and informed consent was obtained.

3. Discussion

During the dialysis period, patients with ESRD become oliguric to anuric. Decreased urine production leads to bladder inactivity, followed by atrophic changes in the bladder wall. Bladder capacity and compliance decrease, becoming more pronounced during a prolonged period of dialysis [4]. After KT, the urine production and bladder function are reestablished. Voiding function typically stabilises within 6 months after a successful KT; however, voiding dysfunction and LUTS might persist long-term [5].

The adaptation of the bladder to the newly established production of urine occurs relatively quickly, and urodynamic parameters, such as maximum flow rate, bladder capacity, and bladder compliance, reach their plateaus within 24 weeks after KT [6]. In that period, the voiding function becomes stabilised. Voiding dysfunction, which was assessed 6 months after transplantation by uroflowmetry and postvoid residual urine, was present in 28% of patients. Its prevalence was not related to age, the period of dialysis, time after transplantation, polyuria, or nocturnal polyuria [7]. In addition, approximately 26% of transplanted patients voided more than twice during their sleeping periods [7]. This nocturia may be caused by functional (overactive bladder, PBNO) or anatomical abnormalities (benign prostatic hyperplasia, BPH) but may be secondary to congestive heart failure, diabetes mellitus, hypertension, or lifestyle patterns, such as night-time drinking. Secondary causes can be treated by restricting fluid intake at night, using pharmacological therapies (desmopressin and diuretics) and better blood pressure control [7].

PBNO as a cause of bladder outlet obstruction can be found in 1–16% of obstructed women [3]. PBNO is characterised by the failure of the bladder neck to open adequately during voiding, resulting in weak urine stream. The exact cause of this condition is still unknown [3]. Because anatomical abnormalities are not present, PBNO is considered to be a functional condition. As such, neurological diseases must be excluded as a possible cause in all patients. As the symptoms of patients with PBNO and of those with other functional causes of bladder outlet obstruction are very similar, an exact diagnosis can be made only using multichannel urodynamics with EMG [8].

In patients with PBNO and minor symptoms, watchful waiting may be recommended. If therapy is necessary, alpha blockers are the first-line treatment. The next treatment possibility is a transurethral incision of the bladder neck [8].

The transurethral incision of the bladder neck is the surgical treatment of choice for patients with PBNO. The standard place of a bladder neck incision is at the 5- and 7-o'clock position, with an overall satisfaction rate of 76–100% [3, 8]. The need for a reoperation depends on the number of initial incisions, from 18% in the single incision to 0% in the four incision technique [3, 8, 9]. Possible complications of procedure include urinary incontinence and perforation of the vaginal wall [3, 8, 9]. Injury to the external urethral sphincter is responsible for urinary incontinence and can be seen in up to 6.2% of operated patients [8, 9].

Significant lower urinary tract symptoms after KT can have severe negative effects on patient quality of life, as what occurred in our patient. More importantly, episodes of retention and urinary infections secondary to BPH may pose a risk for renal allograft, up to graft loss [10]. Dion et al. found that LUTS can be improved up to 1 year after transplantation [4]. In male patients, those authors found moderate to severe LUTS in 39% of patients before transplantation, as well as 33% and approximately 20% at 6 and 12 months after transplantation, respectively. Patients with validated questionnaires and pretransplant urine outputs of less than 250 mL per day had the highest risk for moderate to severe LUTS and voiding dysfunction posttransplant. An adequate urological evaluation of these patients, in most cases, is able to show that BPH and overactive bladder are responsible for these symptoms. Medical therapies (alpha blockers, inhibitors of 5 alpha reductase, and anticholinergics) improve symptoms in most patients. Only in a minority of patients surgical therapy is needed.

Disused bladder dysfunction can be expected after KT. Bladder dysfunction will be cleared during early period in posttransplant; otherwise another cause of LUTS should be checked as this case report of PBNO. To the best of our knowledge, this is the first case of a transurethral incision of the bladder neck in women with primary bladder neck obstruction after KT. In the present case, as in the general population, this procedure is minimally invasive and safe. Additionally, high cure rate can be expected after an endoscopic incision of the bladder neck.

References

[1] J.-L. Chen, M.-C. Lee, and H.-C. Kuo, "Reduction of cystometric bladder capacity and bladder compliance with time in patients with end-stage renal disease," *Journal of the Formosan Medical Association*, vol. 111, no. 4, pp. 209–213, 2012.

[2] H. C. Kuo, "Urodynamic parameters for the: diagnosis of bladder outlet obstruction in women," *Urologia Internationalis*, vol. 72, no. 1, pp. 46–51, 2004.

[3] V. W. Nitti, "Primary bladder neck obstruction in men and women," *Reviews in Urology*, vol. 7, supplement 8, pp. S12–S17, 2005.

[4] M. Dion, O. Cristea, S. Langford, P. P. W. Luke, and A. Sener, "Debilitating lower urinary tract symptoms in the post-renal transplant population can be predicted pretransplantation," *Transplantation*, vol. 95, no. 4, pp. 589–594, 2013.

[5] M. J. A. van der Weide, L. B. Hilbrands, B. L. H. Bemelmans, and L. A. L. M. Kiemeney, "Lower urinary tract symptoms after renal transplantation: are there changes over time?" *Urology*, vol. 63, no. 3, pp. 442–446, 2004.

[6] A. Mizerski, K. Ostrowska Clark, M. Ostrowski et al., "Post-operative adaptation of urinary bladder to variable volume of urine in the initial period following kidney transplantation," *Transplantation Proceedings*, vol. 35, no. 6, pp. 2174–2175, 2003.

[7] T. Mitsui, N. Shimoda, K. Morita, H. Tanaka, K. Moriya, and K. Nonomura, "Lower urinary tract symptoms and their impact on quality of life after successful renal transplantation," *International Journal of Urology*, vol. 16, no. 4, pp. 388–392, 2009.

[8] D. Markić, A. Maričić, R. Oguić et al., "Transurethral bladder neck incision in women with primary bladder neck obstruction," *Wiener Klinische Wochenschrift*, vol. 126, no. 7-8, pp. 217–222, 2014.

[9] X.-B. Jin, H.-W. Qu, H. Liu, B. Li, J. Wang, and Y.-D. Zhang, "Modified transurethral incision for primary bladder neck obstruction in women: a method to improve voiding function without urinary incontinence," *Urology*, vol. 79, no. 2, pp. 310–313, 2012.

[10] F. P. Hurst, R. T. Neff, E. M. Falta et al., "Incidence, predictors, and associated outcomes of prostatism after kidney transplantation," *Clinical Journal of the American Society of Nephrology*, vol. 4, no. 2, pp. 329–336, 2009.

17

Vascular Fluorescence Imaging Control for Complex Renal Artery Aneurysm Repair Using Laparoscopic Nephrectomy and Autotransplantation

Matteo Tozzi,[1] Luigi Boni,[2] Gabriele Soldini,[2] Marco Franchin,[2] and Gabriele Piffaretti[3]

[1] *Vascular Surgery, Department of Surgery and Center for Research on Organ Transplantation, Insubria University School of Medicine, Circolo University Hospital, 21100 Varese, Italy*
[2] *General Surgery 1, Department of Surgery and Center for Research on Organ Transplantation, Insubria University School of Medicine, Circolo University Hospital, 21100 Varese, Italy*
[3] *Vascular Surgery, Department of Surgery and Morphological Sciences, Insubria University School of Medicine, Circolo University Hospital, Via Guicciardini 9, 21100 Varese, Italy*

Correspondence should be addressed to Gabriele Piffaretti; gabriele.piffaretti@uninsubria.it

Academic Editor: Yasuhiko Sugawara

Intraoperative fluorescent imaging using indocyanine green enables vascular surgeons to confirm the location and states of the reconstructed vessels during surgery. Complex renal artery aneurysm repair involving second order branch vessels has been performed with different techniques. We present a case of ex vivo repair and autotransplantation combining the advantages of minimally invasive surgery and indocyanine green enhanced fluorescence imaging to facilitate vascular anatomy recognition and visualization of organ reperfusion.

1. Introduction

Operative repair of renal artery aneurysm (RAA) may be accomplished by different techniques; actually, endovascular stent-grafting or embolization procedures are attractive alternative for the RAAs treatment [1, 2]. However, RAA beyond the renal artery bifurcation may require an open treatment with in vivo or ex vivo surgical repair [1, 3]. In case of ex vivo repair, laparoscopic donor nephrectomy has currently become widely accepted because of the minimally invasiveness and lower morbidity rate if compared to the conventional approach for living renal donation [4, 5].

Intraoperative vascular quality control during renal transplantation is not performed on a routine basis, while duplex ultrasound evaluation of the organ perfusion is generally performed postoperatively [6]. A technical advancement has been recently introduced in general surgery, that is, the intraoperative use of fluorescent imaging using indocyanine green (ICG); this is an intriguing technique for easier intraoperative recognition of vascular anatomy and for evaluating organ perfusion that has been reported also in kidney transplantation [6–9].

We report a case of a complex RAA treatment using laparoscopic nephrectomy, ex vivo aneurysmectomy, and autotransplantation with the intraoperative use of ICG fluorescent imaging to optimize the visualization of vascular anatomy and control the revascularization after vascular repair.

2. Case Report

A 53-year-old man with a history of recurrent right flank pain was referred to our department following the diagnosis of a right renal artery aneurysm. Medical history was relevant for psoriatic arthritis. Preoperative computed tomography-angiography (CT-A) showed a 20 mm juxtahilar RAA, type 5, according to the classification of Henke et al. [10] (Figures 1(a)–1(c)). Baseline serum creatinine level

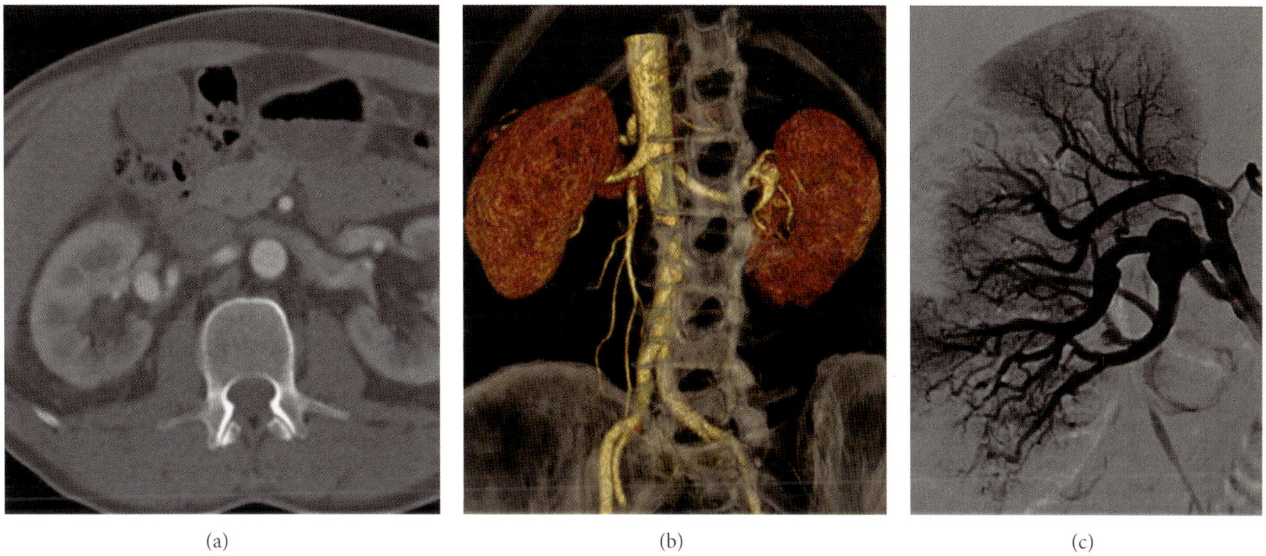

FIGURE 1: Preoperative 3D volume rendering computed tomography scan (a), with volume rendering 3D reconstruction (b) and angiography (c) showing the 20 mm fusiform aneurysm (*arrows*, a-b-c) of the secondary inferior branch of the right renal artery.

was 0.8 mg/dL. A first attempt to treat the RAA with an endovascular stenting using a flow-modulator stent failed. Postoperative CT-A identified the occlusion of another branch artery, while the renal sequential scintigraphy showed two iatrogenic parenchymal ischemic areas with normal perfusion/excretion function. Hence, a decision was made to proceed with an ex vivo repair with an autotransplantation.

2.1. Surgical Technique. Right nephrectomy was performed as previously described [4, 5]; it was completed using a "hockey stick" laparotomy, the same that was subsequently used for autotransplantation. Total time of warm ischemia was 40 seconds. During bench back surgery, the kidney was flushed with hypothermic University of Wisconsin solution; the aneurysm was excised and vascular reconstruction completed with a primary anastomosis with no intervening vein or other grafts. At this time, we identified the thrombosis of a medial branch artery due to a narrowing dissecting flap caused during the endovascular procedure. At the completion of the vascular anastomosis to the external iliac vessels, 5 mL of ICG at a concentration of 0.3 mg/mL/kg was injected intravenously. For ICG fluorescent imaging, we used a laparoscopic system (TELECAM SL II - Storz; Tuttlingen-GER), a 10 mm laparoscope applicable for white light (WL), autofluorescence imaging, and ICG-imaging. Fluorescent imaging confirmed the homogeneous vascular perfusion of the kidney. The ischemic lesions of the lower pole were no longer observed at the completion fluorescent imaging (Figures 2(a)–2(c)). Autotransplantation with a Lich-Gregoir ureteroneocystostomy was then completed in standard fashion [10]. Overall, duration of intervention was 430 minutes and cold ischemia time was 105 minutes. Histological evaluation of the renal aneurysm revealed marked atherosclerotic changes.

2.2. Postoperative Outcome and Follow-Up. No complication occurred. He was ambulatory on postoperative day 3 and then was discharged on postoperative day 10. He was last seen 6 months after the procedure alive and well, asymptomatic with serum creatinine of 0.76 mg/dL; contrast-enhanced magnetic resonance imaging confirmed the successful vascular repair, also confirmed by the fact that the preoperative parenchymal ischemic areas disappeared (Figure 2(d)).

3. Discussion

Current indications for the treatment of RAAs should take into account several factors which are patient and aneurysm related [1–3, 10]. In our case, we had two reasons to recommend RAA repair: a diameter of >20 mm, remarkable if we consider the involvement of a branch artery, and flank pain presumed to be related to the aneurysm [2, 3, 10].

The results of endovascular management of renal artery occlusive disease comparable to those of open repair have led to consider RAAs an attractive target for endovascular therapy [3, 11]. Nevertheless, multiple determinants should influence the decision making process: the aneurysm position and the presence of important branches arising from or in close proximity to the aneurysm are of utmost importance [11–13]. In those circumstances, major concerns remain about the broad applicability of stent-grafting or flow-modulator stent because every attempt should be made to preserve as much of the kidney as possible [10–13]. We also had to deal with the young age in our patient, since the long-term outcomes of endovascular therapies in renal vessels remain uncertain [2, 11]. Having weighed all these factors and following the failed endovascular attempt, open surgery remained our ultimate option.

Anticipated unreconstructable renal artery, ruptures, intraparenchymal location, or irreparable renal ischemia has been treated also with nephrectomy [1–3, 10–12]. This was not an option in our mind because of the young age of the patient, the absence of aneurysm-related hypertension, and last but

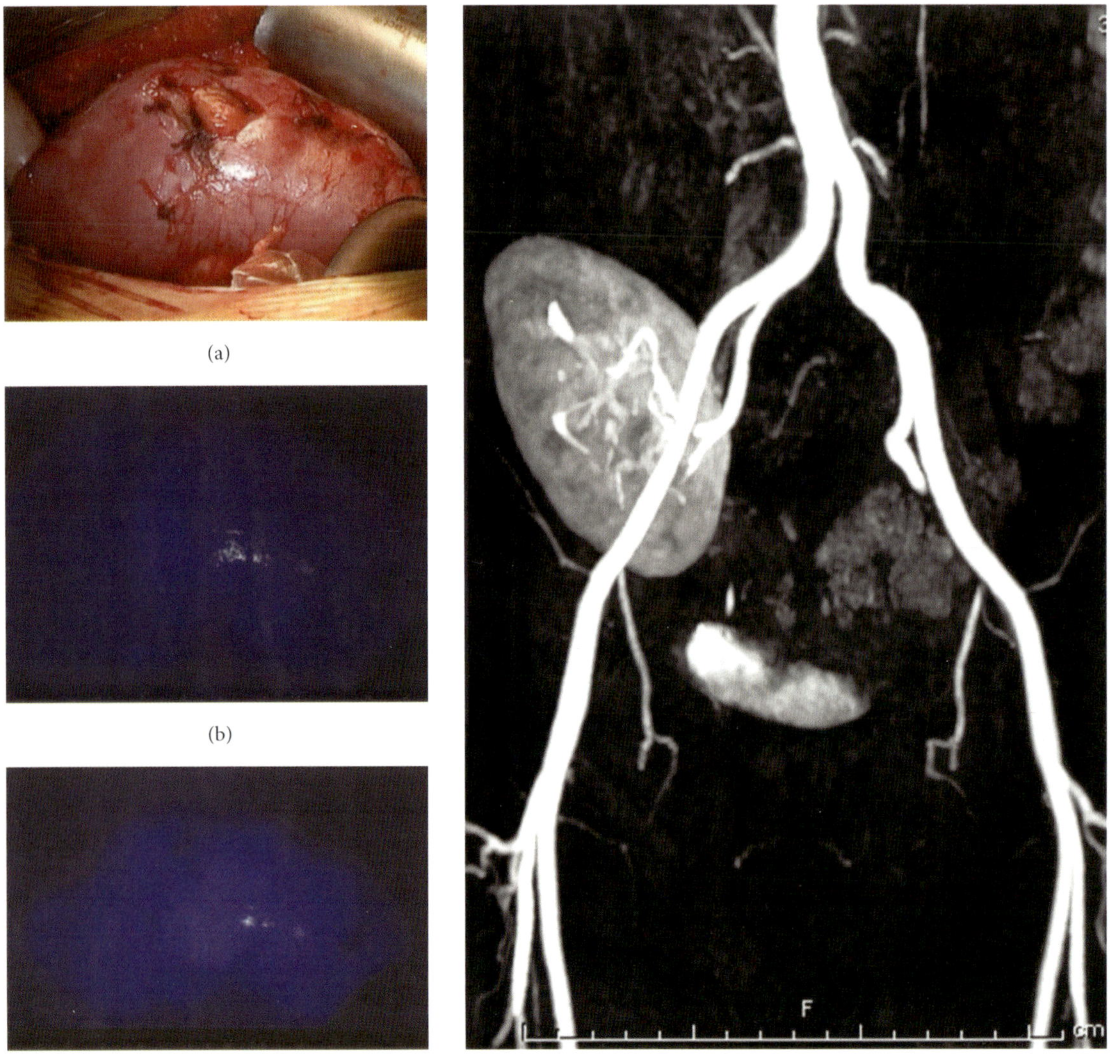

(a) (b) (c) (d)

Figure 2: Intraoperative aspect of the transplanted kidney (a) and visualization of the parenchyma at the time of indocyanine green injection (b) and after the revascularization with real-time fluorescence imaging (c). Follow-up control with magnetic resonance angiography (d).

not the least the satisfactory results of reconstructive surgery in that aneurysm location. Henke et al. [10] reported no major differences in long-term patency or need for secondary interventions between patients who had aneurysmectomy and bypass versus patch closure.

Owing to the complicated renal vascular anatomy operative strategy should be tailored according to the type of lesion and experience of the operator [2–15]. An ex situ repair has been preferred for a complex operation site, such as branch aneurysm with the need of repair at or within the renal hilum [9, 15–19]. This type of operation is generally accomplished with the dissection of the vascular pedicle, while the ureter is mobilized but left intact [13, 14]. We believe this technique is demanding, is associated with significant incisional morbidity, and is time consuming with longer cold ischemia than bench surgery [12, 14]. Further, we believe the best results are obtained with a technique with which surgeon is confident; therefore, we took advantage of the experience we gained in kidney transplantations. Laparoscopic nephrectomy limited the invasiveness of the intervention, and kidney perfusion was optimized with the best available solution, while vascular reconstruction was completed with ease without grafting during the back bench surgery [17, 18].

Complex RAA repair combining laparoscopic nephrectomy and autotransplantation is not new: Gallagher et al. [14] already published a successful case series of seven patients. An interesting aspect added in our case is the use of the fluorescent angiography which has been already adopted during kidney transplantation [6–10]. In our case, major advantages were a reliable real-time roadmap of the renal vessels and ureter anatomy and intraoperative quality control of the vascular reconstruction and kidney perfusion. Further, it is safe because radiations are not requested and the risk of adverse reactions to the ICG injection is very low.

Graft perfusion is of utmost importance since the functions of a transplanted kidney are critically dependent on the quality of blood supply. Although duplex ultrasound may reveal areas of hypoperfusion undetected intraoperatively, currently the assessment of organ reperfusion is left to the visual judgment of the operating surgeon [6–9, 19]. Fluorescent angiography produces a more sensitive real-time assessment of the organ perfusion and may detect other problem areas in the graft [6–9]. Hoffmann et al. [7] emphasized the important role played by ICG fluorescent imaging in providing useful information for intraoperative decisions: ICG dictated a graft repositioning for a large perfusion defect that was unremarkable to visual inspection. This observation finds support in our case: in fact, the perioperative ischemic areas detected in the preoperative scintigraphy were determined by a stenosis of a medial branch artery. The correction of this stenosis was effective and decisive as confirmed by the disappearance of these areas at the completion fluorescent angiography.

There are some limitations with this technique: first and foremost is the limited ability of near-infrared light to penetrate tissues; hence, it is not useful for percutaneous procedure. Second is the absence of well-defined thresholds of the fluorescent signals: the concentration or amount of ICG solution, time and speed of bolus injection, and patient parameters such as body weight all interact with the imaging effect and quality [20]. Apart from these shortcomings, in our case, these disadvantages were partially lessened with the capacity of laparoscopy to be close to the tissues. Nonetheless, it is less invasive, easier to use, and less risky than ionizing radiation using contrast medium to identify the pattern of the vasculature architecture at the end of the vascular anastomosis [6–9]. With regard to the increasing use of marginal grafts that crucially require optimal perfusion conditions, this technique might be useful in the next future to enrich renal transplantation surgery [7].

4. Conclusion

Complex RAA repair using laparoscopic nephrectomy with ex vivo repair and autotransplantation has been shown to be feasible and safe. Indocyanine green mediated fluorescent imaging seems a potentially helpful adjunct for the evaluation of graft reperfusion after transplantation: the application of this technology emphasized the kidney perfusion and confirmed the absence of ischemic areas within the graft.

References

[1] W. P. English, J. D. Pearce, T. E. Craven et al., "Surgical management of renal artery aneurysms," *Journal of Vascular Surgery*, vol. 40, no. 1, pp. 53–60, 2004.

[2] M. K. Eskandari and S. A. Resnick, "Aneurysms of the renal artery," *Seminars in Vascular Surgery*, vol. 18, no. 4, pp. 202–208, 2005.

[3] J. C. Stanley, E. L. Rhodes, B. L. Gewertz, C. Y. Chang, J. F. Walter, and W. J. Fry, "Renal artery aneurysms. Significance of macroaneurysms exclusive of dissections and fibrodysplastic mural dilations," *Archives of Surgery*, vol. 110, no. 11, pp. 1327–1333, 1975.

[4] T. G. Nanidis, D. Antcliffe, C. Kokkinos et al., "Laparoscopic versus open live donor nephrectomy in renal transplantation: a meta-analysis," *Annals of Surgery*, vol. 247, no. 1, pp. 58–70, 2008.

[5] L. Boni, G. Dionigi, F. Rovera et al., "Laparoscopic left nephrectomy for living donor kidney transplant," *Archives of Surgery*, vol. 145, no. 6, pp. 590–591, 2010.

[6] M. Sekijima, T. Tojimbara, S. Sato et al., "An intraoperative fluorescent imaging system in organ transplantation," *Transplantation Proceedings*, vol. 36, no. 7, pp. 2188–2190, 2004.

[7] C. Hoffmann, F. Compton, J. H. Schäfer et al., "Intraoperative assessment of kidney allograft perfusion by laser-assisted indocyanine green fluorescence videography," *Transplantation Proceedings*, vol. 42, no. 5, pp. 1526–1530, 2010.

[8] T. Sawada, M. Solly, J. Kita, M. Shimoda, and K. Kubota, "An alternative tool for intraoperative assessment of renal vasculature after revascularization of a transplanted kidney," *The American Journal of Surgery*, vol. 199, no. 6, pp. e69–e71, 2010.

[9] N. Arichi, Y. Mitsui, K. Ogawa et al., "Intraoperative fluorescence vascular imaging using indocyanine green for assessment of transplanted kidney perfusion," *Transplantation Proceedings*, vol. 46, no. 2, pp. 342–345, 2014.

[10] P. K. Henke, J. D. Cardneau, T. H. Welling III et al., "Renal artery aneurysms: a 35-year clinical experience with 252 aneurysms in 168 patients," *Annals of Surgery*, vol. 234, no. 4, pp. 454–463, 2001.

[11] N. Tsilimparis, J. G. Reeves, A. Dayama, S. D. Perez, E. S. Debus, and J. J. Ricotta II, "Endovascular vs open repair of renal artery aneurysms: outcomes of repair and long-term renal function," *Journal of the American College of Surgeons*, vol. 217, no. 2, pp. 263–269, 2013.

[12] T. Pfeiffer, L. Reiher, K. Grabitz et al., "Reconstruction for renal artery aneurysm: operative techniques and long-term results," *Journal of Vascular Surgery*, vol. 37, no. 2, pp. 293–300, 2003.

[13] T. A. Crutchley, J. D. Pearce, T. E. Craven, M. S. Edwards, R. H. Dean, and K. J. Hansen, "Branch renal artery repair with cold perfusion protection," *Journal of Vascular Surgery*, vol. 46, no. 3, pp. 405–412, 2007.

[14] K. A. Gallagher, M. W. Phelan, T. Stern, and S. T. Bartlett, "Repair of complex renal artery aneurysms by laparoscopic nephrectomy with ex vivo repair and autotransplantation," *Journal of Vascular Surgery*, vol. 48, no. 6, pp. 1408–1413, 2008.

[15] W. P. Robinson III, R. Bafford, M. Belkin, and M. T. Menard, "Favorable outcomes with in situ techniques for surgical repair of complex renal artery aneurysms," *Journal of Vascular Surgery*, vol. 53, no. 3, pp. 684–691, 2011.

[16] S. P. Shirodkar, J. González, J. Parodi et al., "Open or laparoscopic nephrectomy and extracoroporeal repair of complicated renal artery aneurysms: techniques for renal salvage," *Archivos Espanoles de Urologia*, vol. 64, no. 3, pp. 227–236, 2011.

[17] A. R. El Tayar, C. Labruzzo, K. Haritopoulos, and N. S. Hakim, "Renal artery aneurysm: ex vivo repair and autotransplantation: case report and review of the literature," *International Surgery*, vol. 88, no. 2, pp. 61–63, 2003.

[18] F. P. Secin, A. R. Rovegno, R. E. J. Marrugat, R. Virasoro, G. A. Lautersztein, and H. Fernández, "Comparing Taguchi and Lich-Gregoir ureterovesical reimplantation techniques for kidney transplants," *Journal of Urology*, vol. 168, no. 3, pp. 926–930, 2002.

[19] C. Thalhammer, M. Aschwanden, D. Bilecen et al., "Intraoperative color duplex ultrasound during renal transplantation," *Ultraschall in der Medizin*, vol. 29, no. 6, pp. 652–656, 2008.

[20] S. Kim, Y. T. Lim, E. G. Soltesz et al., "Near-infrared fluorescent type II quantum dots for sentinel lymph node mapping," *Nature Biotechnology*, vol. 22, no. 1, pp. 93–97, 2004.

18

Scedosporiosis in a Combined Kidney and Liver Transplant Recipient: A Case Report of Possible Transmission from a Near-Drowning Donor

Rachael Leek,[1] Erika Aldag,[1] Iram Nadeem,[1] Vikraman Gunabushanam,[1] Ajay Sahajpal,[1,2] David J. Kramer,[2,3] and Thomas J. Walsh[4]

[1] *Department of Abdominal Transplant, Aurora St. Luke's Medical Center, Milwaukee, WI, USA*
[2] *University of Wisconsin School of Medicine and Public Health, Madison, WI 53726, USA*
[3] *Department of Critical Care, Aurora St. Luke's Medical Center, Milwaukee, WI, USA*
[4] *Weill Cornell Medicine, Cornell University and New York Presbyterian Hospital, New York, NY, USA*

Correspondence should be addressed to Erika Aldag; erika.aldag@aurora.org

Academic Editor: Graeme Forrest

Scedosporium spp. are saprobic fungi that cause serious infections in immunocompromised hosts and in near-drowning victims. Solid organ transplant recipients are at increased risk of scedosporiosis as they require aggressive immunosuppression to prevent allograft rejection. We present a case of disseminated *Scedosporium apiospermum* infection occurring in the recipient of a combined kidney and liver transplantation whose organs were donated by a near-drowning victim and review the literature of scedosporiosis in solid organ transplantation.

1. Introduction

Scedosporium is a saprobic fungus that naturally occurs in soil, manure, sewage, and water bodies polluted by environmental contaminants. Cases of infections with *Scedosporium* spp. are reported worldwide and can range in severity from colonization or local infection to disseminated disease [1–5]. *S. apiospermum* most commonly infects the lungs as inhalation is often the suspected mode of organism acquisition [6].

The genus *Scedosporium* includes, but is not limited to, three species that cause life-threatening infections in humans: *Scedosporium apiospermum*, *Scedosporium prolificans* (recently renamed *Lomentospora prolificans*), and *Scedosporium aurantiacum* [7]. *Scedosporium* spp. appear as branching septate hyphae when isolated on standard culture media.

Scedosporium spp. have been implicated in near-drowning accidents [8–10]. Indeed *Scedosporium* spp. are the most common cause of fungal pneumonia, infection of the central nervous system, and disseminated disease following near-drowning events. There are few cases of donor to recipient transmission of infection of *Scedosporium* spp. and even fewer reports of near-drowning donor transmission of diseases [11, 12]. We report the clinical course and management of disseminated *S. apiospermum* infection in a combined kidney and liver transplantation case receiving organs from a brain-dead donor who suffered a near-drowning accident; we further review the literature on scedosporiosis in solid organ transplant recipients.

2. Case Presentation: Donor

A 41-year-old male fell into a freshwater lake. Emergency responders pulled him from the lake and return of spontaneous circulation was achieved after twenty minutes of resuscitation. Subsequent chest radiographs showed development and worsening of bilateral opacities suspicious for pneumonia. Brain death was declared three days after hospital admission.

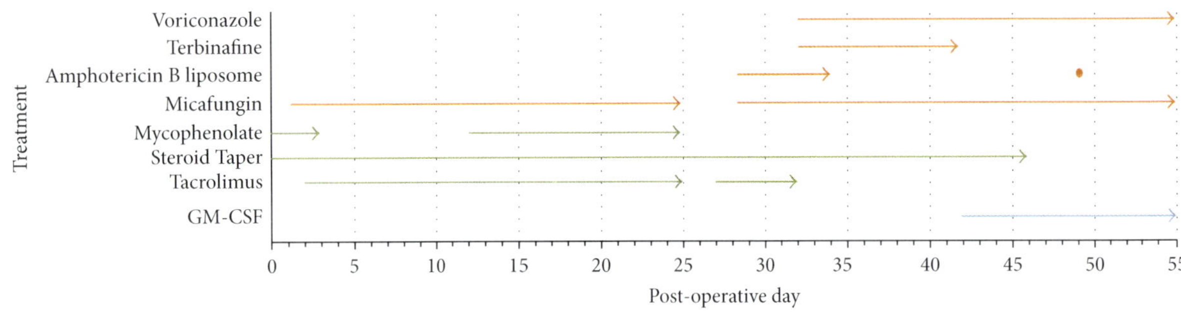

FIGURE 1: Antifungal agents and immunosuppression management.

3. Case Presentation: Recipient

A 66-year-old male actively listed for a kidney and liver transplant presented to the surgical intensive care unit with sepsis and an oxacillin-sensitive *Staphylococcus aureus* bacteremia. He was treated with appropriate antibiotic therapy. He then developed acute tubular necrosis requiring continuous venovenous hemofiltration (CVVH). The patient had a chest X-ray showing mild pulmonary congestion and bronchoscopy was not performed as the patient did not show signs of pneumonia. After two weeks within his admission, the patient was treated for *Escherichia coli* bacteremia with piperacillin-tazobactam. Repeat blood cultures were negative after two days of therapy.

While the patient was hospitalized, a donor became available. The donor kidney and liver were grossly normal. The patient underwent a combined kidney and liver transplant for chronic kidney failure with associated liver cirrhosis caused by the hepatitis C virus and alcoholism. The explanted liver was cirrhotic without any malignancy. At the time of transplantation, the patient's Model for End Stage Liver Disease (MELD) score was 40, having been decompensated in the surgical intensive care unit for the previous month. A summary of the patient's immunosuppression and antifungal management after transplant is provided in Figure 1.

The patient was given methylprednisolone 500 mg and mycophenolate mofetil 1,000 mg intraoperatively as induction immunosuppression. Maintenance immunosuppression protocols were followed after transplant. CVVH was performed intraoperatively and was discontinued on postoperative day (POD) 1 when renal graft function improved. The patient's hospital stay was complicated by a contained urine leak from the ureteroureterostomy which was managed nonoperatively with drains and ureteral stents. On POD 8, the patient was transferred out of the intensive care unit and on POD 14, to the inpatient rehab care unit as graft function continued to improve. The hepatic transaminases fluctuated and, on POD 25, he was transferred back to the surgical intensive care unit with peritonitis. As infection was suspected, immunosuppression was restricted to the use of corticosteroids tapered down to prednisone 5 mg daily. The patient was taken back to the operating room on POD 28 for a peritoneal washout. Cultures obtained during the procedure are presented in Tables 1 and 2. Of most concern was the *S. apiospermum* isolated from the perihepatic, perinephric, and biloma fluid. Endoscopic Retrograde Cholangiopancreatography (ERCP) was performed the following day, which did not reveal any extravasation. Discovery of *S. apiospermum* prompted contact with the Centers for Disease Control and Prevention (CDC), the Disease Transmission Advisory Committee (DTAC) of the United Network for Organ Sharing (UNOS), and the transplant centers treating recipients of allografts from the same donor. Other recipients had no evidence of infection.

On POD 28, due to worsening hemodynamics and peritonitis, another laparotomy and another washout were performed to evacuate an infected hematoma. The entire peritoneal surface was lined with mold. On POD 32, a mold suggestive of *Scedosporium* spp. grew from surgical cultures. Expert opinion for the management of our patient's suspected *S. apiospermum* infection was to use voriconazole targeting a trough of 2–4 mcg/mL, which we started on POD 32. Additionally, terbinafine was started for suspected synergy with voriconazole. A sample of the *S. apiospermum* was sent out for synergy studies which were expected to take a week or more to be conclusive. On POD 41 *S. apiospermum* was identified. Laboratory results suggested terbinafine was not synergistic with voriconazole. Additionally, terbinafine is distributed rapidly to skin and bone and as such is not distributed well into visceral tissue and accumulation of terbinafine may cause hepatotoxicity. In response, terbinafine was discontinued and granulocyte macrophage colony-stimulating factor (GM-CSF) initiated on POD 42. The patient developed neurologic deficits with decreased vision to the right side and blurred vision bilaterally on POD 46. Magnetic resonance imaging (MRI) of the brain, shown in Figure 2, revealed multiple ring-enhancing lesions in the supratentorial compartment consistent with hematogenous central nervous system (CNS) scedosporiosis. We continued treatment with antifungal therapy. He developed septic shock and expired on POD 55.

4. Discussion

Differential diagnoses for opportunistic pathogens causing pneumonia related to near-drowning events include several key pathogenic bacteria and fungi. Gram negative bacteria are most often the causative agents in near-drowning cases [13]. *Aeromonas spp.* have been described most often in near-drowning pneumonia cases. *Aeromonas* spp. naturally thrive in fresh and brackish waters and have been isolated

TABLE 1: Culture results.

Date	Culture site	Source	Result
POD 28	Abdominal fluid	Surgical specimen	*C. tropicalis* *E. faecalis* *E. coli* *M. morganii*
POD 28	Biloma fluid	Surgical specimen	*E. faecium* *E. faecalis* *S. apiospermum* *C. tropicalis*
POD 28	Perihepatic fluid	Surgical specimen	*S. apiospermum* *E. faecium* *C. tropicalis*
POD 28	Perinephric hematoma tissue	Surgical specimen	*S. apiospermum*
POD 32	Abdominal clot	Surgical specimen	*S. apiospermum*
POD 32	Intestinal serosal tissue	Surgical specimen	*S. apiospermum* *E. faecium*
POD 50	LUQ abdominal fluid	Surgical specimen	*C. glabrata* *C. tropicalis*
POD 50	Cerebrospinal fluid	Lumbar puncture	Negative

TABLE 2: Susceptibility testing of fungal isolates.

Isolate	Resistant (MIC)	Intermediate (MIC)	Susceptible (MIC)
Scedosporium apiospermum	5-Fluorocytosine (>64), amphotericin B (>16), caspofungin (>8), micafungin (>8), terbinafine (>2)	None	Voriconazole (1)
Candida tropicalis	None	None	Caspofungin (≤0.25), fluconazole (≤1), voriconazole (≤0.12)
Candida glabrata	None	None	Caspofungin (2), fluconazole (≤1), voriconazole (≤0.12)

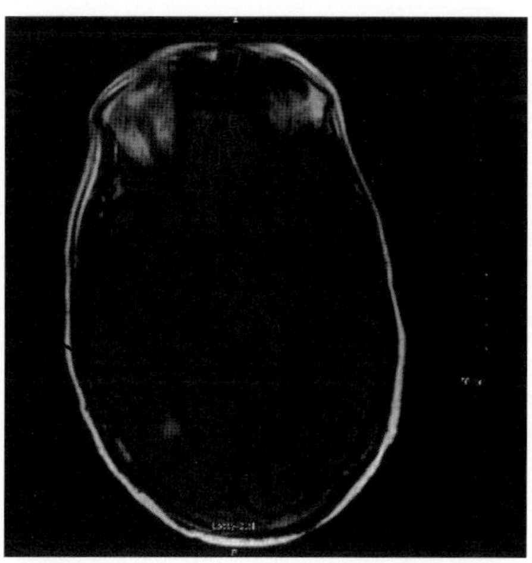

FIGURE 2: MRI of the brain. Multiple ring-enhancing lesions with associated diffusion restriction and T2/FLAIR hyperintensity are present throughout the supratentorial white matter.

in humans in wound and gastrointestinal infections after exposure to contaminated water. Other potential bacterial pathogens include *Pseudomonas aeruginosa*, *Legionella* spp., *Klebsiella* spp., and other Enterobacteriaceae [13]. *Scedosporium* spp. are the most common cause of invasive fungal infection, including pneumonia, CNS disease, and dissemination following near-drowning.

We identified 60 published cases of scedosporiosis after solid organ transplantation between the year 2000 and the present. Few were cases of scedosporiosis after solitary liver transplantation (5/60); most were reported following solitary lung (18/60) or kidney (18/60) transplantation. Table 3 [2, 12, 14–42] provides a summary of the comprehensive literature review performed. *S. apiospermum* was isolated in the majority of cases, though *S. prolificans* and *S. aurantiacum* were also isolated. In four cases, both *S. apiospermum* and *S. prolificans* were identified in the same patient. In patients who had infections with a single isolate of *Scedosporium* spp., the observed mortality rates of *S. apiospermum*, *S. prolificans*, and *S. aurantiacum* were 54.5% (24/44), 70% (7/10), and 100% (3/3), respectively (excluding four cases with combined infections). Observed mortality of all *Scedosporium* spp. infections was 59% (36/61) including our patient case.

Kim et al. reported three fatal and two nonfatal cases of scedosporiosis following solid organ transplantation from

Table 3: Review of solid organ transplant-associated *Scedosporium* infection.

Ref #	Year	Recipient information		Recipient organ(s)	Species of *Scedosporium*	Treatment approach	Outcome
		Age (years)	Gender				
[14]	2000	67	Male	Heart	*apiospermum*	Voriconazole	Deceased
[15]	2001	42	Female	Heart/lung	*apiospermum*	Fluconazole, itraconazole	Deceased
		22	Female	Heart/lung	*prolificans* + *apiospermum*	Fluconazole, itraconazole	Deceased
		42	Male	Heart/lung	*prolificans* + *apiospermum*	Fluconazole, itraconazole	Alive
		49	Male	Lung	*prolificans* + *apiospermum*	Fluconazole, itraconazole	Deceased
		39	Male	Lung	*prolificans* + *apiospermum*	Fluconazole, itraconazole	Alive
		52	Female	Lung	*apiospermum*	Fluconazole, itraconazole	Alive
		38	Female	Heart/lung	*apiospermum*	Fluconazole, itraconazole	Deceased
[16]	2002	58	Female	Liver	*apiospermum*	Itraconazole, miconazole	Alive
		37	Male	Lung	*apiospermum*	Itraconazole	Deceased
		30	Male	Lung	*apiospermum*	Amphotericin B, miconazole	Deceased
		37	Female	Heart/lung	*apiospermum*	Miconazole	Deceased
		39	Male	Liver	*apiospermum*	5-Flucytosine, amphotericin B	Deceased
		67	Male	Heart	*apiospermum*	Itraconazole, voriconazole	Deceased
		36	Male	Kidney	*apiospermum*	Itraconazole, miconazole	Deceased
[17]	2002	49	Male	Kidney	*apiospermum*	Voriconazole	Deceased
[18]	2002	62	Female	Kidney	*apiospermum*	None	Deceased
		58	Male	Kidney	*apiospermum*	Itraconazole, voriconazole	Alive
[19]	2002	64	Female	Lung	*apiospermum*	Amphotericin B, itraconazole	Deceased
[20]	2002	71	Male	Heart	*apiospermum*	Itraconazole	Alive
[21]	2003	24	Male	Lung	*apiospermum*	Voriconazole	Alive
		59	Male	Kidney	*apiospermum*	Voriconazole	Alive
[22]	2004	50	Male	Kidney	*apiospermum*	Voriconazole	Alive
[23]	2004	58	Male	Kidney	*apiospermum*	Amphotericin B, fluconazole, itraconazole, miconazole	Alive
[24]	2004	56	Female	Lung	*prolificans*	Voriconazole	Deceased
[25]	2005	55	Male	Small bowel	*prolificans*	Amphotericin B	Deceased
		40	Male	Kidney/pancreas	*prolificans*	Voriconazole	Alive
		67	Male	Kidney	*apiospermum*	Amphotericin B	Alive
		51	Female	Small bowel	*prolificans*	Amphotericin B, Voriconazole, caspofungin	Deceased
		67	Male	Heart	*apiospermum*	Voriconazole	Deceased
		17	Male	Liver	*prolificans*	Voriconazole	Deceased
		64	Male	Liver	*apiospermum*	None	Deceased
		45	Male	Heart	*apiospermum*	Itraconazole	Deceased
		56	Male	Liver	*apiospermum*	Voriconazole	Deceased
		44	Female	Heart	*prolificans*	Amphotericin B	Deceased
		68	Male	Kidney	*prolificans*	Voriconazole	Alive
		52	Male	Small bowel	*apiospermum*	Amphotericin B, Voriconazole, caspofungin	Alive
		62	Male	Kidney/pancreas	*apiospermum*	Voriconazole	Alive
[26]	2005	26	Female	Lung	*apiospermum*	Miconazole, voriconazole	Deceased
[27]	2006	58	Male	Kidney	*apiospermum*	Miconazole, voriconazole	Alive
[28]	2006	57	Male	Lung	*apiospermum*	Terbinafine, voriconazole	Alive
		63	Male	Lung	*apiospermum*	Liposomal amphotericin B, terbinafine, voriconazole	Alive

TABLE 3: Continued.

Ref #	Year	Recipient information		Recipient organ(s)	Species of *Scedosporium*	Treatment approach	Outcome
		Age (years)	Gender				
[29]	2007	59	Female	Kidney	*apiospermum*	Voriconazole	Alive
[30]	2007	43	Male	Lung	*apiospermum*	Caspofungin, itraconazole, liposomal amphotericin B	Deceased
[31]	2008	70	Male	Kidney	*prolificans*	Terbinafine, voriconazole	Alive
[32]	2009	65	Female	Kidney	*apiospermum*	Voriconazole	Alive
[33]	2010	37	Female	Lung	*apiospermum*	Caspofungin, terbinafine, voriconazole	Deceased
[34]	2011	16	Female	Lung	*apiospermum*	Voriconazole	Alive
[35]	2012	35	Male	Lung/liver	*apiospermum*	Caspofungin, voriconazole	Deceased
[36]	2012	37	Female	Lung	*apiospermum*	Aerosolized amphotericin B, caspofungin, itraconazole, voriconazole	Deceased
[37]	2013	17	Female	Lung	*apiospermum*	Caspofungin, posaconazole, voriconazole	Alive
[38]	2013	70	Female	Lung	*prolificans*	Caspofungin, terbinafine, voriconazole	Deceased
[39]	2014	50	Female	Kidney	*apiospermum*	Voriconazole	Alive
[40]	2014	35	Male	Kidney	*prolificans*	Itraconazole, liposomal amphotericin B, micafungin, voriconazole	Deceased
[41]	2015	70	Male	Heart	*apiospermum*	Posaconazole, terbinafine	Deceased
[12]	2015	19	Male	Heart	*aurantiacum*	Amphotericin B prophylaxis	Deceased
		56	Male	Kidney	*aurantiacum*	Itraconazole, liposomal amphotericin B	Deceased
		57	Female	Kidney	*aurantiacum*	Caspofungin, voriconazole	Deceased
[2]	2015	40	Male	Kidney	*apiospermum*	Voriconazole	Deceased
[42]	2015	18	Female	Lung	*apiospermum*	Terbinafine, voriconazole	Alive

the same donor who was victim to a near-drowning accident [12]. Additionally, they reviewed national Korean data on transplants and found that, among 2600 deceased-donor transplants over thirteen years, 27 (1%) of donors were victims of drowning. We accessed data from the United States Organ Procurement and Transplantation Network and found a similar rate: in 2015, 102/7586 (approximately 1.3%) of solid organ donors died of near-drowning events [43]. While this is a low percentage of all donors, the significance of our case is enhanced by the 58.3% mortality rate of infections involving *Scedosporium* spp. after solid organ transplantation.

At our center, liver transplant recipients are given antifungal prophylaxis based on their risk level. We stratify higher risk patients as those with MELD scores greater than 35, renal failure, requiring hemodialysis or CVVH prior to transplantation, recurrent spontaneous bacterial peritonitis, or preoperative prealbumin less than 10. High risk liver transplant recipients receive micafungin intravenously unless resistant *Candida glabrata*, *Aspergillus* spp., or *Cryptococcus* spp. are suspected; in such cases, amphotericin B lipid complex or voriconazole would be used. Our patient was classified as high risk and given micafungin prophylaxis.

All cases of suspected donor-derived infections should be reported to the DTAC. Communications with the CDC, DTAC, and the centers treating the recipients of the other organs provided by this donor revealed the recipient of the heart was receiving voriconazole prophylaxis, while the recipients of the other kidney and the pancreas were not. To the best of our knowledge, no other recipient of this donor's organs is infected with *Scedosporium* spp. The other centers were advised by the CDC to commence voriconazole prophylaxis for an undetermined duration. Expert opinion for the management of our patient's scedosporiosis was voriconazole targeting a trough of 2–4 mcg/mL. Additionally, immunosuppression was to be limited or discontinued to improve infection clearance.

S. apiospermum is inherently resistant to amphotericin B, including the lipid formulations. Of the newer triazole antifungals, data on the *in vitro* activity of voriconazole is most robust, showing activity against *S. apiospermum* with MICs of 0.12 to 0.5 mcg/mL in clinical isolates [30]. Because of poor activity with single agents, various antifungal combinations have been examined for efficacy against *S. apiospermum*. Strong synergy was found *in vitro* between voriconazole and terbinafine against clinical isolates of *Scedosporium* spp. [30]. Combination of micafungin and voriconazole has demonstrated a synergistic effect against several fungi *in vitro* including *Scedosporium* spp. The synergistic mechanism may include reorganization of the cell wall allowing increased exposure of beta-glucan to the immune system [44].

In addition to antifungal agents, GM-CSF has been studied with some success [44, 45]. While antifungal therapy remains crucial to recovery, the treatment of scedosporiosis infections depends on the function of the host's innate immune system, in particular, polymorphonuclear cells (PMNs). The mechanism of GM-CSF increases the antifungal action of PMNs *in vitro* [45].

Despite good allograft function, our patient did not survive disseminated infection with *S. apiospermum* after combined kidney and liver transplantation. The exact mode of transmission and acquisition of *S. apiospermum* in this patient remains uncertain. We suspect donor to recipient transmission as the donor was the victim of a near-drowning event and had chest radiographs suspicious for pneumonia; however, we cannot rule out recipient colonization or nosocomial infection after the transplant.

Infections caused by *Scedosporium* spp. following solid organ transplant, while not common, are often fatal for recipients. There are no standards of practice for prophylaxis for patients at risk for developing scedosporiosis, such as recipients of organs from nearly drowned donors. Considering our case and the scedosporiosis mortality rate over 50% and the low rate of nearly drowned donors, we recommend screening for *Scedosporium* spp. when donated organs originate from a near-drowning victim.

Competing Interests

The authors declare that there is no significant conflict of interests regarding the publication of this paper.

References

[1] L. S. Johnson, R. K. Shields, and C. J. Clancy, "Epidemiology, clinical manifestations, and outcomes of scedosporium infections among solid organ transplant recipients," *Transplant Infectious Disease*, vol. 16, no. 4, pp. 578–587, 2014.

[2] B. Bose, S. Sharma, P. Derrington, and D. Divi, "Scedosporium apiospermum peritonitis in a patient undergoing peritoneal dialysis," *Nephrology*, vol. 17, no. 5, pp. 521–522, 2012.

[3] A. Malini, N. S. Madhusudan, S. P. Sinhasan, and B. C. Harthimath, "A masquerading subcutaneous swelling caused by Scedosporium apiospermum: an emerging pathogen," *Indian Journal of Pathology and Microbiology*, vol. 58, no. 1, pp. 115–117, 2015.

[4] H. L. Wilson and K. J. Kennedy, "*Scedosporium apiospermum* brain abscesses in an immunocompetent man with silicosis," *Medical Mycology Case Reports*, vol. 2, no. 1, pp. 75–78, 2013.

[5] J. M. Schaenman, D. B. DiGiulio, L. F. Mirels et al., "Scedosporium apiospermum soft tissue infection successfully treated with voriconazole: potential pitfalls in the transition from intravenous to oral therapy," *Journal of Clinical Microbiology*, vol. 43, no. 2, pp. 973–977, 2005.

[6] T. J. Walsh, A. Groll, J. Hiemenz, R. Fleming, E. Roilides, and E. Anaissie, "Infections due to emerging and uncommon medically important fungal pathogens," *Clinical Microbiology and Infection*, vol. 10, supplement 1, pp. 48–66, 2004.

[7] K. J. Cortez, E. Roilides, F. Quiroz-Telles et al., "Infections caused by Scedosporium spp," *Clinical Microbiology Reviews*, vol. 21, no. 1, pp. 157–197, 2008.

[8] P. T. Ender and M. J. Dolan, "Pneumonia associated with near-drowning," *Clinical Infectious Diseases*, vol. 25, no. 4, pp. 896–907, 1997.

[9] A. Katragkou, J. Dotis, M. Kotsiou, M. Tamiolaki, and E. Roilides, "*Scedosporium apiospermum* infection after near-drowning," *Mycoses*, vol. 50, no. 5, pp. 412–421, 2007.

[10] P. A. Kowacs, C. E. Soares Silvado, S. Monteiro de Almeida et al., "Infection of the CNS by *Scedosporium apiospermum* after near drowning. Report of a fatal case and analysis of its confounding factors," *Journal of Clinical Pathology*, vol. 57, no. 2, pp. 205–207, 2004.

[11] M. S. Patel, A. J. Wright, R. Kohn, J. F. Markmann, C. N. Kotton, and P. A. Vagefi, "Successful long-term management of invasive cerebral fungal infection following liver transplantation," *Mycoses*, vol. 58, no. 3, pp. 181–186, 2015.

[12] S.-H. Kim, Y. E. Ha, J.-C. Youn et al., "Fatal scedosporiosis in multiple solid organ allografts transmitted from a nearly-drowned donor," *American Journal of Transplantation*, vol. 15, no. 3, pp. 833–840, 2015.

[13] K. Hoetzenecker, H. J. Ankersmit, G. Lang et al., "Considerations on infectious complications using a drowned lung for transplantation," *Transplant International*, vol. 23, no. 7, pp. e32–e34, 2010.

[14] S. Kusne, S. Ariyanayagam-Baksh, D. C. Strollo, and J. Abernethy, "Invasive *Scedosporium apiospermum* infection in a heart transplant recipient presenting with multiple skin nodules and a pulmonary consolidation," *Transplant Infectious Disease*, vol. 2, no. 4, pp. 194–196, 2000.

[15] M. Tamm, M. Malouf, and A. Glanville, "Pulmonary scedosporium infection following lung transplantation," *Transplant Infectious Disease*, vol. 3, no. 4, pp. 189–194, 2001.

[16] B. Castiglioni, D. A. Sutton, M. G. Rinaldi, J. Fung, and S. Kusne, "Pseudallescheria boydii (Anamorph scedosporium apiospermum) infection in solid organ transplant recipients in a tertiary medical center and review of the literature," *Medicine*, vol. 81, no. 5, pp. 333–348, 2002.

[17] E. L. Campagnaro, K. J. Woodside, M. G. Early et al., "Disseminated Pseudallescheria boydii (Scedosporium apiospermum) infection in a renal transplant patient," *Transplant Infectious Disease*, vol. 4, no. 4, pp. 207–211, 2002.

[18] M. Montejo, M. L. Muñiz, S. Zárraga et al., "Infection due to Scedosporium apiospermum in renal transplant recipients: a report of two cases and literature review of central nervous system and cutaneous infections by Pseudoallescheria boydii/Sc. apiospermum," *Mycoses*, vol. 45, no. 9-10, pp. 418–427, 2002.

[19] R. Raj and A. E. Frost, "Scedosporium apiospermum fungemia in a lung transplant recipient," *Chest*, vol. 121, no. 5, pp. 1714–1716, 2002.

[20] T. R. Talbot, J. Hatcher, S. F. Davis, R. N. Pierson III, R. Barton, and S. Dummer, "*Scedosporium apiospermum* pneumonia and sternal wound infection in a heart transplant recipient," *Transplantation*, vol. 74, no. 11, pp. 1645–1647, 2002.

[21] J. Fortún, P. Martín-Dávila, M. A. Sánchez et al., "Voriconazole in the treatment of invasive mold infections in transplant recipients," *European Journal of Clinical Microbiology and Infectious Diseases*, vol. 22, no. 7, pp. 408–413, 2003.

[22] J. Ahmed, D. M. Ditmars, T. Sheppard, R. Del Busto, K. K. Venkat, and R. Parasuraman, "Recurrence of Scedosporium

apiospermum infection following renal re-transplantation," *American Journal of Transplantation*, vol. 4, no. 10, pp. 1720-1724, 2004.

[23] D. Reimann, E. Büssemaker, and P. Gross, "Successful treatment due to vacuum seal technique of a severe Scedosporium apiospermum skin infection in a renal transplant recipient," *Nephrology Dialysis Transplantation*, vol. 19, no. 1, pp. 245-248, 2004.

[24] M. R. Vagefi, E. T. Kim, R. G. Alvarado, J. L. Duncan, E. L. Howes, and J. B. Crawford, "Bilateral endogenous Scedosporium prolificans endophthalmitis after lung transplantation," *American Journal of Ophthalmology*, vol. 139, no. 2, pp. 370-373, 2005.

[25] S. Husain, P. Muñoz, G. Forrest et al., "Infections due to *Scedosporium apiospermum* and *Scedosporium prolificans* in transplant recipients: clinical characteristics and impact of antifungal agent therapy on outcome," *Clinical Infectious Diseases*, vol. 40, no. 1, pp. 89-99, 2005.

[26] F. Symoens, C. Knoop, M. Schrooyen et al., "Disseminated Scedosporium apiospermum infection in a cystic fibrosis patient after double-lung transplantation," *Journal of Heart and Lung Transplantation*, vol. 25, no. 5, pp. 603-607, 2006.

[27] C. Farina, E. Gotti, F. Suter, and A. Goglio, "*Scedosporium apiospermum* soft-tissue infection: a case report and review of kidney transplant literature," *Transplantation Proceedings*, vol. 38, no. 5, pp. 1333-1335, 2006.

[28] M. Musk, D. Chambers, W. Chin, R. Murray, and E. Gabbay, "Successful treatment of disseminated Scedosporium infection in 2 lung transplant recipients: review of the literature and recommendations for management," *Journal of Heart and Lung Transplantation*, vol. 25, no. 10, pp. 1268-1272, 2006.

[29] P. G. Rogasi, M. Zanazzi, J. Nocentini et al., "Disseminated *Scedosporium apiospermum* infection in renal transplant recipient: long-term successful treatment with voriconazole: a case report," *Transplantation Proceedings*, vol. 39, no. 6, pp. 2033-2035, 2007.

[30] H. Sahi, R. K. Avery, O. A. Minai et al., "Scedosporium apiospermum (Pseudoallescheria boydii) Infection in lung transplant recipients," *Journal of Heart and Lung Transplantation*, vol. 26, no. 4, pp. 350-356, 2007.

[31] J. Y. Z. Li, T. Y. Yong, D. I. Grove, and P. T. H. Coates, "Successful control of *Scedosporium prolificans* septic arthritis and probable osteomyelitis without radical surgery in a long-term renal transplant recipient," *Transplant Infectious Disease*, vol. 10, no. 1, pp. 63-65, 2008.

[32] K. Ezzedine, K. M. Wissing, F. Jacobs, H. Rodriguez, D. Malvy, and T. Simonart, "Recurrent *Scedosporium apiospermum* skin infection in a renal transplant recipient," *Journal of the European Academy of Dermatology and Venereology*, vol. 23, no. 1, pp. 95-96, 2009.

[33] F. Morio, D. Horeau-Langlard, F. Gay-Andrieu et al., "Disseminated *Scedosporium/Pseudallescheria* infection after double-lung transplantation in patients with cystic fibrosis," *Journal of Clinical Microbiology*, vol. 48, no. 5, pp. 1978-1982, 2010.

[34] B. Luijk, M. B. Ekkelenkamp, P. A. De Jong et al., "Effective prolonged therapy with voriconazole in a lung transplant recipient with spondylodiscitis induced by *Scedosporium apiospermum*," *Case Reports in Infectious Diseases*, vol. 2011, Article ID 460313, 4 pages, 2011.

[35] S. Hirschi, V. Letscher-Bru, J. Pottecher et al., "Disseminated *Trichosporon mycotoxinivorans, Aspergillus fumigatus*, and *Scedosporium apiospermum* coinfection after lung and liver transplantation in a cystic fibrosis patient," *Journal of Clinical Microbiology*, vol. 50, no. 12, pp. 4168-4170, 2012.

[36] F. Miraldi, M. Anile, F. Ruberto et al., "*Scedosporium apiospermum* atrial mycetomas after lung transplantation for cystic fibrosis," *Transplant Infectious Disease*, vol. 14, no. 2, pp. 188-191, 2012.

[37] C. Hartmann, C. Müller, H. Weißbrodt et al., "Successful prevention of scedosporiosis after lung transplantation in a cystic fibrosis patient by combined local and systemic triazole therapy," *Medical Mycology Case Reports*, vol. 2, no. 1, pp. 116-118, 2013.

[38] D. M. Sayah, B. S. Schwartz, J. Kukreja, J. P. Singer, J. A. Golden, and L. E. Leard, "Scedosporium prolificans pericarditis and mycotic aortic aneurysm in a lung transplant recipient receiving voriconazole prophylaxis," *Transplant Infectious Disease*, vol. 15, no. 2, pp. E70-E74, 2013.

[39] M. Rathi, S. Gundlapalli, R. Ramachandran et al., "A rare case of cytomegalovirus, scedosporium apiospermum and mycobacterium tuberculosis in a renal transplant recipient," *BMC Infectious Diseases*, vol. 14, article 259, 2014.

[40] K. Uno, K. Kasahara, S. Kutsuna et al., "Infective endocarditis and meningitis due to *Scedosporium prolificans* in a renal transplant recipient," *Journal of Infection and Chemotherapy*, vol. 20, no. 2, pp. 131-133, 2014.

[41] M. E. Clement, E. K. Maziarz, J. N. Schroder, C. B. Patel, and J. R. Perfect, "*Scedosporium apiosermum* infection of the 'Native' valve: fungal endocarditis in an orthotopic heart transplant recipient," *Medical Mycology Case Reports*, vol. 9, pp. 34-36, 2015.

[42] A. Sharma and D. Singh, "*Scedosporium apiospermum* causing brain abscess in a renal allograft recipient," *Saudi Journal of Kidney Diseases and Transplantation*, vol. 26, no. 6, pp. 1253-1256, 2015.

[43] Deceased Donors Recovered in the U.S. by Mechanism of Death: Transplant Data 1988-2015, Department of Health and Human Services, Health Resources and Services Administration, Healthcare Systems Bureau, Division of Transplantation, Rockville, MD; United Network for Organ Sharing, Richmond, VA; University Renal Research and Education Association, Ann Arbor, MI.

[44] C. Goldman, M. J. Akiyama, J. Torres, E. Louie, and S. A. Meehan, "Scedosporium apiospermum infections and the role of combination antifungal therapy and GM-CSF: a case report and review of the literature," *Medical Mycology Case Reports*, vol. 11, pp. 40-43, 2016.

[45] M. J. Abzug and T. J. Walsh, "Interferon-γ and colony-stimulating factors as adjuvant therapy for refractory fungal infections in children," *Pediatric Infectious Disease Journal*, vol. 23, no. 8, pp. 769-773, 2004.

19

Artificially Positive Crossmatches Not Leading to the Refusal of Kidney Donations due to the Usage of Adequate Diagnostic Tools

G. Schlaf,[1] B. Pollok-Kopp,[2] E. Schabel,[1] and W. Altermann[1]

[1] *Tissue Typing Laboratory (GHATT), University Hospital Halle/Saale, Magdeburger Straße 16, 06112 Halle, Germany*
[2] *Department of Transfusion Medicine, University Hospital Göttingen, Robert-Koch-Straße 40, 37075 Göttingen, Germany*

Correspondence should be addressed to G. Schlaf; gerald.schlaf@medizin.uni-halle.de

Academic Editors: P. A. Andrews, C. F. Classen, C. Costa, I. Engelmann, and R. Grenda

Allografting patients with human leukocyte antigens (HLA) which are recognized by preformed antibodies constitutes the main cause for hyper-acute or acute rejections. In order to select recipients without these donor-specific antibodies, the complement-dependent cytotoxicity crossmatch (CDC-CM) assay was developed as a standard procedure about forty years ago. The negative outcome of pretransplant crossmatching represents the most important requirement for a successful kidney graft survival. The artificially positive outcomes of CDC-based crossmatches due to the underlying disease Systemic Lupus Erythematosus (SLE), however, may lead to the unjustified refusal of adequate kidney grafts. Two prospective female recipients destined for a living as well as for a cadaver kidney donation, respectively, exhibited positive CDC-based crossmatch outcomes although for both patients no historical immunizing events were known. Furthermore, solid phase-based screening or antibody differentiation analyses never led to positive results. Immediate reruns of the CDC-based crossmatch assays using the alternative antibody monitoring system (AMS-)crossmatch ELISA resulted in unequivocally negative outcomes. Consequently both transplantations were performed without any immunological complications for the hitherto follow-up time of 25 and 28 months, respectively. We here show two case reports demonstrating an alternative methodical approach to circumvent CDC-based artefacts and point to the urgent need to substitute the CDC-based crossmatch procedure at least for special groups of patients.

1. Introduction

According to the transplantation guidelines of most countries or supranational societies supervising the allocation of kidneys (e.g., Eurotransplant Foundation) the existence of donor-specific anti-HLA antibodies (DSA) is regarded as a contraindication for grafting. This holds true for cadaver as well as for living kidney donations thus requiring the procedure of pretransplant crossmatching. Especially patients characterized by a previous exposure to nonself HLA antigens have (i) to be screened very carefully for anti-HLA antibodies and (ii) to carefully undergo the procedure of crossmatching with a potential kidney donor since DSA have been known for years to be associated with hyperacute or acute rejection episodes up to complete graft loss. To exclude DSA the complement-dependent cytotoxicity crossmatch assay (CDC-CM) was established in the late sixties of the last century as a standard technique by incubating the donors' lymphocytes with sera of the potential recipients in the presence of rabbit complement [1]. As a functional assay the CDC-CM detects only those antibodies which exert their detrimental allogeneic function via the activation of the complement system finally leading to the lysis of donor cells. An alternative approach was introduced with the flow cytometric crossmatch (FACS-CM) leading to the detection of both complement-activating and complement-independent DSA [2, 3]. However, both the CDC- and the FACS-CM do not lead to valid results if only cells of poor quality are available. Due to these methodological drawbacks ELISA-based crossmatch assays which are completely independent of the cell quality have been established in some tissue typing laboratories [4–6]. One of these assays, the antibody monitoring system

(AMS) HLA class I/II ELISA, was implemented by us for special cases of patients not resulting in reliable and valid CDC-based crossmatch outcomes for various reasons. These false outcomes are due to the high susceptibility of the CDC-based crossmatch procedure to apparent disruptive factors which may result from underlying diseases. Based on the examples of two 41- and 43-year-old female recipients, both suffering from systemic lupus erythematosus (SLE) and awaiting a kidney donation, we present data which indicate that an implausible positive CDC-based crossmatch result should not lead to the refusal of the donation without using an alternative methodical crossmatch approach.

2. Case Presentations

2.1. Case 1: Acceptance of a Living Kidney Donation between a Mother and Her Daughter as a Consequence of AMS-ELISA-Based Crossmatching. In the first report a 41-year-old female recipient with end-stage renal insufficiency was HLA-phenotyped and genotyped for HLA-class I antigens HLA-A2; B7,57 (Bw4,6); Cw6,7 and genotyped for HLA-class II antigens HLA-DR7,15; DR51,53; DQ3(9),6. Very soon the decision was reached to perform a living kidney donation from her 60-year-old-mother typed HLA-A1,2; B8,57 (Bw4,6); Cw6,7 for class I and HLA-DR7,17; DR52,53; DQ3(9),2 for class II. Thus, the resulting mismatch scheme of the graft covering only the A-B-DR antigens, which are regarded as the most important, was determined as 1-1-1 (MM A-B-DR). Due to the compatibility of the Cw antigens no additional targets for an immune response against them existed. Concerning the codominant inheritance the degree of HLA matching between the mother as prospective donor and her daughter was as expected. In accordance with different guidelines of the particular kidney transplant centres the crossmatching procedure has to be performed two or three times prior to living kidney grafting, respectively. Any positive outcome of crossmatching, however, leads to the refusal of a living kidney donation. Donor-specific antibodies appeared first to be detectable in October 2010 using the conventional CDC-CM with peripheral blood lymphocytes, as well as isolated T- and B-lymphocytes as this procedure is dictated by the Eurotransplant Foundation and at present represents the standard method to detect alloantibodies in a prospective recipient against HLA antigens of donor cells. For the isolation of T and B cells the tetrameric antibody complex technology crosslinking unwanted cells to red blood cells and their consecutive elimination by density gradient centrifugation was used (System RosetteSep, Stem Cell Technology, Grenoble, France). After their initial isolation the cells were incubated with serum of a chosen recipient before adding complement proteins from a rabbit. In this assay the complement system is activated via the classical activation pathway only by those antibodies which have been bound to the cells in the first incubation step and which belong to the complement-system-activating IgM/IgG (sub)isotypes. The result was determined by two-colour fluorescence microscopy. Dead cells attacked by the complement system were stained red by the intercalating reagent ethidium bromide, whereas vital cells exhibited a green staining pattern due to the active uptake of acridine orange. The intensity of the complement reaction was categorized by indicating the percentage of dead (red) cells using the score system of the National Institute of Health (Washington, USA) as described in the legend of Table 1.

The first CDC-based crossmatch (05/2010) using peripheral blood lymphocytes (PBL) as well as isolated T and B cells was negative (Table 1(a)) in best accordance with a screening ELISA not detecting any anti-HLA antibodies (Table 1(b)). Unexpectedly the second crossmatch (10/2010), performed five months afterwards, was positive for PBL, T, and B cells without any known immunizing event in the meantime (Table 1(a)). The living kidney donation intended for the next day was cancelled. Due to the implausibility of this second CDC-based crossmatch an immediate rerun using the alternative AMS-crossmatch ELISA (GTI, Waukesha, USA; FDA number BK060038 from June 26, 2006) was performed which resulted in an unequivocally negative outcome. The workflow of this procedure is shown in Figure 1. First detergent lysate of a given donor's material was pipetted into the wells of ELISA strips precoated with capture monoclonal antibodies (mAb), directed against a monomorphic epitope on HLA class I or class II molecules, respectively (Figure 1(a)). After the first incubation the strips were washed and incubated with the recipients' sera. These sera may contain DSA to be detected in this assay since they serve as detection antibodies in the case of recognizing the immobilized HLA molecules of a given donor (Figure 1(b)). After additional washing steps the samples were incubated with secondary alkaline phosphatase-conjugated anti-human IgG antibodies to recognize the immobilized donor-specific (detection-) antibodies (Figure 1(c)). This last step was modified in our laboratory through the use of secondary antibodies directed against IgG/M/A isotypes of primary human antibodies. To validate the data three controls had to be performed. (i) The lysate controls (LCRI/II) consist of a second enzyme-labelled mAb for the detection of immobilized HLA class I or class II molecules, respectively, by recognizing a second monomorphic epitope on the immobilized HLA molecules (Figure 1(d)). This control provides evidence that the amount of the donors' HLA molecules is sufficient to get a signal. (ii) The positive control (control of reagents) consists of freeze-dried control lymphocytes and a positive serum sample directed against HLA class I and class II molecules. This control demonstrates the functionality of the reagents, even if the preparation of the donor's material is insufficient to generate a signal. (iii) The negative control corresponds exactly to the positive control of reagents with the difference that an irrelevant human serum which is negative for HLA antigens is used. The value generated by the recipient's serum under investigation has to exceed twofold the background value of the negative control to reach a positive classification. The consequent research for a potential disruptive factor falsifying the outcome of the CDC-based crossmatch led to the formerly unknown diagnosis of lupus disease by the patient's nephrologists. The third conventionally performed CDC-based assay (01/2011) after the acute lupus episode was again negative in best accordance with the AMS-ELISA

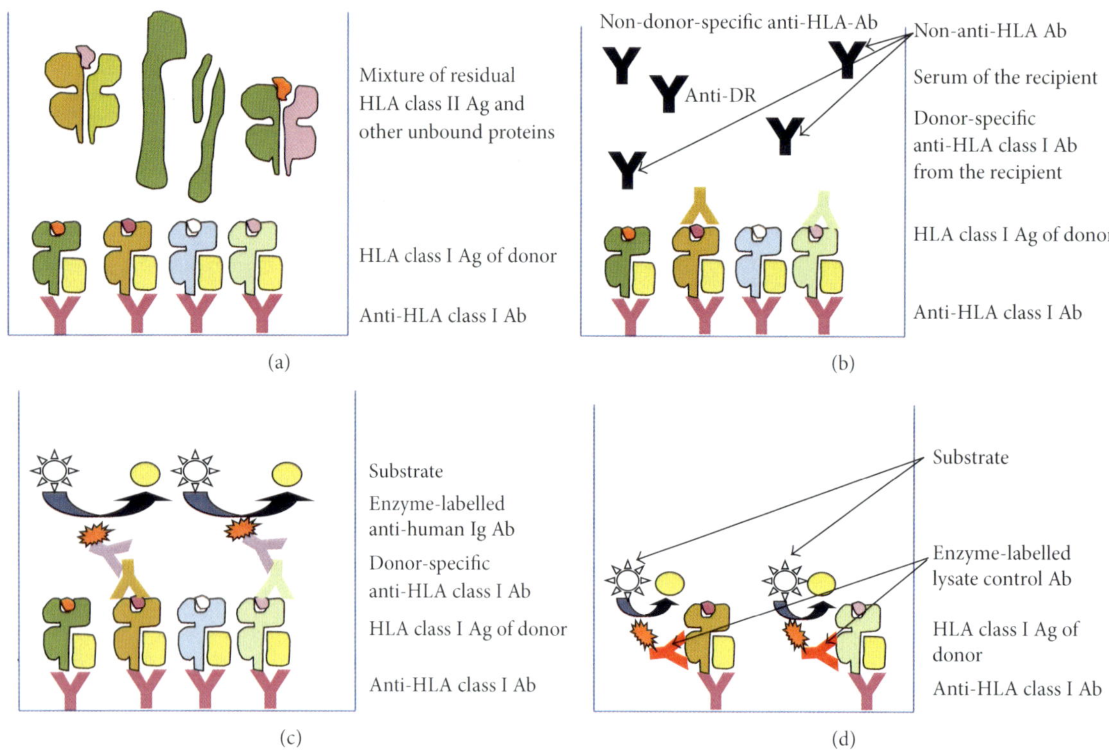

Figure 1: Flow diagram of the AMS-ELISA shown for the detection of HLA class I molecules. (a) Binding of the donor's solubilized HLA class I molecules by monoclonal capture antibodies recognizing a monomorphic epitope on HLA class I molecules. (b) Binding of the donor-specific anti-HLA antibodies out of the recipient's serum to the HLA molecules of the donor. (c) Binding of alkaline phosphatase-conjugated secondary antibodies to the recipient's bound donor-specific anti-HLA class I antibodies and subsequent colour reaction. The original protocol was modified by substituting the human IgG-specific by a human IgG/M/A-specific secondary antibody. (d) Lysate control using an alkaline phosphatase-conjugated monoclonal detection antibody directed against a second monomorphic epitope to confirm the immobilization of a sufficient amount of HLA molecules by the solid-phase-bound capture antibody. The AMS-ELISA variant for the identification of donor-specific antibodies directed against HLA class II molecules is correspondingly designed.

carried out in parallel as a reference assay (Table 1(a)). All sera used for crossmatching were additionally analysed for the detection of anti-HLA class I and anti-HLA class II antibodies using Quik Screen and B-Screen assays (GTI Diagnostics, USA) as shown in Table 1(b), respectively. Furthermore, the sera taken in 10/2010 and 01/2011 were additionally tested using Luminex-based antibody differentiation analyses at the single donor level (Lifecodes class I/II ID, via Inno-Train, Germany) (Table 1(b)). Both Quik Screen (for anti-HLA class I) and B-Screen (for anti-HLA class II) ELISA-based screening assays were modified using secondary antibodies specific for primary antigen-recognizing antibodies of the IgG and IgM isotypes. No screening or differentiation assay resulted in detectable anti-HLA antibodies (Table 1(b)). Consequently the transplantation was performed at the following day without any immunological complication for the follow-up time of about 25 months.

2.2. Case 2: Refusal of an Implausible Positive CDC-Based Crossmatch Result through the Additional Use of the AMS-Crossmatch ELISA with a Negative Outcome during Emergency Duties. In the second report a 43-year-old female cadaver kidney recipient with renal endstage disease was phenotyped and genotyped for HLA class I antigens HLA-A1; B8 (Bw6); Cw7. For HLA-class II antigens she was typed HLA DR17; DR52; DQ2. After 17 months on the kidney waiting list the patient got a kidney offer which was HLA compatible at the low resolution typing level not only for the antigens A-B-DR (resulting mismatch scheme 0-0-0) but also for the HLA class I Cw and the HLA class II DQ antigens. In spite of this high HLA compatibility the CDC-based prior-to-grafting-crossmatch performed in October 2010 was positive using the current serum of the patient taken in October 2010 and a historical serum which had been taken one year ago in October 2009 (Table 2(a)). This second serum had historically been detected to be positive for anti-HLA antibodies in the CDC-based cell tray screening procedure although no distinct specificities had been identifiable. Consequently this historical serum with a panel reactivity (PRA) of 68% had been stored as positive sample (PRA > 5%) to be available for future crossmatching. The current serum taken in October 2010 was as well positive (61% PRA) in the cell tray assay but not in the solid-phase-based screening ELISA (Table 2(b)). Thus, the quarterly performed screening assays to define the degree of anti-HLA preimmunization

TABLE 1: (a) CDC- and AMS-ELISA -based crossmatch results of the 41-year-old recipient and her 60-year-old mother as a prospective living kidney donor. (b) Corresponding analyses for anti-HLA antibody screening/identification.

(a)

Serum sample	CDC-CM (#)			AMS-ELISA-CM	
	PBL	T-cell	B-cell	Class I	Class II
05/2010	1	1	1	n.d.	n.d.
10/2010	2/4	1/2	4	neg.	neg.
01/2011	1	1	1	neg.	neg.

n.d.: not done due to the unequivocally negative outcome of the CDC-CM; neg.: negative; pos.: positive; #: NIH score system of the standard CDC-based crossmatch as a percent of positive/dead (red coloured) cells (%): 1: <10% (negative), 2: 10–20% (doubtfully positive), 4: 20–50% (weakly positive), 6: 50–80% (positive), 8: 80–100% (strongly positive).

(b)

Serum sample	Screening ELISA		Luminex analysis	
	Class I (Quik Screen)	Class II (B-Screen)	Class I	Class II
05/2010	neg.	neg.	n.d.	n.d.
07/2010	neg.	neg.	n.d.	n.d.
10/2010	neg.	neg.	neg.	neg.
01/2011	neg.	neg.	neg.	neg.

n.d.: not done; neg.: negative; the Luminex analysis was not performed using the samples taken in May 2010 and July 2010 due to the unequivocally negative result of the class I and II screening ELISA but was additionally used to analyse the sera taken in October 2010 and January 2011.

resulted in positive outcomes only in the CDC-based cell tray analyses performed in accordance with the guidelines of the European Federation of Immunogenetics (EFI) only once a year during the autumnal screening runs (Table 2(b)). Both cell tray analyses, however, did not lead to definable antibody specificities. Additional identification assays such as the DynaChip solid phase array (Life Technologies/Invitrogen, UK) employed for three times (July 2009, October 2009, 10/2010) never resulted in detectable anti-HLA antibodies (Table 2(b)). These divergent results of solid-phase-based assays on one hand and cell tray-based antibody detection assays on the other hand prompted us to ask the patient's dialysis centre already after the first CDC-based autumnal screening (10/2009) for disruptive factors leading to the formerly unknown information that the patient suffered from lupus disease. Thus, we were prepared that the outcome of any CDC-based prior-to-grafting crossmatch would most probably be positive due to this underlying disease. In accordance with a prior agreement with the transplant centre the obligatory CDC-based pretransplantation crossmatch was performed in parallel to the alternative AMS-crossmatch ELISA (Figure 1) which led to an unequivocally negative outcome. Based on the negative result of the AMS-ELISA the transplantation was performed, and no immunological complications for the hitherto existing follow-up time of about 28 months were observable.

3. Discussion and Conclusions

Based on two exemplary cases it was the aim of the current paper to present data on certain situations of crossmatching which do not lead to reliable results when the conventional CDC-based technique is used. This technique was established as the prototype of crossmatching in the late sixties and unquestionably improved the outcome of transplantations since hyper-acute and acute rejections have highly been reduced after this functional assay's implementation [7, 8]. In spite of this progress the adequate allocation of organs remains a problem if it is solely/mainly based on an assay which is characterized by several drawbacks. In this context the CDC-based crossmatch assay (i) detects only antibodies of complement-activating isotypes, (ii) requires donor cells of a high degree of vitality often not available, and (iii) is obviously highly susceptible to artificially positive reactions as described by us on the basis of two current cases. Although the general phenomenon that the CDC-based crossmatch may be characterized by false-positive outcomes due to autoimmune diseases has sometimes been mentioned [9–11] the literature lacks concrete examples which demonstrate different outcomes of CDC-based and alternative solid-phase-based assays using identical serum samples as exemplarily shown in these reports. As additionally shown by the second case report, the artificially positive reactions hold true both for direct CDC-based crossmatching (Table 2(a)) using cells of a given donor and for CDC-based antibody screening using cell trays with selected panel cells as a basis for virtual crossmatching (Table 2(b)). Using both CDC-based assays without any additional solid-phase-based assay for cross-matching and for anti-HLA antibody detection/identification would presumably not lead to valid results for patients suffering from certain autoimmune diseases such as systemic lupus erythematosus. Thus, the two cases presented here suggest the use of the AMS-ELISA to overcome the general problem of artificially positive CDC-based crossmatch results. However, the results presented are not in accordance with the latest attempts to declare the CDC-based procedures as the leading method for the definition of immunized patients as proposed recently [12]. Quite in contrast they show the general insufficiency of CDC-based assays to lead to valid results under the conditions described demonstrating the urgent need to substitute them at least for special groups of patients. Whether these artificial outcomes of CDC-based assays hold true for other diseases of the immune complex type III such as rheumatoid arthritis will have to be examined.

We present two cases of CDC-based pretransplantation anti-HLA antibody diagnosis completely insufficient to correctly diagnose the existence of DSA in potential kidney allograft recipients due to SLE-based false-positive reactions. Detecting these antibodies has been known for years to be highly important for the survival of kidney allografts. In order to avoid the CDC-based crossmatch artefacts dithiothreitol/dithioerythritol (DTT/DTE) as reducing agents were early introduced to reduce the confounding influence of antibodies of the IgM isotype. Apparently this procedure led to an improvement of CDC-based crossmatch results' interpretability in many cases [13–16]. Hence in

Table 2: (a) CDC- and AMS-ELISA-based pretransplant crossmatch results of the 43-year-old recipient with her completely HLA-matched cadaveric kidney donor. (b) Corresponding analyses for anti-HLA antibody screening/identification.

(a)

Serum sample	CDC-CM (#)			AMS-ELISA-CM	
	PBL	T-cell	B-cell	Class I	Class II
10/2009	6	6	8	neg.	neg.
10/2010	6/8	6	8	neg.	neg.

neg.: negative; pos.: positive; #: NIH score system of the standard CDC-based crossmatch as a percent of positive/dead (red coloured) cells (%) as shown in Table 1(a).

(b)

Serum sample	Screening ELISA/DynaChip (Ø)		CDC cell tray (PBL)
	Class I	Class II	Class I / II
07/2009	neg. (Ø)	neg. (Ø)	n.d.
10/2009	neg. (Ø)	neg. (Ø)	pos. (68% PRA)
01/2010	neg.	neg.	n.d.
04/2010	neg.	neg.	n.d.
07/2010	neg.	neg.	n.d.
10/2010	neg. (Ø)	neg. (Ø)	pos. (61% PRA)

neg.: negative; pos.: positive; n.d.: not done; the CDC-based cell tray analysis was performed during the autumnal screening (i.e., once a year in accordance with the guidelines of the European Federation of Immunogenetics (EFI)) using the samples taken in October 2009 and October 2010 ; Ø: additionally performed DynaChip analyses in all cases exhibiting negative results in accordance with the screening ELISA.

HLA diagnostics these agents are generally used to destroy antibodies of the IgM isotype with the aim to avoid the detection of autoantibodies. However, for more than ten years it has been known that autoantibodies which are generated during autoimmune-mediated diseases such as SLE and which may lead to false-positive CDC-based crossmatches do not necessarily belong to the IgM isotype class but represent lymphocytotoxic, that is, complement-fixing autoantibodies of the IgG-isotype [10]. Additionally some studies demonstrating the detrimental effect of HLA-specific alloantibodies of the IgM isotype have been published, thus clearly showing the benefit to detect and not to destroy them [17]. Unfortunately these alloantibodies of the IgM isotype are as well eliminated using DTT/DTE for CDC-based crossmatching but are detected using our modification of the AMS-ELISA with secondary anti-IgG/M/A antibodies. Taken together the AMS-ELISA is a suitable tool which methodically circumvents false positive crossmatch reactions in the presence of accompanying autoimmune diseases hence clearly improving the outcome for the patients.

Abbreviations

AMS: Antibody monitoring system
CDC: Complement-dependent cytotoxicity
CM: Crossmatch
DTE: Dithioerythritol
DTT: Dithiothreitol
DSA: Donor-specific antibodies
ELISA: Enzyme-linked immunosorbent assay
FACS-CM: Flow cytometric crossmatch
HLA: Human leukocyte antigen
mAb: Monoclonal antibody
SLE: Systemic Lupus Erythematosus
PRA: Panel reactive antibodies.

References

[1] P. I. Terasaki and J. D. McClelland, "Microdroplet assay of human serum cytotoxins," *Nature*, vol. 204, no. 4962, pp. 998–1000, 1964.

[2] M. R. Garovoy, M. A. Rheinschmidt, and M. Bigos, "Flow cytometry analysis: a high technology crossmatch technique facilitating transplantation," *Transplantation Proceedings*, vol. 15, no. 3, pp. 1939–1944, 1983.

[3] M. C. Bittencourt, J. M. Rebibou, Y. Saint-Hillier et al., "Impaired renal graft survival after a positive B-cell flow-cytometry crossmatch," *Nephrology Dialysis Transplantation*, vol. 13, no. 8, pp. 2059–2064, 1998.

[4] B. K. Book, A. Agarwal, A. B. Milgrom et al., "New crossmatch technique eliminates interference by humanized and chimeric monoclonal antibodies," *Transplantation Proceedings*, vol. 37, no. 2, pp. 640–642, 2005.

[5] W. W. Altermann, B. Seliger, S. Sel, D. Wendt, and G. Schlaf, "Comparison of the established standard complement-dependent cytotoxicity and flow cytometric crossmatch assays with a novel ELISA-based HLA crossmatch procedure," *Histology and Histopathology*, vol. 21, no. 10, pp. 1115–1124, 2006.

[6] S. Sel, G. Schlaf, O. Schurat, and W. Altermann, "A novel ELISA-based crossmatch procedure to detect donor-specific anti-HLA antibodies responsible for corneal allograft rejections," *Journal of Immunological Methods*, vol. 31, pp. 23–31, 2012.

[7] F. Kissmeyer-Nielsen and K. E. Kjerbye, "Lymphocytotoxic microtechnique. Purification of lymphocytes by flotation," *Histocompatibility Testing*, pp. 381–384, 1967.

[8] R. Patel and P. I. Terasaki, "Significance of the positive crossmatch test in kidney transplantation," *The New England Journal of Medicine*, vol. 280, no. 14, pp. 735–739, 1969.

[9] G. Ozturk and P. I. Terasaki, "Cytotoxic antibodies against surface immunoglobulin," *Transplantation*, vol. 29, no. 2, pp. 140–142, 1980.

[10] S. Sumitran-Holgersson, "HLA-specific alloantibodies and renal graft outcome," *Nephrology Dialysis Transplantation*, vol. 16, no. 5, pp. 897–904, 2001.

[11] G. Schlaf, B. Pollok-Kopp, T. Manzke, O. Schurat, and W. Altermann, "Novel solid phase-based ELISA assays contribute to an improved detection of anti-HLA antibodies and to an increased reliability of pre-and post-transplant crossmatching," *NDT Plus*, vol. 3, no. 6, pp. 527–538, 2010.

[12] I. I. N. Doxiadis, D. Roelen, and F. H. J. Claas, "Mature wines are better: CDC as the leading method to define highly sensitized patients," *Current Opinion in Organ Transplantation*, vol. 15, no. 6, pp. 716–719, 2010.

[13] B. Barger, T. W. Shroyer, S. L. Hudson et al., "Successful renal allografts in recipients with crossmatch-positive, dithioerythritol-treated negative sera. Race, transplant history, and HLA-DR1 phenotype," *Transplantation*, vol. 47, no. 2, pp. 240–245, 1989.

[14] V. A. Tellis, A. J. Matas, D. Senitzer et al., "Successful transplantation after conversion of a positive crossmatch to negative by dissociation of IgM antibody," *Transplantation*, vol. 47, no. 1, pp. 127–129, 1989.

[15] S. Vaidya and J. Ruth, "Contributions and clinical significance of IgM and autoantibodies in highly sensitized renal allograft recipients," *Transplantation*, vol. 47, no. 6, pp. 956–958, 1989.

[16] S. Barocci, U. Valente, R. Gusmano et al., "Autoreactive lymphocytotoxic IgM antibodies in highly sensitized dialysis patients waiting for a kidney transplant: identification and clinical relevance," *Clinical Nephrology*, vol. 36, no. 1, pp. 12–20, 1991.

[17] P. Stastny, S. Ring, C. Lu, J. Arenas, M. Han, and B. Lavingia, "Role of immunoglobulin (Ig)-G and IgM antibodies against donor human leukocyte antigens in organ transplant recipients," *Human Immunology*, vol. 70, no. 8, pp. 600–604, 2009.

20

Primary Nonfunction of Renal Allograft Secondary to Acute Oxalate Nephropathy

Ravi Parasuraman,[1,2,3] Ping L. Zhang,[4] Dilip Samarapungavan,[1] Krishna Pothugunta,[1] Gampala Reddy,[1] Leslie Rocher,[1] Francis Dumler,[1] Vandad Raofi,[1] Steven Cohn,[1] and Alan Koffron[1]

[1] *Division of Nephrology and Transplantation, William-Beaumont Hospital, Royal Oak, MI 48037, USA*
[2] *Kidney Transplant Outreach Program, William-Beaumont Hospital, Royal Oak, MI 48037, USA*
[3] *Oakland University, William Beaumont School of Medicine, Royal Oak, MI 48037, USA*
[4] *Division of Renal Pathology, William-Beaumont Hospital, Royal Oak, MI 48037, USA*

Correspondence should be addressed to Ravi Parasuraman, ravi.parasuraman@beaumont.edu

Academic Editors: C. Costa, J. Kaneko, and F. Keller

Primary nonfunction (PNF) accounts for 0.6 to 8% of renal allograft failure, and the focus on causes of PNF has changed from rejection to other causes. Calcium oxalate (CaOx) deposition is common in early allograft biopsies, and it contributes in moderate intensity to higher incidence of acute tubular necrosis and poor graft survival. A-49-year old male with ESRD secondary to polycystic kidney disease underwent extended criteria donor kidney transplantation. Posttransplant, patient developed delayed graft function (DGF), and the biopsy showed moderately intense CaOx deposition that persisted on subsequent biopsies for 16 weeks, eventually resulting in PNF. The serum oxalate level was 3 times more than normal at 85 μmol/L (normal <27 μmol/L). Allograft nephrectomy showed massive aggregates of CaOx crystal deposition in renal collecting system. In conclusion, acute oxalate nephropathy should be considered in the differential diagnosis of DGF since optimal management could change the outcome of the allograft.

1. Introduction

Primary Nonfunction (PNF) defined as permanent loss of allograft function starting immediately after transplantation accounts for 0.6% to 8% of all renal graft loss and is significantly associated with poor patient survival [1–4]. The causes of early allograft dysfunction are changing constantly, and recently calcium oxalate (CaOx) crystal deposition has been added to this list. Deposition of CaOx crystal in renal tubules can be seen in >50% of allograft biopsies performed <3 months posttransplant [5]. Although presence of CaOx crystal in allografts can be benign, when present in moderate intensity, it contributes to increased incidence, acute tubular necrosis and poor allograft survival [5, 6]. Here we present a case of extreme complication of CaOx crystal deposition resulting in primary nonfunction of renal allograft that has not been previously reported to our knowledge.

2. Case Report

A-49-year old male with end stage renal disease (ESRD) secondary to autosomal dominant polycystic kidney disease (ADPKD) with past medical history of hypertension, hypothyroidism, secondary hyperparathyroidism, and polycystic liver disease underwent a 6 antigen mismatch, expanded criteria donor (ECD) kidney transplantation. The panel reactive antibody (PRA), donor-specific antibody (DSA), and flow crossmatch (FCX) were negative prior to transplantation. Donor information includes a 75-year-old female with serum creatinine (Scr) of 0.5 mg/dL (44.2 μmol/L) and urine output of 400 mL/hour with negative urinalysis prior to organ recovery. The pre-implant renal biopsy showed 3% glomerulosclerosis without interstitial inflammation or fibrosis. The kidney was on simple cold storage with cold ischemia time of 18 hours. No past history

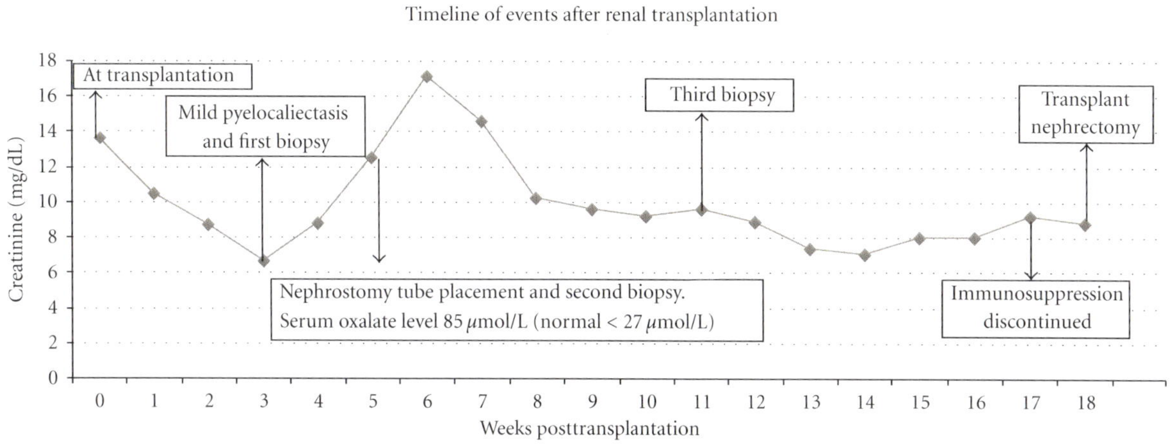

FIGURE 1: Serum creatinine levels and related events during the course of renal transplantation.

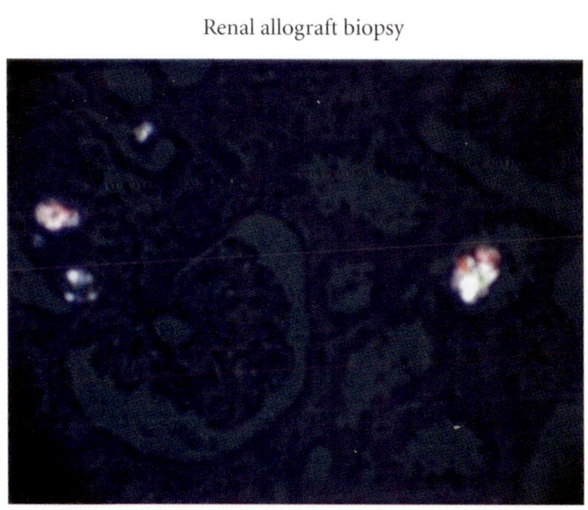

FIGURE 2: Biopsy Shows calcium oxalate crystal deposition in the renal tubules under polarized light microscopy (1st biopsy performed during 3rd week of transplantation).

of renal stones or hypercalcemia either in the donor or in the recipient.

3. Posttransplantation Course

The patient received alemtuzumab (anti-CD52 antibody, Campath, Genzyme Corporation) for induction and tacrolimus and mycophenolate mofetil (MMF) without steroids for maintenance. Other medications included levothyroxine, furosemide, sulfamethoxazole/trimethoprim (Bactrim), and valganciclovir hydrochloride (Valcyte) with dose adjusted for renal function. Posttransplant, the patient developed delayed graft function (DGF) and slow recovery of allograft function with urine volume reaching 2800 mL/day with corresponding decrease in Scr from 13.62 mg/dL (1204.01 μmol/L) to 6.70 mg/dL (592.28 μmol/L) over 2-3-week period. The timeline of clinical events is shown in Figure 1.

An allograft ultrasound (US) and biopsy performed at 3 weeks for slow recovery showed minimal pyelocaliectasis with normal resistive indices (RI; 0.45–0.62) and perfusion. The biopsy was significant for acute tubular necrosis (ATN, confirmed by kidney injury molecule-1 immunostain) and CaOx crystal deposition with no evidence of rejection (Figure 2). In view of CaOx deposition, clinical evaluation performed for secondary hyperoxalosis (enteric hyperoxalosis, MMF-induced diarrhea, excessive oral intake of oxalate-containing foods including vitamin C, ethylene glycol intoxication, or use of methoxyflurane) was found negative. The patient continued his immunosuppression with tacrolimus dose reduction for mildly elevated trough levels days prior to biopsy. Despite tacrolimus dose reduction, the patient showed progressive increase in Scr with subsequent development of microscopic hematuria and moderate fluid overload. Reimaging of the allograft at week 5 showed moderate hydronephrosis with normal RI and perfusion. Because of progression of hydronephrosis, percutaneous nephrostomy and antegrade pyelogram were performed and that showed no ureteral obstruction. A simultaneous biopsy continued to show CaOx deposition and ATN in the absence of rejection or BK virus nephropathy. In view of persistent CaOx deposition, serum oxalate level was measured, and it was 3 times more than normal at 85 μmol/L (normal <27 μmol/L). Due to unrelenting ATN, the dose of tacrolimus was reduced by 50% with addition of prednisone 10 mg/day and cautious increase in furosemide dose to augment urine output hoping to decrease supersaturation of CaOx and crystal formation. Unfortunately Scr remained unchanged despite resolution of hydronephrosis and tacrolimus dose reduction. A third biopsy performed was not significantly different from previous biopsies. Since the patient remained rejection-free, a trial of tacrolimus-free immunosuppression with prednisone and mycophenolate mofetil was attempted for the remaining course of transplantation expecting spontaneous resolution of CaOx-mediated renal injury. Unfortunately, the patient was elected to stay on peritoneal dialysis; otherwise, long duration of daily hemodialysis may have reduced the oxalate burden on the allograft. The patient showed no signs of recovery, and we could not justify the continuation of immunosuppression beyond 15 weeks because of 2 episodes

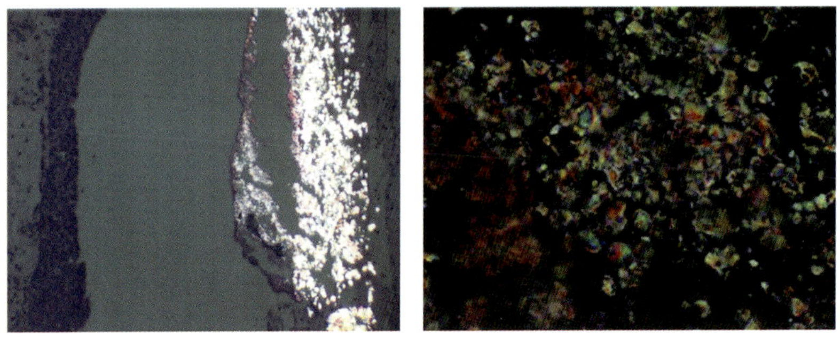

(a) (b)

Figure 3: (a) shows widespread massive aggregate of CaOx crystals in the renal collecting system extending into the parenchyma seen under polarized light. (b) shows a region of (a) under high power showing accumulation of polygonal crystals with multicolored birefringence under polarized light. AON: acute oxalate nephropathy, CaOx: calcium oxalate.

of urinary tract infection. Finally with the diagnosis of PNF, allograft nephrectomy was performed at week 17. The explant showed extensive aggregates of CaOx crystals (multicolored birefringence polygonal crystals under polarized light as shown in Figures 3(a) and 3(b)) in the renal collecting system extending to the parenchyma. In order to exclude the donor origin of CaOx deposition, a review of pre-implant biopsy was performed and showed no CaOx deposition and the mate kidney showed good allograft function with nadir Scr of 1.5 mg% (132.6 μmol/L). The diagnosis of acute oxalate nephropathy (AON) was made based on persistent CaOx deposition in the allograft, high serum oxalate level despite extensive deposition within the kidney, and the explant histology showing extensive CaOx crystal formation in the collecting system in the absence of other causes for allograft dysfunction.

4. Discussion

This case of PNF from AON is an uncommon and extreme manifestation of hyperoxalosis. The defining element of AON in this case is extensive deposition of characteristic crystals in tubules and in the collecting system (Figures 1 and 2). The polygonal, refractile, multicolored birefringence under polarized light identifies them as calcium oxalate [7]. Uremic oxalosis, the most frequent cause of hyperoxalosis in ESRD is likely in our patient in the absence of other causes of hyperoxalosis [5]. The predisposing risk factors included peritoneal dialysis (poor oxalate clearance) as the mode of renal replacement therapy pretransplant, higher serum creatinine level (13.62 mg/dL) at transplantation, and the donor age of 75 years [8, 9]. Although up to 39% of all nephrolithiasis in ADPKD is of CaOx in nature, it is unclear whether ADPKD is an added risk factor [10]. This case was determined to be primary nonfunction since the patient was peritoneal dialysis dependent during the entire period despite early minimal improvement in allograft function.

Both primary and secondary hyperoxaluria are well-recognized causes for renal failure. Primary hyperoxaluria (PH) causing AON in renal allograft has been reported and that rare possibility could not be excluded in our patient in the absence of mutational analysis [11]. Secondary hyperoxalosis causing allograft dysfunction is increasingly recognized in recent years. Normally, dietary calcium binds to oxalate in the intestine and is excreted as CaOx in the stool. Fat malabsorption decreases the availability of intestinal calcium thus increasing oxalate absorption resulting in enteric hyperoxalosis, the most common cause of secondary hyperoxalosis. Fat malabsorption from pancreatic calcification causing AON with resultant loss of first allograft and delayed recovery in the second allograft has been reported in a patient who underwent two renal transplants over 7-month period [12]. Recently, a case of AON secondary to MMF-induced diarrhea was reported in a simultaneous kidney-pancreas transplant recipient [13]. Excessive intake of vitamin C (8 grams/day) causing secondary hyperoxalosis and dialysis-dependent AON in a transplant recipient was reported by our group [14].

Uremic oxalosis of chronic kidney disease results from accumulation of serum oxalate that is 10–30 times above the normal level [15, 16]. Unfortunately, neither hemodialysis nor peritoneal dialysis normalizes Ox level. In a study of 212 recipients with median plasma oxalate level of 35.0 μmol/L (normal: 2.6–11.0) at transplantation, the oxalate level was shown to be negatively associated with absolute GFR and positively to donor age and plasma creatinine at 10 weeks posttransplantation [5, 9]. Excretion of accumulated serum oxalate can cause injury to allograft in the immediate posttransplant period [5, 11, 17]. This may explain the findings of Pinheiro et al. who showed presence of CaOx deposition in 82% and 52.6% of allograft biopsies performed within 3 weeks and 3 months of transplantation [5]. The presence of CaOx deposition in allografts may be nonspecific or truly pathological, and this diagnostic difficulty is not uncommon clinically. Moderate CaOx deposition was shown to be associated with higher ATN (47% versus 24%) in the immediate posttransplant period and poor allograft survival (49.7% versus 74.1%) at 12 years [5]. The intensity of CaOx deposition score proposed by Scheinman et al. adds value in determining pathogenicity [18]. Clinical diagnosis of AON can be made when ATN is associated with moderate to severe CaOx deposition and higher serum oxalate levels in the absence of other causes. Once the diagnosis is made clinically, management strategies may include (1) adequate fluid administration to maintain high urine output to reduce the risk of supersaturation of CaOx [19]. (2) Correction of metabolic acidosis when present to increase urinary citrate and magnesium levels to prevent CaOx crystallization [19], (3) frequent and prolonged hemodialysis treatment to reduce serum oxalate level to near normal levels, and (4) finally, restricting high oxalate-containing diet such as vitamin C treatment of fat malabsorption and diarrhea when present [12, 14].

PNF of renal allograft is significantly associated with poor patient survival with hazard ratio of 2.04 and is further supported by the Canadian organ replacement registry report which shows patient survival to be significantly lower when graft loss occurs <90 days as compared to >90 days posttransplantation [4, 20]. In conclusion, our case reiterates the need for continuous evaluation of DGF patients for all treatable causes. CaOx deposition in renal allograft is an important and probably underrecognized cause of DGF that requires adequate awareness with early intervention to improve the allograft outcome.

Acknowledgment

The authors would like to thank Mrs. Barbara Mulholland for her secretarial assistance during the preparation of this case report.

References

[1] Z. M. El-Zoghby, M. D. Stegall, D. J. Lager et al., "Identifying specific causes of kidney allograft loss," *American Journal of Transplantation*, vol. 9, no. 3, pp. 527–535, 2009.

[2] R. B. Stevens, J. Y. Skorupa, T. H. Rigley et al., "Increased primary non-function in transplanted deceased-donor kidneys flushed with histidine-tryptophan-ketoglutarate solution," *American Journal of Transplantation*, vol. 9, no. 5, pp. 1055–1062, 2009.

[3] A. F. Groenewoud, J. Thorogood, and The HTK Study Group, "Current status of the Eurotransplant randomized multicenter study comparing kidney graft preservation with histidine-tryptophan-ketogluterate, University of Wisconsin, and Euro-Collins solutions," *Transplantation Proceedings*, vol. 25, no. 1, pp. 1582–1585, 1993.

[4] Y. M. Woo, A. G. Jardine, A. F. Clark et al., "Early graft function and patient survival following cadaveric renal transplantation," *Kidney International*, vol. 55, no. 2, pp. 692–699, 1999.

[5] S. H. Pinheiro, N. O. Saraiva Câmara, K. S. Osaki, L. A. Ribeiro De Moura, and A. Pacheco-Silva, "Early presence of calcium oxalate deposition in kidney graft biopsies is associated with poor long-term graft survival," *American Journal of Transplantation*, vol. 5, no. 2, pp. 323–329, 2005.

[6] L. D. Truong, U. Yakupoglu, D. Feig et al., "Calcium oxalate deposition in renal allografts: morphologic spectrum and clinical implications," *American Journal of Transplantation*, vol. 4, no. 8, pp. 1338–1344, 2004.

[7] S. V. Seshan, *Renal Disease: Classification and Atlas of Tubulo-Intestitial and Vascular Diseases*, Williams & Wilkins, Baltimore, Md, USA, 1999.

[8] M. Mydlík and K. Derzsiová, "Renal replacement therapy and secondary hyperoxalemia in chronic renal failure," *Kidney International*, vol. 59, no. 78, pp. S304–S307, 2001.

[9] K. B. P. Elgstoen, L. F. Johnsen, B. Woldseth, L. Morkrid, and A. Hartmann, "Plasma oxalate following kidney transplantation in patients without primary hyperoxaluria," *Nephrology Dialysis Transplantation*, vol. 25, no. 7, pp. 2341–2345, 2010.

[10] V. E. Torres, S. B. Erickson, L. H. Smith, D. M. Wilson, R. R. Hattery, and J. W. Segura, "The association of nephrolithiasis and autosomal polycystic kidney disease," *American Journal of Kidney Diseases*, vol. 11, no. 4, pp. 318–325, 1988.

[11] M. K. Heer, A. Sharma, K. Joshi, and M. Minz, "Early allograft failure in an unrecognized case of primary hyperoxalosis," *Nephrology*, vol. 10, no. 4, pp. 423–424, 2005.

[12] C. Cuvelier, E. Goffin, J. P. Cosyns, M. Wauthier, and C. Y. Strihou, "Enteric hyperoxaluria: a hidden cause of early renal graft failure in two successive transplants: spontaneous late graft recovery," *American Journal of Kidney Diseases*, vol. 40, no. 1, p. E3, 2002.

[13] H. Jahromi, I. S. D. Roberts, C. G. Winearls, and A. Vaidya, "Acute renal failure secondary to oxalosis in a recipient of a simultaneous kidney-pancreas transplant: was mycophenolate the cause?" *Nephrology Dialysis Transplantation*, vol. 23, no. 7, pp. 2409–2411, 2008.

[14] R. Parasuraman and K. K. Venkat, "Crystal-induced kidney disease in 2 kidney transplant recipients," *American Journal of Kidney Diseases*, vol. 55, no. 1, pp. 192–197, 2010.

[15] P. M. Zarembski, A. Hodgkinson, and F. M. Parsons, "Elevation of the concentration of plasma oxalic acid in renal failure," *Nature*, vol. 212, no. 5061, pp. 511–512, 1966.

[16] E. M. Worcester, S. K. Fellner, Y. Nakagawa, and F. L. Coe, "Effect of renal transplantation on serum oxalate and urinary oxalate excretion," *Nephron*, vol. 67, no. 4, pp. 414–418, 1994.

[17] S. M. Bagnasco, B. S. Mohammed, H. Mani et al., "Oxalate deposits in biopsies from native and transplanted kidneys, and impact on graft function," *Nephrology Dialysis Transplantation*, vol. 24, no. 4, pp. 1319–1325, 2009.

[18] J. I. Scheinman, J. S. Najarian, and S. M. Mauer, "Successful strategies for renal transplantation in primary oxalosis," *Kidney International*, vol. 25, no. 5, pp. 804–811, 1984.

[19] A. C. Rankin, S. B. Walsh, S. A. Summers, M. P. Owen, and M. A. Mansell, "Acute oxalate nephropathy causing late renal transplant dysfunction due to enteric hyperoxaluria," *American Journal of Transplantation*, vol. 8, no. 8, pp. 1755–1758, 2008.

[20] D. C. Cattran and S. S. A. Fenton, "Contemporary management of renal failure: outcome of the failed allograft recipient," *Kidney International*, 41, pp. S36–S39, 1993.

21

Severe Necrotizing Adenovirus Tubulointerstitial Nephritis in a Kidney Transplant Recipient

Ravi Parasuraman,[1,2] Ping L. Zhang,[3] Dilip Samarapungavan,[1] Leslie Rocher,[1] and Alan Koffron[1]

[1] *Division of Transplantation and Department of Pathology, Royal Oak, MI 48703, USA*
[2] *Oakland University William Beaumont School of Medicine, William Beaumont Hospital, Royal Oak, MI 48703, USA*
[3] *Beaumont Health System, Royal Oak, MI 48703, USA*

Correspondence should be addressed to Ravi Parasuraman; ravi.parasuraman@beaumont.edu

Academic Editors: P. A. Andrews, A. Beiras-Fernandez, and I. Engelmann

Adenoviruses (AdV) are emerging pathogens with a prevalence of 11% viruria and 6.5% viremia in kidney transplant recipients. Although AdV infection is common, interstitial nephritis (ADVIN) is rare with only 13 biopsy proven cases reported in the literature. We report a case of severe ADVIN with characteristic histological features that includes severe necrotizing granulomatous lesion with widespread tubular basement membrane rupture and hyperchromatic smudgy intranuclear inclusions in the tubular epithelial cells. The patient was asymptomatic at presentation, and the high AdV viral load (quantitative PCR>2,000,000 copies/mL in the urine and 646,642 copies/mL in the serum) confirmed the diagnosis. The patient showed excellent response to a combination of immunosuppression reduction, intravenous cidofovir, and immunoglobulin therapy resulting in complete resolution of infection and recovery of allograft function. Awareness of characteristic biopsy findings may help to clinch the diagnosis early which is essential since the disseminated infection is associated with high mortality of 18% in kidney transplant recipients. Cidofovir is considered the agent of choice for AdV infection in immunocompromised despite lack of randomized trials, and the addition of intravenous immunoglobulin may aid in resolution of infection while help prevention of rejection.

1. Introduction

Adenoviruses (AdV) are emerging pathogens in solid organ transplant recipients with clinical manifestation that ranges from subclinical infection to fatal outcome. The reported prevalence of AdV infection during the first year after kidney transplant (KT) is 11% by urine culture and 6.5% by serum PCR [1, 2]. Manifestations of urinary tract involvement may include hemorrhagic cystitis, ureteral obstruction with hydronephrosis, acute tubular necrosis, interstitial nephritis, or a mass lesion in the kidney [3–5]. Adenovirus interstitial nephritis (ADVIN) is rare in kidney transplant recipients with 13 biopsy proven cases reported in the literature [6–8]. We report a case of severe necrotizing ADVIN with characteristic morphology on biopsy within three weeks after kidney transplantation.

2. Case Report

2.1. Clinical History and Laboratory Data. A 44-year-old African American male with end-stage renal disease from hypertensive nephrosclerosis received a four-antigen mismatch, flow crossmatch negative deceased donor kidney transplantation. The patient received IL-2 receptor antagonist (Basiliximab) for induction and tacrolimus, mycophenolate mofetil (MMF), and prednisone for maintenance immunosuppression. The serological status for cytomegalovirus (CMV) was donor positive/recipient negative, and the patient received trimethoprim-sulfamethoxazole and valganciclovir for infection prophylaxis. After the transplant, the patient developed slow graft function (definition: serum creatinine (SCr) >3.0 mg/dL (265.2 μmol/L) on day 5 without requiring dialysis). Subsequently, allograft function

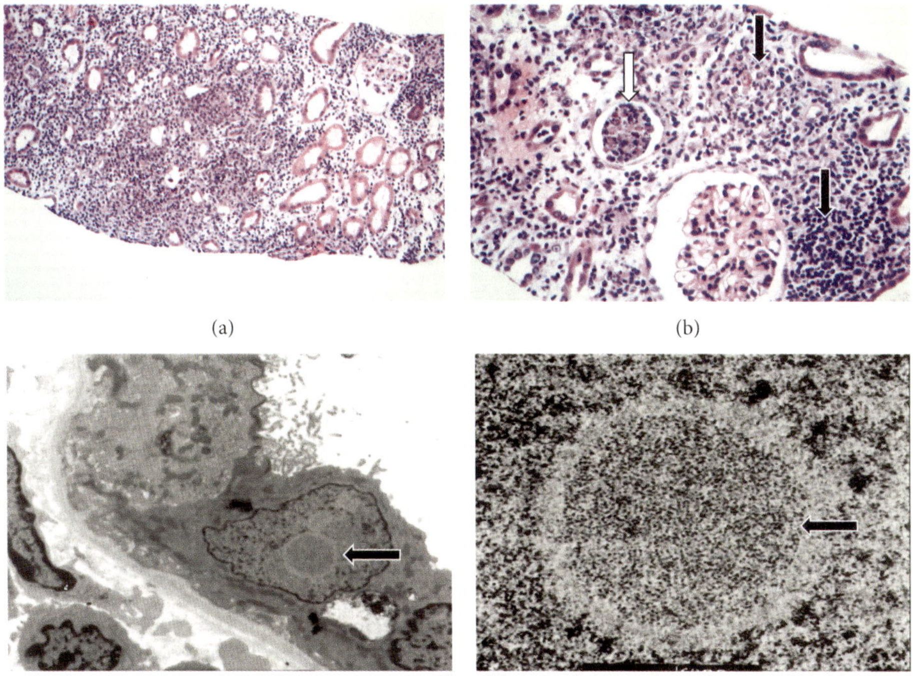

FIGURE 1: Adenovirus tubulointerstitial nephritis. Light microscopy (H&E stain): (a) Severe diffuse interstitial inflammation, (Mag ×200). (b) Granulomatous necrotizing lesions (black arrows). Inflammatory and tubular epithelial cell cast (white arrow) (Mag ×400). Electron microscopy: (c) viral inclusion body in a tubular epithelial cell (×9,500). (d) Viral particles of varying densities (×80,000).

improved with SCr decreasing to 2.33 mg/dL (205.97 μmol/L, eGFR 38 mL/min/1.73 m^2) on day 19. On subsequent followup, SCr increased to 2.81 mg/dL (248.40 μmol/L, eGFR 30 mL/min/1.73 m^2) on day 22 and his urinalysis showed persistent microscopic hematuria (RBC 10–100 cells/μL) with few atypical epithelial cells with no definite decoy cells. Since the rise in SCr could not be attributed clinically to volume status or tacrolimus toxicity (trough levels remained between 8 and 10 ng/mL), allograft ultrasound and biopsy were performed on day 24. The ultrasound showed an unexpected increase in echogenicity with poor corticomedullary differentiation, but the perfusion and resistive indices (from 0.54 to 0.63) were normal.

2.2. Kidney Biopsy. Renal allograft biopsy showed a diffuse severe inflammation consisting of mostly macrophages, neutrophils, and lymphocytes with few noncaseating granulomatous lesions (Figures 1(a) and 1(b)). The most unique feature was the presence of extensive necrosis and basophilic hyperchromatic smudgy intranuclear inclusion bodies in the tubular epithelial cells (Figure 2). Additionally, there was widespread tubular basement membrane disruption. The tubulitis was minimal with no glomerular inflammation or vasculitis. The immunostain for polyoma (BK virus) and CMV were negative. The immunofluorescence (IF) for IgG, IgA, IgM, C3, C1q, fibrinogen, kappa, and lambda in the glomeruli, and C4d stain in the peritubular capillaries were negative. Periodic acid Schiff and Jones stains were negative for bacteria or fungi. Other routine investigations such as blood and urine cultures, routine viral cultures, PCR assay for Epstein-Barr, and CMV and BK viauses were all negative. Electron microscopy (EM) showed several foci of viral particles of varying densities in the nuclei of tubular epithelial cells (Figures 1(c) and 1(d)), but the crystalloid aggregates were atypical for AdV. Because necrotizing granulomatous interstitial nephritis in the presence of smudgy intranuclear viral inclusions is considered characteristic of AdV, additional investigations such as immunohistochemical (IHC) staining, in situ hybridization, and AdV quantitative PCR in the serum and urine were requested. The IHC stain and in situ hybridization for AdV were negative, but the AdV real-time quantitative PCR (QPCR) assay showed

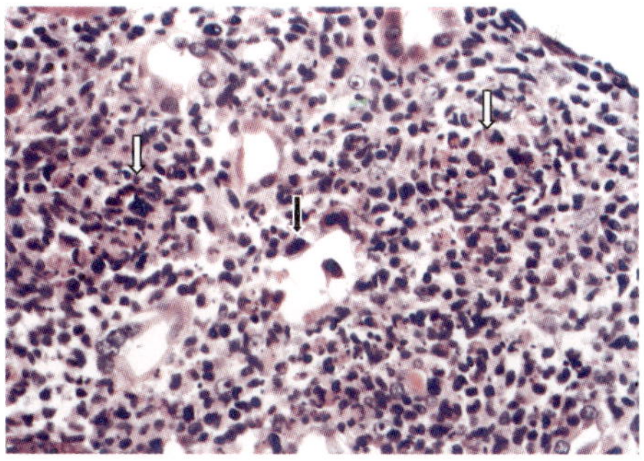

FIGURE 2: Adenovirus tubulointerstitial nephritis. Light microscopy (H&E stain): renal allograft biopsy: shows severe diffuse necrotizing granulomatous interstitial nephritis (white arrows). Basophilic, smudgy nuclear inclusions in the tubular epithelial cells (black arrow) (high power ×400).

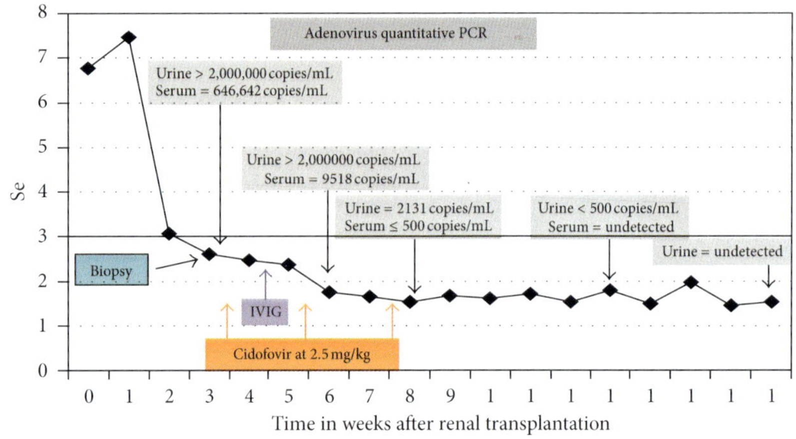

FIGURE 3: Time line and clinical course after transplantation.

>2,000,000 copies/mL in the urine (normal <500 copies/mL, Focus Diagnostics, MICROLAB, Cypress, CA, USA) and 646,642 copies/mL in the serum as shown in Figure 3. A clinical diagnosis of ADVIN was confirmed based on high viral load in the serum and urine with characteristic morphological findings on the biopsy.

2.3. Diagnosis. Necrotizing adenovirus tubulo-interstitial nephritis.

2.4. Clinical Followup. Subsequent to confirmation of AdV interstitial nephritis, immunosuppression was minimized significantly by discontinuation of MMF, reducing prednisone to 5 mg daily with a goal tacrolimus trough level from 4 to 6 ng/mL. Despite reduction in immunosuppression, the hospital course was transiently complicated by development of symptoms of intermittent fever, macroscopic hematuria, diarrhea, and mild shortness of breath. The chest X-ray showed bibasilar patchy opacities likely representing pneumonia. Consequently, a reduced dose intravenous cidofovir at 2.5 mg/kg because of impaired allograft function and intravenous immunoglobulin (IVIG) 500 mg/kg was initiated (Figure 3) for possible early dissemination. The patient responded to therapy with resolution of all systemic symptoms within a week. The patient received two additional doses of cidofovir biweekly which he tolerated without adverse events including nephrotoxicity. Subsequently, a vigilant increase in immunosuppression guided by AdV quantitative PCR was initiated in order to prevent the potential for allograft rejection. The allograft function gradually improved to a final SCr level of 1.53 mg/dL (132.6 μmol/L, eGFR 63 mL/min/1.73 m^2) during his followup. The timeline of interventions, resolution of AdV infection, and the improvement in allograft function are shown in Figure 3.

3. Discussion

Adenoviruses are nonenveloped double-stranded DNA viruses that typically cause self-limiting respiratory and gastrointestinal disease in immunocompetent individuals [9]. Recently, AdV infection is increasingly recognized in immunocompromised with high morbidity and mortality [10]. The incidence of AdV infection ranges from 3% to 47% in stem cell transplant recipients and from 5% to 22% in solid organ transplant recipients [11, 12]. AdV infection is commonly reported early after transplant when the immunosuppression is intense, and in one series 76% of all ADV infection occurred within 3 months after KT [8, 13]. AdV infection in transplant recipients may be a consequence of a primary infection, reactivation of latent infection or acquired through donor organs, and it is believed that majority of the cases are due to reactivation of latent infection [14–17]. Disseminated infection can occur in severely immunocompromised, and has been shown to be associated with poor outcome with a mortality rate of 18% in KT recipients [18].

Asymptomatic AdV infection is common, and the lack of symptoms during viremia has been reported in 58% of AdV infection in SOT recipients [2]. Hemorrhagic cystitis and interstitial pneumonitis are the most common clinical manifestations of AdV infection in kidney transplant recipients [19]. Renal allograft involvement is rare and can manifest as necrotizing tubulointerstitial nephritis and space-occupying lesion with or without ureteral obstruction [5, 6]. The common differential diagnoses for ADVIN include BK and CMV mediated interstitial nephritis for the most part when viral inclusions are present. However, presence of severe necrotizing granulomatous lesions with predominant neutrophilic inflammation would be considered characteristic for ADVIN [20, 21]. Additional features that are more pronounced in AdV interstitial nephritis include presence of mixed cellular infiltration, with macrophages and histiocytes, and tubular basement membrane disruption. Other differential diagnoses that should be considered for granulomatous interstitial nephritis in the absence of viral inclusions include drugs, anti-neutrophil cytoplasmic autoantibody associated vasculitis, tuberculosis, sarcoidosis, and fungal infections. Rarely, ADVIN and cellular rejection may coexist and pose a diagnostic challenge. In such situations, presence of overriding tubulitis, vasculitis, and predominant T-lymphocyte infiltration would favor presence of rejection [7].

Multiple diagnostic modalities may be required to clinch the diagnosis of ADVIN in cases where clinical suspicion is high. Presence of white cell casts with decoy cells on urinalysis may increase the suspicion for AdV infection. Scanning electron microscopy of urinary sediment for viral capsid and quantitative PCR for AdV DNA can confirm presence of viruria. Although tissue diagnosis is ideal for confirmation of ADVIN, not all PCR primers and antibodies used for in situ hybridization and immunohistochemistry provide complete coverage against at least 51 serotypes of adenovirus. Culture for adenovirus usually becomes positive in 2–7 days, but group D strains may take up to 4 weeks, and group F strains (serotypes 40 and 41) may not grow at all [22]. Additionally, because of the focal nature of the disease in the kidney, IHC stain and in situ hybridization may result in false negative tests. The diagnosis of ADVIN can also be confirmed by AdV QPCR assay or by typical electron microscopic finding of crystalline array particles (70–80 nm) in tubular epithelium cells when characteristic histopathological features are present in the biopsy [2, 23].

In contrast to the ADVIN case reported by Keddis et al., we were unable to confirm the presence of adenovirus in the biopsy specimen by IHC or in situ hybridization despite the characteristic morphology, presence of viral particles on EM, and high viral load in the urine and serum. Conversely, the EM did not show the viral particles in that case report, whereas in our case, we were able to find the viral particle on EM after extensive search [24]. These clinical scenarios of inability to demonstrate the virus at times in the pathological specimen are because of uncertainty of commercially available antibodies to capture the genetic diversity of the virus. These findings reiterate the caveats and interpretation of the results and do not essentially exclude the diagnosis when it is negative. In fact, the initial suspicion for ADVIN in our case was based on the characteristic histopathological findings.

The backbone of treatment for AdV infection in transplant recipient is reduction of immunosuppression. Although resolution of infection can occur with minimization of immunosuppression alone, cidofovir, a cytosine nucleotide analogue that inhibits DNA polymerase with greatest in vitro activity against AdV, is considered the agent of choice in immunocompromised despite the lack of randomized trials [25, 26]. However, the side effect profile particularly AKI and tubular dysfunction is a major concern that warrants consideration before its use. A less nephrotoxic new lipid conjugate of cidofovir, Chimerix (CMX001), may be of value in the future when available for commercial use [27].

In summary, AdV is an infrequent cause of tubulointerstitial nephritis in KT recipients and should be considered in the differential diagnosis of interstitial nephritis. Comprehension of characteristic histopathological features of ADVIN, and the caveats in its diagnosis as described in our case may facilitate an early diagnosis and better outcome. Immunosuppression reduction in all and cidofovir therapy in selected cases may significantly alter the outcome of AdV infection. Serial assessment of viral load and lymphocyte recovery are useful in monitoring the course of infection.

Abbreviations

AdV:	Adenoviruses
ADVIN:	Adenovirus interstitial nephritis
QPCR:	Quantitative PCR
KT:	Kidney transplant
IL2-receptor:	Interleukin 2 receptor
MMF:	Mycophenolate mofetil
CMV:	Cytomegalovirus
RBC:	Red blood cells
BK virus:	Polyoma
IF:	Immunofluorescence
Ig:	Immunoglobulins
EM:	Electron microscopy
IHC:	Immunohistochemical
IVIG:	Intravenous immunoglobulin
SOT:	Solid organ transplant
AKI:	Acute kidney injury
BKVN:	BK virus interstitial nephritis
ANCA:	Anti-neutrophil cytoplasmic antibodies
HSCT:	Hematopoietic stem cell transplant
CMX001:	Chimerix.

References

[1] M. G. Ison, "Adenovirus infections in transplant recipients," *Clinical Infectious Diseases*, vol. 43, no. 3, pp. 331–339, 2006.

[2] A. Humar, D. Kumar, T. Mazzulli et al., "A surveillance study of adenovirus infection in adult solid organ transplant recipients," *American Journal of Transplantation*, vol. 5, no. 10, pp. 2555–2559, 2005.

[3] M. Ito, N. Hirabayashi, Y. Uno, A. Nakayama, and J. Asai, "Necrotizing tubulointerstitial nephritis associated with adenovirus infection," *Human Pathology*, vol. 22, no. 12, pp. 1225–1231, 1991.

[4] J. Kapelushnik, A. Verstandig, R. Or et al., "Hydronephrosis in children after bone marrow transplantation: case reports," *Bone Marrow Transplantation*, vol. 17, no. 5, pp. 873–875, 1996.

[5] A. K. H. Lim, S. Parsons, and F. Ierino, "Adenovirus tubulointerstitial nephritis presenting as a renal allograft space occupying lesion," *American Journal of Transplantation*, vol. 5, no. 8, pp. 2062–2066, 2005.

[6] L. M. Kolankiewicz, J. Pullman, M. Raffeld, J. B. Kopp, and D. Glicklich, "Adenovirus nephritis and obstructive uropathy in a renal transplant recipient: case report and literature review," *NDT Plus*, vol. 3, no. 4, pp. 388–392, 2010.

[7] L. Storsley and I. W. Gibson, "Adenovirus interstitial nephritis and rejection in an allograft," *Journal of the American Society of Nephrology*, vol. 22, no. 8, pp. 1423–1427, 2011.

[8] S. P. Watcharananan, R. Avery, A. Ingsathit et al., "Adenovirus disease after kidney transplantation: course of infection and outcome in relation to blood viral load and immune recovery," *American Journal of Transplantation*, vol. 11, no. 6, pp. 1308–1314, 2011.

[9] O. Ruuskanen, O. Meurman, and G. Akusjarvi, "Adenoviruses," in *Clinical Virology*, D. D. Richmann, R. J. Whitley, and F. G. Hayden, Eds., pp. 515–535, ASM Press, Washington, DC, USA, 2002.

[10] M. Echavarria, "Adenoviruses in immunocompromised hosts," *Clinical Microbiology Reviews*, vol. 21, no. 4, pp. 704–715, 2008.

[11] B. Kampmann, D. Cubitt, T. Walls et al., "Improved outcome for children with disseminated adenoviral infection following allogeneic stem cell transplantation," *British Journal of Haematology*, vol. 130, no. 4, pp. 595–603, 2005.

[12] R. H. Rubin, S. A. Kemmerly, D. Conti et al., "Prevention of primary cytomegalovirus disease in organ transplant recipients with oral ganciclovir or oral acyclovir prophylaxis," *Transplant Infectious Disease*, vol. 2, no. 3, pp. 112–117, 2000.

[13] R. R. Razonable and A. J. Eid, "Viral infections in transplant recipients," *Minerva Medica*, vol. 100, no. 6, pp. 479–501, 2009.

[14] T. Kojaoghlanian, P. Flomenberg, and M. S. Horwitz, "The impact of adenovirus infection on the immunocompromised host," *Reviews in Medical Virology*, vol. 13, no. 3, pp. 155–171, 2003.

[15] L. R. Krilov, "Adenovirus infections in the immunocompromised host," *Pediatric Infectious Disease Journal*, vol. 24, no. 6, pp. 555–556, 2005.

[16] N. Singh-Naz, M. Brown, and M. Ganeshananthan, "Nosocomial adenovirus infection: molecular epidemiology of an outbreak," *Pediatric Infectious Disease Journal*, vol. 12, no. 11, pp. 922–925, 1993.

[17] V. Venard, A.-S. Carret, D. Corsaro, P. Bordigoni, and A. Le Faou, "Genotyping of adenoviruses isolated in an outbreak in a bone marrow transplant unit shows that diverse strains are involved," *Journal of Hospital Infection*, vol. 44, no. 1, pp. 71–74, 2000.

[18] J. C. Hierholzer, "Adenoviruses in the immunocompromised host," *Clinical Microbiology Reviews*, vol. 5, no. 3, pp. 262–274, 1992.

[19] T. Umekawa and T. Kurita, "Acute hemorrhagic cystitis by adenovirus type 11 with and without type 37 after kidney transplantation," *Urologia Internationalis*, vol. 56, no. 2, pp. 114–116, 1996.

[20] M. Asim, A. Chong-Lopez, and V. Nickeleit, "Adenovirus infection of a renal allograft," *American Journal of Kidney Diseases*, vol. 41, no. 3, pp. 696–701, 2003.

[21] A. Gaspert, B. Lüthi, N. J. Mueller et al., "Subacute allograft failure with dysuria and hematuria in a kidney transplant recipient," *American Journal of Kidney Diseases*, vol. 54, no. 1, pp. 154–158, 2009.

[22] P. Randhawa, "Adnenovirus nephritis: a pathologicperspective," *eAJKD the Official Blog of AJKD*. In press.

[23] A. C. Lankester, M. J. D. Van Tol, E. C. J. Claas, J. M. Vossen, and A. C. M. Kroes, "Quantification of adenovirus DNA in plasma for management of infection in stem cell graft recipients," *Clinical Infectious Diseases*, vol. 34, no. 6, pp. 864–867, 2002.

[24] M. Keddis, N. Leung, S. Herrmann, Z. El-Zoghby, and S. Sethi, "Adenovirus-induced interstitial nephritis following umbilical cord blood transplant for chronic lymphocytic leukemia," *American Journal of Kidney Diseases*, vol. 59, no. 6, pp. 886–890, 2012.

[25] P. Ljungman, P. Ribaud, M. Eyrich et al., "Cidofovir for adenovirus infections after allogeneic hematopoietic stem cell transplantation: a survey by the Infectious Diseases Working Party of the European Group for Blood and Marrow Transplantation," *Bone Marrow Transplantation*, vol. 31, no. 6, pp. 481–486, 2003.

[26] K. Nagafuji, K. Aoki, H. Henzan et al., "Cidofovir for treating adenoviral hemorrhagic cystitis in hematopoietic stem cell transplant recipients," *Bone Marrow Transplantation*, vol. 34, no. 10, pp. 909–914, 2004.

[27] D. F. Florescu, S. A. Pergam, M. N. Neely et al., "Safety and efficacy of CMX001 as salvage therapy for severe adenovirus infections in immunocompromised patients," *Biology of Blood and Marrow Transplantation*, vol. 18, no. 5, pp. 731–738, 2012.

22

De Novo Renal Cell Carcinoma in a Kidney Allograft 20 Years after Transplant

Masataka Banshodani,[1] Hideki Kawanishi,[1] Seiji Marubayashi,[1] Sadanori Shintaku,[1] Misaki Moriishi,[1] Fumio Shimamoto,[2] Shinichiro Tsuchiya,[1] Kiyohiko Dohi,[3] and Hideki Ohdan[4]

[1] *Department of Artificial Organs, Akane-Foundation, Tsuchiya General Hospital, 3-30 Nakajimacho, Naka-ku, Hiroshima 730-8655, Japan*
[2] *Department of Pathology, Faculty of Human Culture and Science, Prefectural University of Hiroshima, 1-1-71 Ujina-Higashi, Minami-ku, Hiroshima 734-8558, Japan*
[3] *Department of Surgery, Akane-Foundation, Tsuchiya General Hospital, 3-30 Nakajimacho, Naka-ku, Hiroshima 730-8655, Japan*
[4] *Department of Gastroenterological and Transplant Surgery, Applied Life Sciences, Institution of Biomedical & Health Sciences, Hiroshima University, 1-2-3 Kasumi, Minami-ku, Hiroshima 734-8551, Japan*

Correspondence should be addressed to Masataka Banshodani; m-banshodani@tsuchiya-hp.jp

Academic Editor: Marian Klinger

Renal cell carcinoma (RCC) in a kidney allograft is rare. We report the successful diagnosis and treatment of a *de novo* RCC in a nonfunctioning kidney transplant 20 years after engraftment. A 54-year-old man received a kidney transplant from his mother when he was 34 years old. After 10 years, chronic rejection resulted in graft failure, and the patient became hemodialysis-dependent. Intravenous contrast-enhanced computed tomography (CT) for the evaluation of gastrointestinal symptoms revealed a solid 13 mm tumor in the kidney graft. The tumor was confirmed on ultrasound examination. This tumor had not been detected on a surveillance noncontrast CT scan. Needle biopsy showed that the tumor was an RCC. Allograft nephrectomy was performed. Pathological examination showed that the tumor was a Fuhrman Grade 2 RCC. XY-fluorescence hybridization analysis of the RCC showed that the tumor cells were of donor origin. One year after the surgery, the patient is alive and has no evidence of tumor recurrence. Regardless of whether a kidney transplant is functioning, it should periodically be imaged for RCC throughout the recipient's lifetime. In our experience, ultrasonography or CT with intravenous contrast is better than CT without contrast for the detection of tumor in a nonfunctioning kidney transplant.

1. Introduction

Renal cell carcinoma (RCC) is more likely to occur in a native kidney of a transplant recipient than in the general population [1]. On the other hand, RCC in a kidney allograft is rare [2]. In a previous study, kidney carcinomas represented 4.6% of posttransplant cancers, as compared with 3% of tumors in the general population. However, among these carcinomas, only 10% occurred in kidney grafts [3]. Therefore, the management of RCC in a kidney graft has not yet been established. Kidney graft tumors can be carcinomas that are transmitted by donors, metastatic carcinomas from the recipient's native organs, or *de novo* carcinomas that occur after transplant. Identification of the origin of a kidney graft tumor can improve therapeutic safety and certainty. Here, we report the successful diagnosis and treatment of a *de novo* RCC in a nonfunctioning kidney transplant 20 years after engraftment.

2. Case Presentation

A 54-year-old man with a history of immunoglobulin A nephropathy received a sex-mismatched kidney transplant (left kidney graft) from his mother when he was 34 years old.

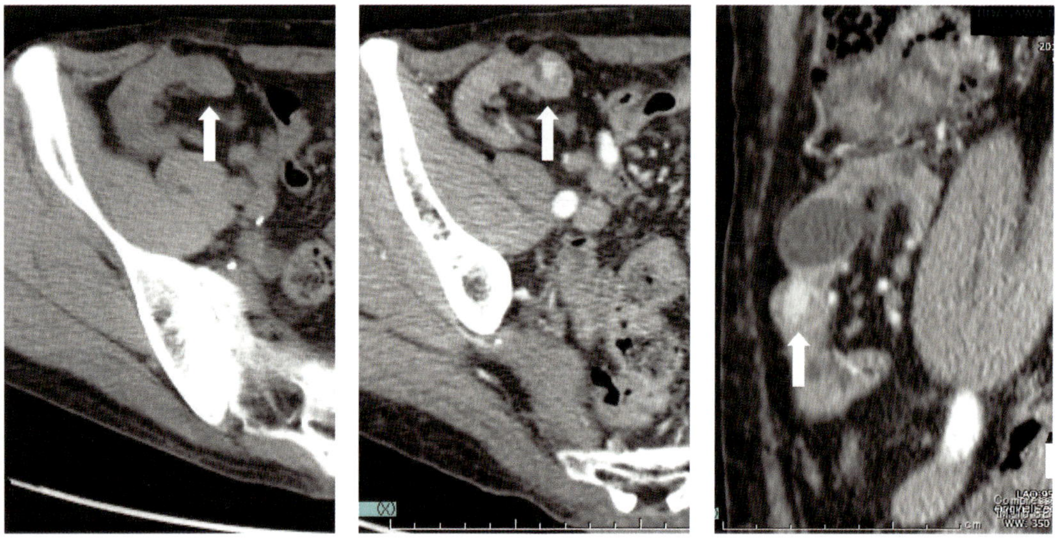

(a) (b) (c)

FIGURE 1: Computed tomography images. (a) A noncontrast computed tomography (CT) scan in the horizontal view, revealing no tumor in the kidney graft. (b) and (c) Intravenous contrast-enhanced CT scans in horizontal (b) and sagittal (c) views showing an enhanced solid tumor in the kidney graft (*white arrows*).

The donor underwent angiographic examination to ensure that there is no tumor stain in the left kidney (i.e., she had not developed a kidney tumor) prior to the transplant. Immunosuppression was induced with cyclosporine, methylprednisolone, mizoribine, and antilymphocyte globulin treatment for 20 days and was maintained with cyclosporine, methylprednisolone, and mizoribine treatment. After 10 years, chronic rejection led to kidney graft failure, and the patient became hemodialysis-dependent. After the transplant, he underwent a noncontrast computed tomography (CT) examination every year, but no tumor became evident in the kidney graft. Twenty years after engraftment, intravenous contrast-enhanced CT for the evaluation of gastrointestinal symptoms revealed an enhanced solid tumor with a diameter of approximately 13 mm in the kidney graft (Figures 1(b) and 1(c)). This tumor was not seen on noncontrast CT performed at the same time (Figure 1(a)). No other abnormal tumor shadows were observed. Ultrasonography revealed a solid 12.9 mm tumor with a hypoechoic rim in the superficial cortex of the kidney graft (Figures 2(a) and 2(b)). The hypervascular nature of the tumor was confirmed on Doppler imaging (Figure 2(c)). Allograft nephrectomy was performed after RCC was identified in a needle biopsy specimen of the graft tumor. Macroscopically, the tumor was a solid nodule, 13 mm wide, and encapsulated with a clear margin (Figures 3(a) and 3(b)). On pathological examination, the tumor was composed almost exclusively of clear cells that exhibited trabecular or papillary growth patterns, and the cells partially involved the capsule surrounding the tumor (Figures 3(c) and 3(d)). The tumor was diagnosed as Grade 2 clear cell carcinoma, according to the Fuhrman classification. XY-fluorescence *in situ* hybridization (XY-FISH) analysis was performed on the graft tumor; an XX genotype was seen in 85% of the tumor cells and an XY genotype was seen in 15% of the tumor cells, including the blood cells from the recipient (Figures 3(e) and 3(f)). These findings showed that the tumor originated from the donor tissue. The patient recovered uneventfully and was discharged 11 days after the operation. One year after the surgery, he is alive and has no evidence of tumor recurrence.

3. Discussion

Cases of RCCs in kidney allografts have rarely been reported. The incidence of *de novo* carcinomas in kidney allografts is reported to be 0.19–0.5% [2, 4]. Periodic ultrasonography and CT are useful for diagnosing kidney graft tumors [5, 6]. The time from kidney transplant to detection of a tumor in the kidney graft has ranged from 9 months to 29 years [4, 6, 7]. In our case, 20 years after engraftment, a tumor was detected in the tumor graft on intravenous contrast-enhanced CT and ultrasonography; however, it was not visible on noncontrast CT.

Kidney graft tumors can be carcinomas that are transmitted by donors, metastatic carcinomas from native recipient organs, or *de novo* carcinomas that occur after transplant. When a kidney graft tumor is detected within a short period after kidney transplant, the tumor is likely transmitted by the donor. However, the growth rate of kidney graft tumors is unknown. One study reported that *de novo* kidney graft carcinoma rapidly developed 9 months after transplant [8]. On the other hand, Tillou et al. concluded that *de novo* kidney graft tumors are predominantly low grade and not aggressive [2]. Therefore, it is difficult to accurately identify the tumor's origin based on the period between kidney transplant and tumor detection. Lotan and Laufer [9] identified the origin of a kidney graft tumor by performing DNA analysis. Moreover,

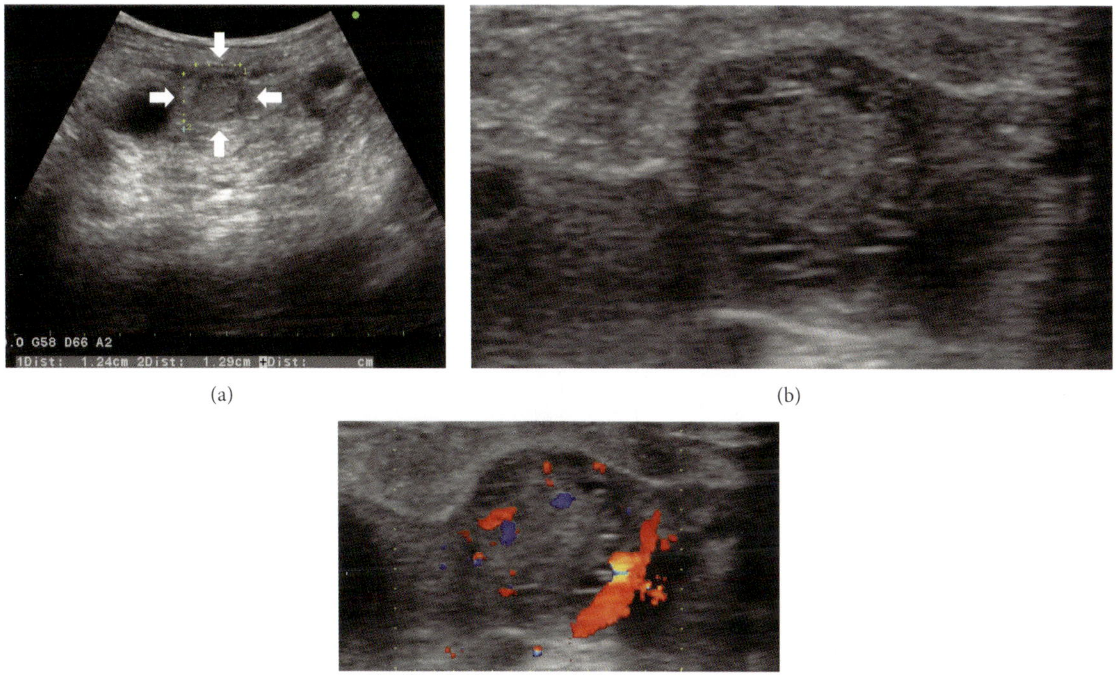

FIGURE 2: Ultrasonography images. (a) and (b) Ultrasonography revealing a solid tumor with a hypoechoic rim in the superficial cortex of the kidney graft (*white arrows*). (c) The hypervascular nature of the kidney graft tumor is confirmed on a Doppler image.

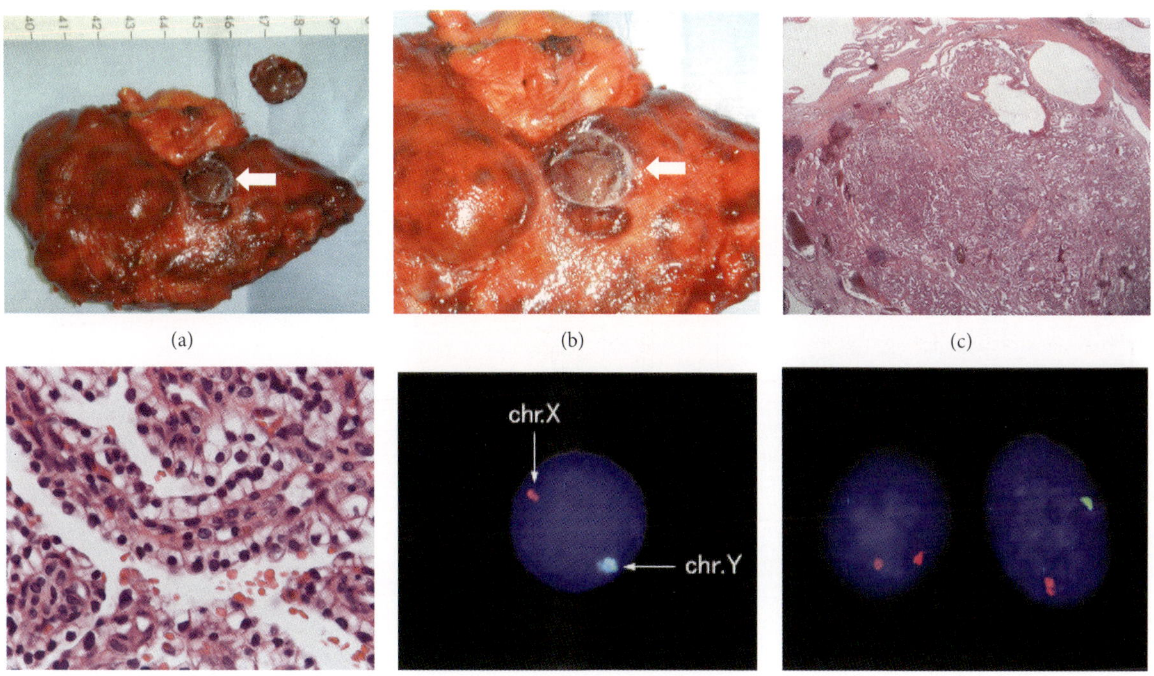

FIGURE 3: Pathological tissue images. (a) and (b) Allograft nephrectomy revealed that the tumor was 13 mm, Grade G2, INFb, v0, ly0, eg, fc1, im0, rc-inf1, rp-inf0, s-inf0, pT1a, pN0, pM0, and stage I. (c) and (d) On pathological examination (hematoxylin and eosin staining), the tumor was composed almost exclusively of clear cells that exhibited trabecular or papillary growth patterns in (c) low-power (10x) and (d) high-power (400x) fields. (e) and (f) An XY-fluorescence *in situ* hybridization (FISH) analysis performed on the kidney graft tumor revealing (e) healthy XX genotype control cells (lymphocytes) as well as (f) XX genotype cells (*left*) and XY genotype cells (*right*) in the tumor, including blood cells from the recipient. chr., chromosome.

another study reported that XY-FISH was useful for identifying the tumor's origin in cases of sex-mismatched kidney transplants [10]. Overall, however, the tumor's origin has been identified in few cases. In our case, the tumor's origin was successfully identified by XY-FISH analysis.

Kidney graft tumors are usually treated surgically. Allograft nephrectomy is justified when a tumor is >40 mm in size, deeply located within the graft, or a recurrence. On the other hand, nephron-sparing surgery can maintain quality of life by retaining kidney graft function and is therefore justified for small tumors with low risks of recurrence [2, 4]. In our case, the kidney graft tumor was treated with allograft nephrectomy because the graft was nonfunctional.

In an analysis of histological types, Tillou et al. [2] reported that papillary carcinomas represented >50% of kidney graft tumors and that low-grade tumors (Fuhrman Grades 1 and 2) accounted for 65% of kidney graft tumors. In our case, the tumor was diagnosed as a Fuhrman Grade 2 clear cell carcinoma.

In the present case, a tumor in a nonfunctional kidney graft was successfully treated with allograft nephrectomy. Further, the tumor's origin was successfully identified by XY-FISH analysis, 20 years after engraftment. To detect RCC, a kidney transplant should be imaged periodically throughout a recipient's lifetime, regardless of whether the kidney transplant is functioning. In our experience, ultrasonography or CT with intravenous contrast is better than CT without contrast for the detection of a tumor in a nonfunctioning kidney transplant.

References

[1] J. R. Chapman, A. C. Webster, and G. Wong, "Cancer in the transplant recipient," *Cold Spring Harbor Perspectives in Medicine*, vol. 3, no. 7, 2013.

[2] X. Tillou, A. Doerfler, S. Collon et al., "De novo kidney graft tumors: results from a multicentric retrospective national study," *American Journal of Transplantation*, vol. 12, no. 12, pp. 3308–3315, 2012.

[3] I. Penn, "Primary kidney tumors before and after renal transplantation," *Transplantation*, vol. 59, no. 4, pp. 480–485, 1995.

[4] A. Barama, G. St-Louis, V. Nicolet, R. Hadjeres, and P. Daloze, "Renal cell carcinoma in kidney allografts: a case series from a single center," *American Journal of Transplantation*, vol. 5, no. 12, pp. 3015–3018, 2005.

[5] M. Claudon, V. Panescu, L. Le Chaffotec et al., "Primary adenocarcinoma of the renal transplant," *Nephrology Dialysis Transplantation*, vol. 13, no. 10, pp. 2667–2670, 1998.

[6] K. Akioka, K. Masuda, S. Harada et al., "How long should we follow the post-transplantation patient after graft loss? A case report of renal cancer in the grafted kidney that occurred 16 years after graft loss," *Transplantation Proceedings*, vol. 46, no. 2, pp. 626–629, 2014.

[7] S. M. Baughman, W. J. Sexton, C. W. Glanton, N. C. Dalrymple, and J. T. Bishoff, "Computerized tomography guided radio frequency ablation of a renal cell carcinoma within a renal allograft," *The Journal of Urology*, vol. 172, no. 4, pp. 1262–1263, 2004.

[8] Y. Gunji, K. Sakamoto, K. Yamada et al., "Successful surgical treatment of renal cell carcinoma in a transplanted kidney from a cadaveric donor: report of a case," *Surgery Today*, vol. 31, no. 4, pp. 374–377, 2001.

[9] D. Lotan and J. Laufer, "Metastatic renal carcinoma in a pediatric recipient of an adult cadaveric donor kidney," *The American Journal of Kidney Diseases*, vol. 26, no. 6, pp. 960–962, 1995.

[10] J. Verine, M. Varna, P. Ratajczak et al., "Human de novo papillary renal-cell carcinomas in a kidney graft: evidence of recipient origin with adenoma-carcinoma sequence," *The American Journal of Transplantation*, vol. 13, no. 4, pp. 984–992, 2013.

23

Successful Treatment of Recurrent Pulmonary Mucormycosis in a Renal Transplant Patient

Morgan S. Martin,[1] Alison A. Smith,[1] Monica Lobo,[2] and Anil S. Paramesh[3]

[1]*Department of Surgery, Tulane University School of Medicine, New Orleans, LA, USA*
[2]*Department of Pathology, Tulane University, School of Medicine, New Orleans, LA, USA*
[3]*Tulane University School of Medicine, Tulane Abdominal Transplant Institute, New Orleans, LA, USA*

Correspondence should be addressed to Alison A. Smith; alison.annette.smith@gmail.com

Academic Editor: David Conti

Background. We describe the unusual case of a recently transplanted cadaveric renal transplant recipient who presented with recurrent pulmonary mucormycosis. *Case Report.* An 18-year-old man with end stage renal disease secondary to congenital renal agenesis status after cadaveric kidney transplant 4 months before presented with acute onset of fever, hemoptysis, and back pain. The patient underwent an emergent left lower lobectomy due to the critical nature of his illness. He was also treated with amphotericin with resolution of his symptoms. One week later, he had evidence of recurrent disease on imaging with a surgical site infection. He underwent reexploration with evacuation of an empyema and debridement of a surgical site infection. He was continued on IV antifungal therapy with isavuconazonium and amphotericin. Radiographic clearance of disease with three months of treatment was apparent with no evidence of recurrence at seven-month follow-up. *Discussion.* Opportunistic infections in solid organ transplant patients represent a significant source of morbidity and mortality. Most patients are treated with prophylactic anti-infective agents. However, rare infections such as pulmonary mucormycosis remain a risk. The transplant physician must be aware of these uncommon infections and their treatment strategies, including the management of uncommon recurrent disease.

1. Introduction

Mucormycosis, which includes fungi in the Mucorales order such as *Rhizopus* and *Mucor,* represents a rare but aggressive infection of immunosuppressed patients. Less than one percent of solid organ transplant patients are infected; however mortality can exceed greater than 80% [1–5]. Rhinocerebral, pulmonary, gastrointestinal, and disseminated disease are the most common sites for infection [6].

Most infections occur within the first year of solid organ transplant [7]. The vast majority of patients infected by mucormycosis are male, older than age of 40 with multiple risk factors, including neutropenia, diabetes, active malignancy, and iron overloaded states. In particular, renal transplant recipients are at even high risk given the presence of comorbid diabetes, use of immunosuppressants, the frequent use of voriconazole and echinocandins to treat fungal infections in transplant patients, and uremia [3, 8]. Pulmonary mucormycosis is the most common site of infection for renal transplant recipients [9]. In addition, the southern United States has the highest incidence of mucormycosis compared to other regions of the country [5].

Mucorales have known resistance to caspofungin and voriconazole. Accordingly, amphotericin B is regarded as the first-line therapeutic agent for mucormycosis [10]. However, the use of amphotericin B usually results in renal injury and concomitant loss of the renal allograft. Use of posaconazole has been proposed in several studies; however it has not shown to be as effective as amphotericin B [11]. Thus, emerging treatment strategies have included extended spectrum azoles with specific activity against Mucorales with improved side effect profiles [12, 13].

Surgical debridement is essential for effective treatment of mucormycosis. Due to the aggressive behavior of this fungus in immunocompromised patients, extensive surgical debridement has appeared to be necessary in successful

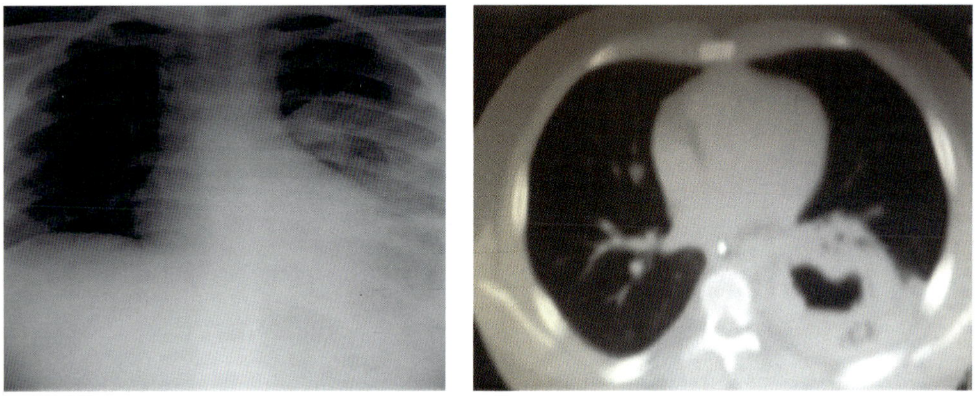

(a) (b)

Figure 1: (a) Initial chest X-ray on initial presentation for an 18-year-old man status after cadaveric kidney transplant demonstrating increased opacification of the mid and lower left lung fields. (b) Computerized topography of chest/thorax for the same patient demonstrating a left lobe cavitary lesion.

clearance of disease reported in various case series [3, 14, 15]. A review of the literature did not identify any studies on the recommended treatment of recurrent pulmonary mucormycosis.

We report the unusual case of a renal transplant recipient with refractory pulmonary mucormycosis. The objective of our study is to describe the management of recurrent lung mucormycosis in a recent cadaveric renal transplant recipient. This case report adds to the growing body of literature surrounding this phenomenon and to elucidating effective treatment algorithms.

2. Case Presentation

An 18-year-old man with history of end stage renal disease secondary to congenital renal agenesis presented to the Emergency Department with an acute onset of hemoptysis, back pain, and fever. He had undergone a cadaveric kidney transplant four months before at a different institution. The transplant was performed without any complications, and the patient had reportedly normal kidney function. He was taking cyclosporine, mycophenolate, and prednisone for maintenance immunosuppression. He was not on any antifungal prophylaxis. The patient was not residing in a house with routine expose to soil and livestock. He denied any weight loss or recent foreign travel. His laboratory values were significant for leukocytosis with a white blood cell count of 21,900/mm^3 and elevated creatinine. His initial chest X-ray demonstrated a consolidation of the left lower lobe (Figure 1(a)). Further imaging on chest CT showed a left lower lobe cavitary lesion (Figure 1(b)). Sputum, bronchoalveolar lavage, and blood cultures were all negative for infectious etiology. His workup was additionally negative for any additional infectious etiology. His renal biopsy showed no evidence of rejection or active infection. He was initially started on broad-spectrum antibiotics and antifungals. His immunosuppressants were held.

He was taken for an open thoracotomy with a left lower lobectomy one week after initial presentation due to the critical nature of his illness. Intraoperatively, he was found to have a solitary consolidated fungal mass surrounded by an area of hemorrhagic necrosis (Figure 2). Final pathology showed *Rhizopus* species (Figure 3). Treatment was initiated with IV liposomal amphotericin B 50 mg daily.

The patient demonstrated overall clinical improvement. However, one week postoperatively, the patient developed a new consolidation of his left upper lobe on chest X-ray. Repeat chest CT demonstrated an empyema. The patient also had *Rhizopus* cultured from his surgical site. He remained febrile with significant leukocytosis. He was taken to the operating room for an evacuation of an empyema and debridement of soft tissue surrounding the incision (Figures 4(a) and 4(b)).

Despite aggressive surgical management of his recurrent disease, the patient continued to remain symptomatic. However, he had evidence of consolidations in both lungs (Figure 5). It was then decided to add isavuconazonium (372 mg daily). The patient improved clinically, and he was discharged home 24 days after his initial presentation.

The patient was maintained on the regimen of amphotericin B (50 mg daily) and isavuconazonium (372 mg daily) after discharge. His follow-up chest X-ray 7 months after treatment showed no evidence of residual disease. His medications were discontinued at this time. To our knowledge, he has had no further issues.

3. Discussion

Mucormycosis is a rare infection with a high likelihood of devastating outcomes in immunocompromised patients. Currently, there is a paucity of data on optimal treatment strategies. In particular, there are no clinical studies that demonstrate successful treatment of patients with recurrent mucormycosis. Our case report demonstrates a strategy to combat recurrent mucormycosis using salvage therapy

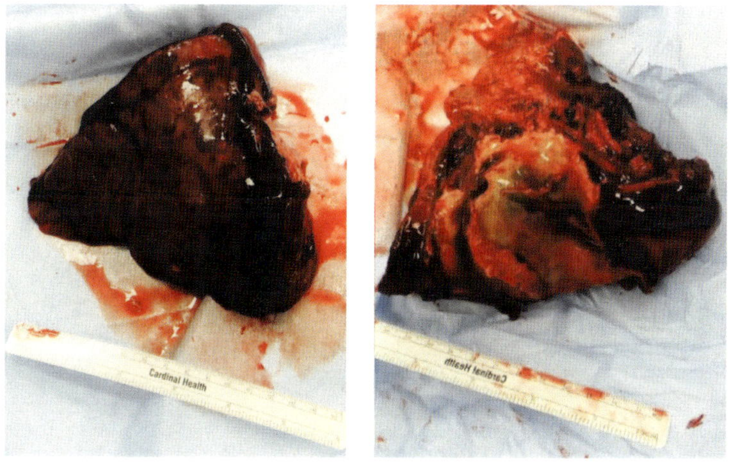

(a) (b)

FIGURE 2: Gross pathology of consolidated fungal mass removed from lung of an 18-year-old male status after cadaveric kidney transplant. (a) Anterior and (b) posterior views of left lower lobe demonstrating a large consolidated fungal mass surrounded by area of hemorrhagic necrosis.

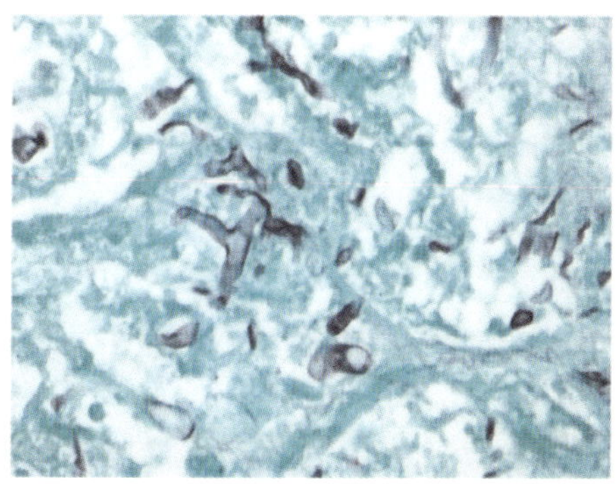

FIGURE 3: Grocott-Gomori methenamine-silver (GMS) stained tissue section of resected lung from an 18-year-old with recent kidney transplant highlighting aseptate hyphae morphologically resembling fungal class *Zygomycetes* (400x).

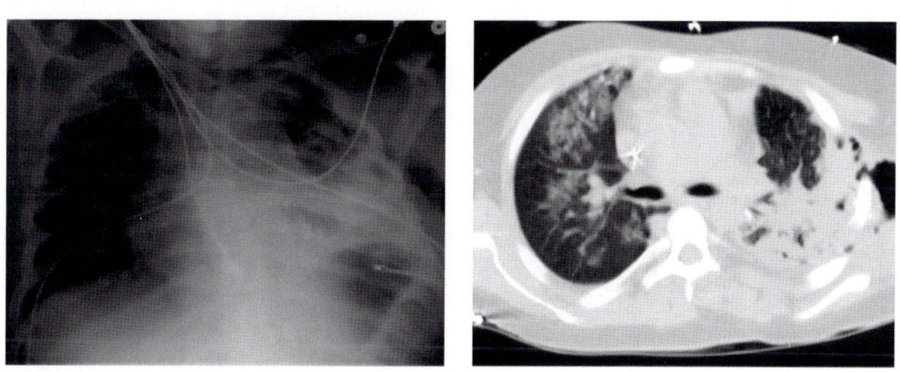

(a) (b)

FIGURE 4: 18-year-old male renal transplant recipient 24 days status after resection of left lower lobe for a fungating mass with (a) chest X-ray demonstrating left upper lobe consolidation and (b) chest computerized topography scan showing consolidation of right upper, middle, and lower lobes.

Table 1: Summary of existing publications on mucormycosis in renal transplant recipients.

Reference	Number of patients	Organ (N)	Treatment	Mortality N (%)
Fisher et al., 1980	1	Skin (1)	AmpB, surgery	1/1 (100)
Nampoory et al., 1996	2	Lungs (1); allograft (1)	AmpB, fluconazole	—
Bakshi and Volk, 2001	1	Lungs (1)	AmpB	0/1 (0)
Godara et al., 2011	16	Rhino (9); lungs (5); allograft (1); disseminated (1)	AmpB, surgery	6/16 (37.5)
Zhao et al., 2012	1	Cutaneous (1)	AmpB, surgery	0/1 (0)
Hatahet et al., 2013	1	Disseminated (1)	AmpB, Mica, surgery	1/1 (100)
Stewart et al., 2014	1	Lungs (1)	Pos, AmpB, Mica, surgery	0/1 (0)
Patel et al., 2014	1	Lungs (1)	Pos, caspofungin	1/1 (100)
Santos et al., 2015	2	Lungs (2)	AmpB, surgery	2/2 (100)
Kursun et al., 2015	1	Rhino (1)	AmpB, surgery	—
Palejwala et al., 2016	2	Rhino (2)	AmpB, Pos, mica, Isa, surgery	2/2 100
Vaezi et al., 2016	20	Rhino (9); lungs (5); cutaneous (3); disseminated (2) pseudoaneurysm (1)	AmpB, Pos	10/20 (50)

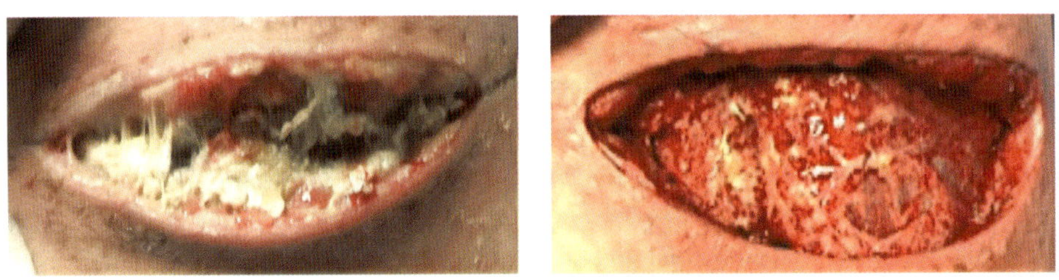

(a) (b)

Figure 5: 18-year-old male renal transplant recipient with pulmonary mucormycosis who developed disseminated skin infection with mucormycosis at thoracotomy site (a) and following debridement (b).

with isavuconazonium. An initial strategy of IV liposomal amphotericin B combined with a newer medication, isavuconazonium, was employed along with aggressive surgical debridement. Despite initial efforts, the patient had evidence of recurrent pulmonary mucormycosis with dissemination of the infection to his surgical incision.

The current gold standard for mucormycosis is IV liposomal amphotericin B, surgical debridement, and, if possible, modification of risk factors [8, 10, 11]. Previous case reports have demonstrated the use of posaconazole for salvage therapy. In our study, we used isavuconazonium. Isavuconazonium is a recently developed extended spectrum azole. Studies have demonstrated clinical response to isavuconazonium with a better side effect profile than amphotericin B and posaconazole [12, 13]. In particular, the incidence of renal injury is significantly lower with isavuconazonium. Aggressive surgical debridement in combination with antifungals has shown to be a mainstay of treatment for mucormycosis. However, despite this knowledge, some case studies reviewed had high mortality rate, approaching 100% in some studies [12–17]. A summary of published reports from previous studies is presented in Table 1.

There are several important limitations to our study. First, we presented evidence from a single patient. High-quality randomized control trials are needed to further elucidate the use of isavuconazonium. Additionally, it is possible to consider that the first pneumonectomy was inadequate and contributed to the spread of the initial disease to the patient's skin.

In conclusion, we present a rare case of recurrent pulmonary mucormycosis with skin dissemination in an immunocompromised patient that was successfully managed with a combination of surgical treatment and aggressive pharmacologic therapy, including amphotericin B and isavuconazonium. It is also important to be aware of this possible diagnosis in all immunosuppressed patients and to be well-versed on potential treatment options for recurrent or refractory disease.

References

[1] A. Chkhotua, A. Yussim, A. Tovar et al., "Mucormycosis of the renal allograft: case report and review of the literature," *Transplant International*, vol. 14, no. 6, pp. 438–441, 2001.

[2] M. R. N. Nampoory, Z. U. Khan, K. V. Johny et al., "Invasive fungal infections in renal transplant recipients," *Journal of Infection*, vol. 33, no. 2, pp. 95–101, 1996.

[3] S. M. Godara, V. B. Kute, K. R. Goplani et al., "Mucormycosis in renal transplant recipients: predictors and outcome," *Saudi Journal of Kidney Diseases and Transplantation*, vol. 22, no. 4, pp. 751–756, 2011.

[4] M. H. Hatahet, M. Narayanan, C. Cleaves, and R. Zreik, "Disseminated mucormycosis in a patient with recent kidney transplantation: a case report and review of the literature," *Case Reports in Nephrology and Urology*, vol. 3, no. 1, pp. 58–63, 2013.

[5] B. J. Park, P. G. Pappas, K. A. Wannemuehler et al., "Invasive non-*Aspergillus*mold infections in transplant recipients, United States, 2001–2006," *Emerging Infectious Diseases*, vol. 17, no. 10, pp. 1855–1864, 2011.

[6] D. F. Florescu and U. Sandkovsky, "Fungal infections in intestinal and multivisceral transplant recipients," *Current Opinion in Organ Transplantation*, vol. 20, no. 3, pp. 295–302, 2015.

[7] G. Hamilos, G. Samonis, and D. P. Kontoyiannis, "Pulmonary mucormycosis," *Seminars in Respiratory and Critical Care Medicine*, vol. 32, no. 6, pp. 693–702, 2011.

[8] N. G. Almyroudis, D. A. Sutton, P. Linden, M. G. Rinaldi, J. Fung, and S. Kusne, "Zygomycosis in solid organ transplant recipients in a tertiary transplant center and review of the literature," *American Journal of Transplantation*, vol. 6, no. 10, pp. 2365–2374, 2006.

[9] J. A. Vazquez, M. H. Miceli, and G. Alangaden, "Invasive fungal infections in transplant recipients," *Therapeutic Advances in Infectious Disease*, vol. 1, no. 3, pp. 85–105, 2013.

[10] N. Singh, J. M. Aguado, H. Bonatti et al., "Zygomycosis in solid organ transplant recipients: a prospective, matched case-control study to assess risks for disease and outcome," *Journal of Infectious Diseases*, vol. 200, no. 6, pp. 1002–1011, 2009.

[11] M. A. Donnelley, E. S. Zhu, and G. R. Thompson, "Isavuconazole in the treatment of invasive aspergillosis and mucormycosis infections," *Infection and Drug Resistance*, vol. 9, pp. 79–86, 2016.

[12] B. Graves, C. O. Morrissey, A. Wei et al., "Isavuconazole as salvage therapy for mucormycosis," *Medical Mycology Case Reports*, vol. 11, pp. 36–39, 2016.

[13] S. E. Nagy-Agren, P. Chu, G. J. W. Smith, H. A. Waskin, and F. L. Altice, "Zygomycosis (mucormycosis) and HIV infection: report of three cases and review," *Journal of Acquired Immune Deficiency Syndromes and Human Retrovirology*, vol. 10, no. 4, pp. 441–449, 1995.

[14] S. Palejwala, T. Zangeneh, S. Goldstein, and G. Lemole, "An aggressive multidisciplinary approach reduces mortality in rhinocerebral mucormycosis," *Surgical Neurology International*, vol. 7, no. 1, pp. 61–64, 2016.

[15] J. Fisher, C. U. Tuazon, and G. W. Geelhoed, "Mucormycosis in transplant patients," *American Surgeon*, vol. 46, no. 5, pp. 315–322, 1980.

[16] T. Santos, B. Aguiar, L. Santos et al., "Invasive fungal infections after kidney transplantation: a single-center experience," *Transplantation Proceedings*, vol. 47, no. 4, pp. 971–975, 2015.

[17] A. Patel, E. Bishburg, and S. Nagarakanti, "Mucormycosis in an HIV-infected renal transplant patient: a case report and review of the literature," *American Journal of Case Reports*, vol. 15, pp. 74–78, 2014.

24

Renal Mucormycosis: A Rare and Potentially Lethal Complication of Kidney Transplantation

SreyRam Kuy,[1] Chun He,[2] and David C. Cronin II[3]

[1] *Division of Vascular Surgery, Department of Surgery, Medical College of Wisconsin, 9200 W Wisconsin Avenue, Milwaukee, WI 53226, USA*
[2] *Department of Pathology, Medical College of Wisconsin, Milwaukee, WI, USA*
[3] *Division of Transplantation, Department of Surgery, Medical College of Wisconsin, Milwaukee, WI, USA*

Correspondence should be addressed to SreyRam Kuy; srkuy@mcw.edu

Academic Editors: P. A. Andrews, G. Forrest, and M. Klinger

Renal mucormycosis is a rare and potentially lethal complication of kidney transplantation. We describe two cases of renal mucormycosis following deceased donor kidney transplantation. This is the second report of renal mucormycosis following kidney transplantation in the United States, and the first case of renal mucormycosis infection presumed to be of recipient origin. Case A had an early presentation of mucormycosis isolated to the kidney allograft. He had an unexpected rise in serum creatinine and leukocytosis necessitating allograft biopsy which showed mucormycosis. He underwent transplant nephrectomy on posttransplant day 11, was treated with amphotericin B, and discharged home on posttransplant day 22. Case B had a late presentation of renal mucormycosis, preceded by a cutaneous manifestation. One year after kidney transplantation he had a nonhealing knee ulcer which on biopsy showed cutaneous mucormycosis. Treatment included aggressive debridement and amphotericin B. Allograft biopsy showed mucormycosis, necessitating transplant nephrectomy. He was discharged to a rehabilitation facility and died from noninfectious causes. Review of the published literature of renal mucormycosis cases following kidney transplantation reveals a mortality rate of more than 50%. The key to successful outcome is early recognition, prompt institution of surgical debridement of all infected tissue, and appropriate antifungal therapy.

1. Introduction

Mucormycosis, previously known as zygomycosis, refers to rare infections caused by fungi of the order of *Mucorales*, which are characterized by the production of aseptate hyphae and asexual spores [1]. The most common clinical isolate of *Mucorales* is *Rhizopus oryzae* (44%), followed by *Rhizopus microsporus* (22%), *Mucor circinelloides* (9.5%), *Mycocladus corymbifer* (5.3%), *Rhizomucor pusillus* (3.7%), *Cunninghamella bertholletiae* (3.2%), *Mucor indicus* (2.6%), *Cunninghamella echinulata* (1%), and *Apophysomyces elegans* (0.5%) [2]. Mortality among patients with mucormycosis is significant. Mortality was as high as 84% in the 1950s and then decreased to approximately 40% in the 2000s, with the drop in mortality attributed to the widespread introduction of amphotericin B in the 1960s [3]. However, from 1940 to 2000, there has been a 70% increase in the number of cases of mucormycosis, with mucormycosis most frequently seen in diabetic patients, followed by neutropenic patients, transplant recipients, patients with hematological disease, patients on deferoxamine therapy, and IV drug users. The most common presentation of mucormycosis is rhinocerebral disease, followed by pulmonary, cutaneous, and disseminated diseases. Less commonly, mucormycosis can involve the GI tract and kidneys [4, 5].

In contrast to the presentation of infection among non-transplant recipients, the majority of infections in solid-organ transplant recipients present as pulmonary (37%), followed by rhinocerebral (16%) and cutaneous (16%) infections. The Transplant-Associated Infection Surveillance Network (Roden) performed prospective surveillance for invasive fungal infections by routine review of monthly logs from a registry of solid organ transplant patients (liver, kidney, lung, pancreas, heart, and small bowel) at 15 US transplant centers from 2001 to 2006 [6]. The most common invasive fungal infections following solid organ transplantation were invasive candidiasis (53%), invasive aspergillosis (19%), cryptococcosis (8%), non-*Aspergillus* molds (8%), endemic fungi (5%), and, least commonly, mucormycosis (2%). The majorities of these mucormycosis cases were pulmonary (56%), with the remainder being sinus (13%), cutaneous (13%), and disseminated (9%). The incidence of invasive fungal infections was the highest among the small bowel transplant recipients (11.6%) and the lowest among kidney transplant recipients (1.3%).

The first reported case of mucormycosis following kidney transplantation was a lethal rhinocerebral form in 1970 [7]. Among kidney transplant recipients, mucormycosis comprises only 2–6% of invasive fungal infections [6, 8]. However, compared with all other fungal infections mucormycosis is associated with the longest duration of hospitalization and highest 2-year mortality among kidney transplant patients [8]. Renal mucormycosis following kidney transplantation has been reported only once before in the United States. Though rare, renal mucormycosis is associated with 50% mortality among kidney transplant patients.

We describe the second report of renal mucormycosis following kidney transplantation in the United States, and the first case of renal mucormycosis infection presumed to be of recipient origin. The remainder of the world literature describes 16 cases of renal mucormycosis following kidney transplantation, nearly all late occurrences of this complication. Overall, mucormycosis is uncommon, mucormycosis of the kidney is even more uncommon, and mucormycosis of the renal allograft specifically is both uncommon and usually a late occurring infection.

2. Two Case Reports

2.1. Case A. Case A, a 36-year-old man whose initial cause of end stage renal disease was Hemolytic uremic syndrome. His history is significant for receiving a deceased donor kidney transplant in 1991. In 1992 he underwent bilateral native nephrectomy and in 2007 a transplant nephrectomy was performed for chronic allograft nephropathy. Significant comorbidities include infection with hepatitis C virus (grade 1, stage 0).

He received zero mismatch, cross match negative, a standard criteria deceased donor kidney transplant after 21 hours of cold preservation. Induction immunosuppression included antithymocyte globulin (rabbit, 1.5 mg/kg) and glucocorticoids. The kidney was implanted into a left lower quadrant retroperitoneal pocket. Due to a short donor ureter an ureteroureterostomy with internal stent provided drainage. After reperfusion the transplanted kidney was pink with firm turgor.

On posttransplant (PT) day 1 there was scant urine output and the patient required hemodialysis. Urine output increased until postoperative day 4 when a decrease in urine output was associated with pain over the left lower quadrant and left groin. On PT 8, ultrasound was obtained due to a rising creatinine, which showed a migrated ureteral stent with hydronephrosis and he underwent cystoscopy with ureteral stent removal. Ultrasound on PT 9 showed persistent hydronephrosis and a nephrostomy tube was placed on PT 10. Nephrostogram on PT 11 showed the nephrostomy tube in proper position, but obstruction of the kidney. He had a persistent leukocytosis and fevers, but blood and urine cultures were negative for growth of aerobes and anaerobes. Due to concerns for rejection, he underwent allograft biopsy which showed mucormycosis and necrosis (Figure 1). He underwent an emergent total transplant nephrectomy including the ureter on PT 11 and was started on a course of amphotericin B. Histology of the explanted graft showed invasive mucormycosis of the transplanted kidney parenchyma and both donor and recipient ureter with an invasion pattern advancing from the luminal surface. There was no invasion of the graft renal vein or artery (Figure 1). This was suggestive of the recipient's urinary tract as the primary source for the mucormycosis. *Rhizomucor* was isolated from the specimen (speciation not identified).

Cystoscopy done 4 days after nephrectomy showed normal appearing bladder with no evidence of necrosis. Due to the known predilection for pulmonary and rhinocerebral manifestations of mucormycosis, CT imaging of the lungs, sinuses, and brain were done which showed no evidence of mucormycosis. The patient was discharged home on PT 21.

Return to clinic on postnephrectomy day 25 revealed drainage from the incision. The patient underwent surgical debridement and wound exploration. Pathology showed no evidence of cutaneous mucormycosis in the wound. The organ procurement organization was promptly notified of this case of renal mucormycosis at the time of initial discovery. Neither the recipient of the partner kidney graft nor liver graft has demonstrated any evidence of mucormycosis.

2.2. Case B. Case B is a 54-year-old man with end-stage renal disease due to diabetes mellitus and hypertension. The patient underwent an expanded criteria deceased-donor, cross match negative kidney transplantation. Induction immunosuppression included antithymocyte globulin (rabbit, 1.5 mg/kg) and glucocorticoids. The initial postoperative course was complicated by delayed graft function, an upper extremity DVT, and a cardiac ischemic episode. One month after transplant the patient was seen for followup in clinic and noted to have a left knee ulcer, which was treated with local wound care. Five months after transplant, the patient underwent work-up for chronic elevated serum creatinine, including an allograft biopsy which showed no evidence of rejection. However, lab studies revealed cytomegalovirus viremia, for which he was appropriately treated. Nine months after transplant he was readmitted with chills, fevers, and an elevated creatinine. The differential included allograft rejection, infection, and/or anatomic obstruction. He underwent a transplant kidney biopsy which showed only acute tubular injury consistent with tacrolimus toxicity. Blood cultures were positive for coagulase-positive staphylococcus, and he was treated for his bacteremia with a two-week course of appropriate antibiotics. Eleven months after transplant he was readmitted with fever, muscle weakness, joint pain, and myalgias. He was found to have a urinary tract infection and bacteremia

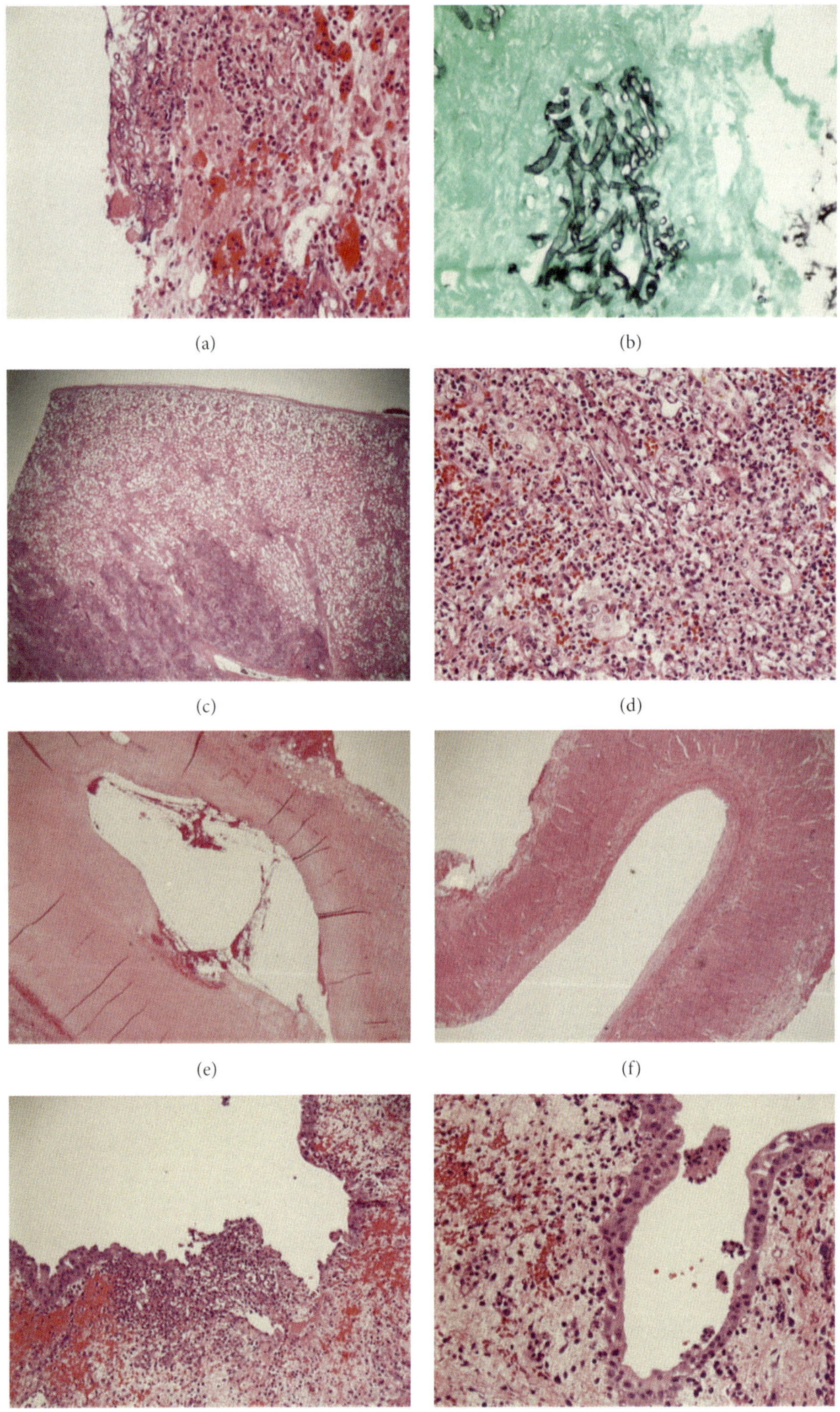

(a) (b) (c) (d) (e) (f) (g) (h)

FIGURE 1: Case A renal allograft histology. Figures 1(a) and 1(b) show renal allograft biopsy indicating broad, pleomorphic, and thin walled fungal small fragments and hyphae with right angle branching and mucoid feature in presence of tissue necrosis consistent with mucormycosis in hematoxylin and eosin stain (a) and Gomori's methenamine silver stain (b). Explanted allograft kidney demonstrates diffuse and invasive mucormycosis predominantly involving the medulla noted by low magnification in (c) and high magnification in (d) on H&E stain; no mucormycetes invasion of renal artery (e) and vein (f); mucormycetes invasion in proximal portion of ureter indicative of donor ureter (g), and no mucormycetes invasion in distal portion of ureter indicative of recipient ureter (h).

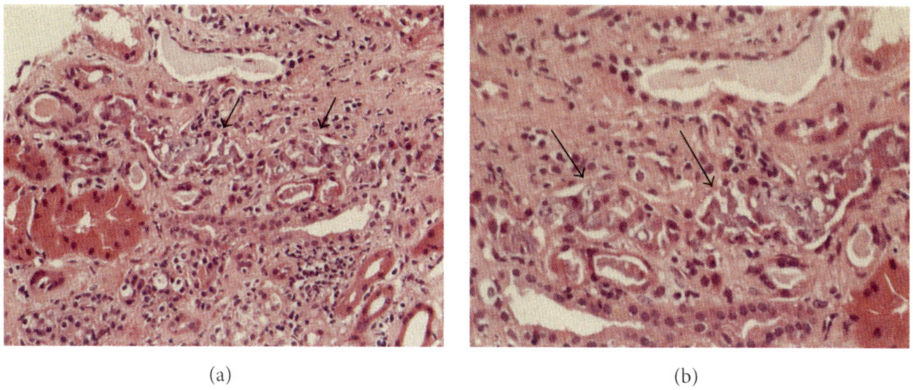

FIGURE 2: Case B renal allograft biopsy. Intratubular small fragments and hyphae of mucormycetes (by arrows) without extratubular invasion are noted by low magnification (a) and high magnification (b) on H&E staining sections.

with coagulase-positive staphylococcus and treated with a course of antibiotics. Rheumatology performed a diagnostic aspiration of his wrist due to concern for crystalline disease, but the aspirate was negative for crystals and the joint pain and myalgias were attributed to his bacteremia and lymphedema. He was discharged to a rehab facility.

Thirteen months after transplant he was seen as an outpatient, the left knee ulcer was noted to not be healing adequately and was biopsied in clinic. The biopsy specimen revealed cutaneous mucormycosis and he was admitted for treatment. He was started on amphotericin B and taken to the operating room for surgical debridement of his left knee lesion. He had an acute rise in his creatinine, which prompted a transplant kidney biopsy three days later, showing renal mucormycosis (Figure 2).

Due to the concern for disseminated mucormycosis, CT imaging of his head, neck, chest, abdomen, and pelvis were done which did not show any evidence mucormycosis in these sites. Due to his significant cardiac history, he first underwent a cardiac catheterization then subsequently underwent transplant nephrectomy. He was also found to have another cytomegalovirus infection which was treated with a course of valganciclovir. He was discharged to a long term care facility on postnephrectomy day 9 on a one month course of amphotericin B and then transitioned to oral posaconazole. He was seen for followup in transplant clinic one month later and was noted to have a healing left knee wound, being treated with a wound vac. He died at the rehabilitation facility from cardiac causes.

3. Discussion

Renal mucormycosis is a rarely described and potentially lethal complication of kidney transplantation. Case A developed isolated renal mucormycosis and was presented early in the posttransplantation course, undergoing transplant nephrectomy eleven days after transplantation. Histopathology showed an invasion of mucormycosis in the transplanted kidney parenchyma and both donor and recipient ureter, but none in the graft artery or vein. This finding, combined with the fact that neither of the other two recipients of grafts from the same donor developed mucormycosis, suggests that this case of renal mucormycosis originated in the recipient rather than donor derived. However, another potential source of the mucormycosis could be from contaminated preservation fluid. Case B, in contrast, was presented late (more than a year after transplantation), initially manifested as cutaneous mucormycosis treated with debridement and amphotericin B, and found to have simultaneous renal mucormycosis, treated with transplant nephrectomy. In both cases, renal mucormycosis was an unanticipated finding, but one that was promptly acted upon with aggressive surgical debridement, including graft removal and appropriate antifungal agents. Prompt surgical intervention combined with appropriate antifungal therapy contributed to successful outcome in Case A. Case B, in contrast, had significant exposure to immunosuppression therapy as indicated by his persistent CMV infection and cutaneous mucormycosis. In addition, he had significant comorbidities known to increase the risk of Mucor infection including poorly managed insulin dependent diabetes mellitus and ischemic cardiomyopathy.

The Literature. The first reported case of renal mucormycosis following kidney transplantation in the United States was in 2010. Alexander et al. described two patients who developed renal mucormycosis following kidney transplant from the same deceased donor [9]. Both patients required nephrectomies and treatment with amphotericin B, with one patient dying at posttransplant day 12 and the other patient surviving to discharge after an 84-day hospitalization. Histopathology of the explanted kidneys revealed vascular invasion with aseptate hyphae and relative sparing of the renal capsules, suggesting a vascular route of contamination. Genotypically indistinguishable strains of *Apophysomyces elegans* were recovered from both recipients but not established in the donor, suggesting either contamination of the organs during recovery or undiagnosed donor infection.

In the world literature there are 14 additional international case reports of renal mucormycosis following renal transplantation, summarized in Table 1 [10–21].

While it is necessary to review the world literature on renal mucormycosis following kidney transplantation, it is important to take into account differences between US and

Table 1: Cases of renal mucormycosis following kidney transplantation.

Case report	R/D age	R/D sex	Donor type	Donor cause of death	Recipient disease	Time to transplant nephrectomy (PT)	Induction agent	Systemic therapy	Geographic location	Speciation	Outcome (PT)
S. Kuy et al.	36/43	M/F	SCD	Intracranial hemorrhage	Hemolytic uremic syndrome	11 days	Thymoglobulin, Solu Medrol	Amphotericin B	US	*Rhizomucor*	Survived
S. Kuy et al.	54/61	M/F	DCD ECD	Stroke	Diabetes mellitus, hypertension	13 months	Thymoglobulin, Solu Medrol	Amphotericin B	US	*Rhizomucor*	Survived
Alexander et al. [9]	61/17	M/F	DCD	MVC, drowning	—	9 days	Thymoglobulin, Solu Medrol	Amphotericin B	US	*Apophysomyces elegans*	Died (12 days)
Alexander et al. [9]	31/17	F/F	DCD	MVC, drowning	—	10 days	Thymoglobulin, Solu Medrol	Amphotericin B	US	*Apophysomyces elegans*	Survived
Mitwalli et al. [10]	18/—	F/—	LURD	—	Polycystic kidney disease	1 month	—	Amphotericin B	India	—	Survived
Nampoory et al. [11]	59/—	F/—	LURD	—	—	1 month	—	—	Kuwait	—	Died (3 months)
Stas et al. [12]	51/—	M/—	LURD	—	Henoch-Schonlein nephritis	2.5 months	—	—	India	*Absidia corymbifera*	Survived
Chkhotua et al. [13]	42/—	M/—	LURD	—	Glomerulonephritis	1.5 months	—	—	Egypt	*Mucorales*	Died (1.5 months)
Nalmas et al. [14]	62	M/—	LURD	—	—	3 weeks	—	—	Pakistan	*Mucor* species	Survived
Armaly et al. [15]	42/—	M/—	LURD	—	Poststreptococcal glomerulonephritis	1 month	—	—	Egypt	—	Died (1.5 months)
Armaly et al. [15]	52/—	F/—	LURD	—	Diabetes mellitus	1 month	—	—	Egypt	—	Survived
Godara et al. [16]	42/—	M/—	—	—	—	1 month		Amphotericin B	India	—	Died (1 month)
Sajiv et al. [17]	14/—	M/—	—	—	Congenital UPJ obstruction	3 months	Methylprednisolone, OKT3	Amphotericin B, Fluconazole	India	*Mucor* species	Died (few days)
Tayyebi et al. [18]	31/—	M/—	DCD	—	UPJ obstruction	2 months	—	—	Iran	*Mucor* species	Survived
Tayyebi et al. [18]	58/—	F/—	LURD	—	Polycystic kidney disease	9 months	—	—	Iran	*Mucor* species	Survived
Tomazic et al. [19]	56/28	M/M	LURD	—	—	2 months	Tacrolimus and Methylprednisolone	—	India	*Mucor* species	Died (2 months)
Minz et al. [20]	52/—	M/—	LURD	—	Chronic glomerulonephritis	8 days	Cyclosporin, azathioprine, prednisolone, Basiliximab	—	India	*Mucor* species	Died (8 days)
Ahmad [21]	49/—	M/M	LRRD	LRRD	Chronic glomerulonephritis	18 months	Cyclosporine, Prednisone, methylprednisolone, ATG	—	India	*Mucor* species	Died

R: recipient; D: donor; M: male, F: female; —: no data available; PT: after transplant; SCD: standard criteria donor; ECD: extended criteria donor, DCD: donor after cardiac death; LURD: living unrelated donor; MVC: motor vehicle crash; yrs: years old; UPJ: ureteropelvic junction; US: United States; ATG: antithymocyte globulin.

worldwide practices in immunosuppression, organ source, recipient surveillance, and graft management. Based on this sum of 18 reported cases worldwide (including our two cases), renal mucormycosis following kidney transplantation carries a staggeringly high 50% mortality rate.

Overall, the majority of renal transplant patients who develop renal mucormycosis are male are diagnosed within the first couple months with the exception of our reported cases, and despite undergoing graft nephrectomy and systemic therapy with Amphotericin B they have a mortality of 50%. The risk factors include the use of immunosuppression drugs, diabetes, environmental factors, and the use of broad spectrum antimicrobial agents. Diagnosis of mucormycosis in transplant patients is extremely difficult and challenging because of rarity, lack of serologic tests, difficulty in isolation, and growth of mucormycetes from infected tissue, blood and body fluid, and often poor staining of mucormycetes with Grocott's methenamine silver stain (GMS) and Periodic Acid Schiff (PAS) due to possible mucoid features and sometimes mimicking acute cellular rejection in clinical presentation.

Although extremely rare, renal mucormycosis is a severe and potentially lethal complication of renal transplantation. The keys to successful outcome are having a high index of suspicion for mucormycosis in the differential to enable early recognition, recognizing over immunosuppression as a risk factor for mucormycosis, and prompt, aggressive institution of surgical resection of infected tissue and appropriate pharmacological therapy in order to salvage patients with renal mucormycosis. A three-point strategy in the treatment of mucormycosis is essential and includes surgery, antifungal therapy, and management of risk factors.

References

[1] D. P. Kontoyiannis, V. C. Wessel, G. P. Bodey, and K. V. I. Rolston, "Zygomycosis in the 1990s in a tertiary-care cancer center," *Clinical Infectious Diseases*, vol. 30, no. 6, pp. 851–856, 2000.

[2] E. Alvarez, D. A. Sutton, J. Cano et al., "Spectrum of zygomycete species identified in clinically significant specimens in the United States," *Journal of Clinical Microbiology*, vol. 47, no. 6, pp. 1650–1656, 2009.

[3] M. M. Roden, T. E. Zaoutis, W. L. Buchanan et al., "Epidemiology and outcome of zygomycosis: a review of 929 reported cases," *Clinical Infectious Diseases*, vol. 41, no. 5, pp. 634–653, 2005.

[4] N. Crum-Cianflone, "Mucormycosis," Emedicine, http://emedicine.medscape.com/article/222551-overview.

[5] J. Brown, "Zygomycosis: an emerging fungal infection," *American Journal of Health-System Pharmacy*, vol. 62, no. 24, pp. 2593–2596, 2005.

[6] P. G. Pappas, B. D. Alexander, D. R. Andes et al., "Invasive fungal infections among organ transplant recipients: results of the transplant-associated infection surveillance network (Transnet)," *Clinical Infectious Diseases*, vol. 50, no. 8, pp. 1101–1111, 2010.

[7] S. Haim, O. S. Better, C. Lichtig, D. Erlik, and A. Barzilai, "Rhinocerebral mucormycosis following kidney transplantation," *Israel Journal of Medical Sciences*, vol. 6, no. 5, pp. 646–649, 1970.

[8] K. C. Abbott, I. Hypolite, R. K. Poropatich et al., "Hospitalizations for fungal infections after renal transplantation in the United States," *Transplant Infectious Disease*, vol. 3, no. 4, pp. 203–211, 2001.

[9] B. D. Alexander, W. A. Schell, A. M. Siston et al., "Fatal apophysomyces elegans infection transmitted by deceased donor renal allografts," *American Journal of Transplantation*, vol. 10, no. 9, pp. 2161–2167, 2010.

[10] A. Mitwalli, G. Hassan Malik, J. Al-Wakeel et al., "Mucormycosis of the graft in a renal transplant recipient," *Nephrology Dialysis Transplantation*, vol. 9, no. 6, pp. 718–720, 1994.

[11] M. R. N. Nampoory, Z. U. Khan, K. V. Johny et al., "Invasive fungal infections in renal transplant recipients," *Journal of Infection*, vol. 33, no. 2, pp. 95–101, 1996.

[12] K. J. F. Stas, P. G. L. H. Louwagie, B. J. C. Van Damme, W. Coosemans, M. Waer, and Y. F. C. Vanrenterghem, "Isolated zygomycosis in a bought living unrelated kidney transplant," *Transplant International*, vol. 9, no. 6, pp. 600–602, 1996.

[13] A. Chkhotua, A. Yussim, A. Tovar et al., "Mucormycosis of the renal allograft: case report and review of the literature," *Transplant International*, vol. 14, no. 6, pp. 438–441, 2001.

[14] S. Nalmas, E. Bishburg, and C. Goldstein, "Mucormycosis in a transplanted kidney," *Transplant Infectious Disease*, vol. 10, no. 4, pp. 269–271, 2008.

[15] Z. Armaly, E. Khankin, R. Ramadan et al., "Two cases of renal mucormycosis in renal transplanted patients," *Clinical Nephrology*, vol. 58, no. 3, pp. 247–249, 2002.

[16] S. M. Godara, V. B. Kute, K. R. Goplani et al., "Mucormycosis in renal transplant recipients: predictors and outcome," *Saudi Journal of Kidney Diseases and Transplantation*, vol. 22, no. 4, pp. 751–756, 2011.

[17] C. Sajiv, B. Pawar, N. Calton et al., "Mucormycosis in renal allograft: a case report," *Indian Journal of Nephrology*, vol. 13, pp. 38–39, 2003.

[18] N. Tayyebi, S. Amouian, N. Mohamadian, and H. R. Rahimi, "Renal allograft mucormycosis: report of two cases," *Surgical Infections*, vol. 8, no. 5, pp. 535–538, 2007.

[19] J. Tomazic, M. Pirs, T. Matos, D. Ferluga, and J. Lindic, "Multiple infections after commercial renal transplantation in India," *Nephrology Dialysis Transplantation*, vol. 22, no. 3, pp. 972–973, 2007.

[20] M. Minz, A. Sharma, R. Kashyap et al., "Isolated renal allograft arterial mucormycosis: an extremely rare complication," *Nephrology Dialysis Transplantation*, vol. 18, no. 5, pp. 1034–1035, 2003.

[21] M. Ahmad, "Graft mucormycosis in a renal allograft recipient," *Journal of Nephrology*, vol. 18, no. 6, pp. 783–786, 2005.

25

Protracted Hypocalcemia following 3.5 Parathyroidectomy in a Kidney Pancreas Recipient with a History of Robotic-Assisted Roux-en-Y Gastric Bypass

Hugo Bonatti,[1,2] Naureen Iqbal,[1,3] Catherine Kling,[1,4] Willie Melvin,[1,5] and James Broome[1,6]

[1] *Department of Surgery, Vanderbilt University Medical Center, Nashville, TN, USA*
[2] *Meritus Surgical Specialists, Hagerstown, MD, USA*
[3] *Geisinger, Wilkes-Barre, PA, USA*
[4] *Surgery, University of Washington, Seattle, WA, USA*
[5] *StoneCrest Medical Center Clinic, Smyrna, TN, USA*
[6] *St. Thomas Endocrine Surgical Specialists, Nashville, TN, USA*

Correspondence should be addressed to Hugo Bonatti; hugo.bonatti@dr.com

Academic Editor: Marian Klinger

Background. Hypocalcemia is a frequent complication of parathyroidectomy for secondary/tertiary hyperparathyroidism. In patients with a history of prior Roux-en-Y gastric bypass (RYGBP), changes in nutritional absorption make management of hypocalcemia after parathyroidectomy difficult. *Case Report.* A 41-old-year morbidly obese female with c-peptide negative diabetes mellitus and renal failure had RYGBP. Following significant weight loss she underwent simultaneous pancreas-kidney transplantation. She had excellent transplant graft function but developed tertiary hyperparathyroidism with calciphylaxis. She underwent resection of 3.5 glands leaving a small, physiologic remnant remaining in situ at the left inferior position. She was discharged on postoperative day one in good condition, asymptomatic with serum calcium of 7.6 mg/dL and intact PTH of 12 pg/mL. The patient had to be readmitted on postoperative day #14 for severe hypocalcemia of 5.0 mg/dl and ionized calcium 2.4 mg/dl. She required intravenous calcium infusion to achieve calcium levels of >6.5 mg/dl. Long-term treatment includes 5 g of elemental oral calcium TID, vitamin D, and hydrochlorothiazide. She remains in the long term on high-dose medical therapy with normal serum calcium levels and PTH levels around 100 pg/mL. *Discussion.* Our patient's protracted hypocalcemia originates from a combination of 3.5 gland parathyroidectomy, altered intestinal anatomy post-RYGBP, and potentially her pancreas transplant causing additional metabolic derangement. Alternative bariatric procedures such as sleeve gastrectomy may be more suitable for patients with renal failure or organ transplants in whom adequate absorption of vitamins, minerals, and drugs such as immunosuppressants is essential.

1. Introduction

Pancreas transplantation (PTx) has evolved as a reliable therapy for insulin-dependent diabetes mellitus (IDDM) and most commonly it is performed as a simultaneous pancreas-kidney transplant (SPK) in the setting of diabetic nephropathy [1, 2]. Only a limited number of patients with non-IDDM have thus far undergone PTx if they were able to lose significant weight and still remain insulin-dependent [3–5]. Obesity has become one of the most common disorders worldwide, and morbid obesity is often a contraindication for kidney and pancreas transplant listing. As nonoperative measures are unsuccessful in the majority of obese individuals, bariatric surgery has gained importance in the therapy of morbid obesity [6]. Currently in the US, the Roux-en-Y gastric bypass (RYGBP) is most commonly performed; the role of adjustable gastric banding (AGB) is declining; and gastric sleeve resection has been gaining importance [7, 8]. One major complication of RYGBP is development of malabsorption of various nutrients, electrolytes, vitamins, and some drugs. Poor absorption of calcium can be of particular concern in patient subsets and may lead to secondary hyperparathyroidism [9–11].

One of the most common secondary complications of DM is renal failure, which commonly is associated with secondary hyperparathyroidism [12]. Although renal transplantation may reverse secondary hyperparathyroidism, commonly tertiary hyperparathyroidism has already developed and, therefore, removal of the parathyroid glands may be required. Most surgeons prefer 3.5 gland resection; however, also total parathyroidectomy with autotransplantation has been suggested [13]. Hypocalcemia is a common complication after parathyroidectomy and in severe cases is also referred to as hungry bone syndrome [14]; it seems to originate from a rapid drop in the PTH levels and may be more common in patients with secondary hyperparathyroidism. The profound hypocalcemia and hypophosphatemia may linger and require high-dose calcium and vitamin D supplementation. Administration of bisphosphonates has been suggested to prevent and/or treat the condition.

We herein report a 35-year-old woman with IDDM, who developed severe hypocalcemia after three-and-a-half-gland parathyroidectomy for tertiary hyperparathyroidism in the setting of being status post-RYGBP and SPK.

2. Case Report

A 35-year-old female was diagnosed with type I DM at the age of 9 years. During childhood her DM was poorly controlled and the patient gained significant weight. At the age of 25 years her weight was 105 kg with a body mass index (BMI) of 40 kg/m2 and her renal function started to deteriorate with progression to requiring hemodialysis by age 30. With development of renal failure, secondary hyperparathyroidism was noted. Due to her obesity, she was not eligible for a renal transplant or a SPK. At this point it was decided to offer her bariatric surgery, and, after extensive discussion, it was felt that a RYGBP was the best option for her in terms of weight loss. At the age of 32 years, she underwent uneventful robotic-assisted surgery; the stomach remnant was attached to the abdominal wall for potential future access.

Over the next 2 years she lost 60 kg and underwent SPK during which the donor duodenal segment was diverted to a bowel loop distal to her Roux loop implant site into the common channel. Induction immunosuppression with alemtuzumab was followed by maintenance with tacrolimus (trough levels 5-7 ng/mL), mycophenolate-mofetil (2 g daily), and a steroid taper. She was CMV seronegative and received a graft from a CMV positive donor and received standard prophylaxis with oral ganciclovir (GCV) for 100 days. Within 100 days posttransplant, she was readmitted to the hospital with acute CMV disease, which was successfully treated with intravenous ganciclovir.

Shortly after this episode the patient was found to have skin lesions on her right leg, which were diagnosed as calciphylaxis. Her serum calcium at that time was 14 mg/dl and the diagnosis of tertiary hyperparathyroidism was made. A three-and-a-half-gland resection together with subtotal thymectomy was done without any complications; the left lower parathyroid gland was the only normal appearing and half of it was preserved taking care that blood supply remained intact. Intraoperative parathyroid hormone levels dropped from >1500 to 150. Calcium serum levels within 24 hours postoperatively were 9 mg/dl with ionized calcium of 3.5 mg/dl. She was discharged in good condition within 24 hours postoperatively with daily calcium supplementation of 4.5 g/day divided into three doses.

During the following week her calcium levels started to drop and on day 10 postoperatively at an outside hospital serum calcium was found to be critically low at 5.5 mg/dl with an ionized fraction of 2.1 mg/dl. However, the patient had remained clinically symptom free. She was admitted for intravenous calcium replacement. Pushes of calcium were unable to appropriately raise her calcium levels and, therefore, a calcium drip (85 mg/h) was started. Her calcium levels came up to 7.1 mg/dl. Oral calcium dose was raised to 15 g/day and hydrochlorothiazide was started. The calcium drip was stopped and the patient was discharged home in good condition.

Intense calcium supplementation was continued. Gradually the patient's gastrointestinal tract started to adapt and after two years her calcium levels started to stabilize. She has not experienced any additional complications from her transplant or gastric bypass. She is currently alive with excellent function of both grafts, normal calcium levels, stable weight, and an excellent quality of life almost five years after her last surgery.

3. Discussion

We report a patient with a complex medical history and multiple surgical interventions involving bariatric, transplant, and endocrine surgeons. The patient benefited from each of these interventions and all were clearly indicated. However, better communication between the various involved teams may have resulted in an even better outcome and prevention of the severe hypocalcemia following her three-and-a-half-gland parathyroidectomy. She was cured from her type 1 and type 2 DM and since her successful SPK she is off any antidiabetic medication and is off dialysis and has regained an excellent quality of life having maintained a normal weight after bariatric surgery.

Development of obesity in patients with type I DM is rare and is associated with an excessive risk for secondary complications due to the superimposed peripheral insulin resistance [15]. Escalating amounts of exogenous insulin may be required in these patients in order to maintain acceptable blood glucose control. In combination with other comorbidities, development of secondary complications including renal failure is common such as in our patient. Once on dialysis, renal transplant was discussed but her obesity was considered a contraindication. Therefore, bariatric surgery was suggested and RYGBP seemed to be the most promising intervention to rapidly achieve the necessary weight loss.

Hypocalcemia is more common after RYGBP than after AGB or gastric sleeve resection as calcium absorption takes place mainly in the proximal gastrointestinal tract which is excluded in patients with RYGBP [16]. However, sleeve gastrectomy also may cause secondary metabolic complications with low calcium and elevated PTH levels [17]. Successful AGB has been reported in a SPK recipient who developed significant weight gain [18] and another SPK recipient underwent placement of a gastric pacemaker for gastroparesis associated with significant weight gain [19]. Limited data on sleeve gastrectomy in PTx are available but the procedure seems promising and appealing in this patient population [20–22]. Small series of patients with NIDDM undergoing PTx have been published; the treatment is reserved for patients who have lost significant weight and remain insulin-dependent [23].

In our patient, management of hypocalcemia was challenging [24]. Hungry bone syndrome may have been an important component leading to the very low serum calcium levels [14]. It is unclear if a RYGBP or a SPK transplant may exacerbate hungry bone syndrome. Even with 15 g of oral calcium and administration of vitamin D, the patient had difficulties to maintain normal calcium levels due to limited calcium absorption. Vitamin D levels were kept above 50 ng/ml throughout the postoperative course. Palal et al. reported on life-threatening hypocalcemia after parathyroidectomy in a renal failure patient with previous RYGBP [24]. Hydrochlorothiazide increases calcium reabsorption and decreases renal calcium loss; however, use of diuretics in SPK recipients is controversial.

If the patient would not have been able to maintain adequate calcium levels in the long term, placing a gastrostomy tube into the stomach remnant under fluoroscopic guidance may have been an option. Calcium could be delivered directly into her proximal gastrointestinal tract, with improved absorption and resolution of hypocalcemia. Recently, recombinant parathyroid hormone has been introduced in clinical practice [25] for refractory cases of hypoparathyroidism but is reluctantly used in patients like ours. In fact PTH levels recovered in our patient and ultimately she was able to adjust to her unique metabolic challenge with high-dose oral calcium and vitamin D administration. This complication of severe hypocalcemia after parathyroidectomy should be considered in patients with a history of RYGBP [26, 27].

References

[1] A. C. Gruessner and R. W. G. Gruessner, "Long-term outcome after pancreas transplantation: A registry analysis," *Current Opinion in Organ Transplantation*, vol. 21, no. 4, pp. 377–385, 2016.

[2] A. C. Gruessner and R. W. G. Gruessner, "Pancreas transplant outcomes for United States and non United States cases as reported to the United Network for Organ Sharing and the International Pancreas Transplant Registry as of December 2011," *Clinical Transplantation*, pp. 23–40, 2012.

[3] C. Fourtounas, "Transplant options for patients with type 2 diabetes and chronic kidney disease," *World Journal of Transplantation*, vol. 4, no. 2, pp. 102–110, 2014.

[4] A. C. Gruessner, M. R. Laftavi, O. Pankewycz, and R. W. G. Gruessner, "Simultaneous Pancreas and Kidney Transplantation—Is It a Treatment Option for Patients With Type 2 Diabetes Mellitus? An Analysis of the International Pancreas Transplant Registry," *Current Diabetes Reports*, vol. 17, no. 6, article no. 44, 2017.

[5] C. Margreiter, T. Resch, R. Oberhuber et al., "Combined pancreas-kidney transplantation for patients with end-stage nephropathy caused by type-2 diabetes mellitus," *Transplantation*, vol. 95, no. 8, pp. 1030–1036, 2013.

[6] J. L. Colquitt, K. Pickett, E. Loveman, and G. K. Frampton, "Surgery for weight loss in adults," *Cochrane Database of Systematic Reviews*, vol. 8, Article ID CD003641, 2014.

[7] W. J. English, E. J. DeMaria, S. A. Brethauer, S. G. Mattar, R. J. Rosenthal, and J. M. Morton, "American Society for Metabolic and Bariatric Surgery estimation of metabolic and bariatric procedures performed in the United States in 2016," *Surgery for Obesity and Related Diseases*, vol. 14, no. 3, pp. 259–263, 2018.

[8] D. A. Hirth, E. L. Jones, K. B. Rothchild, B. C. Mitchell, and J. A. Schoen, "Laparoscopic sleeve gastrectomy: Long-term weight loss outcomes," *Surgery for Obesity and Related Diseases*, vol. 11, no. 5, pp. 1004–1007, 2015.

[9] J. Jin, A. V. Robinson, P. T. Hallowell, J. J. Jasper, T. A. Stellato, and S. M. Wilhem, "Increases in parathyroid hormone (PTH) after gastric bypass surgery appear to be of a secondary nature," *Surgery*, vol. 142, no. 6, pp. 914–920, 2007.

[10] P. Toelle, R. Peterli, I. Zobel, C. Noppen, C. Christoffel-Courtin, and T. Peters, "Risk factors for secondary hyperparathyroidism after bariatric surgery: a comparison of 4 different operations and of vitamin D-receptor-polymorphism," *Experimental and Clinical Endocrinology & Diabetes*, vol. 120, no. 10, pp. 629–634, 2012.

[11] S. Hewitt, T. T. Søvik, E. T. Aasheim et al., "Secondary hyperparathyroidism, vitamin D sufficiency, and serum calcium 5 years after gastric bypass and duodenal switch," *Obesity Surgery*, vol. 23, no. 3, pp. 384–390, 2013.

[12] T. Amin, PT. Coates, J. Barbara, P. Hakendorf, and N. Karim, "Prevalence of Hypercalcaemia in a Renal Transplant Population: A Single Centre Study," *International Journal of Nephrology*, vol. 2016, Article ID 7126290, p. 2016, 2016.

[13] H. Gilat, R. Feinmesser, Y. Vinkler et al., "Clinical and operative management of persistent hyperparathyroidism after renal transplantation: A single-center experience," *Head & Neck*, vol. 29, no. 11, pp. 996–1001, 2007.

[14] N. Jain and R. F. Reilly, "Hungry bone syndrome," *Current Opinion in Nephrology and Hypertension*, vol. 26, no. 4, pp. 250–255, 2017.

[15] V. M. da Costa, P. de Carvalho Padilha, G. C. de Lima et al., "Overweight among children and adolescent with type I diabetes mellitus: prevalence and associated factors," *Diabetology & Metabolic Syndrome*, vol. 8, no. 1, 2016.

[16] V. Newcombe, A. Blanch, G. H. Slater, A. Szold, and G. A. Fielding, "Laparoscopic adjustable gastric banding prior to renal transplantation," *Obesity Surgery*, vol. 15, no. 4, pp. 567–570, 2005.

[17] N. Zarshenas, M. Nacher, K. W. Loi, and J. O. Jorgensen, "Investigating Nutritional Deficiencies in a Group of Patients 3 Years Post Laparoscopic Sleeve Gastrectomy," *Obesity Surgery*, vol. 26, no. 12, pp. 2936–2943, 2016.

[18] H. Bonatti, T. Schmitt, J. Northup et al., "Laparoscopic gastric banding in a kidney-pancreas transplant recipient with new

onset type II diabetes mellitus associated with morbid obesity," *Clinical Transplantation*, vol. 22, no. 6, pp. 829–832, 2008.

[19] H. Bonatti, G. Brandacher, E. Hoeller et al., "Laparoscopically implanted gastric pacemaker after kidney-pancreas transplantation: Treatment of morbid obesity and diabetic gastroparesis," *Obesity Surgery*, vol. 17, no. 1, pp. 100–103, 2007.

[20] E. F. Elli, R. Gonzalez-Heredia, L. Sanchez-Johnsen, N. Patel, R. Garcia-Roca, and J. Oberholzer, "Sleeve gastrectomy surgery in obese patients post-organ transplantation," *Surgery for Obesity and Related Diseases*, vol. 12, no. 3, pp. 528–534, 2016.

[21] M. Porubsky, J. A. Powelson, D. J. Selzer et al., "Pancreas transplantation after bariatric surgery," *Clinical Transplantation*, vol. 26, no. 1, pp. E1–E6, 2012.

[22] J. Zelones, O. Biswas, and A. Mehran, "Laparoscopic sleeve gastrectomy after simultaneous pancreas-kidney transplant," *The American Surgeon*, vol. 78, no. 5, pp. 613-614, 2012.

[23] D. J. Lo, B. A. Sayed, and N. A. Turgeon, "Pancreas transplantation in unconventional recipients," *Current Opinion in Organ Transplantation*, vol. 21, no. 4, pp. 393–398, 2016.

[24] B. Palal, M. Sinsakul, and S. Reutrakul, "Life-Threatening Hypocalcemia following Subtotal Parathyroidectomy in a Patient with Renal Failure and Previous Roux-en-Y Gastric Bypass Surgery," *Case Reports in Endocrinology*, vol. 2011, Article ID 370583, p. 2011, 2011.

[25] G. Marcucci, G. Della Pepa, and M. L. Brandi, "Drug safety evaluation of parathyroid hormone for hypocalcemia in patients with hypoparathyroidism," *Expert Opinion on Drug Safety*, vol. 16, no. 5, pp. 617–625, 2017.

[26] S. M. Pietras and M. F. Holick, "Refractory hypocalcemia following near-total thyroidectomy in a patient with a prior roux-en-y gastric bypass," *Obesity Surgery*, vol. 19, no. 4, pp. 524–526, 2009.

[27] J. A. Gross, S. M. Olsen, C. A. Koch, and E. J. Moore, "Severe symptomatic hypocalcemia following total thyroidectomy in a patient with a history of Roux-en-Y gastric bypass surgery," *Ear, Nose & Throat Journal*, vol. 93, no. 1, p. E6, 2014.

26

Differing Tales of Two Patients after Receiving a Kidney Transplant from a Donor with Disseminated Intravascular Coagulation

Pradeep V. Kadambi,[1] Ann K. Gamilla-Crudo,[1] Mohammad Almiani,[2] Michelle A. Josephson,[2] and W. James Chon[2]

[1] *University of Texas Medical Branch, 301 University Boulevard, Galveston, TX 77555, USA*
[2] *University of Chicago, 5841 S Maryland Avenue, MC 5100, Chicago, IL 60637, USA*

Correspondence should be addressed to Pradeep V. Kadambi; pkadambi@email.arizona.edu

Academic Editor: Mariano Ferraresso

In order to decrease the time on the deceased donor kidney wait list and to have more organs available, criteria for acceptable organs for transplant could be made less stringent. There are reports of successful recipient outcomes using kidney donors presenting with disseminated intravascular coagulation (DIC). We report a unique circumstance where two patients received kidneys from the same deceased donor who had DIC; one patient developed thrombotic microangiopathy (TMA) while the other did not. This difference in outcome may indicate that both donor and recipient factors contribute to the development of posttransplant TMA.

1. Introduction

Kidney transplantation is the treatment of choice for end stage kidney disease (ESKD). Unfortunately, the wait time for a deceased donor kidney continues to increase every year as the number of potential recipients on the waiting list has far surpassed the number of kidney donors available for transplantation [1]. Over the past decade, initiatives such as the addition of Expanded Criteria Donors [2] and Donation after Cardiac Death [3] have had minimal impact on the number of available organs. Other strategies to increase organ availability are being undertaken. For example, a number of organs which were once thought unusable have been transplanted. We report our experience where at the time of recovery the donor had DIC, and the kidneys had TMA. Despite the microscopic findings, both kidneys were transplanted into different recipients with very different short-term clinical outcomes.

2. Case Report

The donor was a 24-year-old African American male with no significant medical history who sustained a gunshot wound to the head and subsequently developed DIC and multiorgan failure. The terminal serum creatinine was 6.0 mg/dL. Preimplantation biopsy of the donor's right kidney showed 27 glomeruli with no sclerosis; fibrin thrombi were present in 8 glomeruli; there was no interstitial fibrosis and tubular atrophy (IFTA), acute tubular necrosis (ATN), or infiltrates; mild (<25%) arterial sclerosis was identified but there was no arteriolar hyalinosis. Preimplantation biopsy of the left donor kidney revealed 34 glomeruli with 1 sclerosed glomerulus (2.9%); fibrin thrombi were present in 1 glomerulus; no IFTA, ATN, infiltrate, arterial, or arteriolar hyalinosis were observed.

The first recipient was a 55-year-old Caucasian male with ESKD secondary to hypertension who had been on hemodialysis for 6 years. There were 4 HLA mismatches with the donor, and the panel reactive antibody (PRA) titer at the time of transplant was 0%. He received the donor's right kidney. The cold ischemia time (CIT) was 18 hours and 10 minutes. The patient was induced with antithymocyte globulin and maintained on tacrolimus, mycophenolate sodium, and prednisone. He had an uncomplicated postoperative course with a serum creatinine of 3.1 mg/dL at time of

discharge. A month later, the serum creatinine improved to 1.2 mg/dL.

The second recipient was a 39-year-old African American, nonobese female with body mass index of 28.7, with ESKD presumed to be due to hypertension, and had been on peritoneal dialysis for 9 years. She received the donor's left kidney and there were 4 HLA mismatches and the PRA was 0%. The CIT was 22 hours and 17 minutes. She was also induced with antithymocyte globulin. She had delayed graft function (DGF) requiring peritoneal dialysis for about 10 days after transplant.

As shown in Table 1, 48 hours after the transplant, she developed severe thrombocytopenia and anemia even before the calcineurin inhibitor (CNI) was started. A clinical diagnosis of thrombotic thrombocytopenic purpura-hemolytic uremic syndrome (TTP-HUS) was made based on the peripheral blood smear findings which revealed schistocytes and the laboratory values (high lactate dehydrogenase, low fibrinogen, and high fibrin split products). The ADAMTS13 activity was measured at 59%. On further questioning, the patient denied prior use of oral contraceptives or hormone replacement therapy.

She was treated with daily therapeutic plasma exchanges (total of 11 treatments) and four doses of rituximab (375 mg/m^2 of body surface area or 700 mg per dose) on postoperative days 14, 21, 28, and 35. Her blood parameters improved with subsequent recovery of her kidney allograft as noted in Table 1.

3. Discussion

TMA refers to blood vessel wall thickening (mainly arterioles or capillaries) with swelling or detachment of the endothelial cell from the basement membrane, accumulation of fluffy material in the subendothelial space, intraluminal platelet thrombosis, and partial or complete obstruction of the vessel lumina [4]. Depending on whether kidney or brain lesions prevail, two pathologically indistinguishable but clinically separate entities occur: the hemolytic uremic syndrome (HUS) and the thrombotic thrombocytopenic purpura (TTP), respectively [5]. After kidney transplantation, TMA may be either recurrent or de novo. Among patients with ESKD due to TMA who undergo transplantation, the risk of recurrence depends upon the underlying etiology. Less commonly, patients who undergo renal transplantation for other causes of ESKD may also develop TMA; this is termed de novo TMA. Antibody mediated rejection (AMR) is a well-recognized cause of TMA after transplantation. It would be appropriate to check donor specific antibodies (DSA) upon recognition of clinical findings suggestive of TTP-HUS as TMA may often be found in the renal allograft.

The recurrence rate of TMA after kidney transplantation is reported between 25 and 50 percent [6, 7]. Most cases of recurrence are probably due to HUS and as previously mentioned the risk depends on the underlying cause of TMA. For example, recurrence among patients who had infection related variant of TMA (typical HUS) seems low. On the other hand, higher rates of recurrence are associated with the noninfection related or atypical variant of HUS (aHUS), where a clear link has been established to defects in regulation of the alternate complement pathway [8]. Mutations have been identified in complement factor H (CFH), complement factor I (CFI), matrix cofactor protein, and thrombomodulin [9]. In the right setting, these mutations may trigger TMA. While checking for complement factor mutations is ideal, the long turnaround time (~ 3 months) makes it impractical for rapid therapeutic decisions. In the appropriate clinical setting, empiric treatment with plasmapheresis is initiated as soon as the possibility of TTP-HUS is raised. Moreover specific genetic susceptibility mutations are identified in only about 60% of affected individuals.

De novo TMA after kidney transplantation is far less common with a reported incidence of only 0.8% in the analysis of United States Renal Data Systems [10]. Typically, it develops in the early posttransplant period; however, it may also be recognized years after transplant [11]. One of the most important risk factors for developing de novo TMA is the use of CNI as maintenance immunosuppression [12, 13]. The disease triggering effects of CNI seem multifactorial and are related to vasoconstriction, endothelial toxicity, and prothrombotic and antifibrinolytic actions. Other risk factors include viral infections (BK virus, parvovirus B19, and cytomegalovirus), use of Expanded Criteria Donor kidneys, presence of antiphospholipid antibodies, antibody mediated rejection, and other medications (clopidogrel and valacyclovir) [14–18].

DIC is characterized by activation of the coagulation pathway which results in the intravascular formation of fibrin [19]. This causes thrombotic occlusion of small and midsize vessels which can lead to multiple organ failure, including the kidneys [19]. This condition has been well described in patients with traumatic brain injury [20] who serve as a large source of deceased donors. Whether or not to accept kidneys for transplantation from donors with DIC, even from those who had normal kidney function prior to the DIC, is controversial. However, over the past few years, there is growing evidence of successful use of kidneys from such donors [21–23].

Supporting this approach were findings from a retrospective cohort of 162 kidney transplants in which donor DIC was not associated with suboptimal graft function in the short term [24].

The role of ADAMTS13 deficiency for identifying patients who have a clinical diagnosis of TTP has not been well defined. In one study, the presenting features and clinical outcomes of 16 patients with idiopathic TTP-HUS who had severe ADAMTS13 deficiency were variable and not distinctively different from the 32 patients with idiopathic TTP-HUS who did not have ADAMTS13 deficiency [25]. Regardless of ADAMTS13 activity, many patients responded to treatment with plasma exchange [25]. Patients described as having HUS were not [26] or were rarely [27] severely deficient in ADAMTS13 activity. Our patient had ADAMTS13 activity of 59%. Since there are no explicit criteria to distinguish patients with TTP from patients with HUS, the initial role of ADAMTS13 activity measurement remains unknown.

TABLE 1: Pertinent laboratory values of the second patient describing the postoperative clinical course.

Labs	Before surgery	48 hours after transplant	4 weeks later/at discharge	2 years after transplant
WBC (×1000/L)	10	8.6	5.2	6
Hemoglobin (gm/dL)	8.6	7.1	11	11.2
Platelets (×1000/L)	289	35	239	188
Prothrombin time (sec)	14	16		
Partial thromboplastin time (sec)	30	32		
Lactate dehydrogenase (mg/mL)		622		
Haptoglobin (mg/dL)		<20		
Coombs' test		Negative		
ADAMTS13 activity		59%		
HIT antibody PF-4 assay*		Negative		
Creatinine (mg/dL)	14	12.5	1.4	1.3

*HIT: heparin induced thrombocytopenia; PF-4: platelet factor 4.

Our report indicates that both donor and recipient factors are important in posttransplant TMA as the first recipient did not manifest the disease while the second recipient did. Since the underlying cause of ESKD was reported as hypertension in the second recipient, donor DIC perhaps played an important role in causing TMA.

Organ transplantation by itself can cause microvascular injury in numerous ways and thus may trigger TMA [28]. Endothelial lesions in the graft, caused by prolonged warm ischemia, might increase antigenic presentation giving rise to acute rejection and TMA [14]. In a study of 24 patients with de novo posttransplant TMA, 7 (29%) carried mutations in CFH, CFI, or combined CFH/CFI indicating that undiagnosed complement abnormalities may represent important risk factors [29]. However, we did not check the second patient for complement mutations.

In general, the prognosis of de novo TMA is better than that of recurrent TMA. However, it may depend on the severity of clinical features and histological lesions. Patients with isolated glomerular TMA usually have a good outcome while patients with systemic signs and symptoms of TMA are more likely to need renal replacement therapy with associated loss of allograft function [11].

While there are no guidelines for treatment of de novo TMA after kidney transplantation, withdrawal of the offending agent is mandatory. Switching from a CNI based immunosuppressive regimen to a non-CNI based regimen can be helpful in some cases [30, 31]. Main therapeutic options include plasma exchange, intravenous immunoglobulin (IVIg), and rituximab [32–34].

Our second patient developed posttransplant TTP-HUS even before the initiation of CNI. The syndrome was recognized early and with aggressive treatment her clinical course improved. She was maintained on mycophenolate mofetil and prednisone and was started on tacrolimus after completion of plasma exchange with close monitoring of her clinical course. A biopsy was not performed after the intervention as the patient's kidney function remained stable. She did not have any subsequent episodes of TTP/HUS and her serum creatinine at 4 years after transplant was stable at 1.3 mg/dL.

More recently, there is evidence that eculizumab (anti-C5a) may be effective in treating and preventing recurrence of aHUS after kidney transplantation [35, 36].

4. Conclusion

TMA in either the kidney recipient or the donor is generally associated with a poor prognosis. While donor kidneys with TMA should not be automatically discarded, reasonable caution should be exercised as to whom these kidneys should be transplanted into. For example, they should not be used in recipients who have had previous episodes of TMA needing therapy or those who currently have thrombocytopenia for unknown reasons. Needless to say, informed consent is critical. Recipients should be informed about the potential risk of developing TMA after transplant with associated loss of the allograft. Patients should be monitored closely after transplant and therapy instituted as soon as possible if there are signs or symptoms of TMA, either clinically or on the allograft biopsy. While conventional therapies of plasma exchange, IVIg and rituximab, are frequently used, the anti-C5a antibody eculizumab offers promise.

References

[1] Organ Procurement and Transplantation Network (OPTN) and Scientific Registry of Transplant Recipients (SRTR), OPTN/SRTR 2011 Annual Data Report, Department of Health and Human Services, Health Resources and Services Administration, Healthcare Systems Bureau, Division of Transplantation, Rockville, Md, USA, 2012.

[2] A. O. Ojo, "Expanded criteria donors: process and outcomes," *Seminars in Dialysis*, vol. 18, no. 6, pp. 463–468, 2005.

[3] D. M. Summers, R. J. Johnson, J. Allen et al., "Analysis of factors that affect outcome after transplantation of kidneys donated after cardiac death in the UK: a cohort study," *The Lancet*, vol. 376, no. 9749, pp. 1303–1311, 2010.

[4] G. Remuzzi, P. Ruggenenti, and T. Bertani, *Renal Pathology: With Clinical and Functional Correlations*, J.B. Lipppincott, Philadelphia, Pa, USA, 1994.

[5] P. Ruggenenti, M. Noris, and G. Remuzzi, "Thrombotic microangiopathy, hemolytic uremic syndrome, and thrombotic thrombocytopenic purpura," *Kidney International*, vol. 60, no. 3, pp. 831–846, 2001.

[6] D. Hebert, R. K. Sibley, and S. M. Mauer, "Recurrence of hemolytic uremic syndrome in renal transplant recipients," *Kidney International*, vol. 29, supplement 19, pp. S51–S58, 1986.

[7] M. A. Artz, E. J. Steenbergen, A. J. Hoitsma, L. A. H. Monnens, and J. F. M. Wetzels, "Renal transplantation in patients with hemolytic uremic syndrome: high rate of recurrence and increased incidence of acute rejections," *Transplantation*, vol. 76, no. 5, pp. 821–826, 2003.

[8] M. Noris and G. Remuzzi, "Atypical hemolytic-uremic syndrome," *The New England Journal of Medicine*, vol. 361, no. 17, pp. 1676–1687, 2009.

[9] M. Salvadori and E. Bertoni, "Update on hemolytic uremic syndrome: diagnostic and therapeutic recommendations," *The World Journal of Nephrology*, vol. 2, no. 3, pp. 56–76, 2013.

[10] J. C. Reynolds, L. Y. Agodoa, C. M. Yuan, and K. C. Abbott, "Thrombotic microangiopathy after renal transplantation in the United States," *The American Journal of Kidney Diseases*, vol. 42, no. 5, pp. 1058–1068, 2003.

[11] C. Ponticelli and G. Banfi, "Thrombotic microangiopathy after kidney transplantation," *Transplant International*, vol. 19, no. 10, pp. 789–794, 2006.

[12] A. Zarifian, S. Meleg-Smith, R. O'Donovan, R. J. Tesi, and V. Batuman, "Cyclosporine-associated thrombotic microangiopathy in renal allografts," *Kidney International*, vol. 55, no. 6, pp. 2457–2466, 1999.

[13] C. Lin, K. King, Y. Chao, A. H. Yang, C. Chang, and W. Yang, "Tacrolimus-associated hemolytic uremic syndrome: a case analysis," *Journal of Nephrology*, vol. 16, no. 4, pp. 580–585, 2003.

[14] A. Jumani, K. Hala, S. Tahir et al., "Causes of acute thrombotic microangiopathy in patients receiving kidney transplantation," *Experimental and Clinical Transplantation*, vol. 2, no. 2, pp. 268–272, 2004.

[15] L. Murer, G. Zacchello, D. Bianchi et al., "Thrombotic microangiopathy associated with parvovirus B19 infection after renal transplantation," *Journal of the American Society of Nephrology*, vol. 11, no. 6, pp. 1132–1137, 2000.

[16] T. Petrogiannis-Haliotis, G. Sakoulas, J. Kirby et al., "BK-related polyomavirus vasculopathy in a renal-transplant recipient," *The New England Journal of Medicine*, vol. 345, no. 17, pp. 1250–1255, 2001.

[17] H. H. Balfour Jr., "Antiviral drugs," *The New England Journal of Medicine*, vol. 340, pp. 1255–1268, 1999.

[18] A. A. Satoskar, R. Pelletier, P. Adams et al., "*De novo* thrombotic microangiopathy in renal allograft biopsies—role of antibody-mediated rejection," *American Journal of Transplantation*, vol. 10, no. 8, pp. 1804–1811, 2010.

[19] M. Levi and H. Ten Cate, "Disseminated intravascular coagulation," *The New England Journal of Medicine*, vol. 341, no. 8, pp. 586–592, 1999.

[20] S. C. Stein and D. H. Smith, "Coagulopathy in traumatic brain injury," *Neurocritical Care*, vol. 1, no. 4, pp. 479–488, 2004.

[21] M. Pastural, B. Barrou, A. Delcourt, M. Bitker, S. Ourahma, and F. Richard, "Successful kidney transplantation using organs from a donor with disseminated intravascular coagulation and impaired renal function: case report and review of the literature," *Nephrology Dialysis Transplantation*, vol. 16, no. 2, pp. 412–415, 2001.

[22] L. Sibulesky, G. Reginald, K. Charpentier, and P. Morrissey, "Kidney transplantation from donors with severe disseminated intravascular coagulation," *ISRN Transplantation*, vol. 2013, Article ID 646310, 4 pages, 2013.

[23] P. P. Ghuge, V. B. Kute, A. V. Vanikar et al., "Successful renal transplantation from a brain-dead deceased donor with head injury, disseminated intravascular coagulation and deranged renal functions," *Indian Journal of Nephrology*, vol. 23, no. 6, pp. 448–451, 2013.

[24] C. J. Wang, S. Shafique, J. McCullagh, D. A. Diederich, F. T. Winklhofer, and J. B. Wetmore, "Implications of donor disseminated intravascular coagulation on kidney allograft recipients," *Clinical Journal of the American Society of Nephrology*, vol. 6, no. 5, pp. 1160–1167, 2011.

[25] S. K. Vesely, J. N. George, B. Lämmle et al., "ADAMTS13 activity in thrombotic thrombocytopenic purpura-hemolytic uremic syndrome: relation to presenting features and clinical outcomes in a prospective cohort of 142 patients," *Blood*, vol. 102, no. 1, pp. 60–68, 2003.

[26] M. Furlan, R. Robles, M. Galbusera et al., "Von Willebrand factor-cleaving protease in thrombotic thrombocytopenic purpura and the hemolytic-uremic syndrome," *The New England Journal of Medicine*, vol. 339, no. 22, pp. 1578–1584, 1998.

[27] A. Veyradier, B. Obert, A. Houllier, D. Meyer, and J. Girma, "Specific von Willebrand factor-cleaving protease in thrombotic microangiopathies: a study of 111 cases," *Blood*, vol. 98, no. 6, pp. 1765–1772, 2001.

[28] G. W. Burke, G. Ciancio, R. Cirocco et al., "Microangiopathy in kidney and simultaneous pancreas/kidney recipients treated with tacrolimus: evidence of endothelin and cytokine involvement," *Transplantation*, vol. 68, no. 9, pp. 1336–1342, 1999.

[29] M. le Quintrec, A. Lionet, N. Kamar et al., "Complement mutation-associated de novo thrombotic microangiopathy following kidney transplantation," *The American Journal of Transplantation*, vol. 8, no. 8, pp. 1694–1701, 2008.

[30] O. Oyen, E. H. Strom, K. Midtvedt et al., "Calcineurin inhibitor-free immunosuppression in renal allograft recipients with thrombotic microangiopathy/hemolytic uremic syndrome," *The American Journal of Transplantation*, vol. 6, no. 2, pp. 412–418, 2006.

[31] A. Yango, P. Morrissey, A. Monaco, J. Butera, and R. Y. Gohh, "Successful treatment of tacrolimus-associated thrombotic microangiopathy with sirolimus conversion and plasma exchange," *Clinical Nephrology*, vol. 58, no. 1, pp. 77–78, 2002.

[32] A. Ahmad, A. Aggarwal, D. Sharma et al., "Rituximab for treatment of refractory/relapsing thrombotic thrombocytopenic purpura (TTP)," *The American Journal of Hematology*, vol. 77, no. 2, pp. 171–176, 2004.

[33] S. Jasti, T. Coyle, T. Gentile, L. Rosales, and B. Poiesz, "Rituximab as an adjunct to plasma exchange in TTP: a report of 12

cases and review of literature," *Journal of Clinical Apheresis*, vol. 23, no. 5, pp. 151–156, 2008.

[34] V. Karthikeyan, R. Parasuraman, V. Shah, E. Vera, and K. K. Venkat, "Outcome of plasma exchange therapy in thrombotic microangiopathy after renal transplantation," *The American Journal of Transplantation*, vol. 3, no. 10, pp. 1289–1294, 2003.

[35] J. Zuber, M. Le Quintrec, S. Krid et al., "Eculizumab for atypical hemolytic uremic syndrome recurrence in renal transplantation," *American Journal of Transplantation*, vol. 12, no. 12, pp. 3337–3354, 2012.

[36] C. M. Legendre, C. Licht, P. Muus et al., "Terminal complement inhibitor eculizumab in atypical hemolytic-uremic syndrome," *The New England Journal of Medicine*, vol. 368, no. 23, pp. 2169–2181, 2013.

Early Focal Segmental Glomerulosclerosis as a Cause of Renal Allograft Primary Nonfunction

Emma J. Griffin,[1] Peter C. Thomson,[2] David Kipgen,[3] Marc Clancy,[2] and Conal Daly[2]

[1] *University of Glasgow Medical School, Glasgow G12 8QQ, UK*
[2] *Renal Unit, Western Infirmary, Dumbarton Road, Glasgow G11 6NT, UK*
[3] *Department of Pathology, Southern General Hospital, Glasgow G51 4TF, UK*

Correspondence should be addressed to Peter C. Thomson; peter.thomson@nhs.net

Academic Editors: D. Capone, R. Grenda, and R. L. Heilman

Background. Primary focal segmental glomerulosclerosis (FSGS) is one of the commonest causes of glomerular disease and if left untreated will often progress to established renal failure. In many cases the best treatment option is renal transplantation; however primary FSGS may rapidly recur in renal allografts and may contribute to delayed graft function. We present a case of primary nonfunction in a renal allograft due to biopsy-proven FSGS. *Case Report.* A 32-year-old man presented with serum albumin of 22 g/L, proteinuria quantified at 12 g/L, and marked peripheral oedema. Renal biopsy demonstrated tip-variant FSGS. Despite treatment, the patient developed progressive renal dysfunction and was commenced on haemodialysis. Cadaveric renal transplantation was undertaken; however this was complicated by primary nonfunction. Renal biopsies failed to demonstrate evidence of acute rejection but did demonstrate clear evidence of FSGS. The patient was treated to no avail. *Discussion.* Primary renal allograft nonfunction following transplantation is often due to acute kidney injury or acute rejection. Recurrent FSGS is recognised as a phenomenon that drives allograft dysfunction but is not traditionally associated with primary nonfunction. This case highlights FSGS as a potentially aggressive process that, once active in the allograft, may prove refractory to targeted treatment. Preemptive therapies in patients deemed to be at high risk of recurrent disease may be appropriate and should be considered.

1. Background

A well-recognised cause of renal allograft dysfunction is recurrence of the primary glomerular disease. Primary focal glomerulosclerosis (FSGS) is one of the commonest causes of glomerular disease [1], and in those who have subsequently undergone successful transplantation, its contribution to progressive renal allograft dysfunction and eventual allograft loss is well described [2]. The clinical picture of recurrent primary FSGS usually takes two main forms: early graft dysfunction which is characterised by the emergence of significant proteinuria through the graft within the first few weeks following transplantation [3] with subsequent loss of excretory function, and late graft dysfunction where there is a progressive rise in urinary protein excretion and serum creatinine many months or years following transplantation.

We describe a case where biopsy has proven that early recurrence of FSGS is the cause of primary nonfunction in the renal allograft.

2. Case Report

A 32-year-old man presented to renal services in early 2009 with a 3-week history of facial puffiness. He was found to have nephrotic syndrome with an initial serum albumin of 22 g/L, proteinuria quantified at 12 g/L, and marked peripheral oedema. He proceeded to renal biopsy which demonstrated focal segmental glomerulosclerosis with no evidence of immune complex deposition, only mild to moderate chronic arteriopathy, and minimal chronic tubulointerstitial damage. Whilst his renal excretory function was well preserved at presentation, he experienced a relatively rapid subsequent decline in function in the context of persisting nephrotic syndrome despite treatment with both high-dose prednisolone and ciclosporin. He commenced haemodialysis nine months after his initial presentation.

In July 2011 a kidney from a 27-year-old donor who died following an intracerebral haemorrhage became available.

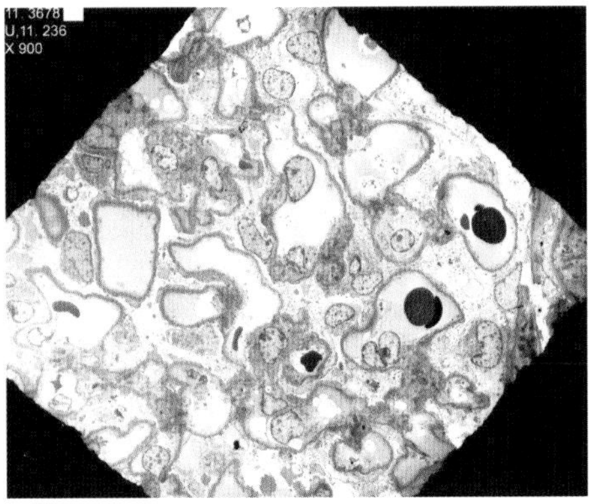

Figure 1: Electron micrograph (×900).

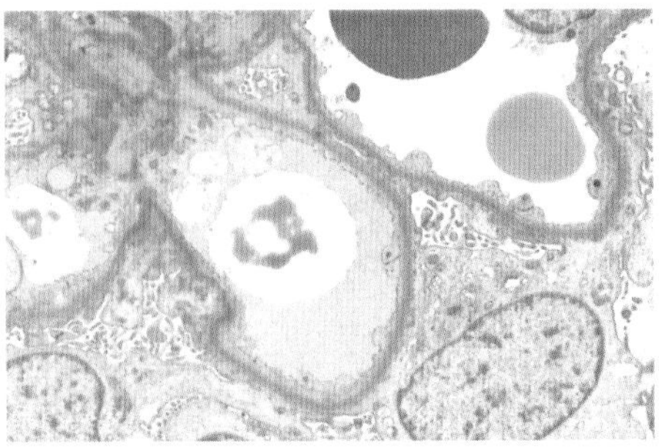

Figure 2: Electron micrograph (×1100). These EM appearances were consistent with early recurrent FSGS. The presence of neutrophils in tubules raised a possibility of ascending bacterial urinary tract infection.

The kidney provided a 1 HLA A, 1 HLA B, and 0 HLA DR mismatch and negative T cell and B cell cross-matches. Successful surgical transplantation of the kidney occurred following a total cold ischaemic time of 8.5 hours and anastomosis time of 31 minutes. The patient received alemtuzumab (CAMPATH) induction followed by low-dose tacrolimus (target trough levels 5–7 ng/mL) and mycophenolic acid (Myfortic) 360 mg twice daily. Cotrimoxazole 480 mg prophylaxis was given, and as both donor and recipient were noted to be CMV antibody positive, valganciclovir prophylaxis was commenced. The EBV status of both donor and recipient was negative.

Over the ensuing days there was persistent proteinuria of 18 g/L prior to the patient becoming oligoanuric and required regular haemodialysis. Throughout the perioperative and postoperative periods he remained haemodynamically stable with a proteinuria of 7.1 g/L and minimal urine output. Serial ultrasonography of the allograft consistently demonstrated no evidence of hydronephrosis and adequate perfusion. On postoperative days 4, 5, and 6 he received daily 500 mg intravenous methylprednisolone on the presumption that the cause of delayed graft function was acute rejection, proceeding to renal allograft biopsy on day 6. This demonstrated mild to moderate flattening and loss of tubular epithelial cell cytoplasm consistent with expected acute ischaemic injury related to transplantation. There was also moderate arterial intimal oedematous thickening. There was no arteritis and no evidence of other cell mediated or antibody mediated rejection. Immunoperoxidase staining for C4d was negative in glomerular and peritubular capillaries. There were no glomerular abnormalities and no chronic tubulointerstitial damage.

He remained oligoanuric and a subsequent biopsy on day 15 showed similar features with moderate acute tubular injury and minimal chronic inflammation involving less than 5% of the tubulointerstitium. In this biopsy the arterial intimal oedema had decreased; again there was no arteritis and no other features diagnostic of cell mediated or antibody mediated acute rejection. Immunoperoxidase staining for C4d remained negative.

The clinical picture persisted and a transplant biopsy on day 35 demonstrated neutrophil polymorph casts in about 15% of tubules, together with predominantly acute inflammation in about 15% of the interstitium. Apart from this, light microscopy was very similar to the previous biopsy, with moderate features of acute tubular injury. There was no evidence of cell mediated or antibody mediated rejection. Staining for C4d was negative. On immunofluorescence, no significant staining was seen. Electron microscopy revealed widespread visceral epithelial cell (podocyte) foot process effacement, involving more than 90% of the glomerulus examined (Figures 1 and 2). There was mild patchy glomerular basement membrane folding. No endothelial cell tubuloreticular inclusions and no electron dense deposits were seen. The mesangium appeared normal. The general consensus was a recurrence of FSGS causing delayed graft function.

A 3-week course of alternate day plasma exchange was undertaken in conjunction with oral prednisolone and continued tacrolimus and mycophenolic acid. These interventions were of little effect and the patient remained anuric and continued his dependency on regular haemodialysis.

Six months following transplantation the patient attended otolaryngology with recurrent sore throat. CT of his head/neck was performed reported as "bilateral ulcerating lesions of both tonsils with excess parapharyngeal tissue and small cervical lymph nodes." Bilateral tonsillectomy was performed with pathology demonstrating an Epstein Barr Virus (EBV) driven posttransplant diffuse large B cell lymphoma involving both tonsils.

No CNS or marrow involvement of the disease was found on imaging. Ann-Arbour stage was 2AE and the patient has since undergone R-CHOP chemotherapy followed by field radiotherapy. He continues on haemodialysis 3x/week and will not be reactivated on the transplant list until his lymphoma has been successfully treated and there is no subsequent evidence of recurrent disease for a minimum of 5-year period.

3. Discussion

Primary FSGS with rapid renal decline is not uncommon and in many patients renal function continues to deteriorate despite treatment with steroids and immunosuppressants [4]. Studies have shown that if FSGS is left untreated, it will often follow a progressive course to established renal failure and in only about 10% of cases there will be spontaneously complete remission [5]. Previously, prognosis for FSGS was poor despite treatment; currently with longer courses of treatment prognosis has been improved significantly [6]. Factors contributing to a less favorable outcome include the degree of proteinuria, histological findings, and response to therapy [7]. Our patient had a poor renal prognosis from the outset with persistent proteinuria that proved refractory to treatment. In such patients renal transplantation is considered the treatment of choice [8]; however recurrent FSGS is always a concern.

The pathogenesis of recurrent FSGS is still not completely understood however. In animal models early onset recurrence has been associated with a circulating permeability factor thought to be released from abnormal clonal T cells [9]. This factor significantly increases permeability to albumin and is thought to cause podocyte injury classifying FSGS as a podocyte disease. A bioassay is now available to quantify the glomerular permeability factor in patients prior to renal transplant. Although higher levels are associated with the development of recurrent FSGS, the predictive value of an abnormal test result is limited [9] and this is not used routinely to identify "at risk" patients who are proceeding to transplantation. Another circulating factor that has recently been identified is the soluble form of the urokinase receptor (suPAR) which has been shown to activate podocyte β_3 integrin which can lead to recurrent FSGS pathology. In two thirds of patients presenting with FSGS suPAR levels were found to be elevated [10].

Recurrent FSGS following transplantation has been shown to develop in up to 30% of renal transplant patients [11]. Factors which influence the risk of recurrence include a second transplant after loss from recurrence, childhood transplantation, rapid progression to uraemia, and being of white ethnicity [12, 13]. Neither posttransplant duration of dialysis nor choice of immunosuppression has any influence over graft survival or recurrence of FSGS. Early recurrence is more common and presents with massive proteinuria hours to days following transplant. Graft biopsies at first can appear normal on light microscopy but show effacement of foot processes on electron microscopy. After some time biopsies show a more "cellular" quality which includes foam cell accumulation, endocapillary proliferation, and thickened podocytes, in the later stages and these then appear as sclerosing lesions [14]. Late recurrence develops over months to years following transplantation and presents similarly to early recurrence. Outcomes are much the same but late recurrence is insidious compared with early recurrence.

Following transplantation our patient developed primary nonfunction with initial renal transplant biopsy appearances consistent demonstrating acute tubular injury.¡?ehlt?¿ The transplant biopsy on day 35 demonstrated evidence of recurrent FSGS on electron microscopy which appears to have compounded the overall renal injury to this transplant and ultimately led to primary nonfunction and a lack of renal recovery following tubular injury. This case highlights FSGS as a potentially aggressive process that, once active in the allograft, may subsequently prove refractory to targeted treatment. This raises the question of whether Preemptive therapies in patients deemed to be at high risk of recurrent disease may be appropriate and should be considered. Current practice has been based on the role of plasmapheresis or immunoadsorption with protein A in conjunction with steroid and calcineurin inhibition. Sustained beneficial effects have been reported with the use of the chimeric monoclonal anti-CD20 antibody Rituximab although this has not always been successful [15, 16]. Whether Preemptive treatment with plasmapheresis and/or anti-CD20 antibodies could offer an improved likelihood of successful transplantation in such patients remains unproven [17].

Our patient developed posttransplant lymphoproliferative disease (PTLD) 6 months after transplantation which pathology reported as a diffuse large B cell lymphoma. PTLD is an increasingly important complication following transplantation as it is unpredictable, can lead to graft loss, and is at times fatal [18]. The majority of cases are associated with Epstein Barr Virus (EBV) which drives tumour formation in B cells and are a consequence of the negative effects of immunosuppressants given following solid organ transplantation and the decreased T cell surveillance which alters the body's control of EBV [19]. Clinical presentation is extremely varied and includes fever, lymphadenopathy, and gastrointestinal symptoms. Most common sites for involvement are lymph nodes (59%), liver (31%), lung (29%), and kidneys (25%) with tonsillar presentation being down at 10% [20]. Increased incidence has been noted to occur with more intense immunosuppression. To our knowledge, the recurrence of FSGS following transplantation does not increase the chances of developing PTLD and both are thought to be mutually exclusive.

When considering subsequent transplantation in patients who have previously lost an allograft through recurrent FSGS, outcomes remain poor. A retrospective paediatric study of 29 patients who received a graft for FSGS was conducted; 3 received a second transplant for recurrent FSGS. Of these, all 3 experienced severe proteinuria and had biopsy proven recurrent FSGS [21]. Other studies have quoted figures of over 80% for the development of FSGS following previous transplant and previous recurrence [22, 23]. We therefore suggest that in such cases targeted Preemptive therapies may have a role and should be considered.

References

[1] G. L. Braden, J. G. Mulhern, M. H. O'Shea, S. V. Nash, A. A. Ucci, and M. J. Germain, "Changing incidence of glomerular diseases in adults," *American Journal of Kidney Diseases*, vol. 35, no. 5, pp. 878–883, 2000.

[2] E. M. Briganti, G. R. Russ, J. J. McNeil, R. C. Atkins, and S. J. Chadban, "Risk of renal allograft loss from recurrent glomerulonephritis," *The New England Journal of Medicine*, vol. 347, no. 2, pp. 103–109, 2002.

[3] D. M. Cibrik, B. Kaplan, D. A. Campbell, and H. U. M. Kriesche, "Renal allograft survival in transplant recipients with focal segmental glomerulosclerosis," *American Journal of Transplantation*, vol. 3, no. 1, pp. 64–67, 2003.

[4] C. B. Brown, J. S. Cameron, and D. R. Turner, "Focal segmental glomerulosclerosis with rapid decline in renal function ('malignant FSGS')," *Clinical Nephrology*, vol. 10, no. 2, pp. 51–61, 1978.

[5] J. K. J. Deegens, K. J. M. Assmann, E. J. Steenbergen et al., "Idiopathic focal segmental glomerulosclerosis: a favourable prognosis in untreated patients?" *Netherlands Journal of Medicine*, vol. 63, no. 10, pp. 393–398, 2005.

[6] S. Troyanov, C. A. Wall, J. A. Miller, J. W. Scholey, and D. C. Cattran, "Focal and segmental glomerulosclerosis: definition and relevance of a partial remission," *Journal of the American Society of Nephrology*, vol. 16, no. 4, pp. 1061–1068, 2005.

[7] J. J. Rydel, S. M. Korbet, R. Z. Borok, and M. M. Schwartz, "Focal segmental glomerular sclerosis in adults: presentation, course, and response to treatment," *American Journal of Kidney Diseases*, vol. 25, no. 4, pp. 534–542, 1995.

[8] C. Ponticelli, "Recurrence of focal segmental glomerular sclerosis (FSGS) after renal transplantation," *Nephrology Dialysis Transplantation*, vol. 25, no. 1, pp. 25–31, 2010.

[9] W. Couser, "Recurrent glomerulonephritis in the renal allograft: an update of selected areas," *Experimental and Clinical Transplantation*, vol. 3, no. 1, pp. 283–288, 2005.

[10] C. Wei, S. El Hindi, J. Li et al., "Circulating urokinase receptor as a cause of focal segmental glomerulosclerosis," *Nature Medicine*, vol. 17, no. 8, pp. 952–960, 2011.

[11] C. G. Newstead, "Recurrent disease in renal transplants," *Nephrology Dialysis Transplantation*, vol. 18, no. 6, pp. vi68–vi74, 2003.

[12] A. Tejani and D. H. Stablein, "Recurrence of focal segmental glomerulosclerosis posttransplantation: a special report of the North American pediatric renal transplant cooperative study," *Journal of the American Society of Nephrology*, vol. 2, no. 12, pp. S258–S263, 1992.

[13] R. R. Verani and E. P. Hawkins, "Recurrent focal segmental glomerulosclerosis. A pathological study of the early lesion," *American Journal of Nephrology*, vol. 6, no. 4, pp. 263–270, 1986.

[14] V. J. Savin, R. Sharma, M. Sharma et al., "Circulating factor associated with increased glomerular permeability to albumin in recurrent focal segmental glomerulosclerosis," *The New England Journal of Medicine*, vol. 334, no. 14, pp. 878–883, 1996.

[15] V. R. Dharnidharka, E. Kenneth Sullivan, D. M. Stablein, A. H. Tejani, and W. E. Harmon, "Risk factors for posttransplant lymphoproliferative disorder (PTLD) in pediatric kidney transplantation: a report of the North American pediatric renal transplant cooperative study (NAPRTCS)," *Transplantation*, vol. 71, no. 8, pp. 1065–1068, 2001.

[16] A. L. Taylor, R. Marcus, and J. A. Bradley, "Post-transplant lymphoproliferative disorders (PTLD) after solid organ transplantation," *Critical Reviews in Oncology/Hematology*, vol. 56, no. 1, pp. 155–167, 2005.

[17] R. Y. Gohh, A. F. Yango, P. E. Morrissey et al., "Preemptive plasmapheresis and recurrence of FSGS in high-risk renal transplant recipients," *American Journal of Transplantation*, vol. 5, no. 12, pp. 2907–2912, 2005.

[18] A. Raut, J. Huryn, A. Pollack, and I. Zlotolow, "Unusual gingival presentation of post-transplantation lymphoproliferative disorder: a case report and review of the literature," *Oral Surgery, Oral Medicine, Oral Pathology, Oral Radiology, and Endodontics*, vol. 90, no. 4, pp. 436–441, 2000.

[19] S. H. K. Oertel, E. Verschuuren, P. Reinke et al., "Effect of anti-CD 20 antibody rituximab in patients with post-transplant lymphoproliferative disorder (PTLD)," *American Journal of Transplantation*, vol. 5, no. 12, pp. 2901–2906, 2005.

[20] R. Dall'Amico, G. M. Ghiggeri, and M. Carraro, "Prediction and treatment of recurrent focal segmental glomerulosclerosis after renal transplantation in children," *American Journal of Kidney Diseases*, vol. 34, no. 6, pp. 1048–1055, 1999.

[21] L. J. Hickson, M. Gera, H. Amer et al., "Kidney transplantation for primary focal segmental glomerulosclerosis: outcomes and response to therapy for recurrence," *Transplantation*, vol. 87, no. 8, pp. 1232–1239, 2009.

[22] N. Kamar, S. Faguer, L. Esposito et al., "Treatment of focal segmental glomerular sclerosis with rituximab: 2 case reports," *Clinical Nephrology*, vol. 67, no. 4, pp. 250–254, 2007.

[23] A. El-Firjani, S. Hoar, J. Karpinski, R. Bell, M. J. Deschenes, and G. A. Knoll, "Post-transplant focal segmental glomerulosclerosis refractory to plasmapheresis and rituximab therapy," *Nephrology Dialysis Transplantation*, vol. 23, no. 1, p. 425, 2008.

28

Angiosarcoma Developing in an Arteriovenous Fistula after Kidney Transplantation

Bruna Natacha Leite Costa,[1] Constantino Fernández Rivera,[1] Maria Calvo Rodríguez,[1] Teresa Hermida Romero,[2] Andrés López Muñiz,[1] Tamara Ferreiro Hermida,[1] Felipe Sacristán Lista,[2] Pilar Iglesias Díaz,[2] and Ángel Alonso Hernández[1]

[1]*Department of Nephrology, Xerencia de Xestión Integrada A Coruña, A Coruña, Spain*
[2]*Department of Pathological Anatomy, Xerencia de Xestión Integrada A Coruña, A Coruña, Spain*

Correspondence should be addressed to Bruna Natacha Leite Costa; natacha.costa@hotmail.com

Academic Editor: Mohammed Rafique Moosa

After transplantation, the main concerns involve immunosuppression, the prevention and treatment of infections and graft rejection, and tumor prevention. Sometimes the complications that may appear in the arteriovenous fistula are neglected following kidney transplantation. This is the reason why we are presenting the case of an angiosarcoma developing in an arteriovenous fistula after kidney transplantation. It is a very rare case and our goal is to create an alarm so that after kidney transplantation clinicians do not lose sight of the patients' previous history.

1. Introduction

Kidney transplantation is considered the best treatment in patients with end stage renal disease [1]. Graft survival has improved in the last years [2] although graft loss after the first year remains constant [3]. The main cause of renal loss is death from tumors, cardiovascular disease, and infections with a functioning graft [4, 5]. Skin, kidney, lung, colorectal, and thyroid cancers are the most reported tumors affecting transplanted patients [6]. Arteriovenous fistula is the best vascular access for hemodialysis when renal failure occurs [7]. After transplantation, the AV fistula should not be closed except in the case of clinical indications such as hand ischemia, recurrent infections, and aneurysmal complications [8]

Here, we report the case of a renal transplant recipient with a high-grade epithelioid angiosarcoma presenting with lung metastasis.

2. Case Report

A 70-year-old white woman with a renal transplant performed nine years ago arrived at the emergency room with a dry cough and minimal activity dyspnea. She had no fever, expectoration, or chest pain.

She had been diagnosed with hypertension and dyslipidemia and the origin of the kidney disease was unknown. Before transplantation in 2007, she received hemodialysis for two years due to a right brachiocephalic fistula. In 2012, the brachiocephalic fistula was closed as a consequence of an aneurysm and during the last year she suffered from local pain which was treated with pregabalin and opiates, with no local complications observed. The immunosuppression drugs administered to the patient were tacrolimus, mycophenolate mofetil, and steroids. The renal function remained stable with a serum creatinine level of 1.4 mg/dL (normal range: 0.6–1.2 mg/dL). After transplantation, she suffered from continuous urinary tract infections that were treated with antibiotics, and after a urologic evaluation in 2012, a left kidney nephrectomy was performed because of a pyelonephritis. In March 2015, an anterior colporrhaphy and posterior perineoplasty were also performed to correct a cystocele.

In March 2016, at admission, blood pressure was 159/92 mmHg, temperature was 36°C, and arterial oxygen saturation was 94%. A clinical examination revealed 20 breaths per minute, wheezing and basal hypoventilation, fistula pain, and ankle swelling. The rest of the physical examination was strictly normal with no local findings in the AV-fistula area. Lab tests showed normal C-reactive protein level of 0.77 mg/dL (normal range: 0.0–1.0 mg/dL), serum creatinine of 1.38 mg/dL, and leucocytes count of 7670 (normal range: 4000–11500); PCR herpes viruses 6, 7, and 8 were negative and so were galactomannan antigen, H1N1, and influenza B virus smear. Blood and urine culture were negative as well as cytomegalovirus PCR.

The initial workup showed a diffuse interstitial-alveolar pattern in the chest radiography and hence a piperacillin-tazobactam and a bronchodilator treatment was initiated. The first CT revealed peripheral bilateral infiltrates and minimum pleural effusion. After completing antibiotic therapy, the patient did not improve and a bronchoscopy was performed which showed no atypical cells or signs of infection. BAL and pleural effusion were also tested and were negative for infection and showed no malignancy. A second CT revealed worsening of the infiltrates and pleural thickening which suggested neoplasia. A pulmonary biopsy by videothoracoscopy was performed. It was of an excellent quality and revealed a good representation of the pleura (parietal and visceral), pulmonary parenchyma, vascular areas, and airways.

A first examination of the histologic sections showed a tumor characterized by atypical cells with vascular affectation that invaded the visceral pleura. There were multiple nodular neoformations with hemorrhagic areas showing a circumferential growth that affected blood vessels and bronchioles, which extended to adjacent areas and to the subpleural pulmonary interstitium. Vimentin stain, CD34, CD31, and VIII factor all resulted to be positive. The expression of herpes virus 8 was negative. These results suggested a metastatic mesenchymal tumor. Subsequently, a right arm arteriography revealed a 7 cm mass in the brachiocephalic fistula (Figures 1 and 2) and a biopsy was performed that was compatible with epitheliod angiosarcoma (Figure 3). The diagnosis of an arteriovenous fistula angiosarcoma with pulmonary metastasis was carried out.

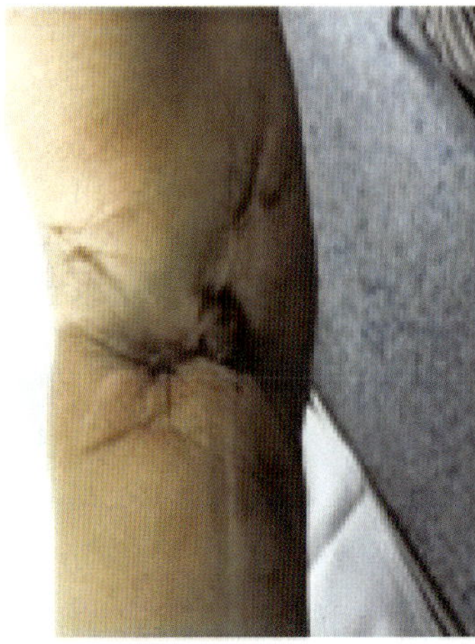

Figure 1: Macroscopic image of the right arm.

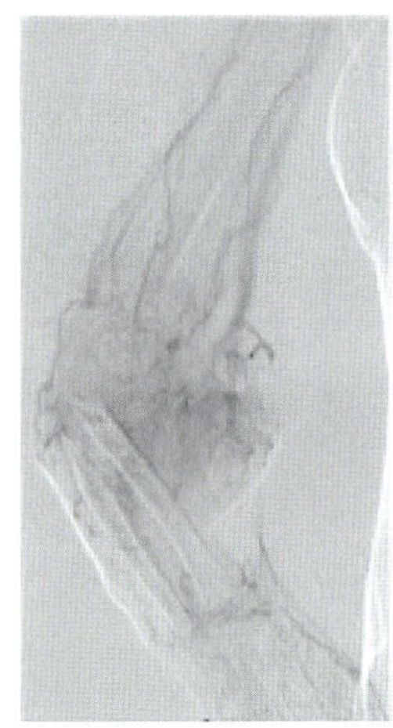

Figure 2: Arteriography of the right arm that revealed a 7 cm mass on the arteriovenous fistula.

3. Discussion

Tumors, along with cardiovascular disease and infections, are the main causes of death with functioning kidney graft [4, 5]. The incidence of cancer increases after transplantation, but there are some tumors that are more frequent than others. Nonmelanoma skin cancer predominates as the most frequent cancer, followed by lymphoproliferative disorders, especially non-Hodgkin's lymphoma and genitourinary tumors [9]. Colon cancer risk is also higher, and so are several other types of cancer. There has been no demonstrated increased risk for prostate or breast cancer among transplantation recipients compared with the general population [9, 10].

The highest associated risk factors are age, oncogenic virus, and immunosuppressant drugs, most commonly azathioprine, cyclosporin, and steroids [11]. Our patient received tacrolimus, mycophenolate mofetil, and steroids.

Angiosarcomas comprise less than 1% of all sarcomas. They typically arise from endothelial cells in blood or lymph vessels [12]. They are aggressive tumors with median survival of between 11 and 15 months when metastatic disease is presented [13].

Despite angiosarcoma usually having a local affectation of between 20% and 45% present with distant metastatic disease most frequently to the lung [14, 15], there were no local findings in 2012 when the AV fistula was closed.

The prognosis is not related to the chemotherapy response, which suggests that survival depends mostly on histological type, mass size, and presence of metastatic

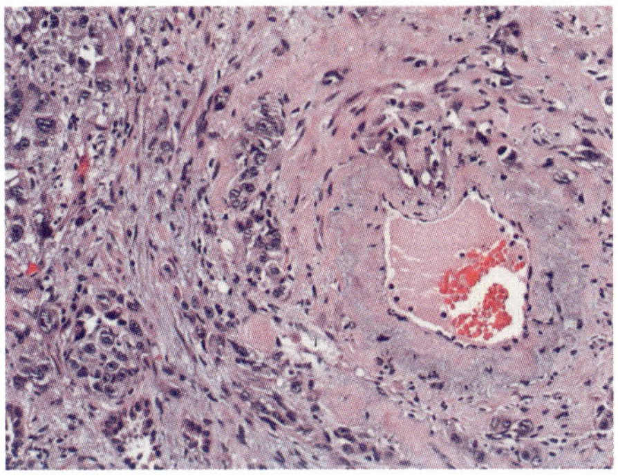

FIGURE 3: H-E staining of the fistula with large and irregular cells with prominent nucleoli and mitosis.

disease [16, 17]. In a recent report of 22 cases of angiosarcoma developing in a fistula, they were all epithelioid sarcomas.

In patients with unresectable metastasis, palliative treatment should be set to prevent symptoms and rapid progression of the disease and to prolong survival. Paclitaxel in monotherapy is ineffective except in the case of angiosarcomas [18]. Our patient survived 6 months after the diagnosis following treatment with paclitaxel.

Although angiosarcoma is rare, it is aggressive and should be suspected when there are clinical changes in the vascular access such as pain, mass, lymphedema, and neurovascular symptoms.

References

[1] R. A. Wolfe, V. B. Ashby, E. L. Milford et al., "Comparison of mortality in all patients on dialysis, patients on dialysis awaiting transplantation, and recipients of a first cadaveric transplant," *The New England Journal of Medicine*, vol. 341, no. 23, pp. 1725–1730, 1999.

[2] OPTN & SRTR Annual data report 2012.

[3] S. A. Lodhi and H.-U. Meier-Kriesche, "Kidney allograft survival: the long and short of it," *Nephrology Dialysis Transplantation*, vol. 26, no. 1, pp. 15–17, 2011.

[4] J. R. Chapman, P. J. O'Connell, and B. J. Nankivell, "Chronic renal allograft dysfunction," *Journal of the American Society of Nephrology*, vol. 16, no. 10, pp. 3015–3026, 2005.

[5] Z. M. El-Zoghby, M. D. Stegall, D. J. Lager et al., "Identifying specific causes of kidney allograft loss," *American Journal of Transplantation*, vol. 9, no. 3, pp. 527–535, 2009.

[6] E. A. Engels, R. M. Pfeiffer, and J. F. Fraumeni Jr., "Spectrum of cancer risk among US solid organ transplant recipients," *The Journal of the American Medical Association*, vol. 306, no. 17, pp. 1891–1901, 2011.

[7] R. Navuluri and S. Regalado, "The KDOQI 2006 vascular access update and fistula first program synopsis," *Seminars in Interventional Radiology*, vol. 26, no. 2, pp. 122–124, 2009.

[8] H. C. Yaffe and S. M. Greenstein, "Should functioning AV fistulas be ligated after renal transplantation?" *The journal of vascular access*, vol. 13, no. 4, pp. 405–408, 2012.

[9] E. C. Hall, R. M. Pfeiffer, D. L. Segev, and E. A. Engels, "Cumulative incidence of cancer after solid organ transplantation," *Cancer*, vol. 119, no. 12, pp. 2300–2308, 2013.

[10] W. S. Asch and M. J. Bia, "Oncologic issues and kidney transplantation: a review of frequency, mortality, and screening," *Advances in Chronic Kidney Disease*, vol. 21, no. 1, pp. 106–113, 2014.

[11] J. D. Briggs, "Causes of death after renal transplantation," *Nephrology Dialysis Transplantation*, vol. 16, no. 8, pp. 1545–1549, 2001.

[12] Y. A. Qureshi, D. C. Strauss, K. Thway, C. Fisher, and J. M. Thomas, "Angiosarcoma developing in a non-functioning arteriovenous fistula post-renal transplant," *Journal of Surgical Oncology*, vol. 101, no. 6, pp. 520–523, 2010.

[13] M. van Glabbeke, A. T. van Oosterom, J. W. Oosterhuis et al., "Prognostic factors for the outcome of chemotherapy in advanced soft tissue sarcoma: an analysis of 2,185 patients treated with anthracycline-containing first-line regimens—a European organization for research and treatment of cancer soft tissue and bone sarcoma group study," *Journal of Clinical Oncology*, vol. 17, no. 1, pp. 150–157, 1999.

[14] N. Naka, M. Ohsawa, Y. Tomita, H. Kanno, A. Uchida, and K. Aozasa, "Angiosarcoma in Japan: a review of 99 cases," *Cancer*, vol. 75, no. 4, pp. 989–996, 1995.

[15] R. C. Ramanathan, R. A'Hern, C. Fisher, and J. M. Thomas, "Modified staging system for extremity soft tissue sarcomas," *Annals of Surgical Oncology*, vol. 6, no. 1, pp. 57–69, 1999.

[16] G. K. Zagars, M. T. Ballo, P. W. T. Pisters et al., "Prognostic factors for patients with localized soft-tissue sarcoma treated with conservation surgery and radiation therapy: an analysis of 1225 patients," *Cancer*, vol. 97, no. 10, pp. 2530–2543, 2003.

[17] K. M. Skubitz and P. A. Haddad, "Paclitaxel and pegylated-liposomal doxorubicin are both active in angiosarcoma," *Cancer*, vol. 104, no. 2, pp. 361–366, 2005.

[18] R. J. Young, N. J. Brown, M. W. Reed, D. Hughes, and P. J. Woll, "Angiosarcoma," *The Lancet Oncology*, vol. 11, no. 10, pp. 983–991, 2010.

29

Successful Kidney Transplantation for End-Stage Renal Disease in Marfan's Syndrome

Makoto Ryosaka, Kazuya Omoto, Taiji Nozaki, Kazuhiko Yoshida, Yugo Sawada, Hajime Hirano, Tomokazu Shimizu, Hideki Ishida, and Kazunari Tanabe

Department of Urology, Tokyo Women's Medical University, 8-1 Kawada-cho, Shinjuku-ku, Tokyo 162-8666, Japan

Correspondence should be addressed to Kazunari Tanabe; k-tanabe@k3.dion.ne.jp

Academic Editors: C. F. Classen and R. L. Heilman

Marfan's syndrome is a systemic disorder of the connective tissue caused by mutations in the extracellular matrix protein fibrillin-1, with aortic dissection and aneurysm being its most life-threatening manifestations. Kidney transplantation for end-stage renal disease (ESRD) in patients with Marfan's syndrome has not been reported in the literature, and the rate of the incidence of dissection or aneurysm in the iliac artery is unknown. Here, we present a patient with Marfan's syndrome with ESRD due to severe renal ischemia caused by massive bleeding from thoracoabdominal aortic dissection leading to transplant surgery of a living kidney procured from the patient's mother. After kidney transplantation, the renal function normalized without vascular complications, and stable graft function along with negative results for both microhematuria and proteinuria continued for two years. Also, vascular complication such as aneurysm or dissection of the iliac artery was not observed using ultrasonography during the follow-up period. ESRD patients with Marfan's syndrome might be suitable for kidney transplantation, but long-term and careful observations are needed.

1. Introduction

Marfan's syndrome is an autosomal dominant condition with a reported incidence of one in 3,000 to 5,000 individuals [1]. It is caused by mutations in the gene encoding fibrillin-1 (*FBN1*). *FBN1* mutations cause connective tissue disorder in terms of classic ocular, cardiovascular, and musculoskeletal abnormalities. Manifestations include involvement of the lung, skin, and central nervous system. One of the most important clinical problems is the occurrence of thoracoabdominal aortic aneurysm and/or dissection. Most commonly, the dilation of the ascending aorta at the level of the aortic sinus is a cardiovascular manifestation of the disease. Progressive aortic sinus enlargement leading to aortic aneurysm is present in 50%–60% of adults and in 50% of children with Marfan's syndrome. Recent data suggest that Marfan's syndrome is present in 50% of patients presenting with aortic dissection under the age of 40 and accounts for only 2% of dissections in older patients [2, 3]. Because of this, the lifespan of patients with Marfan's syndrome is often shortened. A report in the early 1970s describes that life expectancy for affected individuals was about two-thirds that of individuals without Marfan's syndrome [4]. However, a recent assessment of outcome in Marfan's syndrome describes a nearly normal life expectancy by virtue of aortic replacement and cardiac transplantation. In general, Marfan's syndrome in itself will not cause renal dysfunction. Some of these patients, however, develop ESRD because of aortic dissection, abdominal aortic aneurysm, or/and the operations for them. Enlargement of the distal aorta and its branches is less common than an ascending aortic enlargement. A previous report recommended graft replacement of the aortic segment involved if the expansion rate accelerates to ≧1 cm/year, or when symptoms occur, or the aorta reaches 6.0–6.5 cm in diameter [5]. In tandem with abdominal aortic dissection, renal function is sometimes severely injured by impairment of blood flow to the renal arteries, which induces end-stage renal disease (ESRD).

As far as we can ascertain, the techniques and problems of kidney allograft transplantation in Marfan's syndrome have not been described previously. Here, we report a case of living

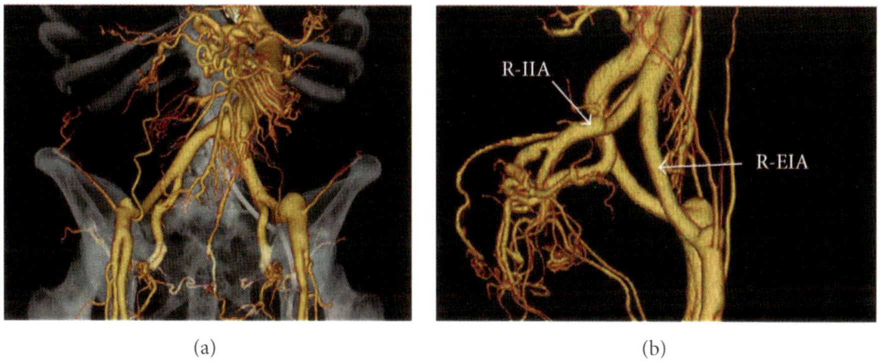

FIGURE 1: Three-dimensional computed tomography scan demonstrating no dissection or aneurysm in the iliac and external iliac arteries. (a) Anterior to posterior imaging. (b) Right-to left-sided imaging. R-IIA: right internal iliac artery; R-EIA: right external iliac artery.

kidney transplantation in an ESRD patient with Marfan's syndrome.

2. Case Report

A pregnant 33-year-old woman with Marfan's syndrome was found to have an abdominal aortic aneurysm approximately 7 × 6 cm in diameter, stretching from the bilateral renal arteries to the common iliac arteries. After Caesarean section, she underwent a composite graft replacement for abdominal aortic aneurysm that bypassed her celiac, superior mesenteric, and bilateral renal arteries with a branched graft. Two weeks later, a thoracoabdominal aortic dissection suddenly occurred. This prompted the emergency replacement of her endovascular stent graft. The replacement of the stent and massive bleeding led to severe ischemic renal injury in both kidneys. Her renal function gradually decreased, and four months later, maintenance hemodialysis was required due to ESRD induced by irreversible ischemic renal damage.

She and her family had been considering a living kidney transplantation ever since she began maintenance hemodialysis. The donor was her 60-year-old mother, because her father had been diagnosed with Marfan's syndrome and had also undergone a composite graft replacement for thoracoabdominal aortic aneurysm.

For treatment of annuloaortic ectasia and preparation for kidney transplantation, our patient underwent aortic root replacement using the David aortic valve-sparing reimplantation technique two years after the commencement of maintenance hemodialysis. Her cardiac function has been stable since the aortic valve-sparing operation.

Although the patient had many anti-human leukocyte antigens (HLA) antibodies due to repeated blood transfusions, donor-specific HLA antibodies were not found. Blood type of donor and recipient were types B and O, respectively. The titer of anti-blood type B antibody was 64 : 1. The preoperative, 3-dimensional CT scan showed that there was no aneurysm or dissection of the iliac arteries (Figure 1).

The patient received a living kidney transplantation from her mother 3 years and 5 months after the onset of hemodialysis. The initial immunosuppression consisted of tacrolimus, mycophenolate mofetil, methylprednisolone, basiliximab, and rituximab. Before transplantation, she underwent double filtration plasma pheresis twice to reduce the anti-blood type B antibody. We transplanted a left-sided kidney into the right iliac fossa. Although we had predicted severe adhesion around the external iliac artery and vein because of previous surgery for graft replacement, it was comparatively easy to dissect those vessels. The renal vein was anastomosed to the external iliac vein (Figure 2(a)). The renal artery was then anastomosed to the external iliac artery (Figure 2(b)). We could not anastomose the renal artery to her internal iliac artery end-to-end because the vessel diameters were very different (Figure 2(c)). After the declamping of vessels, a good blood supply was established to the transplanted kidney (Figure 2(d)). Operating time was 234 minutes, and the estimated blood loss was 117 mL. After surgery an ultrasonography showed that there was no dissection or aneurysm of the iliac artery. The serum creatinine level was 1.37 mg/dL at day four after transplantation. Two months after transplantation, we performed a protocol biopsy, which indicated that the specimen showed no signs of rejection. Eight months after transplantation, renal function remained stable, and the serum creatinine level was 1.0 mg/dL. Microhematuria and proteinuria were not detected. In addition, neither dissection nor aneurysm was observed by ultrasonography two years after the kidney transplantation.

3. Discussion

The incidence of acute renal injury after thoracoabdominal aortic aneurysm and aortic dissection repair has been reported to be about 30%, with renal failure that requires hemodialysis occurring in about 3% of patients with or without Marfan's syndrome [6]. In terms of kidney transplantation, a report of successful preservation of threatened renal function by renal autotransplantation, following dissection of the descending aorta, has been published in a patient with Marfan's syndrome [7]. There is also a report of kidney transplantation from a deceased donor with Marfan's syndrome [8]. As far as we know, however, there are no reports in the literature of successful living-related kidney transplantation in a patient with Marfan's syndrome. It seems to be difficult to anastomose blood vessels because of their connective

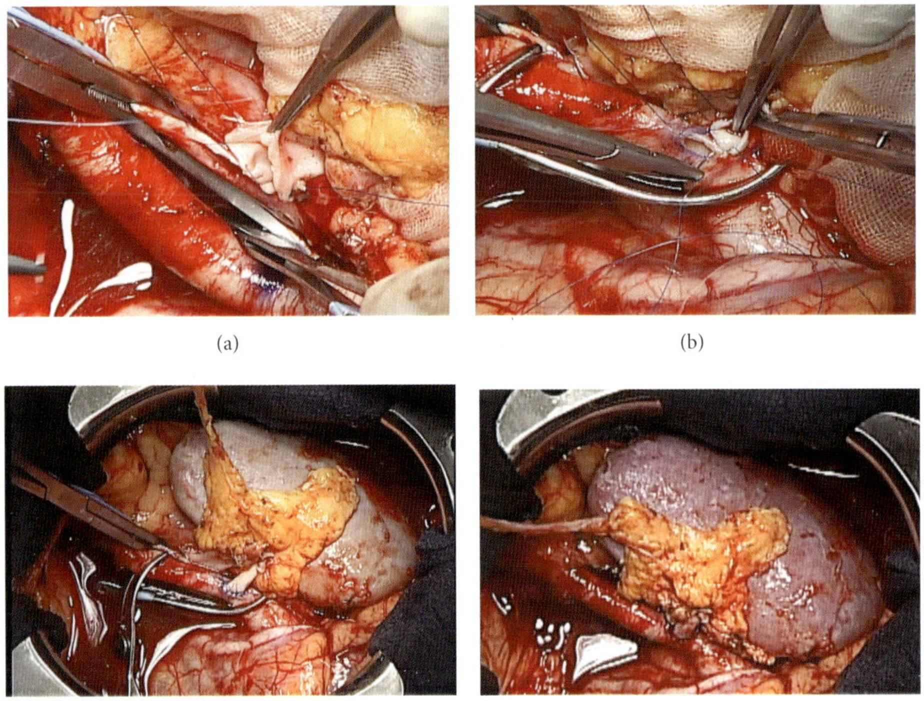

(a) (b) (c) (d)

FIGURE 2: (a) The left renal vein of donor kidney anastomosed to the right external iliac artery end-to-side with a continuous suture. (b) The renal artery anastomosed to the right iliac artery by end-to-side, continuous and interrupted sutures. (c) All anastomoses completed right before the declamping of vessels. (d) There was no bleeding at the anastomoses, and blood flow to the renal artery was stable.

tissue disorder. In the present case, we performed a kidney transplantation in a patient with Marfan's syndrome without any complications. After transplantation, although there was a small hematoma near the upper pole of the transplanted kidney, vascular complications of the kidney graft did not occur, and blood flow in the peripheral areas of the graft was clearly stable.

Immunosuppressive treatment for patients of Marfan's syndrome needs to be discussed. The use of immunosuppressive therapy in patients with Marfan's syndrome is a matter of controversy, as hypertension induced by calcineurin inhibiters and steroid therapy may reduce the integrity of the venous connective tissue. We do not know whether it is safe to use tacrolimus because, as far as we know, there has been no report of administration of tacrolimus to a patient with Marfan's syndrome. Furthermore, it is reported that long-term use of prednisolone leads to aneurysm [9, 10]. However, some reports suggest that there was no problem in using immunosuppressive drugs (cyclosporine, mycophenolate mofetil, and prednisolone) for cardiac recipients with Marfan's syndrome as compared with similar doses in normal recipients [11]. As there are no reports for kidney transplantation, we should administer these drugs carefully. For our patient, we administered a dose of 4 mg/day methylprednisolone from day eight after transplantation. One animal study showed that administration of tacrolimus does not appear to exacerbate graft arterial aneurysm [12]. But this was only a 30-day followup, so further study should be aimed at confirming whether administration of tacrolimus and mycophenolate mofetil to patients with Marfan's syndrome contributes to the exacerbation of aortic aneurysm.

After cardiac transplantation, the incidence of aortic dissection in patients with Marfan's syndrome is about 30%–40% [13]. Some medications may slow expansion of the vessels. Until now, β-receptor antagonists were thought to cause exacerbation of the ascending aorta, but recently it was reported that angiotensin receptor blockers result in a significant reduction of the rate of change in aortic root diameter as compared with β-blocker therapy [14, 15]. Beta-blockade may reduce the onset of graft problems and new arterial aneurysms.

We revealed that a living-related kidney transplantation to a patient of Marfan's syndrome was successful. However, the guidelines recommend taking a CT scan or MRI periodically [16], and there is a report about a case of a second retrograde common iliac artery dissection in a Marfan's patient after delivery of her child [17]. For this reason, we suggest that patients with Marfan's syndrome receive a CT scan or MRI at least once a year. Two years after transplantation, graft function remains normal, there is no rejection, and abdominal CT scan shows no exacerbation of an aneurysm. However, there are some unclear points regarding complications and graft survival. Because cases of Marfan's syndrome with advanced iliac artery dissection are rare, we need to evaluate and follow up more carefully transplant patients with Marfan's syndrome.

Abbreviations

ESRD: End-stage renal disease
HLA: Human leukocyte antigen
TGFβ: Transforming growth factor β.

Acknowledgments

The authors thank Ms. Makiko Fujiwara for data collection. The authors also thank Ms. Elizabeth Kiritani for English language assistance in the preparation of the paper.

References

[1] D. P. Judge and H. C. Dietz, "Marfan's syndrome," *Lancet*, vol. 366, no. 9501, pp. 1965–1976, 2005.

[2] J. L. Januzzi, F. Marayati, R. H. Mehta et al., "Comparison of aortic dissection in patients with and without Marfan's syndrome (results from the International Registry of Aortic Dissection)," *American Journal of Cardiology*, vol. 94, no. 3, pp. 400–402, 2004.

[3] J. L. Januzzi, E. M. Isselbacher, R. Fattori et al., "Characterizing the young patient with aortic dissection: results from the international registry of aortic dissection (IRAD)," *Journal of the American College of Cardiology*, vol. 43, no. 4, pp. 665–669, 2004.

[4] J. L. Murdoch, B. A. Walker, B. L. Halpern, J. W. Kuzma, and V. A. McKusick, "Life expectancy and causes of death in the Marfan syndrome," *New England Journal of Medicine*, vol. 286, no. 15, pp. 804–808, 1972.

[5] S. A. LeMaire, M. M. Jones, L. D. Conklin et al., "Randomized comparison of cold blood and cold crystalloid renal perfusion for renal protection during thoracoabdominal aortic aneurysm repair," *Journal of Vascular Surgery*, vol. 49, no. 1, pp. 11–19, 2009.

[6] M. S. Kalkat, I. Rahman, K. Kotidis, B. Davies, and R. S. Bonser, "Presentation and outcome of Marfan's syndrome patients with dissection and thoraco-abdominal aortic aneurysm," *European Journal of Cardio-thoracic Surgery*, vol. 32, no. 2, pp. 250–254, 2007.

[7] S. D. Thomson, A. M. Chmura, and M. Slapak, "Renal auto-transplantation for aortic dissection in Marfan's syndrome," *Journal of the Royal Society of Medicine*, vol. 88, no. 9, pp. 532–533, 1995.

[8] S. Farese, B. Vogt, F. J. Frey, and U. Huynh-Do, "Successful kidney transplantation from donor with Marfan's syndrome," *American Journal of Transplantation*, vol. 6, no. 8, pp. 1972–1974, 2006.

[9] M. P. Stern, O. G. Kolterman, and J. F. Fries, "Adrenocortical steroid treatment of rheumatic diseases: effects on lipid metabolism," *Archives of Internal Medicine*, vol. 132, no. 1, pp. 97–101, 1973.

[10] B. H. Bulkley and W. C. Roberts, "The heart in systemic lupus erythematosus and the changes induced in it by corticosteroid therapy: a study of 36 necropsy patients," *American Journal of Medicine*, vol. 58, no. 2, pp. 243–264, 1975.

[11] C. Knosalla, Y.-G. Weng, R. Hammerschmidt et al., "Orthotopic Heart Transplantation in Patients With Marfan Syndrome," *Annals of Thoracic Surgery*, vol. 83, no. 5, pp. 1691–1695, 2007.

[12] M. Rigol, N. Solanes, A. Sionis et al., "Effects of cyclosporine, tacrolimus and sirolimus on vascular dhanges related to immune response," *Journal of Heart and Lung Transplantation*, vol. 27, no. 4, pp. 416–422, 2008.

[13] P. S. Chaggar, M. Greaves, and S. G. Williams, "Aortic dissection and cytomegalovirus activation: a possible link?" *British Journal of Hospital Medicine*, vol. 72, no. 1, pp. 50–51, 2011.

[14] B. S. Brooke, J. P. Habashi, D. P. Judge, N. Patel, B. Loeys, and H. C. Dietz III, "Angiotensin II blockade and aortic-root dilation in marfan's syndrome," *New England Journal of Medicine*, vol. 358, no. 26, pp. 2787–2795, 2008.

[15] J. P. Habashi, J. J. Doyle, T. M. Holm et al., "Angiotensin II type 2 receptor signaling attenuates aortic aneurysm in mice through ERK antagonism," *Science*, vol. 332, no. 6027, pp. 361–365, 2011.

[16] N. M. Ammashu, T. M. Sundt, and H. M. Connolly, "Marfan syndrome-diagnosis and management," *Current Problems in Cardiology*, vol. 33, no. 1, pp. 361–365, 2008.

[17] S. G. E. Barker and K. G. Burnand, "Retrograde iliac artery dissection in Marfan's syndrome. A case report," *Journal of Cardiovascular Surgery*, vol. 30, no. 6, pp. 953–954, 1989.

30

Diagnosis and Treatment of Status Epilepticus in a Pediatric Renal Recipient

Gao Hongjun, Luo Xiangdong, Liang Taisheng, Lu Shangguang, Liang FangFang, Dong Yu, Tan Zhen, and Wu Zhen

RuiKang Hospital, Affiliated to GuangXi Chinese Traditional Medicine College, Nanning 530011, China

Correspondence should be addressed to Gao Hongjun, gao4056@163.com

Academic Editors: D. Capone, C. F. Classen, and Y. Sugawara

We elaborate on the retrospective analysis of clinical data on a patient afflicted with grand mal seizures following a kidney transplant. The 16-year-old female patient was hospitalized for chronic glomerulonephritis. She experienced an epileptic seizure and was treated with carbamazepine. Renal transplantation was performed; the function of the transplant kidney was normal. However, grand mal seizures, which required intravenous and luminal intramuscular diazepam injections for control, began on the fourth postoperative day and lasted for 3 days, occurring approximately 10 to 20 times per day. On the sixth day, the patient fell into a deep comatose state and developed the inability to move the right side of her body, hypomyotonia, type 1 respiratory failure, and a pulmonary infection. She was given a breathing machine to assist with respiration. At the same time, she was given protection from infection, tranquilization, treatment for dehydration and diuresis, supportive therapy for the right side of her body, and adjustment of her immunosuppressants. On the 12th postoperative day, the patient's consciousness gradually returned; on the 15th day, the breathing machine was removed with recovery of myodynamia; on the 27th day, she was fully cured with no neurological sequelae.

1. Introduction

Under the effect of immunosuppression and other factors, renal transplant recipients are likely to be afflicted with epilepsy, the attack rate of which can reach almost 20% among pediatric patients. However, at present, there are insufficient statistics to explain the cause of this danger [1]. Status epilepticus, also called grand mal seizures, can have a serious effect on the prognosis of renal transplant recipients. In particular, the first few attacks after kidney transplantation may have a serious effect on renal transplant recipients.

2. Briefing of Case History

2.1. Object. A 17-year-old female patient was hospitalized because of dizziness and fatigue of more than 2 months' duration and with no obvious precipitating factor. Without timely treatment, she soon experienced syncope. She was hospitalized and examined, judged to have high blood pressure and a serum creatinine (SCr) level of 1374.9 μmmol/L, diagnosed with chronic glomerulonephritis and uremia, and treated with hemodialysis.

2.2. Preoperative Diagnosis and Treatment. After being hospitalized, the patient was treated with regular hemodialysis and underwent a series of preoperative therapeutic measures including blood pressure control, anemia improvement, and weight control. On the 40th preoperative day, the patient developed acute loss of consciousness, expressionless eyes, foaming at the mouth, and convulsion of the limbs, all of which lasted for about 5 min. Cerebral MRI was performed, but no abnormalities were detected. The patient was then diagnosed with symptomatic epilepsy. Carbamazepine was initially administered at a dosage of 0.1 g twice a day; the concentration was checked at regular intervals to adjust the dosage. After 2 weeks, the patient was treated with maintenance therapy at a dosage of 0.1 g once a day. This therapy was successful, and the patient was never again afflicted with epilepsy. The patient confirmed that there had been no record of epilepsy in her previous case history.

2.3. Surgery. Renal transplantation was performed. The transplanted kidney secreted urine normally during establishment of its blood supply, but the postoperative urine amount gradually decreased until it reached a low of only 368 mL at the 14th postoperative hour. Ten hours postoperatively, reversed blood flow was observed in the transplant renal vein by color Doppler ultrasound, which suggested the presence of renal vein thrombosis (RVT). Thus, removal of the RVT was immediately implemented. After the operation, the patient was treated with urokinase thrombolysis and heparin anticoagulant therapy. As a result, transplant renal function rapidly returned to normal with urine volume maintaining a level of 4000 to 5000 mL/d and no worsening of the creatinine level. The patient was not disturbed and experienced no discomfort.

2.4. The Patient's Postoperative Condition

2.4.1. Conditions on Postoperative Days 3 and 4. During these 2 days, the general condition of the patient was well, and she was able to perform the Q & A. With the exception of pain associated with the surgical incision, the patient reported no discomfort. Urine volume was normal, being maintained at approximately 5000 mL/d. The heparin anticoagulant therapy was performed with a continuous infusion of liquaemin for 24 h. On the fourth postoperative day, anticoagulation therapy was stopped on the basis of PT and APTT levels, and conventional postoperative antirejection therapy was implemented.

2.4.2. Conditions on Postoperative Days 5 to 11. At 4:30 a.m. on the fifth day, the patient experienced acute paroxysmal convulsions of her lower right extremity with no obvious precipitating factor; the convulsions subsequently spread to both upper and lower extremities. Her entire body was afflicted with persistent tonic convulsions, and she experienced loss of consciousness, expressionless eyes, frothing at the mouth, and gatism, all of which lasted approximately 2 min. The patient was given a pressure pad to protect her tongue and was treated with intravenous and luminal intramuscular injections of diazepam and oral carbamazepine, which had no obvious effect. The patient experienced the aforementioned typical signs of epilepsy at intervals ranging from 30 min to 2 h. These typical epileptic seizures occurred 10 times in 24 h. Given the frequency of status epilepticus and the unusually severe drug effect, the patient underwent a neurological consultation and was treated with a continuous intravenous drip of 500 mL 5% glucose plus 100 mg diazepam at 10 mL/h. The patient fell into somnolence, and her symptoms improved. During treatment with diazepam, although no typical epileptic attacks occurred, atypical epileptic seizures occurred 10 times in the form of twitching of the corners of the mouth and right upper extremity. On the sixth postoperative day, there were still no typical epileptic attacks with continuous use of diazepam. With a decreasing dose of diazepam, the patient was in a superficial coma, afflicted with hypomyotonia, and had an inability to move the right side of her body. A head CT scan revealed a nodule with an unclear outline in the left frontal lobe, around which patches of edema were observed. Patches of edema were also observed in the right semioval center, and the left tricorn was narrowed by the pressure. The midline shifted toward the left, resulting in edema of the brain tissue (Figures 1, 2, and 3).

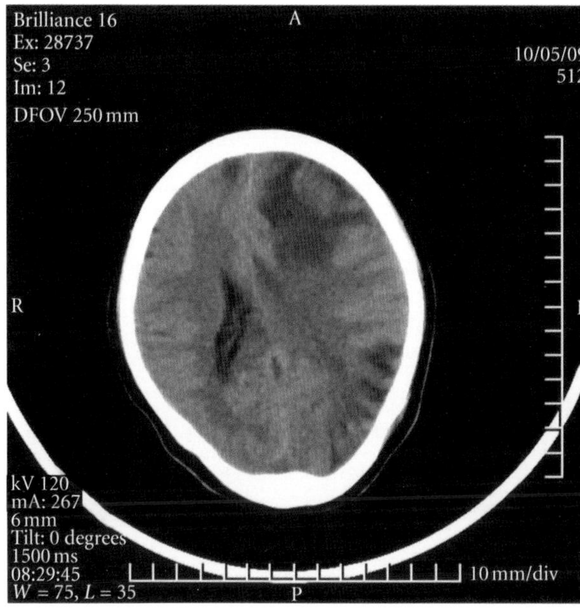

Figure 1: The frist day CT scan.

The patient's tranquilization was continued, and she was treated for dehydration and diuresis and given supportive therapy for the right side of her body. From the seventh postoperative day, the patient was in a lighter comatose state but was afflicted with type 1 respiratory failure and pulmonary infection. Thus, she was given a breathing machine and anti-infective treatment.

2.4.3. Conditions on Postoperative Days 12 to 30. On the 12th postoperative day, the patient's condition improved with a gradual recovery of consciousness and myodynamia of the extremities. The muscular tension level of the left extremities was low, while that of the right was zero. On the 15th postoperative day, the breathing machine was removed; the muscular tension level of the left extremities returned to normal, and that of the right was five. Head CT revealed large patches of low-density areas in the semioval center of the left frontal lobe, and the left ventricle was under a small amount of pressure (Figures 4 and 5). The patient was able to perform early ambulation, but discordance of the right extremities was still observed. Head CT on the 27th postoperative day revealed the persistence of irregular low-density areas in the left frontal lobe, and the left frontal angle had moved back slightly. With normal movement of the extremities, an almost-normal muscular tension level of the left extremities, and elimination of the pulmonary infection, the patient was cured and discharged from the hospital.

2.4.4. Followups from Hospital Discharge to Present. At present, the general health condition, spirit, and appetite are

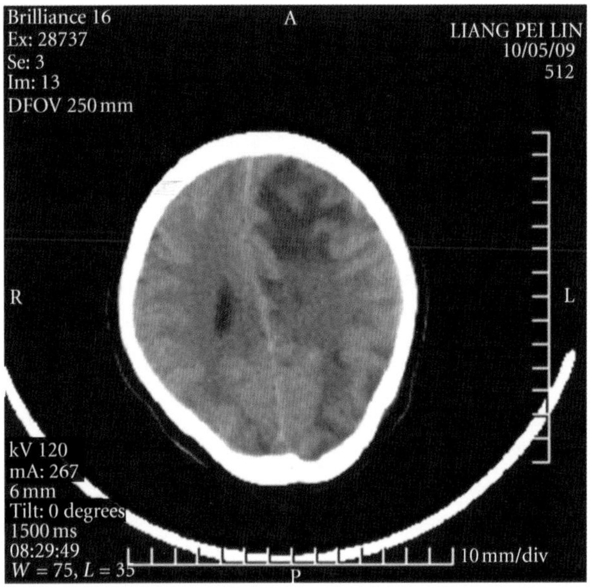

Figure 2: The frist day CT scan.

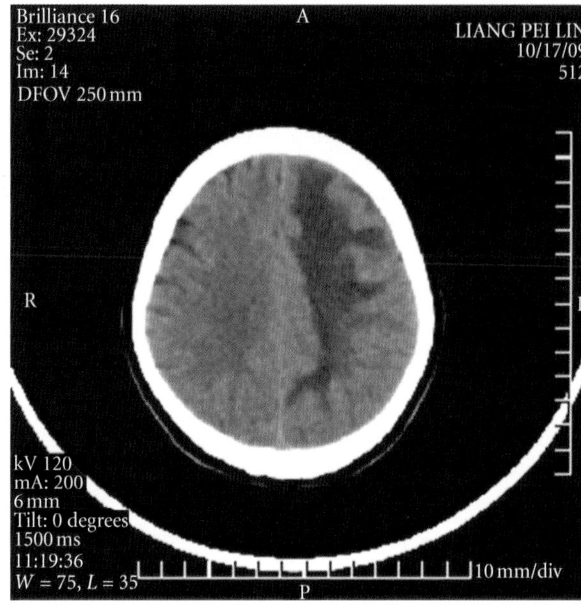

Figure 4: The 12th day CT scan.

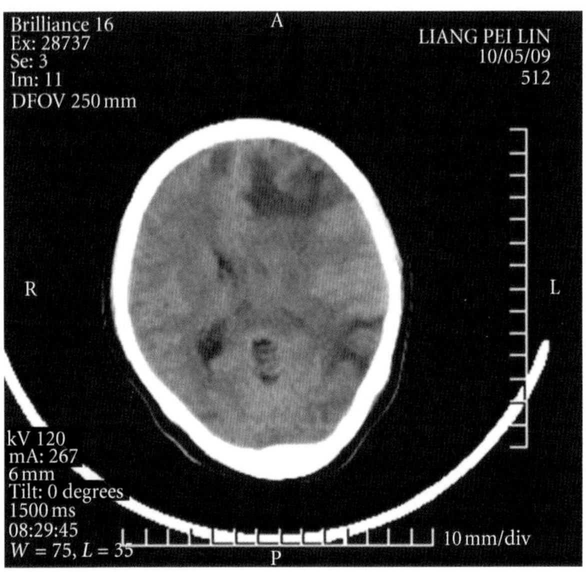

Figure 3: The frist day CT scan.

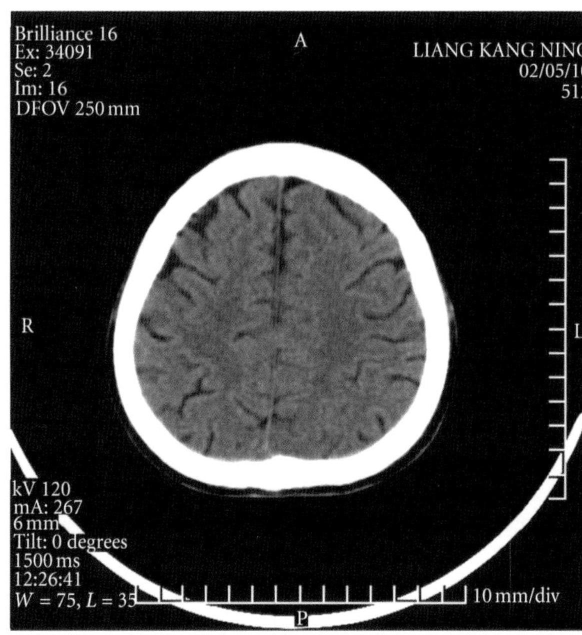

Figure 5: The 30th day CT scan.

good; the transplant kidney functions well; no neurological sequelae remain; no abnormalities exist on head CT.

2.5. The Application of Immunosuppressive Agents. During the operation, 350 mg methylprednisolone was administered *via* intravenous injection, and in the following 3 days, the use of methylprednisolone was continued at a dosage of 350 mg in the first 2 days and 200 mg on the third day. tacrolimus (FK506) plus mycophenolate mofetil (MMF) plus prednisone was implemented postoperatively. Oral administration of FK506 at a dosage of 5 to 7 mg/kg/d and MMF at a dosage of 0.5 mg twice daily was begun one day preoperatively. Because of carbamazepine's effect on FK506, the amount of FK506 was increased to achieve the target concentration.

3. Discussion

Status epilepticus is a pathological condition characterized by continuous and frequent seizures and is classified as a neurological emergency. According to conventional standards, status epilepticus consists of attacks lasting more than 30 min or repeated attacks during which consciousness is lost. New diagnostic criteria have recently been proposed by

Lowenstein and other experts [1], and among adults and children older than 5 years of age, generalized convulsive status epilepticus refers to a continuous seizure of more than 5 minutes in duration or more than 2 seizures at a time; during the seizure, the patient's consciousness is lost. A common clinical, and the most dangerous, form is the persistent state of the generalized tonic-clonic seizure. Symptoms are a sudden loss of consciousness, muscle twitching, foaming (sometimes with blood) at the mouth, frequent apnea, cyanosis, dilated pupils, a diminishing papillary light response, and gatism. The seizure is long in duration or occurs repeatedly. If not quickly controlled, it may be life threatening or cause perpetual brain damage. Status epilepticus is mainly caused by improper drug decrease and withdrawal, sudden changes in medication, or nonstandard times of antiepileptic treatment administration; it may also be induced by infection, mental factors, fatigue, pregnancy, drinking, and other causes. Infection, birth injury, and congenital malformation are the main causes in infancy and childhood. Common causes in young adults include traumatic brain injury, intracranial masses, and parasitic diseases, while stroke, brain tumors, trauma, and degenerative diseases are the main causes in the elderly.

Neural complications in renal transplant recipients are likely to occur at any stage of the postoperative period and have an incidence of 30% to 60%. Both the neural complication incidence and the mortality have a great effect on renal transplant recipients [2–4]. The characteristics of neural complications caused by renal transplants are distinct from those caused by other organ transplants and include limb tremors, insomnia, dysphoria, coma, and convulsions. Epilepsy also occurs among renal transplant recipients [5], and the incidences among adults and children are 11.4% and 17.6%, respectively [6]. In cats with end-stage renal failure that have undergone renal transplants, the incidence of epilepsy may reach 28.9% [7].

Many factors can lead to epilepsy after transplantation, among which electrolyte disturbance is the most common [8]. Characteristics include early epileptic attacks, usually in the 72nd postoperative hour, a high urine volume at 10 000 mL/d, rapid recovery of renal function, and the return of SCr to a normal level at the first epileptic attack. Epilepsy can be easily controlled by correction of electrolyte disturbances with supplementation of blood calcium, magnesium, and sodium and intramuscular injections of diazepam. However, the causes of status epilepticus might be linked to withdrawal of antiepileptic drugs (AEDs) and intoxication [9] of the calcineurin inhibitors cyclosporine and tacrolimus. Epilepsy can be caused by intoxication of cyclosporine and tacrolimus [10], the incidences of which are 2% to 6% [11–14] and 5.6% to 11.6% [15]. Antirejection therapy can be impacted by the use of larger doses of hormones, by which the patient's mental state can be changed and epilepsy can be easily triggered. This type of epilepsy has more severe symptoms, easily causes acute respiratory distress syndrome, and maintains a high mortality; it is also very difficult to cure, often requiring tracheal cannulation and positive end-expiratory pressure with a breathing machine. The aforementioned patient was afflicted by epilepsy once during the month before the transplant. Because of AED withdrawal, the impact of MMP, and the use of tacrolimus, children and young adults with a history of epilepsy are afflicted with epilepsy more frequently, and its persistent state is caused by neurological diseases under the combined action of hormones and physiological changes. It was found by Gleeson through 3-year followups of patients with epileptic seizures during the perioperative period during AED withdrawal that the patients were never afflicted with epilepsy [16].

The grand mal seizures after renal transplantation were usually serious. However, the patient was cured without neurological sequelae, and the transplant kidney recovered very well. Experience with this diagnosis and treatment regimen has been gained in the following 4 respects. First, while the patient's life must be saved, transplant renal function must be maintained, and delayed graft function (DGF) must be prevented, which is the core of successful treatment. Changes in the patient's blood pressure and heart rate can be caused by epileptic seizures. In particular, status epilepticus has a more serious effect on the circulatory system, easily triggering DGF because of the adverse effect on transplant renal function. Once DGF has been triggered, the whole treatment will be more difficult. Second, accurate judgment of the causes of epilepsy is critical to effective diagnosis and treatment. Different causes, such as brain tumors, cerebrovascular accident, and drug-induced factors, require different treatments. However, the treatment should be simplified in case the patient's condition is complicated. Third, when epilepsy occurs during the perioperative period, immunosuppressive agents [17, 18] should be appropriately adjusted. Because of the interaction between AEDs and antirejection drugs, blood concentrations of cyclosporine and tacrolimus can be dramatically lowered by the carbamazepine. Thus, blood concentrations of carbamazepine and tacrolimus should be monitored so that the adjustment of immunosuppressive agents can be performed in time. Finally, comprehensive measures should be taken to prevent other complications and reduce adverse effects in the therapeutic process. Aspiration can easily be caused by seizures, and status epilepticus requires patients to stay in bed; both increase the possibility of pulmonary infection. In addition, central respiratory problems can be caused by severe cerebral problems. The importance of prevention and cure of pulmonary infection is determined by the complexity, refractory characteristics, and high mortality of pulmonary infection after transplant.

The improvement of surgical techniques of organ transplantation and specific nursing practices that can reduce mortality and morbidity make it possible to perform many organ transplantations. The postoperative period of organ transplantation mostly focuses on infection prevention and antirejection treatment. Most neural complications are atypical and have not been given enough attention. However, a certain amount of morbidity and mortality is still attributed to serious neural complications. On one hand, neural complications in some renal transplant recipients are caused by postoperative diseases. On the other hand, neurotoxicity caused by immunotherapy medication can also lead to a series of complications. The adverse effects of the immune overreaction to cyclosporine and tacrolimus should be noted

[17]. Many factors, acting alone or in combination, can cause epileptic seizures after renal transplantation. Thus, for prevention and cure, great importance should be attached to comprehensive treatment. Drugs that can trigger epileptic seizures should be avoided. If epileptic seizures take place, the pathogenesis should be determined and symptomatic therapy begun.

References

[1] D. H. Lowenstein, T. Bleck, and R. L. Macdonald, "It's time to revise the definition of status epilepticus," *Epilepsia*, vol. 40, no. 1, pp. 120–122, 1999.

[2] A. Bruno and H. P. Adams Jr., "Neurologic problems in renal transplant recipients," *Neurologic Clinics*, vol. 6, no. 2, pp. 305–325, 1988.

[3] A. J. Martínez, "The neuropathology of organ transplantation: comparison and contrast in 500 patients," *Pathology Research and Practice*, vol. 194, no. 7, pp. 473–486, 1998.

[4] K. Schwechheimer and A. Hashemian, "Neuropathologic findings after organ transplantation. An autopsy study," *General & Diagnostic Pathology*, vol. 141, no. 1, pp. 35–39, 1995.

[5] L. D. Hamiwka, J. P. Midgley, and L. A. Hamiwka, "Seizures in children after kidney transplantation: has the risk changed and can we predict who is at greatest risk?" *Pediatric Transplantation*, vol. 12, no. 5, pp. 527–530, 2008.

[6] A. Q. Awan, M. A. Lewis, R. J. Postlethwaite, and N. J. A. Webb, "Seizures following renal transplantation in childhood," *Pediatric Nephrology*, vol. 13, no. 4, pp. 275–277, 1999.

[7] K. G. Mathews and C. R. Gregory, "Renal transplants in cats: 66 cases (1987–1996)," *Journal of the American Veterinary Medical Association*, vol. 211, no. 11, pp. 1432–1436, 1997.

[8] R. Wanjun, L. Zidong, and W. Xiaoping, "After renal transplantation epilepsy tonic—clonic seizure two cases," *China Organ Transplantation*, vol. 23, no. 4, pp. 235–237, 2002.

[9] R. A. Patchell, "Neurological complications of organ transplantation," *Annals of Neurology*, vol. 36, no. 5, pp. 688–703, 1994.

[10] B. A. Appignani, R. A. Bhadelia, S. C. Blacklow, A. K. Wang, S. F. Roland, and R. B. Freeman, "Neuroimaging findings in patients on immunosuppressive therapy: experience with tacrolimus toxicity," *American Journal of Roentgenology*, vol. 166, no. 3, pp. 683–688, 1996.

[11] L. C. Racusen, L. M. Famiglio, B. A. Fivush, D. S. Olton, and K. Solez, "Neurologic abnormalities and mortality in rats treated with cyclosporine A," *Transplantation Proceedings*, vol. 20, supplement 3, pp. 934–936, 1988.

[12] R. M. Graham, "Cyclosporine: mechanisms of action and toxicity," *Cleveland Clinic Journal of Medicine*, vol. 61, no. 4, pp. 308–313, 1994.

[13] J. M. M. Gijtenbeek, M. J. van den Bent, and C. J. Vecht, "Cyclosporine neurotoxicity: a review," *Journal of Neurology*, vol. 246, no. 5, pp. 339–346, 1999.

[14] R. W. Walker and J. A. Brochstein, "Neurologic complications of immunosuppressive agents," *Neurologic Clinics*, vol. 6, no. 2, pp. 261–278, 1988.

[15] S. Sevmis, H. Karakayali, R. Emiroglu, H. Akkoc, and M. Haberal, "Tacrolimus-related seizure in the early postoperative period after liver transplantation," *Transplantation Proceedings*, vol. 39, no. 4, pp. 1211–1213, 2007.

[16] J. G. Gleeson, A. J. DuPlessis, P. D. Barnes, and J. J. Riviello, "Cyclosporin A acute encephalopathy and seizure syndrome in childhood: clinical features and risk of seizure recurrence," *Journal of Child Neurology*, vol. 13, no. 7, pp. 336–344, 1998.

[17] N. Yardimci, T. Colak, S. Sevmis, S. Benli, T. Zileli, and M. Haberal, "Neurologic complications after renal transplant," *Experimental and Clinical Transplantation*, vol. 6, no. 3, pp. 224–228, 2008.

[18] S. Marco, F. Cecilia, and B. Patrizia, "Neurologic complications after solid organ transplantation," *Transplant International*, vol. 22, no. 3, pp. 269–278, 2009.

31

De Novo Fibrillary Glomerulonephritis (FGN) in a Renal Transplant with Chronic Hepatitis C

Edward J. Filippone,[1,2] Christine Chmielewski,[1] Rakesh Gulati,[1,2] Eric Newman,[1,2] and John L. Farber[3]

[1] *Department of Medicine, Thomas Jefferson University, 2228 South Broad Street, Philadelphia, PA 19145, USA*
[2] *Division of Nephrology, Thomas Jefferson University, Philadelphia, PA 19107, USA*
[3] *Department of Pathology, Thomas Jefferson University, Philadelphia, PA 19107, USA*

Correspondence should be addressed to Edward J. Filippone; kidneys@comcast.net

Academic Editors: P. A. Andrews, M. L. Coppage, R. L. Heilman, F. Keller, and S. Pinney

Chronic hepatitis C viremia (HepC) has been associated with numerous renal manifestations both in native kidneys and in the setting of renal transplantation. Glomerulonephritis (GN) of the renal allograft in the setting of HepC most commonly manifests as type 1 membranoproliferative GN (MPGN), either representing recurrence of the original disease or arising *de novo*. Other GNs were reported after transplantation in the patient with HepC including membranous nephropathy and thrombotic microangiopathy, as well as an enhanced susceptibility to transplant glomerulopathy. We describe the first case of *de novo* fibrillary GN in a renal transplant patient with HepC where the primary renal disease was biopsy proven type 1 MPGN. We discuss this relationship in detail.

1. Introduction

Chronic hepatitis C (HepC) affects 170 million persons worldwide and is a leading cause of cirrhosis and hepatocellular carcinoma. Renal disease is a prominent extrahepatic complication of HepC, typically manifesting as membranoproliferative glomerulonephritis (MPGN) in the setting of cryoglobulinemia (cryo) [1]. In addition, HepC remains a major concern after renal transplantation, affecting both patient and graft survival [2]. A strong association is documented with development of posttransplant diabetes mellitus, *de novo* glomerulonephritis, and possibly transplant glomerulopathy. Here we report a patient with HepC and biopsy proven MPGN, who progressed to end-stage, and after 2 years on dialysis received a deceased donor renal transplant. Eight years later, in the setting of proteinuria and declining renal function, transplant biopsy revealed *de novo* FGN.

2. Case Report

A 56-year-old Caucasian male with HepC presented in 1994 with an elevated serum creatinine and nephrotic-range proteinuria. He had a history of hypertension, nephrolithiasis, and diverticulitss. Renal biopsy revealed type 1 MPGN. Symptomatic cryoglobulinemic vasculitis (cryoV) developed, which was treated in 1995 with plasmapheresis, intravenous cyclophosphamide, and steroids. Renal function progressively deteriorated necessitating dialysis in 1996. Treatment with interferon was curtailed, owing to severe psychiatric symptoms, and the patient remained viremic and on dialysis. A deceased donor renal transplant was performed in April 2003. An early Banff 1A rejection was treated with a course of IV methylprednisolone with resolution. Immunosuppressive therapy included cyclosporine and sirolimus. A biopsy in June 2003 showed no signs of rejection. In July 2003 cryoV reappeared with asthenia, severe arthralgias, purpura, and

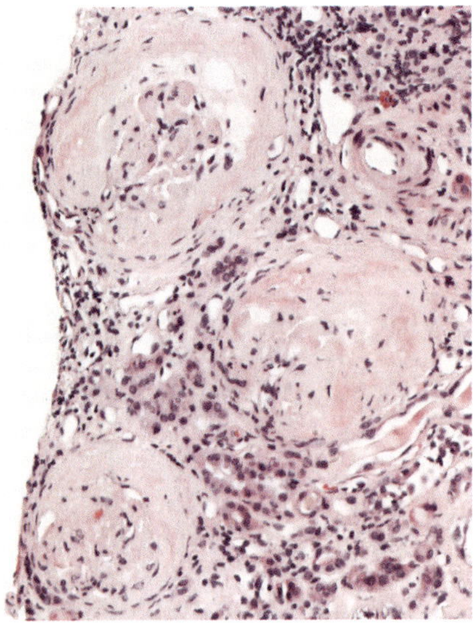

FIGURE 1: Photomicrograph of the kidney biopsy showing 3 glomeruli with prominent and advanced accumulation of amorphous, eosinophilic material (H & E, 40x).

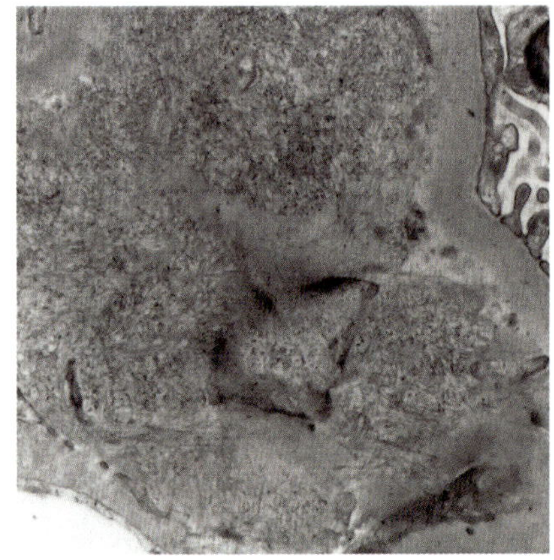

FIGURE 2: Electron micrograph showing an accumulation of randomly oriented, 18 nm in diameter fibrils in the subendothelial space between the lamina densa (upper right) and the endothelial cell (bottom left). Magnification: 20,000x.

abdominal pain. The patient was viremic and hypocomplementemic with a cryocrit from 2 to 5%. Treatment included plasmapheresis and a 4-week course of rituximab, which produced symptomatic improvement. The serum creatinine ranged from 1.8 to 2.5 mg/dL from 2003 until 2010, when it increased to 4.5 mg/dL. A biopsy in June 2010 showed moderate acute tubular damage and mild chronic calcineurin inhibitor toxicity. Electron microscopy revealed a mild glomerulopathy consistent with calcineurin inhibitor toxicity. No evidence of recurrent MPGN was present. Dialysis was required for several weeks, but renal function spontaneously improved, and creatinine stabilized around 2.5 mg/dL. Over the course of the next year, creatinine slowly increased and proteinuria became nephrotic range. The protein/creatinine ratio was 4991 mg/g; SPEP showed decreased albumin and UPEP a pattern consistent with glomerular proteinuria. Both serum and urine immunofixation were negative. ANA was negative. HCV RNA PCR revealed 17,369,084 IU/mL. Serum cryo was negative, although they had been intermittently positive at 1-2%. C3 was normal and C4 was undetectable. A biopsy in December 2011 showed prominent and advanced accumulation of amorphous, eosinophilic material in glomeruli, interstitial fibrosis, tubular atrophy, and vascular intimal sclerosis (Figure 1). Electron microscopy showed 10–15 nm fibrils in the mesangium and glomerular capillary walls (Figure 2). A Congo red stain was negative. Renal function progressively deteriorated and dialysis was initiated in March 2012.

Our patient is the first reported case of FGN in a renal transplant developing in the setting of HepC. The morphologic features of the final transplant biopsy are clearly different from those of the native kidney (type I MPGN) and, thus, indicate a *de novo* process.

3. Discussion

HepC has been associated with various renal manifestations in both native and transplant kidneys. HepC is the cause of the large majority of cases of essential mixed cryo (EMC), whether due to type II (monoclonal IgM against polyclonal IgG) or type III (polyclonal IgM against polyclonal IgG) cryo [3]. This B-cell proliferative disorder is frequently complicated by glomerulonephritis (GN). About 75% of cases of GN complicating EMC are found with type II cryo and about 25% with type III [4]. Histologically, the lesions are a type 1 MPGN. Features that suggest an EMC etiology include prominent monocytic inflammation, large hyaline thrombi, and organization of deposits by electron microscopy (EM). Our patient's initial clinical presentation and native kidney biopsy clearly fit this description of cryo GN.

In a seminal report Johnson et al. found MPGN in all 8 HepC positive patients referred for evaluation of proteinuria [5]. Only 5 of the 8 had detectable cryo, although all 8 had low serum complement and positive RF. Organized deposits consistent with cryo were found in 3 of 4 examined specimens. In a follow-up study involving 34 HepC patients with proteinuria, 31 had MPGN and 3 had an acute proliferative and exudative GN [6]. Only 20 of 34 had cryo detectable on presentation. Over time, however, 9 more became positive (29 of 34 total). Twenty of the 29 positive patients had symptoms of EMC. Others have confirmed the association of HepC with MPGN [7, 8]. Most but not all of the reported cases had detectable cryo. In a series of 105 biopsies of native kidneys, Cosio at al. did not find an increased incidence of HepC in noncryo MPGN and concluded that the relationship between HepC and MPGN only holds in the presence of EMC [8].

Other glomerulopathies have been associated with HepC. Membranous nephropathy (MN) is documented in case reports [9]. Unlike MPGN, cryo and RFs are usually not found, and serum complement is usually normal. FGN or immunotactoid GN has been associated with HepC in several case reports [10–12]. In a series of 6 patients (4 with FGN and 2 with ITGN) reported in 1998, all were negative for cryo on presentation [13]. One patient, however, did develop them over time. This is somewhat analogous to our patient who had intermittent positivity. In a follow-up report in 2003, of 67 patients (61 with FGN and 6 with ITGN), HepC was found in 17% [14]. By contrast, however, in another series of 66 patients with FGN, only 3% had HepC [15]. In the report from Cosio et al. [8], HepC was significantly more frequent in patients with focal segmental glomerulosclerosis (FSGS) than in controls, but this was only true for intravenous drug users. In a series of 303 Egyptian patients presenting with GN, HepC was found in 38% [16]. This contrasts with a rate of 16% in the general Egyptian population. Of the 50 HepC patients from this series, 18 had type I MPGN, 9 type II MPGN, 12 FSGS, 2 MN, and 9 mesangioproliferative GN. Cryo were found in 27 of these 50 patients.

In order to establish the causality of HCV in these various disorders, numerous groups have sought evidence in renal tissue of HCV RNA by polymerase chain reaction (RCR) or *in situ* hybridization (ISH), as well as detection of viral proteins by indirect immunofluorescence (IIF) or immunohistochemistry (IH). In the Egyptian series noted above, IH for viral proteins was negative in all patients studied [16]. Electron microscopy detected particles consistent with HCV in 50% of cases, and PCR detected RNA in 4 of 21 cryo patients and 5 of 21 noncryo ones. Sansonno et al. studied 12 HepC patients with MPGN and type II cryo [17]. After electroelution, HCV-related proteins were detected in 8 of 12 patients by IH; all 8 HCV negative patients with MPGN had no positive reactions. Using laser capture microdissection to extract glomeruli from 20 HepC patients with various histologic types, the same group found HCV detectable RNA in 65% of glomeruli [18]. Positivity ranged from 33% of glomeruli in patients with IgA nephropathy to 83% of glomeruli in those with MPGN; HCV core protein was detected in an equal number of glomeruli as was RNA within each histologic type. Okada et al. detected HCV core protein by IIF in 2 patients with MN (both negative for RF and cryo) [19]. Cao et al. used IH to detect the NS3 protein in 21 HCV antibody positive patients with various types of GN [20]. This antigen was detected in 6 of the 21 (3 MPGN, 1 IgAN, 1 MN, and 1 amyloid); only 4 of the 6 were serum RNA positive. Immunoelectron microscopy showed that the antigen was localized mainly in electron dense deposits and in amyloid fibrils. Finally, in a study of 9 HepC MN patients, viral RNA (both genomic and replicative) and protein were detected in the perinuclear area of tubular epithelial cells by ISH and IH and were associated with greater interstitial inflammation/fibrosis compared to HCV negative MN patients [21]. It remains unclear if HCV has a causal role in these various glomerulopathies, with the exception of type 1 MPGN in the setting of EMC.

The incidence of HCV in patients on dialysis varies between 10 and 50% [22]. The same rate applies to patients who have received a renal transplant. Numerous studies have shown reduced patient survival after renal transplantation in case of HepC. This increased mortality may be due to post-transplant diabetes (strongly linked to HepC), cardiovascular disease, liver disease, and/or infection [2, 22]. Graft survival is also shortened by HepC. It still remains beneficial to receive a transplant as opposed to remaining on dialysis.

Proteinuria and the development of *de novo* glomerulopathy have been ascribed to HepC in renal transplantation. In a 1998 study of 322 consecutive transplants, Hestin et al. showed by multivariable analysis that HepC conferred a significant relative risk of 5.36 on the development of persistent proteinuria (>1 g/day for 3 months) [23]. Roth et al. studied 8 patients with proteinuria exceeding 1 g/day from a cohort of 98 HepC renal transplants [24]. Three had what was previously termed as chronic allograft nephropathy (CAN), but the other 5 had *de novo* development of type 1 MPGN. All 5 had undetectable cryo, but 2 did have low complement levels and positive RFs, and 2 patients also had organized deposits on EM. Cruzado et al. found 9 patients with >1.5 g/day proteinuria from a series of 94 HepC renal transplants [25]. One patient had MN, 2 CAN, and the remaining 6 *de novo* type 1 MPGN. All 6 did have detectable cryo, but none were symptomatic. IgM-RFs were detectable in the cryoglobulins, but 5 of the 6 had negative serum RF. HCV RNA was concentrated in the cryoglobulins, with enrichment of up to 18,000%. The same group evaluated 96 transplant biopsies performed at least 3 months after transplantation that did not show acute rejection [26]. Forty-four of the 96 (46%) were from HepC patients, and 63% of these showed *de novo* glomerulopathy (20 MPGN and 8 MN). This compares to 14% in those negative for HCV (3 MPGN, 4 MN). Similarly, Özdemir et al. studied 165 renal transplants of whom 44 were HCV antibody positive [27]. Of the 24 RNA+ patients, 15 developed *de novo* glomerulopathy (11 MPGN, 4 MN); only 8 of the 121 HCV negative patients did so. No case had detectable cryo. However, in a series of 2000 renal transplants (400 HepC), 15 cases of MN were detected, 10 of which were clearly *de novo*; no MPGN was apparently detected in this large series [28].

Other glomerular manifestations of HCV have been reported in renal transplants. Cosio et al. noted HCV in 29% of 41 patients with acute transplant glomerulitis and 33% of 27 patients with transplant glomerulopathy (TG) compared to 1.8% of 105 transplant patients with neither one [8]. Baid et al. studied 18 HepC transplants out of 339 total transplants [29]. Five of these 18 developed a thrombotic microangiopathy (TMA) a mean of 14 days after transplantation. All 5 had detectable anticardiolipin antibodies, as opposed to 1 of the 13 without TMA and 0 of 7 TMA patients without HCV. In a series of 209 indication biopsies for chronic renal allograft dysfunction from the same institution, 25 cases of TG were detected [30]. HepC was detected in 36% of these compared to 7% in a control group with calcineurin inhibitor nephrotoxicity and 3.6% in their overall transplant population. A TMA was detectable in 32% of the TG patients as well, and there was significant overlap between HCV and TMA in the setting of TG.

Glomerular organized deposits detected by EM as in our patient may be nonspecific findings or may be diagnostic of various conditions [31, 32]. Amyloid fibrils of any etiology are randomly oriented, nonbranching, and usually measure about 10 nm in diameter. Congo red positivity with green birefringence under polarized light is diagnostic, as is staining with thioflavin T. Cryoglobuins are frequently organized, as noted above, and may take various shapes depending on the type involved; interestingly, EM examination of cryoglobulins obtained from serum may mimic the morphology of those deposited in tissues [33]. The immune complexes of systemic lupus may occasionally be organized, appearing to resemble fingerprints [32].

The lesion termed as FGN, found in about 1% of renal biopsies, is characterized by the EM findings of randomly oriented, nonbranching fibrils about twice the diameter of amyloid (about 20 nm) [14, 15, 31, 32]. They are usually found in the glomerular basement membrane or paramesangial area. Tubular deposits are distinctly unusual, and except for isolated case reports they are not found outside the kidney. They are Congo red and thioflavin T negative but regularly stain for immunoglobulins, usually IgG (especially subclass IgG4), and complement by immunofluorescence (IF). Various light microscopic features may be obtained, including MPGN, mesangial proliferative GN, MN, and diffuse sclerosis. Patients present with hematuria, proteinuria, and renal impairment, and about half progress to ESRD in 2–4 years. It may recur following renal transplantation in about 50% of cases, but it tends to progress at a much slower rate in the transplant [34]. The largest series reported to date found an underlying paraproteinemia (PP) in 15–17% of such cases [15]. Some authors feel that detection of a PP excludes a diagnosis of idiopathic FGN, suggesting that the fibrils are a manifestation of the underlying plasma or B-cell disorder [35]. This remains an area on contention.

Related to FGN, but occurring about one-tenth as frequently, is ITG. This has a similar clinical presentation, light microscopic findings, and IF (except more commonly monoclonal) but differs by EM. Here, the fibrils are larger (usually, but not always, >30 nm), hollow (when viewed under 30,000x power or less), and/or organized (at least focally) into bundles. Patients with such deposits are more likely than those with the fibrils of FGN to have an underlying PP and/or B-cell neoplasm, occurring in over 50% of cases. This has led to the argument that FGN and ITG should be viewed as discreet entities. Others feel, however, that after excluding PPs, there would be no difference between them other than the diameter of the fibrils [34]. Neither FGN nor ITG frequently occurs *de novo* in renal allografts. Besides our case, we know of one case of *de novo* ITG associated with CMV infection [36] and another in a patient with systemic lupus [37]. One case of FGN from a large series was presumed to be *de novo*, although there was no native kidney biopsy [14].

As noted above, hepatitis C has been associated with FGN and is clearly associated with cryo. Since cryoglobulins are frequently organized, the fibrils detected in our patient, and other cases with HCV, may simply be cryoglobulin deposits. Indeed, it has been hypothesized that FGN may represent a forme fruste of cryo [13, 34]. Although our patient's initial biopsy had the more characteristic lesion of type 1 MPGN, the final transplant biopsy clearly did not. It is possible that after transplantation, due to immunosuppressive medications and/or effects of the allograft itself, the antigen/antibody ratio or other features of the immune complexes have been altered such that fibril formation was fostered. Perhaps in some patients with HepC this may occur from the outset, resulting in typical FGN in the native kidney. Finally, HCV-related EMC is definitively a B-cell proliferative disorder [38]. Considering the known association of such neoplastic disorders and PP with FGN and/or ITG [39], it may be that through the development of a neoplasm that HepC is linked to fibrillogenesis, independent of its ability to induce cryoglobulin formation.

In conclusion, we present the first documented case of FGN developing *de novo* in a renal transplant patient chronically infected with HCV.

References

[1] G. D'Amico, "Renal involvement in hepatitis C infection: cryoglobulinemic glomerulonephritis," *Kidney International*, vol. 54, no. 2, pp. 650–671, 1998.

[2] B. Domínguez-Gil and J. M. Morales, "Transplantation in the patient with hepatitis C," *Transplant International*, vol. 22, no. 12, pp. 1117–1131, 2009.

[3] O. Trejo, M. Ramos-Casals, M. García-Carrasco et al., "Cryoglobulinemia: study of etiologic factors and clinical and immunologic features in 443 patients from a single center," *Medicine*, vol. 80, no. 4, pp. 252–262, 2001.

[4] D. Roccatello, A. Fornasieri, O. Giachino et al., "Multicenter study on hepatitis C virus-related cryoglobulinemic glomerulonephritis," *The American Journal of Kidney Diseases*, vol. 49, no. 1, pp. 69–82, 2007.

[5] R. J. Johnson, D. R. Gretch, H. Yamabe et al., "Membranoproliferative glomerulonephritis associated with hepatitis C virus infection," *The New England Journal of Medicine*, vol. 328, no. 7, pp. 465–470, 1993.

[6] R. J. Johnson, D. R. Gretch, W. G. Couser et al., "Hepatitis C virus-associated glomerulonephritis. Effect of α-interferon therapy," *Kidney International*, vol. 46, no. 6, pp. 1700–1704, 1994.

[7] H. Yamabe, R. J. Johnson, D. R. Gretch et al., "Hepatitis C virus infection and membranoproliferative glomerulonephritis in Japan," *Journal of the American Society of Nephrology*, vol. 6, no. 2, pp. 220–223, 1995.

[8] F. G. Cosio, Z. Roche, A. Agarwal, M. E. Falkenhain, D. D. Sedmak, and R. M. Ferguson, "Prevalence of hepatitis c in patients with idiopathic glomerulopathies in native and transplant kidneys," *The American Journal of Kidney Diseases*, vol. 28, no. 5, pp. 752–758, 1996.

[9] C. Stehman-Breen, C. E. Alpers, W. G. Couser, R. Willson, and R. J. Johnson, "Hepatitis C virus associated membranous glomerulonephritis," *Clinical Nephrology*, vol. 44, no. 3, pp. 141–147, 1995.

[10] E. Coroneos, L. Truong, and J. Olivero, "Renal biopsy case: fibrillary glomerulonephritis associated with hepatitis C viral infection," *The American Journal of Kidney Diseases*, vol. 29, no. 1, pp. 132–135, 1997.

[11] G. Guerra, G. Narayan, H. G. Rennke, and B. L. Jaber, "Crescentic fibrillary glomerulonephritis associated with hepatitis C viral infection," *Clinical Nephrology*, vol. 60, no. 5, pp. 364–368, 2003.

[12] S. Ray, K. Rouse, A. Appis, R. Novak, and N. A. Haller, "Fibrillary glomerulonephritis with hepatitis C viral infection and hypocomplementemia," *Renal Failure*, vol. 30, no. 7, pp. 759–762, 2008.

[13] G. S. Markowitz, J.-T. Cheng, R. B. Colvin, W. M. Trebbin, and V. D. D'Agati, "Hepatitis C viral infection is associated with fibrillary glomerulonephritis and immunotactoid glomerulopathy," *Journal of the American Society of Nephrology*, vol. 9, no. 12, pp. 2244–2252, 1998.

[14] J. L. Rosenstock, G. S. Markowitz, A. M. Valeri, G. Sacchi, G. B. Apple, and V. D. D'Agati, "Fibrillary and immunotactoid glomerulonephritis: distinct entities with different clinical and pathologic features," *Kidney International*, vol. 63, no. 4, pp. 1450–1461, 2003.

[15] S. Nasr, A. M. Valeri, L. D. Cornell et al., "Fibrillary glomerulonephritis: a report of 66 cases from a single institution," *Clinical Journal of the American Society of Nephrology*, vol. 6, no. 4, pp. 775–784, 2011.

[16] A. A. Sabry, M. A. Sobh, W. L. Irving et al., "A comprehensive study of the association between hepatitis C virus and glomerulopathy," *Nephrology Dialysis Transplantation*, vol. 17, no. 2, pp. 239–245, 2002.

[17] D. Sansonno, L. Gesualdo, C. Manno, F. P. Schena, and F. Dammacco, "Hepatitis C virus-related proteins in kidney tissue from hepatitis C virus-infected patients with cryoglobulinemic membranoproliferative glomerulonephritis," *Hepatology*, vol. 25, no. 5, pp. 1237–1244, 1997.

[18] D. Sansonno, G. Lauletta, M. Montrone, G. Grandaliano, F. P. Schena, and F. Dammacco, "Hepatitis C virus RNA and core protein in kidney glomerular and tubular structures isolated with laser capture microdissection," *Clinical and Experimental Immunology*, vol. 140, no. 3, pp. 498–506, 2005.

[19] K. Okada, Y. Takishita, H. Shimomura et al., "Detection of hepatitis C virus core protein in the glomeruli of patients with membranous glomerulonephritis," *Clinical Nephrology*, vol. 45, no. 2, pp. 71–76, 1996.

[20] Y. Cao, Y. Zhang, S. Wang, and W. Zou, "Detection of the hepatitis C virus antigen in kidney tissue from infected patients with various glomerulonephritis," *Nephrology Dialysis Transplantation*, vol. 24, no. 9, pp. 2745–2751, 2009.

[21] K. Kasuno, T. Ono, A. Matsumori et al., "Hepatitis C virus-associated tubulointerstitial injury," *The American Journal of Kidney Diseases*, vol. 41, no. 4, pp. 767–775, 2003.

[22] B. J. G. Pereira, S. N. Natov, B. A. Bouthot et al., "Effect of hepatitis C infection and renal transplantation on survival in end-stage renal disease," *Kidney International*, vol. 53, no. 5, pp. 1374–1381, 1998.

[23] D. Hestin, F. Guillemin, N. Castin, A. Le Faou, J. Champigneulles, and M. Kessler, "Pretransplant hepatitis C virus infection: a predictor of proteinuria after renal transplantation," *Transplantation*, vol. 65, no. 5, pp. 741–744, 1998.

[24] D. Roth, R. Cirocco, K. Zucker et al., "*De novo* membranoproliferative glomerulonephritis in hepatitis C virus- infected renal allograft recipients," *Transplantation*, vol. 59, no. 12, pp. 1676–1682, 1995.

[25] J. M. Cruzado, S. Gil-Vernet, G. Ercilla et al., "Hepatitis C virus-associated membranoproliferative glomerulonephritis in renal allografts," *Journal of the American Society of Nephrology*, vol. 7, no. 11, pp. 2469–2475, 1996.

[26] J. M. Cruzado, M. Carrera, J. Torras, and J. M. Grinyó, "Hepatitis C virus infection and *de novo* glomerular lesions in renal allografts," *The American Journal of Transplantation*, vol. 1, no. 2, pp. 171–178, 2001.

[27] B. H. Özdemir, F. N. Özdemir, S. Sezer, T. Çolak, and M. Haberal, "*De novo* glomerulonephritis in renal allografts with hepatitis C virus infection," *Transplantation Proceedings*, vol. 38, no. 2, pp. 492–495, 2006.

[28] J. M. Morales, J. Pascual-Capdevila, J. M. Campistol et al., "Membranous glomerulonephritis associated with hepatitis C virus infection in renal transplant patients," *Transplantation*, vol. 63, no. 11, pp. 1634–1639, 1997.

[29] S. Baid, M. Pascual, W. W. Williams Jr. et al., "Renal thrombotic microangiopathy associated with anticardiolipin antibodies in hepatitis C-positive renal allograft recipients," *Journal of the American Society of Nephrology*, vol. 10, no. 1, pp. 146–153, 1999.

[30] S. Baid-Agrawal, A. B. Farris, M. Pascual et al., "Overlapping pathways to transplant glomerulopathy: chronic humoral rejection, hepatitis C infection, and thrombotic microangiopathy," *Kidney International*, vol. 80, no. 8, pp. 879–885, 2011.

[31] D. N. Howell, X. Gu, and G. A. Herrera, "Organized deposits in the kidney and look-alikes," *Ultrastructural Pathology*, vol. 27, no. 5, pp. 295–312, 2003.

[32] G. A. Herrera and E. A. Turat-Herrera, "Renal diseases with organized deposits," *Archives of Pathology and Laboratory Medicine*, vol. 134, pp. 512–531, 2010.

[33] D. Cordonnier, H. Martin, P. Groslambert, C. Micouin, F. Chenais, and P. Stoebner, "Mixed IgG IgM cryoglobulinemia with glomerulonephritis. Immunochemical, fluorescent and ultrastructural study of kidney and in vitro cryoprecipitate," *The American Journal of Medicine*, vol. 59, no. 6, pp. 867–872, 1975.

[34] P. H. Pronovost, H. R. Brady, M. E. Gunning, O. Espinoza, and H. G. Rennke, "Clinical features, predictors of disease progression and results of renal transplantation in fibrillary/immunotactoid glomerulopathy," *Nephrology Dialysis Transplantation*, vol. 11, no. 5, pp. 837–842, 1996.

[35] S. M. Korbert, M. M. Schwartz, B. F. Rosenberg, R. K. Sibley, and E. J. Lewis, "Immunotactoid glomerulopathy," *Medicine*, vol. 64, no. 4, pp. 228–243, 1985.

[36] K. V. Rao, G. P. Hafner, G. S. Crary, W. R. Anderson, and J. T. Crosson, "*De novo* immunotactoid glomerulopathy of the renal allograft: possible association with cytomegalovirus infection," *The American Journal of Kidney Diseases*, vol. 24, no. 1, pp. 97–103, 1994.

[37] J. Isaac, G. A. Herrara, and F. S. Shihab, "*De novo* fibrillary glomerulopathy in the renal allograft of a patient with systemic lupus erythematosus," *Nephron*, vol. 87, no. 4, pp. 365–368, 2001.

[38] G. Geri, B. Terrier, O. Semoun et al., "Surrogate markers of B cell non-Hodgkin's lymphoma in patients with hepatitis C virus-related cryoglobulinaemia vasculitis," *Annals of the Rheumatic Diseases*, vol. 69, no. 12, pp. 2177–2180, 2010.

[39] P. G. Czarnecki, D. J. Lager, N. Leung, A. Dispenzieri, F. G. Cosio, and F. C. Fervenza, "Long-term outcome of kidney transplantation in patients with fibrillary glomerulonephritis or monoclonal gammopathy with fibrillary deposits," *Kidney International*, vol. 75, no. 4, pp. 420–427, 2009.

A Case of Continuous Negative Pressure Wound Therapy for Abdominal Infected Lymphocele after Kidney Transplantation

Marco Franchin,[1,2] Matteo Tozzi,[1,2] Gabriele Soldini,[2,3] and Gabriele Piffaretti[1]

[1] *Vascular Surgery, Department of Surgery and Morphological Sciences, Insubria University School of Medicine, Circolo University Teaching Hospital, Via Guicciardini 9, 21100 Varese, Italy*
[2] *Center for Research on Organ Transplantation, Insubria University School of Medicine, Circolo University Teaching Hospital, 21100 Varese, Italy*
[3] *General Surgery 1, Department of Surgery and Morphological Sciences, Insubria University School of Medicine, Circolo University Teaching Hospital, 21100 Varese, Italy*

Correspondence should be addressed to Gabriele Piffaretti; gabriele.piffaretti@uninsubria.it

Academic Editor: David Conti

Lymphocele is a common complication after kidney transplantation. Although superinfection is a rare event, it generates a difficult management problem; generally, open surgical drainage is the preferred method of treatment but it may lead to complicated postoperative course and prolonged healing time. Negative pressure wound therapy showed promising outcomes in various surgical disciplines and settings. We present a case of an abdominal infected lymphocele after kidney transplantation managed with open surgery and negative pressure wound therapy.

1. Introduction

Lymphocele is a common complication after kidney transplantation [1–3]. Although it is a rare event, superinfection may complicate the postoperative course or even threaten survival [4, 5]. It also generates a difficult management problem whose resolution is not made easier by the lack of literature data [6]. Up to now, infected lymphocele has been preferentially treated with open surgical drainage; however, these wounds often caused subsequent complications requiring prolonged healing time [5, 7]. Moreover, it increases the financial burden in transplanted recipients [8]. Negative pressure wound therapy (NPWT) was developed to promote healing of open wounds and actually has found wide application in various surgical disciplines and settings [9–12].

The aim of this paper is to report a case of an infected lymphocele after kidney transplantation managed with surgical drainage and subsequent application of NPWT.

2. Case Report

He is a 65-year-old male, Rh positive group B, with a medical history significant for hypertension, dyslipidemia, obesity (body mass index = 32), chronic obstructive pulmonary disease, ischemic heart disease treated with percutaneous transluminal coronary angioplasty, and end-stage renal disease due to glomerulonephritis. Kidney transplantation was performed using a retroperitoneal approach on common iliac vessels, while ureteral implantation was accomplished with the Lich-Gregoir technique. Kidney donor was a Rh positive group B 60-year-old male, died for cerebral hemorrhage: his serology (HBcAb, VDRL, TPHA, HIV, HCV, and HBsAg) and cultures for active infections were negative. HLA-A, HLA-B, and HLA-DR loci presented a single mismatch, evenly. Induction immunosuppressive treatment consisted of monoclonal antibodies (Basiliximab, Simulectm; Novartis, Basel; Switzerland), whereas maintenance immunosuppressive therapy included cyclosporine (Sandimun Neoral, Novartis, Basel; Switzerland) and Everlomus (Certican, Novartis, Basel; Switzerland), in association with steroid. Postoperative course was uneventful; he was discharged on day 12th with a serum creatinine level of 1.2 mg/dL. Two months after intervention a magnetic resonance angiography (MR-A) was performed accordingly to our follow-up protocol: a 150 mm × 20 mm lymph collection was detected between the graft and the abdominal wall (Figures 1(a) and 1(b)). At that time, clinical signs of infection were absent and blood tests were in normal range (C-reactive protein (CRP) = 12 mg/L, leukocytes = 8.230/mm^3, serum creatinine = 1.17 mg/dL). It was asymptomatic; hence, we decided to continue with close renal function surveillance, delaying any percutaneous procedures. On day 46 after intervention, fever (38.5°C) and oliguria abruptly developed, with local signs of infection: blood tests showed an increase of CRP (206 mg/L), serum creatinine (2.2 mg/dL), and leukocytes count (15.220/mm^3). Soon after, a broad spectrum antibiotic therapy with (Cefotaxime, Max Farma; Castel San Giorgio, IT) was started and urgent surgical drainage was performed. Intraoperative cultures were positives for *Escherichia coli, Staphylococcus haemolyticus,* and *Enterococcus faecalis*; therefore, we modified the antibiotic regimen adding daptomicine (Cubicin, Novartis Europharm; Horsham, UK). Systemic sepsis resolved but a 99^{m}-technetium renal scan showed an abnormal lymphatic leakage in the right iliac fossa (Figure 1(c)). A change in immunosuppressive therapy was not considered. The remaining lymphatic cavity was large, scar margins were widely dehiscent and the graft exposed. We decided to use a NPWT (Renasys, Smith & Nephew; London, UK) medication to assist wound healing: the cavity was then filled with polyurethane foam dressing connected via a tubing system to a portable device using continuous 80 mmHg negative pressure. He was discharged twelve days later, on oral antibiotic therapy with amoxicillin/clavulanic acid: at that time, creatinine was 1.63 mg/dL; leukocytes count 9.300/mm^3. This system was subsequently renewed every five days (Figure 1(d)). Forty-five days later, lymphocele was sealed and skin closed. Wound cultures were negative. Ultrasound evaluation confirmed the complete resolution of the lymphatic collection. He was last seen 6 months after the intervention asymptomatic with stable serum creatinine at 1.32 mg/dL. No ventral hernia developed.

3. Discussion

Lymphocele incidence rate is reported in the range from 0.6% to 49% [1–3]. This broad limit may be determined at different levels: it may be explained by the variety of lymphocele definition, as well as an underestimation in reporting results, and also because of different follow-up to which this complication has been reported [4]. Infected lymphocele is even more rarely described in literature [6]. The case report we are presenting is the only one in our experience which means an incidence rate of 0.5%. This data is consistent with the literature: out of 11.497 kidney transplantations in thirteen studies which reported the operative management of posttransplant lymphocele, we found only five papers with a total amount of 22 cases and an incidence rate of 0.2% (Table 1) [4, 5, 13–23]. We cannot assure if it happens because of low infection rate or it was an author omission; nonetheless, in these studies, information was incompletely reported (Table 2) [6]. This goes at the expense of the fact that, though loss of graft was never reported, septic complication should have been ascribed to lymphocele superinfection.

Once the diagnosis is established, uncertainty coming from these data opens the equally important debate of the best treatment for an infected lymphocele [5, 19, 23, 24]. Percutaneous drainage and/or sclerotherapy, open evacuation, and surgical fenestration into peritoneal cavity have been proposed in the past for symptomatic lymphocele: unfortunately, precise and widely adopted strategies are missing and results have been described with mixed success [5, 7, 22, 23, 25–27]. Percutaneous drainage is a minimally invasive option which does not preclude subsequent surgery; however, it has been associated with a high risk of recurrence and superinfection also because it has been used alone [6, 28]. This is the main reason why Hamza et al. [5] in their treatment algorithm advocated the use of systemic antibiotic therapy and continuous internal-external drainage in every case of suspected infection or confirmed microbiological determination. In the present case, the risk of potential iatrogenic superinfection in such a sensitive recipient led us to prefer a conservative approach. Instrumental diagnosis confirmed the nature of the collection without the need of biochemical confirmation on aspirated liquid. We agree with most of the authors that large lymphocele should be treated with open surgery [6, 19], first and foremost because it is effective on an active infection and limits the potential superinfection. Furthermore, the persistence of a lymphatic drainage or residual debris and fluid collection could be a dangerous gateway to the graft or a favourable soil for other infective agents. These latter are the main reason to take advantage of the NPWT qualities: it removes excessive or contaminated fluids and assists wound closure [9, 29, 30]. Moreover, the presence of an adhesive vapour-permeable plastic drape facilitates gas exchange, thus working against the development of anaerobic organisms and preventing access to external agents [11, 31].

Several studies have documented the appropriateness of the NPWT use in the treatment of lymphocele and lymphocutaneous fistula; however, the application of NPWT for abdominal injuries is still debated [9–13]. Accordingly to Mendez-Eastman et al. [31] the exposure of intra-abdominal organs and blood vessels is a contraindication to NPWT because of the risk of tissue damage due to subatmospheric pressure. Precise guidelines in this latter circumstance are missing: up to now, few data are available on the use of NPWT for dehiscent wounds after organ transplantation: Shrestha et al. [32] first presented a case series of 9 kidney recipients treated with NPWT for infection-related wound dehiscence. None of these patients had lymphocele or deep wounds in continuity with the iliac vessels such as in our case; nevertheless, in their cases NPWT assisted wound healing in a significantly shorter time. In similar circumstances, Heap et al. [11] treated with NPWT two complex urinary fistulas. Although literature is sporadic and heterogeneous, these reports encouraged us about the possibility to use NPWT. This is the reason why we did not change the ongoing immunosuppressive therapy: in fact, responsibility of mTOR inhibitor in the genesis of lymphocele is widely recognized [33, 34]. We have to point out that literature did not help us with practically guidelines for the application of NPWT: hence, type and intensity of negative pressure applied to the

Table 1: 14-year literature review on posttransplant lymphocele: 15 cases operatively managed at least.

Author	N of transplant	Lymphoceles (n)	Incidence (%)	Symptomatic lymphoceles (n)	Presentation days median (range)	Diameter (cm) mean (range)	Volume (mL) mean (range)	Graft loss (n)	Infection (n)	Conservative management n (recurrence)	Percutaneous treatment n (recurrence)	Laparoscopic fenestration n (recurrence)	Open surgery n (recurrence)	Surgical compli-cation (n)
Duepree et al. [13]	1502	90	5.9	90	52 (13–1398)	ND	ND	0	0	0	0	56 (4)	34	4
Hamed et al. [12]	480	31	6.4	31	66 (19–111)	ND	200 (45–2000)	0	0	0	31 (19)	19 (4)	4	0
Bailey et al. [14]	1863	60	3.2	60	ND	ND	ND	0	0	0	0	20 (2)	42 (2)	0
Øyen et al. [15]	385	34	8.8	34	147 (18–1110)	ND	ND	0	0	34	0	26 (2)	10 (1)	0
Florian Fuller et al. [16]	138	36	26.1	36	ND	ND	480 (ND)	0	6	0	20 (6)	8	14	0
Hamza et al. [5]	620	42	6.8	42	ND	ND	250 (80–125)	0	8	0	42 (24)	17 (3)	10 (1)	0
Atray et al. [17]	1289	24	1.9	24	121 (35–631)	ND	977 (200–2000)	0	4	3 (0)	7 (5)	3	17 (3)	1
Smyth et al. [18]	386	24	6.2	13	29 (17–40)	ND	354 (ND)	0	3	0	13	0	3 (0)	0
Król et al. [19]	2147	17	7.9	17	42 (10–90)	ND	ND	0	0	0	11 (7)	0	13 (0)	0
Ulrich et al. [4]	426	42	9.9	24	ND (2–4)	7.8 (ND)	ND	0	0	18	7 (7)	26 (2)	0	0
Zargar-Shoshtari et al. [20]	744	36	4.8	14	ND (10–182)	ND	ND	0	0	ND	14 (7)	5 (1)	3 (0)	0
Lee et al. [21]	154	9	5.8	9	19 (6–28)	5 (1.5–8)	ND	0	1	5 (3)	7 (4)	1 (0)	3 (0)	0
Choudhrie et al. [22]	1363	35	2.5	35	29 (7–3670)	ND	ND	0	0	ND	25 (7)	17 (0)	0	0

n: number; ND: not determined.

Table 2: Literature data on infected lymphocele.

Author	Infection (*n*)	Systemic complication (*n*)	Fluid culture positivity Gram negative *Klebsiella* spp.	Treatment Gram positive *Staphylococcus* spp.	Antibiotic first *Enterococcus*	Sclerotherapy	External drainage	Fenestration	
Florian Fuller et al. [16]	6	ND							
Hamza et al. [5]	8	0	ND	8	0	8	0		
Atray et al. [17]	4	0	ND						
Smyth et al. [18]	3	0	0	2	1	3	1	1	1
Lee et al. [21]	1	0	1	0	0	0	0	0	1

n: number.

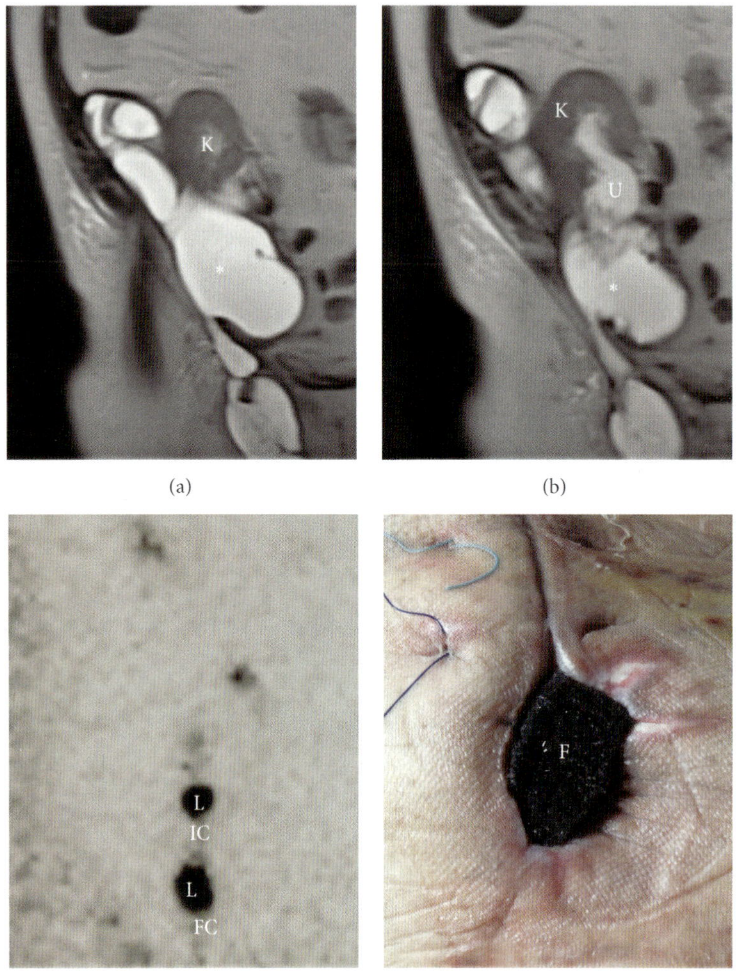

(a) (b) (c) (d)

Figure 1

cavity were borrowed from our experience on NPWT in open abdomen [35].

In our case, major concerns were related to the fact that NPWT would have been needed for a long time even at home, which meant poor medical control in a patient with an open abdominal wound and a transplanted kidney. Surprisingly, we were impressed by the fact that this system was well tolerated by the patient: on our behalf, we established a rigorous outpatient reevaluation every three days to assess dressing integrity and efficiency of the machine. Honestly, we recognize the limitation of our case report which lends itself to have an anecdotal value. Further, this type of treatment may not be used in uncooperative or not motivated patients, and question about the financial burden of this therapy can be an obstacle to its broad application [36]. Nevertheless, it was very easy to guarantee an accurate control of either local infection or lymphatic leak. The cost-effectiveness analysis of the Medicare charges and providers confirmed a lower long-term costs when using NPWT if compared with standard wound care methods [8, 37].

4. Conclusion

Our case showed NPWT was effective to assist the treatment of a symptomatic infected lymphocele; it also proved to be a safe management alternative for a complex deep infected wound in a transplant recipient too. We hope our case will find further confirmation in future studies.

Authors' Contribution

Marco Franchin was responsible for research design, writing of the paper, and data analysis. Matteo Tozzi was responsible for performance of the research, writing the paper. Corrado Chiappa contributed to performance of the research, literature research. Gabriele Soldini contributed to performance of the research, literature research. Gabriele Piffaretti contributed to writing of the paper, data analysis.

References

[1] W. E. Braun, L. H. Banowsky, R. A. Straffon et al., "Lymphoceles associated with renal transplantation. Report of 15 cases and review of the literature," *The American Journal of Medicine*, vol. 57, no. 5, pp. 714–729, 1974.

[2] J. V. Thomalla, J. E. Lingeman, S. B. Leapman, and R. S. Filo, "The manifestation and management of late urological complications in renal transplant recipients: use of the urological armamentarium," *The Journal of Urology*, vol. 134, no. 5, pp. 944–948, 1985.

[3] M. L. de Lima, C. A. C. Cotrim, J. C. Moro, R. Miyaoka, and C. A. L. D'Ancona, "Laparoscopic treatment of lymphoceles after renal transplantation," *International Braz J Urol*, vol. 38, no. 2, pp. 215–221, 2012.

[4] F. Ulrich, S. Niedzwiecki, P. Fikatas et al., "Symptomatic lymphoceles after kidney transplantation—multivariate analysis of risk factors and outcome after laparoscopic fenestration," *Clinical Transplantation*, vol. 24, no. 2, pp. 273–280, 2010.

[5] A. Hamza, K. Fischer, E. Koch et al., "Diagnostics and therapy of lymphoceles after kidney transplantation," *Transplantation Proceedings*, vol. 38, no. 3, pp. 701–706, 2006.

[6] A. Lucewicz, G. Wong, V. W. T. Lam et al., "Management of primary symptomatic lymphocele after kidney transplantation: a systematic review," *Transplantation*, vol. 92, no. 6, pp. 663–673, 2011.

[7] D. L. García, J. M. J. Pais, J. G. Dacal et al., "Giant lymphocele after renal transplantation. Case report and bibliographic review," *Archivos Españoles de Urología*, vol. 62, no. 5, pp. 399–403, 2009.

[8] Weinberg Group, *Technology Assessment of the V.A.C. for in-Home Treatment of Chronic Wounds*, Weinberg Group, Washington, DC, USA, 1999.

[9] D. T. Ubbink, S. J. Westerbos, E. A. Nelson, and H. Vermeulen, "A systematic review of topical negative pressure therapy for acute and chronic wounds," *British Journal of Surgery*, vol. 95, no. 6, pp. 685–692, 2008.

[10] M. P. Tocco, A. Costantino, M. Ballardini et al., "Improved results of the vacuum assisted closure and Nitinol clips sternal closure after postoperative deep sternal wound infection," *European Journal of Cardio-thoracic Surgery*, vol. 35, no. 5, pp. 833–838, 2009.

[11] S. Heap, S. Mehra, A. Tavakoli, T. Augustine, H. Riad, and R. Pararajasingam, "Negative pressure wound therapy used to heal complex urinary fistula wounds following renal transplantation into an ileal conduit," *American Journal of Transplantation*, vol. 10, no. 10, pp. 2370–2373, 2010.

[12] O. Hamed, P. E. Muck, J. M. Smith, K. Krallman, and N. M. Griffith, "Use of vacuum-assisted closure (VAC) therapy in treating lymphatic complications after vascular procedures: new approach for lymphoceles," *Journal of Vascular Surgery*, vol. 48, no. 6, pp. 1520–1523, 2008.

[13] H.-J. Duepree, P. Fornara, J.-C. Lewejohann, J. Hoyer, H.-P. Bruch, and T. H. K. Schiedeck, "Laparoscopic treatment of lymphoceles in patients after renal transplantation," *Clinical Transplantation*, vol. 15, no. 6, pp. 375–379, 2001.

[14] S. H. Bailey, M. C. Mone, J. M. Holman, and E. W. Nelson, "Laparoscopic treatment of postrenal transplant lymphoceles," *Surgical Endoscopy and Other Interventional Techniques*, vol. 17, no. 12, pp. 1896–1899, 2003.

[15] O. Øyen, V. Siwach, P.-D. Line et al., "Improvement of post-transplant lymphocele treatment in the laparoscopic era," *Transplant International*, vol. 15, no. 8, pp. 406–410, 2002.

[16] T. Florian Fuller, S.-M. Kang, R. Hirose, S. Feng, P. G. Stock, and C. E. Freise, "Management of lymphoceles after renal transplantation: laparoscopic versus open drainage," *Journal of Urology*, vol. 169, no. 6, pp. 2022–2025, 2003.

[17] N. K. Atray, F. Moore, F. Zaman et al., "Post transplant lymphocele: a single centre experience," *Clinical Transplantation, Supplement*, vol. 18, no. 12, pp. 46–49, 2004.

[18] G. P. Smyth, G. Beitz, M. P. Eng, N. Gibbons, D. P. Hickey, and D. M. Little, "Long-term outcome of cadaveric renal transplant after treatment of symptomatic lymphocele," *Journal of Urology*, vol. 176, no. 3, pp. 1069–1072, 2006.

[19] R. Król, A. Kolonko, J. Chudek et al., "Did volume of lymphocele after kidney transplantation determine the choice of treatment modality?" *Transplantation Proceedings*, vol. 39, no. 9, pp. 2740–2743, 2007.

[20] M. A. Zargar-Shoshtari, M. Soleimani, H. Salimi, and K. Mehravaran, "Symptomatic lymphocele after kidney transplantation: a single-center experience," *Urology Journal*, vol. 5, no. 1, pp. 34–36, 2008.

[21] H. S. Lee, D. J. Joo, K. H. Huh et al., "Laparoscopic fenestration versus percutaneous catheter drainage for lymphocele treatment after kidney transplantation," *Transplantation Proceedings*, vol. 45, no. 4, pp. 1667–1670, 2013.

[22] A. V. Choudhrie, S. Kumar, L. Gnanaraj, A. Devasia, N. Chacko, and N. S. Kekre, "Symptomatic lymphocoeles post renal transplant," *Saudi Journal of Kidney Diseases and Transplantation*, vol. 23, no. 6, pp. 1162–1168, 2012.

[23] A. Sim, L. G. Ng, and C. Cheng, "Occurrence of a lymphocele following renal transplantation," *Singapore Medical Journal*, vol. 54, no. 5, pp. 259–262, 2013.

[24] D.-Y. Han, M.-F. Cheng, R.-F. Yen, K.-Y. Tzen, and Y.-W. Wu, "Postoperative lymphocele demonstrated by lymphoscintigraphy SPECT/CT," *Clinical Nuclear Medicine*, vol. 37, no. 4, pp. 374–376, 2012.

[25] I. Iwan-Zietek, Z. Zietek, T. Sulikowski et al., "Minimally invasive methods for the treatment of lymphocele after kidney transplantation," *Transplantation Proceedings*, vol. 41, no. 8, pp. 3073–3076, 2009.

[26] D. D. Nghiem and I. Beckman, "Intraperitoneal catheter drainage of lymphocele: an outpatient procedure," *Transplant International*, vol. 18, no. 6, pp. 721–723, 2005.

[27] W. M. Chen and H. C. Ho, "Management of recurrent lymphocele after renal tranplantation using the Tenckhoff catheter," *Urology*, vol. 74, no. 5, pp. 1150–1151, 2009.

[28] M. R. Ebadzadeh and M. Tavakkoli, "Lymphocele after kidney transplantation: where are we standing now?" *Urology Journal*, vol. 5, no. 3, pp. 144–148, 2008.

[29] P. Vikatmaa, V. Juutilainen, P. Kuukasjarvi, and A. Malmivaara, "Negative pressure wound therapy: a systematic review on effectiveness and safety," *The European Journal of Vascular and Endovascular Surgery*, vol. 36, no. 4, pp. 438–448, 2008.

[30] P. Stevens, "Vacuum-assisted closure of laparostomy wounds: a critical review of the literature," *International Wound Journal*, vol. 6, no. 4, pp. 259–266, 2009.

[31] S. Mendez-Eastman, "Guidelines for using negative pressure wound therapy," *Advances in Skin & Wound Care*, vol. 14, no. 6, pp. 314–323, 2001.

[32] B. M. Shrestha, V. C. Nathan, M. S. Delbridge et al., "Vacuum-assisted closure (VAC) therapy in the management of wound infection following renal transplantation," *Kathmandu University Medical Journal*, vol. 5, no. 17, pp. 4–7, 2007.

[33] Kidney Disease: Improving Global Outcomes (KDIGO) Transplant Work Group, "KDIGO clinical practice guideline for the care of kidney transplant recipients," *American Journal of Transplantation*, vol. 9, supplement 3, pp. S1–155, 2009.

[34] M. Cooper, A. C. Wiseman, G. Zibari et al., "Wound events in kidney transplant patients receiving de novo everolimus: a pooled analysis of three randomized controlled trials," *Clinical Transplantation*, vol. 27, no. 6, pp. E625–E635, 2013.

[35] A. Bruhin, F. Ferreira, M. Chariker, J. Smith, and N. Runkel, "Systematic review and evidence based recommendations for the use of negative pressure wound therapy in the open abdomen," *International Journal of Surgery*, vol. 12, no. 10, pp. 1105–1114, 2014.

[36] D. Upton, D. Stephens, and A. Andrews, "Patients' experiences of negative pressure wound therapy for the treatment of wounds: a review," *Journal of Wound Care*, vol. 22, no. 1, pp. 34–39, 2013.

[37] J. M. de Leon, S. Barnes, M. Nagel, M. Fudge, A. Lucius, and B. Garcia, "Cost-effectiveness of negative pressure wound therapy for postsurgical patients in long-term acute care," *Advances in Skin & Wound Care*, vol. 22, no. 3, pp. 122–127, 2009.

De Novo Postinfectious Glomerulonephritis Secondary to Nephritogenic Streptococci as the Cause of Transplant Acute Kidney Injury

Alexander Bullen and Mita M. Shah

Division of Nephrology-Hypertension, University of California San Diego, San Diego, CA, USA

Correspondence should be addressed to Mita M. Shah; mshah@ucsd.edu

Academic Editor: Ryszard Grenda

Acute kidney injury is common among kidney transplant recipients. Postinfectious glomerulonephritis secondary to nephritogenic streptococci is one of the oldest known etiologies of acute kidney injury in native kidneys but rarely reported among kidney transplant recipients. This report is of a biopsy-proven case of acute kidney injury in a renal allograft recipient caused by de novo poststreptococcal glomerulonephritis.

1. Introduction

Acute kidney injury (AKI) is common in kidney transplant recipients (KTR) [1] and it has been identified as a risk factor for graft failure [1, 2] and death with a functioning transplant [2]. Postinfectious glomerulonephritis (PIGN) secondary to nephritogenic streptococci is a well-recognized cause of native kidney AKI. In a seminal paper in 1812, Wells detailed the complications of scarlet fever and described this glomerulonephritis as the "dropsy that follows scarlet fever" [3]. He noted that it mainly occurred in children, approximately three weeks after a mild fever and it consisted of edema starting in the face, decreased urine output, red urine, nausea, and vomiting, which would "recede after no long stay" [3].

PIGN secondary to nephritogenic streptococci has a heterogeneous clinical presentation ranging from asymptomatic to nephrotic syndrome [4]. Diagnosis is based on clinical findings in addition to documentation of a recent GAS infection by positive throat or skin culture or serologic tests, such as anti-streptolysin O (ASO) antibodies [5].

Few reports of PIGN secondary to nephritogenic streptococci as the cause of AKI in KTR are currently available in the literature. We present a biopsy-proven rare cause of AKI in a KTR as PIGN secondary to nephritogenic streptococci.

2. Case Presentation

The patient was a 45-year-old Hispanic male who had end-stage renal disease of unknown etiology, hypertension, and hyperlipidemia. His HLA typing was A 2,- B 7, 35, Cw 4, 7, DR 4,- DQ 8,-. His donor was a 46-year-old Hispanic female with history of hyperlipidemia with a measured 24-hour urine creatinine clearance of 151 ml/min. Her HLA typing was A 2,31, B 35,44, Cw 4,5, DR 4,-, DQ 7,8. The patient had been on intermittent hemodialysis for two years prior to undergoing living related kidney transplant. Induction therapy consisted of basiliximab and solumedrol. Maintenance therapy was with tacrolimus, mycophenolate mofetil, and prednisone. His two-year course after transplant had been unremarkable, with a baseline serum creatinine of 1.5–1.7 mg/dL (134–150 μmol/L), without proteinuria or hematuria.

Two years after transplant he presented to the renal transplant clinic with complaints of lower extremity edema that had appeared over the previous three days. He stated he had experienced a flu-like illness a week prior. In addition, he admitted to inadvertently taking tacrolimus 1 mg q12h, rather than his prescribed dose of 3 mg twice a day for almost one month. He had corrected the dose approximately 3 weeks prior to presentation. On examination, he was normotensive

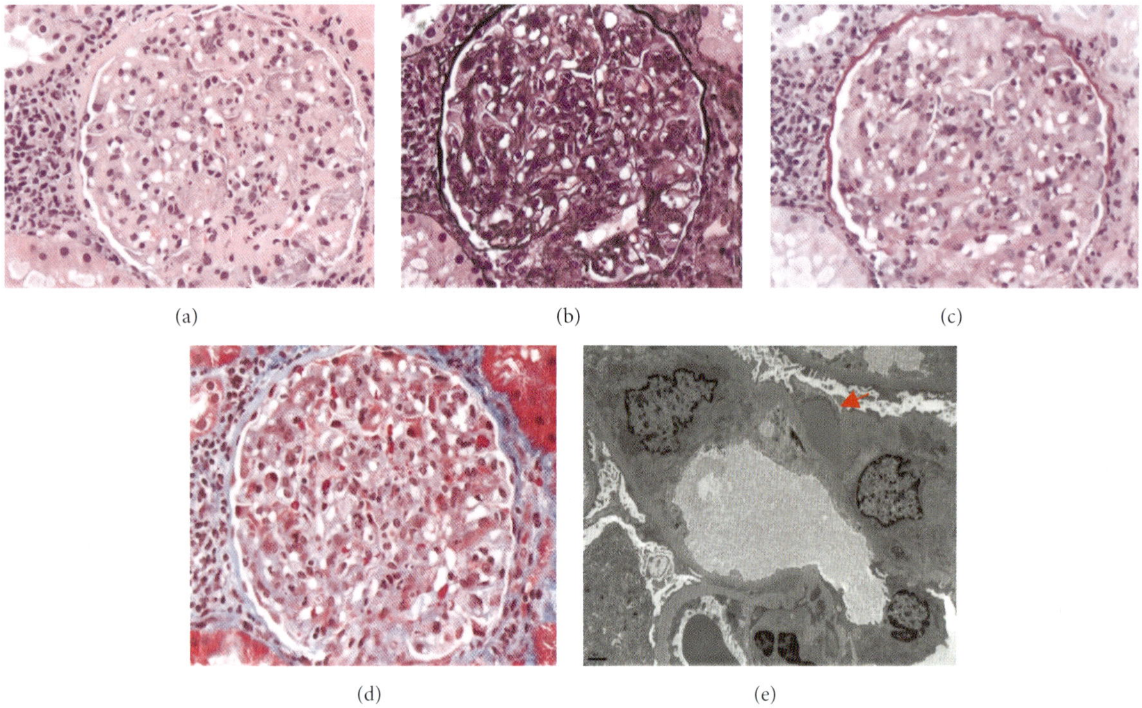

FIGURE 1: (a) Light microscopy. Hematoxylin and stain. Significant endocapillary proliferation with neutrophils and swollen endothelial cells. (b) Jones stain with occasional double contour. No evidence of significant crescents noted. (c) Periodic acid-Schiff stain revealed mild mixed interstitial inflammation with lymphocytes, plasma cells, and neutrophils. (d) Trichrome stain with focal mild interstitial fibrosis and tubular atrophy. (e) Electron microscopy. Large subepithelial electron dense deposits (arrow) consistent with "humps".

and afebrile. Cardiovascular and respiratory examinations were normal. He had periorbital edema and 6 mm pitting edema in lower extremities. He did not have graft tenderness or bruit.

Laboratory data was remarkable for creatinine of 2.2 mg/dL (194 μmol/L). Urinalysis showed moderate blood and 3+ protein (previously no proteinuria), urinary sediment of more than 50 red blood cells (RBCs), 11–20 white blood cells (WBCs) per high power field (HPF), and urine protein/creatinine ratio of 8.2 g (previously 100 mg). Tacrolimus trough was 4.9 ng/mL.

Due to acute kidney injury, proteinuria, and hematuria in the setting of suboptimal immunosuppression, there was a high concern for acute rejection versus rapidly progressive glomerulonephritis perhaps due to recurrence of the unknown primary disease. Renal ultrasound and a renal biopsy were ordered. Given the risk of acute rejection due to inadvertent medication noncompliance, prednisone was increased from 10 mg daily to 50 mg daily, tacrolimus was increased from 3 mg twice a day to 5 mg twice a day, and mycophenolate mofetil was increased to 1500 mg twice a day. Of note, BK virus and donor specific antibodies were negative a month prior.

The renal US was negative for hydronephrosis or calculi. Three days later, a biopsy was performed.

Preliminary biopsy report was consistent with postinfectious glomerulonephritis (Figure 1). Due to the recent infection, anti-streptolysin O (ASO) antibodies, C3, and C4 were ordered. Since initial biopsy did not have any glomeruli for immunofluorescence (IF), he was scheduled for repeat biopsy.

In the interim, C3 and C4 were reported. C3 was low at 59 mg/dL with a normal C4 at 35 mg/dL (Table 1). Tacrolimus trough was 8.6 ng/mL.

Second kidney biopsy one week later revealed minimal residual subendothelial electron dense deposits, but no evidence of large subepithelial electron dense deposits (Figure 2). IF showed nonspecific patchy staining with C3 in glomeruli and some tubules. All other reagents were negative, including C4d in peritubular capillaries, BK, and SV40 in tubular cells. There is no evidence of cell-mediated or antibody mediated glomerulonephritis. Overall, biopsy was consistent with resolving postinfectious glomerulonephritis. Anti-streptolysin O (ASO) was elevated at 603 IU/mL (Table 1), highly indicative of *Streptococcus* being the causative agent.

Given that his AKI did not appear to be due to rejection, tacrolimus was decreased back to his basal dose of 3 mg twice a day and prednisone was tapered to 10 mg daily. Fluid management was achieved with furosemide. He was not prescribed any antibiotics. A month later, creatinine had decreased to 1.9 mg/dL (168 μmol/L), and in a 3-month period, it had returned to baseline and proteinuria and hematuria had completely resolved (Figure 3 and Table 1).

3. Discussion

AKI is common in renal allograft recipients [1] due to multiple risk factors including single kidney, use of calcineurin

TABLE 1: Laboratory parameters during clinical course.

Day	0	1	5	10	15	55	85
Creatinine (mg/dL)	1.6	2.2	2.1	2.3	1.9	1.8	1.7
Protein/creat ratio	0.1	8.3	4.4	2	1.6	0.4	0.2
Urine RBCs	0–2	0–2	>50	21–50	11–20	11–20	0–2
Urine WBCs	0–2	0–2	11–20	11–20	11–20	3–5	0–2
C3 (mg/dL)*			59		93		146
C4 (mg/dL)**			34		36		42
ASO Ab***			603				359

*C3 normal range: 90–180; **C4 normal range: 10–40 mg/dL; ***ASO Ab = anti-streptolysin O antibodies.

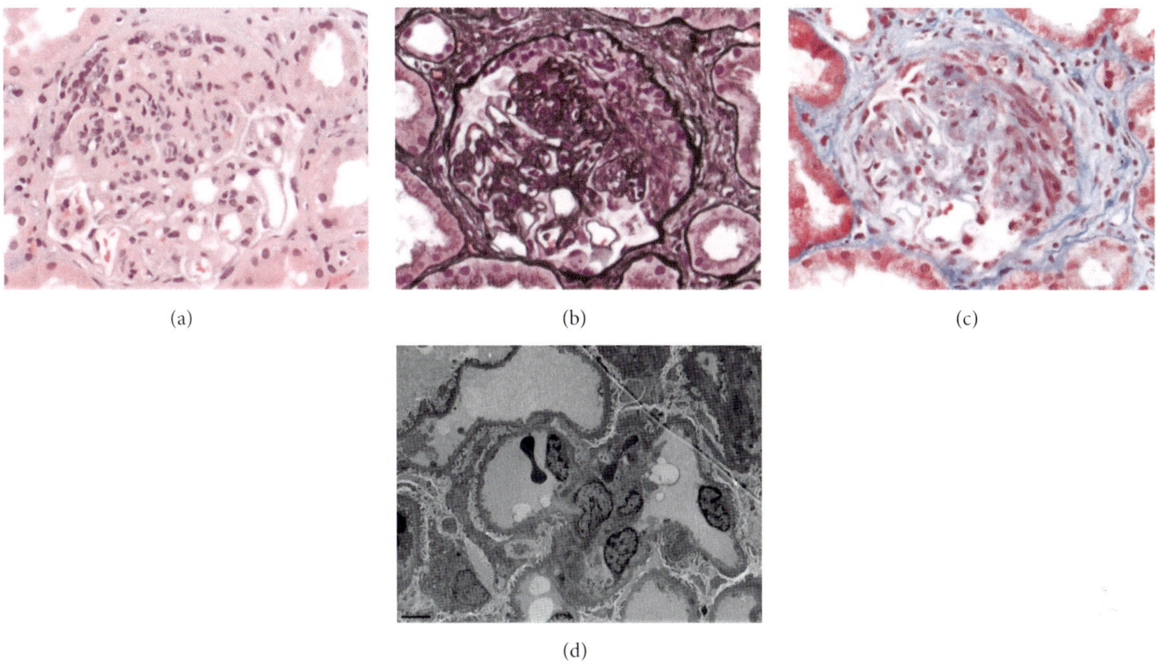

FIGURE 2: (a) Light microscopy. Hematoxylin and Eosin stain with decreased endocapillary proliferation of neutrophils with some karyorrhectic debris and moderate crescents. (b) Jones stain with an early fibroepithelial crescent. (c) Trichrome stain with crescent and focal mild interstitial fibrosis and tubular atrophy. (d) Electron microscopy. Minimal residual subendothelial electron dense deposits but no evidence of large subepithelial electron dense deposits "humps".

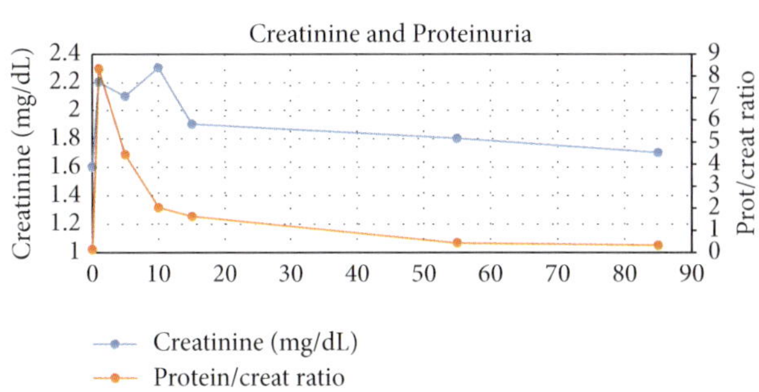

FIGURE 3: Creatinine and spot urine protein/creatinine ratio during clinical course.

inhibitors, and increasing use of marginal donor kidneys, among others. AKI in this population has been identified as a risk factor for graft failure [1, 2] and death with a functioning transplant [2]. Infections are the second most common cause of death in kidney transplants recipients due to multiple factors including immunosuppressed status, donor-derived infection, and underlying comorbidities [6]. CMV disease, Epstein-Barr virus infection, and BK polyomavirus infection are among the most common infections in kidney transplant recipients [7]. Glomerular disease because of infection has been described in KTR in the case of cryoglobulinemic and noncryoglobulinemic membranoproliferative GN secondary to hepatitis C; however, there are only seven reported cases of postinfectious glomerulonephritis [8], with only one reported case to our knowledge of poststreptococcal glomerulonephritis occurring in a pediatric transplant recipient [9]. Three cases were due to *Staphylococcus aureus*, none of which had recovery of their graft function and one died.

PIGN secondary to nephritogenic streptococci is caused by nephritogenic strains of group A beta-hemolytic *Streptococcus*, which cause skin and throat infections. Two of the primary antigens are the nephritis-associated plasmin receptor (NAPlr) [10] and the streptococcal pyrogenic exotoxin B (SPEB) [11]. They both activate the alternative complement pathway [12]. The plasmin-binding capacity of NAPlr plays a key role in the immune complex deposition and local inflammation [13]. SPEB is found in the subepithelial electron dense deposits (humps) which are a characteristic finding of this disease [14]. Over thirty years ago, HLA-DRw4 was found to be associated with increased susceptibility to poststreptococcal glomerulonephritis [15]. Currently, genomics studies with microarray technology and proteomic analysis are being performed to better understand GAS pathogenesis and thus develop targeted therapies [16].

Although poststreptococcal glomerulonephritis is typically thought of as a disease affecting children, it has a bimodal distribution, also affecting patients older than 60 years of age. The clinical spectrum is varied, ranging from asymptomatic disease with microscopic hematuria to acute nephritic syndrome. Patients develop nephrotic range proteinuria, edema, and acute kidney injury. Laboratory studies reveal low C3 and CH50 early in the disease course with typically normal C4 [17, 18]. Nonetheless, there are some cases with low C4, suggestive of activation of classical pathway as well [19].

Some have postulated that PIGN is a self-limiting form of C3 glomerulopathy [20], based on the presence of low levels of C3. However, it is important to denote some key differences between the two diseases. First, in accordance with the hypothesis that C3 glomerulopathy is secondary to an abnormality in the alternative complement pathway, there is bright C3 staining and lack of significant immunoglobulin staining, whereas in PIGN there is bright staining of both C3 and IgG [21]. It is important to note that there are the so called cases of "atypical" PIGN, in which the IgG may not be present in the IF and clinically, there is persistent hematuria and proteinuria and sometimes progression to end-stage renal disease. When Sethi et al. evaluated eleven of such cases; they found an abnormality in the alternative pathway, leading them to speculate that those cases represented undiagnosed C3 glomerulonephritis [22]. Another key difference is found in the electron microscopy where in C3 glomerulopathy, there are mesangial, subendothelial, or sometimes subepithelial or intramembranous deposits which are lobular and amorphous [21]. However, in PIGN, one typically finds clearly demarcated subepithelial humps. Furthermore, C3 glomerulopathy tends to be a progressive disease [23] and it is known to recur in transplant kidneys [24, 25] and in the patient described in this case, the C3 levels returned to normal and he has remained with stable renal function without proteinuria, hematuria, or hypocomplementemia for the past five years. Certainly, as the C3 glomerulopathy consensus report noted in 2013 [26] and the study from Sethi et al. suggests [22], further investigation for C3 glomerulopathy is warranted if any atypical clinical or histological features are present.

De novo acute postinfectious glomerulonephritis is not a commonly reported etiology of AKI in KTRs, but in the few cases that have been reported, some peculiarities have been noted [8]. First, a heterogeneous etiology of bacterial, fungal, viral, and parasitic infections triggering an acute glomerulonephritis is sometimes seen in transplant patients. Second, when the glomerulonephritis was triggered by etiologies other than *Streptococcus*, such as *Staphylococcus* and *E. coli*, the most common urinary pathogen in KTRs [9], patients required renal replacement therapy. Interestingly, of the three cases described by Moroni et al., none were caused by *Streptococcus*. Plumb et al. also reported three cases of PIGN caused by *S. aureus*, CMV infection, and a presumed urinary tract infection [27]. It is important to note that all the cases they reported of PIGN were in patients with type 1 DM, leading to the speculation that these patients may be at higher risk of developing this glomerular disease as others have suggested [28]. None of the cases that Plumb et al. reported were caused by nephritogenic streptococci. To our knowledge there is only one other case of posttransplant acute PIGN secondary to nephritogenic streptococci in the literature and it was in a 12-year-old male, 1 year after receiving a transplant [9].

Treatment for this disease is mainly supportive, although methylprednisolone and even plasmapheresis have been used, especially when caused by *S. aureus* and *E. coli* [19, 29]. Unfortunately, of the seven cumulative cases reviewed by Moroni et al., four ultimately were restarted on dialysis and one died [8], illustrating the severity of this disease.

4. Conclusions

This case reveals the importance of having a prompt and thorough evaluation of acute kidney injury. Although the most common etiologies of AKI in KTRs are calcineurin inhibitor toxicity, recurrence of the primary disease, and acute rejection, relatively uncommon entities such as PIGN secondary to nephritogenic streptococci may cause acute kidney injury.

Acknowledgments

Dr. Alexander Bullen was supported by a Ruth L. Kirschstein training grant from the National Institute of Diabetes and Digestive and Kidney Diseases (NIDDK; T32DK104717).

References

[1] M. Nakamura, G. Seki, K. Iwadoh et al., "Acute kidney injury as defined by the RIFLE criteria is a risk factor for kidney transplant graft failure," *Clinical Transplantation*, vol. 26, no. 4, pp. 520–528, 2012.

[2] A. Mehrotra, C. Rose, N. Pannu, J. Gill, M. Tonelli, and J. S. Gill, "Incidence and consequences of acute kidney injury in kidney transplant recipients," *American Journal of Kidney Diseases*, vol. 59, no. 4, pp. 558–565, 2012.

[3] W. C. Wells, "Observations on the dropsy which succeeds scarlet fever," *Transactions of a Society for the Improvement of Medical and Chirurgical Knowledge*, vol. 3, pp. 167–186, 1812.

[4] J. E. Lewy, L. Salinas-Madrigal, P. B Herdson, C. L. Pirani, and J. Metcoff, "Clinico-pathologic correlations in acute poststreptococcal glomerulonephritis. A correlation between renal functions, morphologic damage and clinical course of 46 children with acute poststreptococcal glomerulonephritis," *Medicine*, vol. 50, no. 6, pp. 453–501, 1971.

[5] T. M. Eison, B. H. Ault, D. P. Jones, R. W. Chesney, and R. J. Wyatt, "Post-streptococcal acute glomerulonephritis in children: clinical features and pathogenesis," *Pediatric Nephrology*, vol. 26, no. 2, pp. 165–180, 2011.

[6] K. S. Ko, D. O. Cho, and J. H. Ahn, "Infections after renal transplantation," *Transplantation proceedings*, vol. 26, no. 4, pp. 2072–2074, 1994.

[7] S. Karuthu and E. A. Blumberg, "Common infections in kidney transplant recipients.," *Clinical journal of the American Society of Nephrology : CJASN*, vol. 7, no. 12, pp. 2058–2070, 2012.

[8] G. Moroni, D. Papaccioli, G. Banfi, A. Tarantino, and C. Ponticelli, "Acute Post-Bacterial Glomerulonephritis in Renal Transplant Patients: Description of Three Cases and Review of the Literature," *American Journal of Transplantation*, vol. 4, no. 1, pp. 132–136, 2004.

[9] J. M. Sorof, N. Weidner, D. Potter, and A. A. Portalel, "Acute post-streptococcal glomerulonephritis in a renal allograft," *Pediatric Nephrology*, vol. 9, no. 3, pp. 317–319, 1995.

[10] N. Yoshizawa, K. Yamakami, M. Fujino et al., "Nephritis-associated plasmin receptor and acute poststreptococcal glomerulonephritis: Characterization of the antigen and associated immune response," *Journal of the American Society of Nephrology*, vol. 15, no. 7, pp. 1785–1793, 2004.

[11] G. Parra, B. Rodríguez-Iturbe, S. Batsford et al., "Antibody to streptococcal zymogen in the serum of patients with acute glomerulonephritis: A multicentric study," *Kidney International*, vol. 54, no. 2, pp. 509–517, 1998.

[12] B. Rodríguez-Iturbe and S. Batsford, "Pathogenesis of post-streptococcal glomerulonephritis a century after Clemens von Pirquet," *Kidney International*, vol. 71, no. 11, pp. 1094–1104, 2007.

[13] T. Oda, K. Yamakami, F. Omasu et al., "Glomerular plasmin-like activity in relation to nephritis-associated plasmin receptor in acute poststreptococcal glomerulonephritis," *Journal of the American Society of Nephrology*, vol. 16, no. 1, pp. 247–254, 2005.

[14] B. Rodriguez-Iturbe and J. M. Musser, "The current state of poststreptococcal glomerulonephritis," *Journal of the American Society of Nephrology*, vol. 19, no. 10, pp. 1855–1864, 2008.

[15] Z. Layrisse, B. Rodríguez-Iturbe, R. García-Ramírez, A. Rodríguez, and J. Tiwari, "Family studies of the HLA system in acute post-streptococcal glomerulonephritis," *Human Immunology*, vol. 7, no. 3, pp. 177–185, 1983.

[16] A. H. Tart, M. J. Walker, and J. M. Musser, "New understanding of the group A *Streptococcus pathogenesis* cycle," *Trends in Microbiology*, vol. 15, no. 7, pp. 318–325, 2007.

[17] E. J. Lewis, C. B. Carpenter, and P. H. Schur, "Serum complement component levels in human glomerulonephritis.," *Annals of Internal Medicine*, vol. 75, no. 4, pp. 555–560, 1971.

[18] J. S. Cameron, R. M. Vick, C. S. Ogg, W. M. Seymour, C. Chantler, and D. R. Turner, "Plasma C3 and C4 Concentrations in Management of Glomerulonephritis," *British Medical Journal*, vol. 3, no. 5882, pp. 668–672, 1973.

[19] R. J. Wyatt, J. Forristal, C. D. West, S. Sugimoto, and J. G. Curd, "Complement profiles in acute post-streptococcal glomerulonephritis," *Pediatric Nephrology*, vol. 2, no. 2, pp. 219–223, 1988.

[20] H. T. Cook, "C3 glomerulopathy," *F1000Research*, vol. 6, article no. 248, 2017.

[21] *Fervenza FCSS. Clinical presentation, classification, and causes of membranoproliferative glomerulonephritis*, https://www.uptodate.com/contents/clinical-presentation-classification-and-causes-of-membranoproliferative-glomerulonephritis.

[22] S. Sethi, F. C. Fervenza, Y. Zhang et al., "Atypical postinfectious glomerulonephritis is associated with abnormalities in the alternative pathway of complement," *Kidney International*, vol. 83, no. 2, pp. 293–299, 2013.

[23] A. Servais, L.-H. Noël, L. T. Roumenina et al., "Acquired and genetic complement abnormalities play a critical role in dense deposit disease and other C3 glomerulopathies," *Kidney International*, vol. 82, no. 4, pp. 454–464, 2012.

[24] M. D. Denton and A. K. Singh, "Recurrent and de novo glomerulonephritis in the renal allograft," *Seminars in Nephrology*, vol. 20, no. 2, pp. 164–175, 2000.

[25] J. Floege, "Recurrent glomerulonephritis following renal transplantation: An update," *Nephrology Dialysis Transplantation* , vol. 18, no. 7, pp. 1260–1265, 2003.

[26] M. C. Pickering, V. D. D'agati, C. M. Nester et al., "C3 glomerulopathy: consensus report," *Kidney International*, vol. 84, no. 6, pp. 1079–1089, 2013.

[27] T. J. Plumb, A. Greenberg, S. R. Smith et al., "Postinfectious glomerulonephritis in renal allograft recipients," *Transplantation*, vol. 82, no. 9, pp. 1224–1228, 2006.

[28] S. H. Nasr, G. S. Markowitz, J. D. Whelan et al., "IgA-Dominant Acute Poststaphylococcal Glomerulonephritis Complicating Diabetic Nephropathy," *Human Pathology*, vol. 34, no. 12, pp. 1235–1241, 2003.

[29] H. G. Nebeker, G. Hercz, G. K. Feld, T. M. Stanley, J. W. Coburn, and K. Kurokawa, "Postinfectious glomerulonephritis in a renal allograft associated with a mycotic aneurysm of a coronary artery," *American Journal of Medicine*, vol. 76, no. 5, pp. 940–942, 1984.

34

Preserved Renal Function in Kidney Transplantation over a Thrombosed Aortobifemoral Bypass Graft: The Role of Retrograde Flow and Early Thrombolysis

Saúl Pampa-Saico,[1] Sara Jiménez-Alvaro,[1] Fernando Caravaca-Fontán,[1] Ana Fernández-Rodríguez,[1] Maite Rivera-Gorrín,[1,2] Juan Sánchez,[3] Antonio Chinchilla,[4] and Roberto Marcén[1]

[1]*Department of Nephrology, Hospital Universitario Ramón y Cajal, Carretera de Colmenar Viejo Km. 9.100, 28034 Madrid, Spain*
[2]*Department of Medicine, Universidad de Alcalá, 28805 Madrid, Spain*
[3]*Department of Radiology, Hospital Universitario Ramón y Cajal, 28034 Madrid, Spain*
[4]*Department of Vascular Surgery, Hospital Universitario Ramón y Cajal, 28034 Madrid, Spain*

Correspondence should be addressed to Saúl Pampa-Saico; saups5@hotmail.com

Academic Editor: Marian Klinger

Aortobifemoral bypass (ABFB) thrombosis is not uncommon, and when the artery of a renal graft is implanted on a bypass the risk of graft loss is high. We report the case of a 48-year-old woman with a previous history of ABFB under antiplatelet therapy and a kidney allograft implanted on the vascular prosthesis, who presented with acute limb ischemia and severe renal impairment. Imaging techniques revealed a complete thrombosis of the proximal left arm of the ABFB. However, a faint retrograde flow over the graft was observed thanks to the recanalization of distal left bypass by collateral native arteries. This unusual situation not previously reported in a kidney transplant setting, together with an early diagnosis, allowed graft survival until an early local thrombolysis resolved the problem. Two years later, renal function remains normal.

1. Introduction

Thrombosis of an aortobifemoral bypass (ABFB) graft is a common complication that may occur in about 10–15% of the cases within the first five years after surgery [1]. Moreover, when a renal allograft artery is implanted on a vascular prosthesis there is a higher risk of thrombosis and subsequent graft loss [2].

Here, we report the case of a patient presenting a complete occlusion of the arterial bypass in which renal graft perfusion was partially maintained by retrograde flow from collateral arteries in the distal end of the aortobifemoral bypass. Early diagnosis and preemptive treatment with local fibrinolysis allowed the resolution of thrombosis and complete recovery of kidney graft function.

2. Case Report

A 48-year-old woman with a previous history of chronic kidney disease secondary to type IV lupus nephritis (negative lupus anticoagulant and negative antiphospholipid antibodies) was diagnosed with Leriche syndrome in July 2012. Thus, a 14 mm × 7 mm expanded polytetrafluoroethylene (ePTFE) ABFB graft was successfully implanted and the patient was later discharged with antiplatelet therapy (acetylsalicylic acid 100 mg/day).

Four months later, the patient received a kidney transplant from a deceased donor. An end-to-side arterial anastomosis to the left branch of the ABFB was performed and an end-to-side venous anastomosis to the external iliac vein with no significant complications was performed. The patient

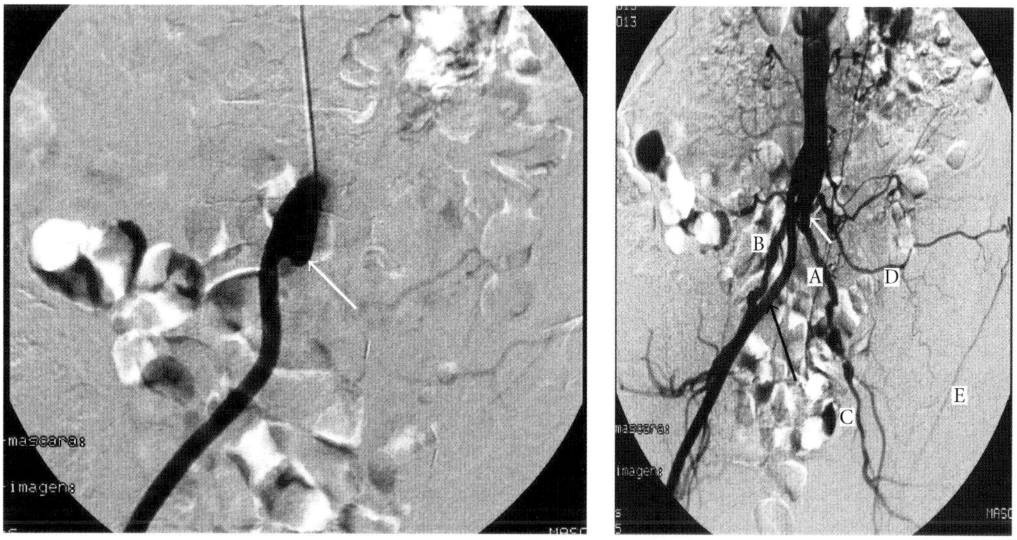

(a) (b)

Figure 1: (a) Early image of abdominal angiogram showing a complete occlusion of the left arm of the ABFB (arrow). (b) The right arm of the ABFB is patent (black arrow); proximal button of the left ABFB (white arrow); primitive iliac arteries (A, B); collateral circulation: left hypogastric (C), left lumbar (D), and circumflex iliac (E) arteries.

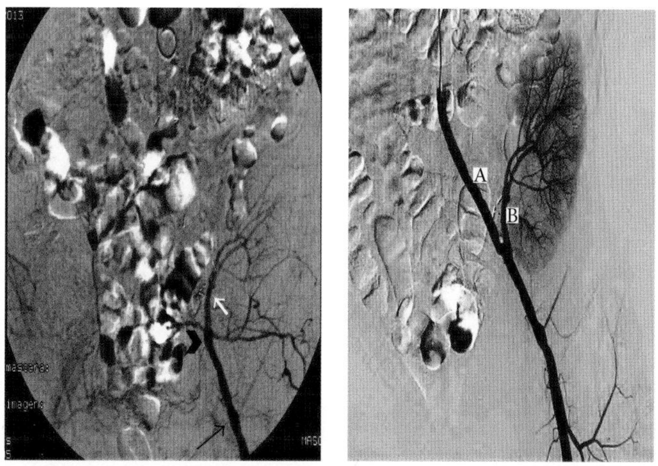

(a) (b)

Figure 2: (a) Recanalization of both the distal branch of the left ABFB (head arrow) and renal artery of the graft (white arrow) and femoral common artery (black arrow). (b) Angiographic control showing both patency of the left arm of the ABFB (A) and the artery of kidney graft (B).

was started on tacrolimus, mycophenolic acid, and steroids, reaching normal renal graft function over the next months (mean serum creatinine of 1 mg/dL).

Nine months later, the patient presented to the emergency room complaining of pain and coldness in the left lower limb and progressive decrease of diuresis in the last two days. Blood pressure was 185/105 mmHg, and physical examination revealed absence of popliteal and pedal pulses in the left lower limb and normal peripheral perfusion of the contralateral leg. Initial laboratory data revealed a serum creatinine of 4.1 mg/dL; lactate dehydrogenase 228 U/L (normal range: 140–240 U/L); creatine kinase 44 IU/L (normal range: 24–174 IU/L); hemoglobin 9.3 g/dL; leukocyte count 4.9 per 10^9/L; serum tacrolimus concentration 4.6 ng/mL (reference range: 4–8 ng/mL). Urinalysis showed a sodium concentration of 55 mmol/L, with negative proteinuria and normal urinary sediment.

She was admitted to the hospital and an abdominal angiography performed through the right humeral artery revealed a complete thrombosis of the proximal left branch of the ABFB (Figure 1(a)), along with an important collateral circulation (Figure 1(b)). However, late-phase angiogram showed a retrograde filling of the distal prosthesis with only faint perfusion of the kidney (Figure 2(a)). Local fibrinolytic therapy with 10 mg of alteplase (recombinant tissue plasminogen activator-rtPA) was initiated, followed by systemic sodium heparin (250 IU/Kg) to achieve a target activated thromboplastin time between 1.5-fold and 2.0-fold over the normal range. A control angiogram 8 hours after that showed a successful restoration of patency of the bypass, together with both a normal nephrogram and arterial vascular tree of the kidney (Figure 2(b)).

The patient was discharged 14 days after admission under treatment with oral anticoagulation (acenocoumarol), with a complete resolution of ABFB thrombosis and recovery of kidney graft function (serum creatinine concentration of 1.2 mg/dL).

3. Discussion

This case report highlights the risk of development of acute renal allograft failure in kidneys transplanted over vascular grafts. A myriad of case reports documenting the recovery of renal function after thrombolysis have been published; however, to the best of our knowledge, this is the first case of a kidney allograft implanted on a vascular bypass graft.

Kidney transplantation on prosthetic vascular grafts was described first by Sterioff in 1974 [1], although it is not a frequent procedure nowadays according to case series (0.2–1.7% of renal transplants) [2, 3].

The etiology of vascular graft thrombosis may be related to progressive fibrosis and development of stenosis or aneurysms at the site of implantation which could eventually lead to abnormal vascularization [2–4].

Clinically, the presence of coldness and/or lower limb pain with no peripheral pulses in patients with ABFB suggests a thrombosis of the bypass graft. In our patient, the coexistence of reduced urine output pointed out that the perfusion of the kidney graft could also be compromised.

Peripheral arterial occlusions are usually associated with increased leukocyte count and increased serum levels of lactate dehydrogenase [5], although our patient had normal values. It has been reported that, in the setting of renal artery thrombosis, there may be a great variability in laboratory values depending on the number and size of segmental arteries affected, the intensity of ischemic injury, the time of development, and the presence of collateral circulation. As expected, thrombosis of the main renal artery in patients with only one functioning kidney is associated with impaired renal function. However, urinary parameters may vary depending on the stage of arterial occlusion [5, 6].

In our case, the patient had severe renal impairment and oliguria at presentation, but retrograde filling of the distal vascular graft permitted a partial perfusion of the transplanted kidney. This was probably the result of a high blood pressure in collateral arteries and relatively low intra-arterial resistance in renal graft with respect to the limb, and we believe that this phenomenon played a pivotal role in the allograft viability.

Finally, early recognition and initiation of thrombolytic therapy restore the circulation. We initiated therapy with rtPA due to the low side-effect profile and ease of use. Moreover, it is less aggressive than surgical thrombectomy, and it is associated with a lower average length of stay in hospital [7–9].

In conclusion, thrombosis of an ABFB with an implanted kidney allograft may not result in graft loss if early diagnosed and treated. The presence of collateral circulation together with retrograde filling of the vascular prosthesis played an important role in maintaining the viability of the organ.

Competing Interests

The authors declare that there is no conflict of interests regarding the publication of this paper.

References

[1] H. Önder, L. Oguzkurt, G. Tekbaş, S. Gür, and M. Gedikoglu, "Successful treatment of delayed aortobifemoral graft thrombosis with manual aspiration thrombectomy," *Diagnostic and Interventional Radiology*, vol. 18, no. 1, pp. 142–145, 2012.

[2] D. Patrono, R. Verhelst, A. Buemi et al., "Renal allograft implantation on prosthetic vascular grafts: short- and long-term results," *World Journal of Surgery*, vol. 37, no. 7, pp. 1727–1734, 2013.

[3] W. Coosemans, A. Nevelsteen, J. Pirenne, and Y. Vanrenterghem, "Renal transplantation in patients with a vascular aortoiliac prosthesis," *Transplantation Proceedings*, vol. 31, no. 4, pp. 1925–1927, 1999.

[4] G. Andros and L. Lee, "Bypass grafts: the state of the art," *Scandinavian Journal of Surgery*, vol. 101, no. 2, pp. 100–106, 2012.

[5] F. Liaño, C. Gámez, J. Pascual et al., "Use of urinary parameters in the diagnosis of total acute renal artery occlusion," *Nephron*, vol. 66, no. 2, pp. 170–175, 1994.

[6] H. R. Sosa Barrios, S. Jiménez Álvaro, A. Gomis Couto et al., "Oclusión de arteria renal y fibrinolisis local intravascular," *NefroPlus*, vol. 6, no. 1, pp. 57–60, 2014.

[7] O. Rouvière, P. Berger, C. Béziat et al., "Acute thrombosis of renal transplant artery: graft salvage by means of intra-arterial fibrinolysis," *Transplantation*, vol. 73, no. 3, pp. 403–409, 2002.

[8] C. Gallego-Ferreiroa, E. de Sá, B. Torrón-Casal et al., "Análisis critico del tratamiento fibrinolítico en la thrombosis del Bypass femoropopliteo," *Angiologia*, vol. 59, no. 2, pp. 129–138, 2007.

[9] A. M. Schrijver, M. M. P. J. Reijnen, J. A. Van Oostayen et al., "Initial results of catheter-directed ultrasound-accelerated thrombolysis for thromboembolic obstructions of the aortofemoral arteries: a feasibility study," *CardioVascular and Interventional Radiology*, vol. 35, no. 2, pp. 279–285, 2012.

35

Successful Renal Transplantation after Presumed Cyanide Toxicity Treated with Hydroxocobalamin

Ryan J. Hendrix,[1] Paulo N. Martins,[1] Jeffrey S. Stoff,[2] Aaron Ahearn,[1] Adel Bozorgzadeh,[1] and Babak Movahedi[1]

[1]University of Massachusetts Medical School, Department of Surgery, Division of Organ Transplantation, USA
[2]University of Massachusetts Medical School, Department of Medicine, Division of Nephrology, USA

Correspondence should be addressed to Ryan J. Hendrix; ryan.hendrix@umassmemorial.org

Academic Editor: Ryszard Grenda

We report two cases of successful renal transplantation with allografts from donors who suffered anoxic brain injury as the primary cause of death from house fires. Each was treated prophylactically with hydroxocobalamin (Cyanokit) for suspected cyanide toxicity. During organ procurement, gross examination was notable for deep discoloration of the parenchymal tissues. Approximately 6 and 18 months after transplantation, both recipients have excellent renal graft function and remain independent from hemodialysis (HD). Hydroxocobalamin is the antidote for suspected acute cyanide toxicity. While largely tolerated by the recipient, there is concern over the potential functional implications of the associated side effects of dramatic tissue discoloration and development of oxalate crystals. Furthermore, difficulties performing hemodialysis in patients treated with hydroxocobalamin have been reported due to discoloration of the effluent fluid impacting the colorimetric sensor, causing false alarms and repetitive interruptions. As such, many transplant centers in the United States (US) continue to reject these organs. We seek to highlight two cases of successful transplantation following donor administration of hydroxocobalamin (Cyanokit) and present the first documented case of successful perioperative intermittent hemodialysis following transplantation of an allograft exposed to hydroxocobalamin. Furthermore, we emphasize the importance of optimal organ utilization and caution against unnecessary refusal.

1. Introduction

End stage renal disease (ESRD) is a devastating medical condition representing the most advanced form of chronic kidney disease (CKD). Five-year survival rates for patients undergoing renal transplantation are 85.5%, while those on hemodialysis (HD) are significantly reduced at 35.8% [1–3]. Of the 10,286 deceased donor kidney transplant operations performed in 2017, asphyxiation was the documented mechanism of death for 6% of donors [2]. While the etiology of asphyxia is multifactorial and diverse, house fires are a major contributor [2, 4].

Annually, there are approximately 16,000 domestic fire related injuries and 3,000 deaths [4]. Greater than 75% of these fatalities are directly attributed to smoke inhalation toxicity from carbon monoxide (CO) and hydrogen cyanide (CN) gases [4–6]. CN can be liberated during the combustion of products containing both carbon and nitrogen, notably wool, silk, polyurethane (insulation/upholstery), polyacrylonitriles (plastics), melamine resins (household goods), and synthetic rubber [5, 6].

Cyanide is an extremely toxic poison. Mechanistically, cyanide binds rapidly with cytochrome a3, a component of the cytochrome c oxidase complex in mitochondria. Inhibition of cytochrome a3 prevents the cell from using oxygen and forces anaerobic metabolism, resulting in lactate production, cellular hypoxia and metabolic acidosis [7, 8]. Untreated, this cascade can lead to death within minutes. The presence and extent of cyanide poisoning are often initially unknown given the absence of a rapid, confirmatory cyanide blood test. Thus, treatment decisions must be made on the basis of clinical history, mechanism of injury, and suspicion of cyanide intoxication.

The antidote, hydroxocobalamin, classically induces an abnormal reddish discoloration of renal allografts, and oxalate crystals on histologic examination are common. Despite these disconcerting physical features, no evidence suggests an effect on short- or long-term renal function. The only issue lies in the potential need for perioperative HD following renal transplantation. Discoloration of the dialysate can lead to altered refractive properties as detected by the HD machine photodetector. Ultimately, this results in the repetitive triggering of the blood leak alarm initiating a cascade which halts the blood pump and pauses the dialysis cycle.

Here we present two cases of successful renal transplantation utilizing organs that were severely discolored due to prior administration of hydroxocobalamin to the donor and therefore declined by the majority of other centers in our region. For both cases, our standard institutional protocols were followed which specify all patients receive depleting antibodies as part of their induction regimen. Patients that are considered immunologically high risk such as those receiving a second transplant, the presence of donor specific antibodies (DSA), or high calculated panel reactive antibodies (cPRA) receive anti-thymocyte globulin. Low immunologic risk patients receive alemtuzumab.

2. Case 1

A 58-year-old female was found unresponsive after a house fire, with the primary cause of death anoxic brain injury. Despite a short period of asystole, her renal function was preserved with an admission creatinine of 0.88, peak creatinine of 1.24, and a final creatinine of 1.04. The Kidney Donor Profile Index (KDPI) was 64%. On gross examination, severe organ discoloration was noted (Figure 1), and biopsy results were significant for the presence of oxalate crystals. Kidney pump pressure was set at 35 mmHg, resulting in a flow of 133 mL/min with a resistance of 0.23 (Table 1). The organ recipient was a 53-year-old male with end stage renal disease secondary to hypertensive nephrosclerosis on hemodialysis three times per week for a total duration of 52 months. His cPRA was 0% with no evidence of gray zone DSA (Table 2). A complement dependent cytotoxicity (CDC) T cell cross match was performed and negative.

Following transplantation, induction immunosuppression consisted of alemtuzumab 30 mg and solumedrol 500 mg, followed by a maintenance regimen of tacrolimus, mycophenolate 500mg twice daily and prednisone 10 mg daily. Early in the perioperative period, the patient's hospital course was complicated by severe hyperkalemia and delayed graft function requiring HD on postoperative day (POD) 1, 2, 4, and 6. Each session was performed without incident. On POD 7, in the setting of ongoing oliguria and worsening abdominal distention, laboratory and imaging studies revealed a large pelvic fluid collection consistent with an acute perinephric hematoma. The patient was taken emergently to the operating room for reexploration and evacuation of the hematoma. Subsequently, the patient's urine output began to improve and serum creatinine started to decrease. Ultimately, the patient was discharged to home on POD 13.

Approximately 3 weeks after transplant, the patient presented with an elevated creatinine to 4.70 mg/dL (previous nadir 2.60 mg/dL). A biopsy of the renal allograft revealed acute T cell mediated rejection (Banff category 2A) as well as acute antibody-mediated rejection. A C4D stain was positive in more than 30% of the peritubular capillaries. A Human Leukocyte Antigen (HLA) antibody screen revealed a class II (DQ) DSA at 8000 mean fluorescence intensity (MFI). Institutional protocols for rejection were followed, and the patient was initially treated with solumedrol 500 mg x3 doses. Despite this, his creatinine continued to rise and he remained oliguric. Subsequently, anti-thymocyte globulin 1 mg/kg x 3 doses was administered, followed by plasmapheresis and IVIG x 5 doses (2g/kg ideal body weight). During this 2-week hospital readmission for rejection, 4 additional sessions of HD were required, and again, there were no complications. A repeat biopsy 6 weeks later did not reveal any signs of ongoing rejection, and all prior oxalate crystals had disappeared. The patient's creatinine improved and plateaued in the 1.9-2.0 range. Eighteen months after transplant, the patient has a stable graft function with creatinine levels near 2 mg/dL (Figure 2).

3. Case 2

A 57-year-old male found unresponsive after a house fire subsequently developed pulseless electrical activity (PEA) arrest with the primary cause of death documented as anoxic brain injury. The donor met criteria to be considered public health services (PHS) high risk given his recent history of incarceration. Overall, renal function was preserved with a creatinine on admission of 1.60, peak creatinine of 1.60, and final creatinine of 1.40. The KDPI was 75%. On gross examination, severe organ discoloration was noted (Figure 1), however, renal biopsy did not reveal the presence of oxalate crystals. Kidney pump pressure was set at 35 mmHg, resulting in a flow of 94 mL/min with a resistance of 0.30 (Table 1). The organ recipient was a 78-year-old male with ESRD secondary to hypertension and diabetes undergoing HD three times a week for a total duration of 25 months. The cPRA was 0%, however, a single gray zone DSA against HLA A29 was identified (Table 2). All crossmatch tests were negative.

Induction immunosuppression consisted of anti-thymocyte globulin (total dose of 5mg/kg) administered over 5 doses and solumedrol 500 mg, followed by a maintenance regimen of tacrolimus, mycophenolate 500 mg twice daily and prednisone 10 mg daily. The patient had an overall uneventful postoperative course with immediate graft function and progressive downtrend in creatinine levels. On POD 7, the patient was discharged to a short-term rehabilitation facility. Six months after organ transplantation, the patient continues to experience a stable graft function with baseline creatinine of 1.14 (Figure 2).

TABLE 1: Donor demographics and organ parameters.

	Donor 1	Donor 2
Age (yrs)	58	57
Sex	Female	Male
Weight (kg)	94.4	60.8
KDPI* (%)	64	75
Cause of Death	Anoxia	Anoxia
Mechanism	House Fire	House Fire
Creatinine (mg/dL)		
First	0.88	1.60
Peak	1.24	1.60
Last	1.04	1.40
Biopsy at Procurement		
Glomerulosclerosis (%)	0	1
Tubular Fibrosis (%)	1-10	1-10
Vessel Atherosclerosis	Absent	Mild
Oxalate Crystals	Positive	Negative
Serology		
CMV	Negative	Positive
EBV	Negative	Positive
HBV	Negative	Positive
HCV	Negative	Negative
HIV	Negative	Negative
NAT**, HBV, HCV, HIV	Negative	Negative
PHS*** Increased Risk	Negative	Positive
Final Pump Parameters		
Pressure (mmHg)	35	35
Flow (mL/min)	133	94
Resistance	0.23	0.30
Organ Laterality	Right	Right

*KDPI: Kidney Donor Profile Index.
**NAT: Nucleic Acid Testing.
***PHS: U.S. Public Health Service.

TABLE 2: Recipient demographics.

	Recipient 1	Recipient 2
Age (yrs)	53	78
Sex	Male	Male
Disease Etiology	Hypertension	Type II Diabetes
Dialysis Duration (months)	52	25
Sequence Match	9	470
cPRA* (%)	0	House Fire
Gray zone Antibody	Negative	A29
CMV	Negative	Negative
EBV	Positive	Positive
HBV/HCV	Negative	Negative
Cold Ischemia Time (hrs)	22	21.65
Warm Ischemia Time (mins)	48	25

*cPRA: Calculated Panel Reactive Antibody.

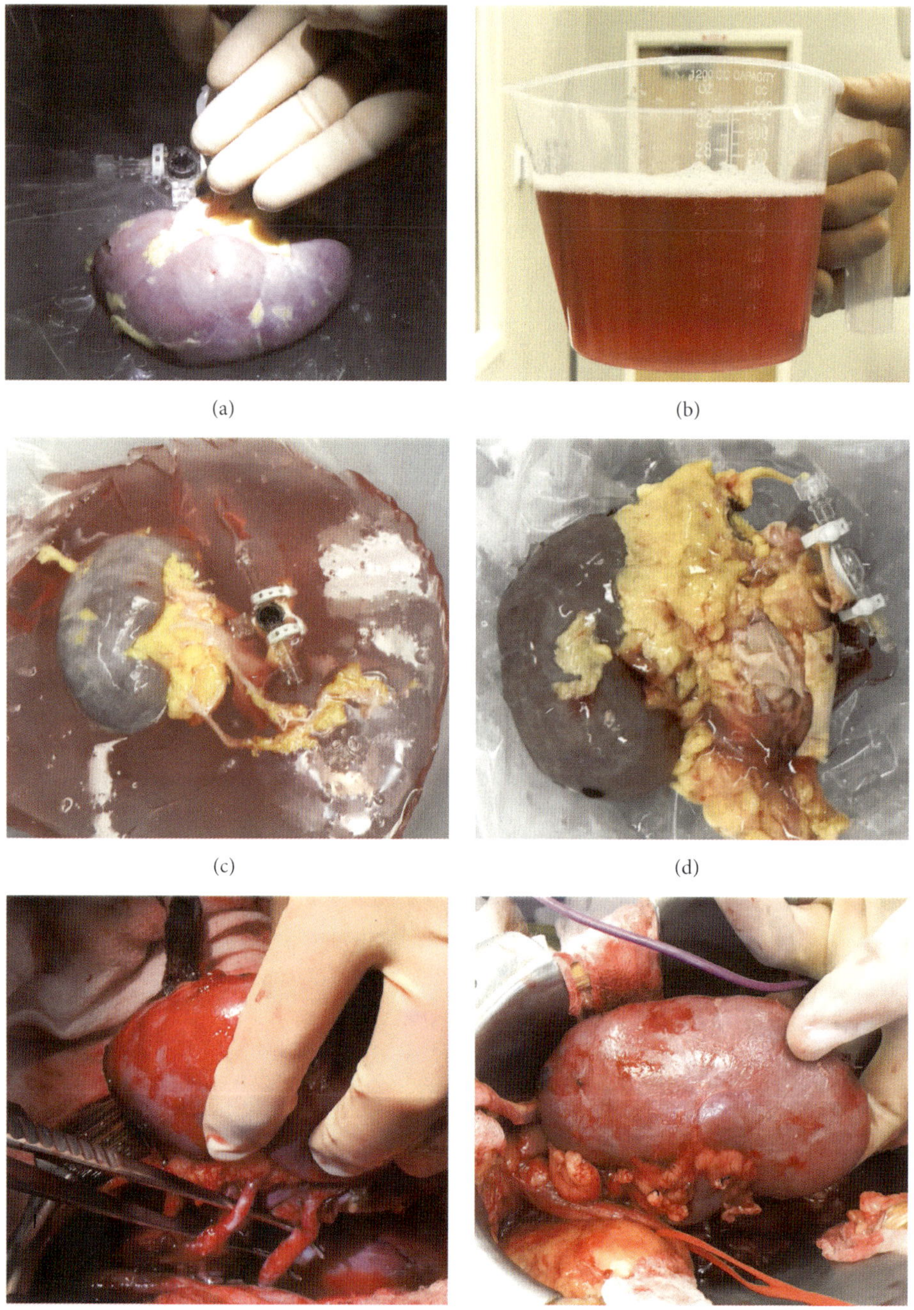

FIGURE 1: (a) Allograft #1 at time of procurement. (b) Discoloration of effluent. (c) Allograft #1 on pump. (d) Allograft #2 on pump. (e) Allograft #1 in vivo. (f) Allograft #2 in vivo.

4. Discussion

Cyanide is a lethal toxin which uncouples mitochondrial oxidative phosphorylation; preventing aerobic metabolism and initiating a cascade of acidosis and hypoxia. Hydroxocobalamin, the gold standard treatment for cyanide toxicity, was FDA-approved in the United States in 2006 but has been formally licensed in Europe since 1996 to treat known or suspected cyanide poisoning [9]. The initial dose of hydroxocobalamin for adults is 5 grams administered as an intravenous (IV) infusion over fifteen minutes. Intravenous administration of hydroxocobalamin leads to interaction and binding to plasma proteins and low molecular weight physiologic compounds generating various cobalamin-(III) complexes. These molecules can then bind cyanide ions through a substitution for the hydroxo ligand linked to the

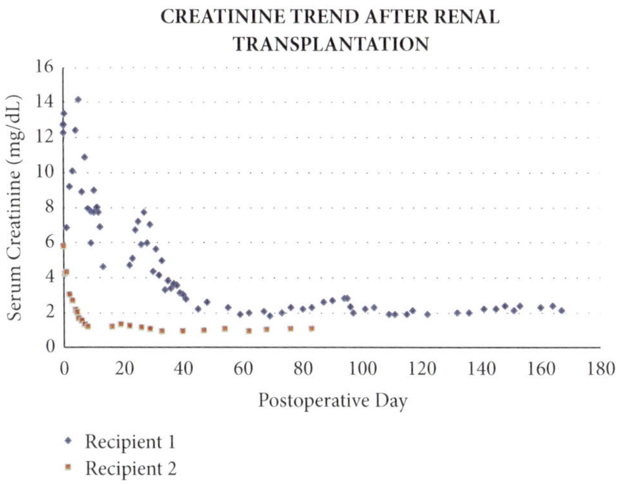

FIGURE 2: Serum creatinine (mg/dL) following renal transplantation. Above demonstrates the significant improvement in renal function after renal transplantation and the sustained viability of each organ.

trivalent cobalt ion. End product is cyanocobalamin, which is then excreted in the urine.

Pharmacodynamic effects include an increase in blood pressure and variable effects on heart rate. Dose-proportional pharmacokinetics has been observed following administration of hydroxocobalamin with total urinary excretion calculated to be 60-70% of a given dose of hydroxocobalamin. Discoloration of urine has been noted to occur for up to 35 days after administration. Mean half-life of free cobalamins-(III) was 26 hours at the 5g dosage. Most common adverse reactions include chromaturia, erythema, and oxalate crystal formation. These crystals have been observed in the urine of both healthy subjects given hydroxocobalamin and patients treated with hydroxocobalamin following suspected cyanide poisoning [10]. Interestingly, oxalate crystals were observed in donor 1's kidney biopsy performed at the time of organ recovery. Most patients will experience a reversible red/orange discoloration of the skin, urine and mucous membrane secretions which can contribute to alterations in colorimetric tests and co-oximetry measurements [11, 12].

The first published case report of a successful organ transplant from a donor, whose cause of death was cyanide toxicity, was published in 1987 [13]. Several additional case reports and small series echoed the findings that cyanide toxicity itself was not a contraindication to transplant [14–17]. Since 2006, hydroxocobalamin has established itself as the gold standard antidote for cyanide toxicity replacing amyl nitrate and sodium thiosulfate. Initial reports suggested Cyanokit administration was safe prior to organ transplantation [18]. However, more recent reports have found hydroxocobalamin to be associated with failure of intermittent hemodialysis, thus limiting the opportunity to provide life-saving treatment should a transplanted allograft fail or experience delayed function [19, 20]. The presumed mechanism for this phenomenon is the discoloration of bodily fluids triggering a "pseudo-blood leak" [21]. This triggering of the colorimetric sensor of the dialysis machine subsequently causes false alarms and repetitive interruptions of the dialysis cycle.

While it is not possible to determine the exact reasoning for neighboring transplantation centers to decline the organs, discussions with the Organ Procurement Organization (OPO) highlighted genuine concern regarding the feasibility of perioperative dialysis. A recent study postulated that hemodialysis machines employing a photodetector consisting of a single optical emitter designed to detect light scatter and signal drop off are unlikely to be affected by hydroxocobalamin whereas those using a dual LED array that depends on light absorption are susceptible [22, 23]. In congruence with this explanation, a multidisciplinary discussion was held at our institution prior to transplantation at which time it was confirmed the dialysis machine leak alarm could be overridden should dialysis be required.

5. Conclusion

Although we present only two cases, our experience reiterates that kidneys from donors treated with hydroxocobalamin can be used with good long-term outcome. Furthermore, we present the first documented case of successful perioperative intermittent HD following transplantation of an allograft exposed to hydroxocobalamin.

References

[1] A. Hart, J. M. Smith, and M. A. Skeans, "OPTN/SRTR 2013 Annual Data Report: Kidney," *American Journal of Transplantation*, vol. 17, Supplement 1, no. 21, 2017.

[2] "Organ Procurement and Transplantation Network of the United States Department of Health and Human Services," https://optn.transplant.hrsa.gov/data/view-data-reports/national-data/#.

[3] "National Institute of Digestive, Diabetes and Kidney Diseases," https://www.niddk.nih.gov/health-information/health-statistics/Pages/kidney-disease-statistics-united-states. aspxs.

[4] H. Haynes, "Fire Loss in the United States During 2016 Report of the National Fire Protection Association," https://www.nfpa.org/News-and-Research/Fire-statistics-and-reports/Fire-statistics/Fires-in-the-US.

[5] S. N. Vogel, T. R. Sultan, and R. P. Ten Eyck, "Cyanide poisoning," *Clinical Toxicology*, vol. 18, no. 3, pp. 367–383, 1981.

[6] C. Bismuth, F. J. Baud, H. Djeghout, A. Astier, and D. Aubriot, "Cyanide poisoning from propionitrile exposure," *The Journal of Emergency Medicine*, vol. 5, no. 3, pp. 191–195, 1987.

[7] "CYANOKIT® Hydroxocobalamin. Product monograph," 2016, http://www.medical-information.ca/wp-content/uploads/2015/07/CYANOKIT-HCP.pdf.

[8] G. Shepherd and L. I. Velez, "Role of hydroxocobalamin in acute cyanide poisoning," *Annals of Pharmacotherapy*, vol. 42, no. 5, pp. 661–669, 2008.

[9] H. L. Williams, D. J. Johnson, J. S. McNeil, and D. G. Wright, "Studies of cobalamin as a vehicle for the renal excretion of

cyanide anion," *Journal of Laboratory and Clinical Medicine*, vol. 116, pp. 37–44, 1990.

[10] M. Legrand, T. Michel, M. Daudon et al., "Risk of oxalate nephropathy with the use of cyanide antidote hydroxocobalamin in critically ill burn patients," *Intensive Care Medicine*, vol. 42, no. 6, pp. 1080-1081, 2016.

[11] S. C. Curry, D. A. Connor, and R. A. Raschke, "Effect of the Cyanide Antidote Hydroxocobalamin on Commonly Ordered Serum Chemistry Studies," *Annals of Emergency Medicine*, vol. 24, no. 1, pp. 65–67, 1994.

[12] P. V. A. Pamidi, M. DeAbreu, D. Kim, and S. Mansouri, "Hydroxocobalamin and cyanocobalamin interference on co-oximetry based hemoglobin measurements," *Clinica Chimica Acta*, vol. 401, no. 1-2, pp. 63–67, 2009.

[13] P. W. G. Brown, J. A. C. Buckels, A. B. Jain, and P. Mcmaster, "Successful cadaveric renal transplantation from a donor who died of cyanide poisoning," *British Medical Journal (Clinical Research ed.)*, vol. 294, no. 6583, p. 1325, 1987.

[14] D. M. Wood, P. I. Dargan, and A. L. Jones, "Poisoned patients as potential organ donors: Postal survey of transplant centres and intensive care units," *Critical Care*, vol. 7, no. 2, pp. 147–154, 2003.

[15] M. G. Hebert, A. Coucher, G. Beaucage et al., "Transplantation of kidneys from a donor with carbon monoxide poisoning," *The New England Journal of Medicine*, vol. 326, Article ID 1571, 1992.

[16] P. Hantson, M.-C. Vekemans, J.-P. Squifflet, and P. Mahieu, "Outcome following organ removal from poisoned donors: experience with 12 cases and a review of the literature," *Transplant International*, vol. 8, no. 3, pp. 185–189, 1995.

[17] T. J. Barkoukis, C. A. Sarbak, D. Lewis, and F. C. Whittier, "Multiorgan procurement from a victim of cyanide poisoning: A case report and review of the literature," *Transplantation*, vol. 55, no. 6, pp. 1434–1436, 1993.

[18] J. L. Fortin, M. Ruttimann, G. Capellier, A. Bigorie, S. Ferlicot, and E. Thervet, "Successful organ transplantation after treatment of fatal cyanide poisoning with hydroxocobalamin," *Clinical Toxicology*, vol. 45, no. 5, pp. 468–471, 2007.

[19] M. Sutter, N. Tereshchenko, R. Rafii, and G. P. Daubert, "Hemodialysis Complications of Hydroxocobalamin: A Case Report," *Journal of Medical Toxicology*, vol. 6, no. 2, pp. 165–167, 2010.

[20] J. Abdelmalek, S. Thornton, J. Nizar, A. Schneir, and A. P. Sanchez, "Successful use of continuous renal replacement therapy after hydroxocobalamin administration," *Dialysis & Transplantation*, vol. 40, no. 9, pp. 415–417, 2011.

[21] J. Avila, D. Prasad, L. S. Weisberg, and R. Kasama, "Pseudo-blood leak? A hemodialysis mystery," *Clinical Nephrology*, vol. 79, no. 4, pp. 323–325, 2013.

[22] K. Lim, E. Heher, D. Steele et al., "Hemodialysis Failure Secondary to Hydroxocobalamin Exposure," *Baylor University Medical Center Proceedings*, vol. 30, no. 2, pp. 167-168, 2017.

[23] M. E. Sutter, M. E. Clarke, J. Cobb et al., "Blood leak alarm interference by hydoxocobalamin is hemodialysis machine dependent," *Clinical Toxicology*, vol. 50, no. 10, pp. 892–895, 2012.

36

False Positive B-Cells Crossmatch after Prior Rituximab Exposure of the Kidney Donor

Judith Desoutter, Marie-Joëlle Apithy, Ségolène Bartczak, and Nicolas Guillaume

Department of Histocompatibility, Amiens University Medical Center, 80000 Amiens, France

Correspondence should be addressed to Nicolas Guillaume; guillaume.nicolas@chu-amiens.fr

Academic Editor: Gerald Schlaf

Crossmatching is essential prior to kidney transplantation to confirm compatibility between the donor and the recipient, particularly to prevent acute antibody-mediated rejection. An unexpected positive crossmatch may be obtained in recipients with an autoimmune disease or preexisting antibodies not detected by single-antigen bead array due to complement interference or who have been previously treated by desensitization protocols such as rituximab, antithymocyte globulin, or intravenous immunoglobulins. We report donor and recipient investigations that revealed unexpected positive B-cells crossmatch, probably due to donor cells, as the donor had received rituximab therapy shortly before organ harvesting, in a context of severe idiopathic thrombocytopenic purpura. We consequently detected unexpected Class II IgG complement-dependent cytotoxicity for all sera tested. Other laboratory investigations failed to elucidate the reasons for this recipient-related positivity.

1. Introduction

The presence of preformed donor-specific antibodies (DSA) directed against human leukocyte antigens (HLA) interferes with kidney transplantation, as it is associated with all types of antibody-mediated rejection. Prior to transplantation, recipients are therefore routinely screened for preformed anti-HLA antibodies and prospective crossmatches are performed by conventional complement-dependent cytotoxicity crossmatch (CDC-XM) techniques, but also by flow-cytometry-based methods [1, 2].

The CDC-XM method is based on incubation of donor isolated B- and T-lymphocytes with recipient serum. The presence of anti-HLA antibodies in serum, targeting donor HLA antigens, induces donor cells complement-dependent cytotoxicity. Positive T-cells IgG-CDC-XM constitutes a contraindication for transplantation. Some centers have extended this contraindication to positive B-cells IgG-CDC-XM.

Positive CDC-XM can be observed in other situations, notably in recipients with an autoimmune disease [3] or preexisting antibodies not detected by single-antigen bead array due to complement interference [4] or previously treated by desensitization protocols such as rituximab (RTX), antithymocyte globulin, and intravenous immunoglobulins [5]. In the prospective setting, an unexpected positive CDC-XM must be rapidly documented to avoid nonaccessibility to the transplant.

We report donor and recipient investigations revealing unexpected positive B-cells crossmatch, probably due to donor cells.

2. Case Report

A 46-year-old woman with end-stage kidney disease was considered for first kidney transplantation.

HLA-A*30, HLA-B*13, HLA-B*40, HLA-DRB1*04, HLA-DRB1*13, HLA-DQB1*03, and HLA-DQB1*06 genotyping was performed with PCR-SSO genotyping test (One Lambda, Canoga Park, CA). A high-definition LABScreen® single-antigen Class I and Class II assay (One Lambda, Canoga Park, CA) was prospectively performed on the LABScan100® flow cytometer (Luminex Corporation, Austin, TX) to determine the specificity of anti-HLA IgG antibodies. A positive result was defined as mean fluorescence intensity (MFI) greater than 1,000. This assay

Table 1: Prospective crossmatch performed by complement-dependent cytotoxicity for pretransplantation screening.

Sera collected months before CDC-XM	Class I results (ASHI score)		Class II results (ASHI score)	
	Without DTT	With DTT	Without DTT	With DTT
50	1	1	*1*	*6*
35	1	1	*4*	*6*
26	1	1	*4*	*8*
18	1	1	*4*	*8*
11	1	1	*2*	*8*
8	1	2	*2*	*4*
3	1	2	*4*	*8*
Day of organ harvesting	1	2	*1*	*8*

revealed the presence of anti-A2, anti-A10, anti-A24, anti-A25, anti-A26, anti-A28, anti-A29, anti-A32, anti-A34, anti-A43, anti-A66, anti-A68, anti-A69, anti-A74, anti-B8, anti-B14, anti-B17, anti-B38, anti-B48, anti-B55, anti-B57, anti-B58, anti-B59, anti-B60, anti-B64, anti-B65, anti-B70, anti-B71, anti-B72, anti-B81, anti-B82, anti-Cw7, anti-Cw17, and anti-DR7 antibodies.

A potentially suitable ABO-compatible organ was found with HLA-A*03, HLA-A*30, HLA-B*35, HLA-B*49, HLA-C*03, HLA-C*04, HLA-DRB1*04, HLA-DRB1*13, HLA-DQB1*03, HLA-DQB1*03, HLA-DPB1*03, and HLA-DPB1*15 status. The recipient had no identified donor-specific antibodies (DSA). A prospective CDC-XM was performed with selected nodal T- and B-donor cells (Fluorobeads® T and B, One Lambda) to distinguish anti-HLA Class I and II antibodies, with or without recipient serum pretreated by dithiothreitol (DTT) to distinguish IgG and IgM antibodies. We used as positive controls anti-HLA Class I (# hla-c1, Invivogen, San Diego, USA) and anti-HLA Class II (# hla-c2, Invivogen, San Diego, USA) controls to highlight the quality of the cell suspension, respectively, enriched for T- or B-cells in the corresponding well.

We detected an unexpected Class II IgG complement-dependent cytotoxicity for all sera tested, enhanced by DTT treatment according to the ASHI scoring system (1 and 2 as negative, 4 as 30–49%, 6 as 50–79%, and 8 as 80–100% lysed lymphocytes (see Table 1)) and also in the B-cells negative control well (serum pool from donors which shows no cytotoxic reactions in the lymphocytotoxicity test, Bio-Rad, CA). Because of the unexplained strongly positive Class II IgG, transplantation was not performed by our center.

To test the hypothesis that positive CDC-XM reflects the presence of unidentified antibodies directed against the donor, we performed investigations on the recipient, which failed to provide any explanation for the positive CDC-XM:

(i) No treatment to prevent acute rejection before transplantation.

(ii) Negative auto-CDC-XM between cells (B- and T-lymphocytes) and recipient serum in accordance with the lack of a documented autoimmune disease.

(iii) Absence of detection of preexisting antibodies due to a complement interference phenomenon by testing sera after EDTA pretreatment, as previously described (0.1 M solution of disodium EDTA, Sigma-Aldrich, St. Louis, MI, at pH = 7.4 diluted 1:10 in serum and incubated for 10 min before LABScreen single-antigen testing) [4].

We also performed a donor auto-CDC-XM with donor serum collected on the day of organ harvesting. This assay was positive for B-cells negative control well again, for B-cells with donor serum, and was also enhanced by sera DTT pretreatment. Detailed review of the donor's medical history revealed a diagnosis of severe idiopathic thrombocytopenic purpura, refractory to treatment by corticosteroids, IV immunoglobulins, splenectomy (performed six months before organ harvesting), eltrombopag, and romiplostim. RTX therapy (only one injection) was initiated 12 days before the donor's death.

3. Discussion

CDC-XM reveals the functional potential of anti-HLA antibodies to activate complement and can be used to guide the decision to perform transplantation. We report a case of false-positive B-cells CDC-XM due to donor RTX therapy prior to organ harvesting.

In the case of RTX therapy, CDC-XM positivity is restricted to B-cells [6]. False-positive CDC-XM may be detected at low RTX concentrations (0.02 μg/mL) corresponding to blood concentrations observed several months after the last infusion [5]. Moreover, pretreatment of serum by DTT reduced lysis triggered by adding RTX. However, in this case of donor (and not recipient) RTX therapy revealed an opposite effect with complement-dependent cytotoxicity enhanced by DTT treatment, whereas DTT deleted serum interference. Unfortunately, no more donor cells were available to perform flow-cytometry crossmatch, especially to detect RTX adsorption onto donor lymphocytes after a pronase treatment that removes CD20 from B-cells and so the RTX binding [7].

RTX, a CD20 monoclonal antibody, has been shown to be beneficial in some diseases such as hematopoietic malignancies, rheumatoid arthritis, autoimmune disease, and organ acute rejection. Via its Fab fragment, RTX is able to link with CD20, the receptor present on the surface of the majority of B-cells. This RTX-CD20 complex is not internalized inside the cells and the RTX Fc fragment can generate immune effect functions, leading to B-cells lysis secondary after binding a C1q fragment. RTX is also slowly eliminated from the blood circulation (half-life about 20–30 days) [8]. These pharmacokinetic properties can explain the positive CDC-XM observed in this case.

In conclusion, this case highlights the fact that recent donor RTX therapy can induce false-positive Class II CDC-XM on pretransplantation screening and reminds us that a positive crossmatch may be due to reasons related to the donor and not only to the recipient.

Competing Interests

The authors declare that there is no conflict of interests regarding the publication of this paper.

References

[1] N. Guillaume, H. Mazouz, V. Piot, C. Presne, and P.-F. Westeel, "Correlation between Luminex donor-specific crossmatches and levels of donor-specific antibodies in pretransplantation screening," *Tissue Antigens*, vol. 82, no. 1, pp. 16–20, 2013.

[2] M. Alheim, P. K. Paul, D.-M. Hauzenberger, and A.-C. Wikström, "Improved flow cytometry based cytotoxicity and binding assay for clinical antibody HLA crossmatching," *Human Immunology*, vol. 76, no. 11, pp. 849–857, 2015.

[3] G. Schlaf, B. Pollok-Kopp, E. Schabel, and W. Altermann, "Artificially positive crossmatches not leading to the refusal of kidney donations due to the usage of adequate diagnostic tools," *Case Reports in Transplantation*, vol. 2013, Article ID 746395, 6 pages, 2013.

[4] J. Visentin, M. Vigata, S. Daburon et al., "Deciphering complement interference in anti-human leukocyte antigen antibody detection with flow beads assays," *Transplantation*, vol. 98, no. 6, pp. 625–631, 2014.

[5] D. Milongo, G. Vieu, S. Blavy et al., "Interference of therapeutic antibodies used in desensitization protocols on lymphocytotoxicity crossmatch results," *Transplant Immunology*, vol. 32, no. 3, pp. 151–155, 2015.

[6] B. K. Book, A. Agarwal, A. B. Milgrom et al., "New crossmatch technique eliminates interference by humanized and chimeric monoclonal antibodies," *Transplantation Proceedings*, vol. 37, no. 2, pp. 640–642, 2005.

[7] C. M. Bearden, A. Agarwal, B. K. Book et al., "Pronase treatment facilitates alloantibody flow cytometric and cytotoxic crossmatching in the presence of rituximab," *Human Immunology*, vol. 65, no. 8, pp. 803–809, 2004.

[8] P. Feugier, "A review of rituximab, the first anti-CD20 monoclonal antibody used in the treatment of B non-Hodgkin's lymphomas," *Future Oncology*, vol. 11, no. 9, pp. 1327–1342, 2015.

37

Duodenal Graft Perforation after Simultaneous Pancreas-Kidney Transplantation

Akihito Sannomiya, Ichiro Nakajima, Yuichi Ogawa, Kotaro Kai, Ichiro Koyama, and Shohei Fuchinoue

Department of Surgery, Kidney Center, Tokyo Women's Medical University, Tokyo, Japan

Correspondence should be addressed to Akihito Sannomiya; san@rb3.so-net.ne.jp

Academic Editor: Luca Cicalese

A 45-year-old woman with type 1 diabetes and chronic renal failure on dialysis underwent simultaneous pancreas-kidney transplantation from a brain dead donor. On postoperative day 15, acute generalized peritonitis was diagnosed and emergency laparotomy was performed. Perforation of the donor duodenum was found, which had apparently resulted from duodenal compression by the tip of the intestinal fistula tube placed for decompression. The perforation was sutured and the intestinal fistula tube was exchanged. Following this, perforation repeatedly recurred at the same site and open repair at laparotomy was required a total of four times. The fourth operation involved both suturing the perforation and covering it with ileum, after which there was no further recurrence. The patient was discharged on posttransplantation day 219, with the pancreas and kidney grafts both functioning well. This report presents a rare complication of simultaneous pancreas-kidney transplantation.

1. Introduction

In Japan, the Organ Transplant Act was revised in July 2010, leading to an increase of patients undergoing simultaneous pancreas and kidney transplantation from brain dead donors, which has been established as surgical treatment for diabetes [1]. Common complications of pancreatic transplantation include graft thrombosis, graft pancreatitis, and rejection, but perforation of the associated duodenal graft is rare [2]. Nath et al. described late anastomotic leaks with bladder drainage as not uncommon [3]. Here we report a patient who required open repair four times for perforation of the donor duodenum due to compression by an intestinal tube after simultaneous pancreas-kidney transplantation. Eventually, both grafts were preserved and remained functional.

2. Case Report

A 45-year-old woman was diagnosed with type I diabetes at the age of 16 years and hyperthyroidism at age 20, as well as acute pancreatitis at 22 years, caesarean section at 30 years, and gastric ulcer at the age of 38.

She received insulin therapy for diabetes. At the age of 33 years, she started hemodialysis due to chronic renal failure caused by diabetic nephropathy. Hypoglycemic episodes were frequent. She was admitted to our department for simultaneous pancreas and kidney transplantation from a brain dead donor (a 39-year-old man with cerebral hemorrhage).

On admission, she was 156 cm tall, weighed 54.0 kg, and had a body mass index of 22.2 kg/m^2. Her total insulin dose was 27 units/day (ultra-long-acting insulin: 10 units in the morning, ultrarapid insulin: 17 units). Hemoglobin A1c (HbA1c) was 8.2% (National Glycohemoglobin Standardization Program value), glycoalbumin was 34.1%, and C-peptide was <0.0099 nmol/L. In addition, anti-insulin antibodies were <0.4 kU/L, antiglutamic acid decarboxylase antibodies were 6.5 kU/L, and anti-islet antigen-2 antibodies were <0.4 kU/L.

Surgery. The pancreas was transplanted into the right iliac fossa and the kidney was transplanted into the left iliac fossa. To drain exocrine secretions, a Y-limb was created at the terminal ileum by the Roux-en-Y method and was anastomosed side-to-side to the donor duodenum following vascular

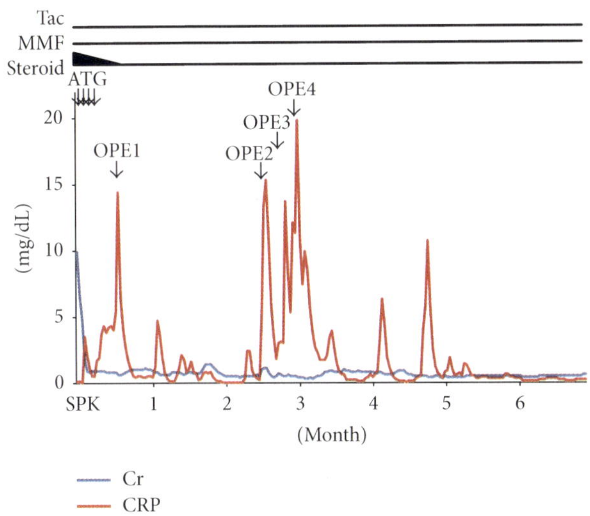

Figure 1: Postoperative course. The pancreas graft was salvaged by four laparotomies to repair duodenal perforation after pancreas-kidney transplantation.

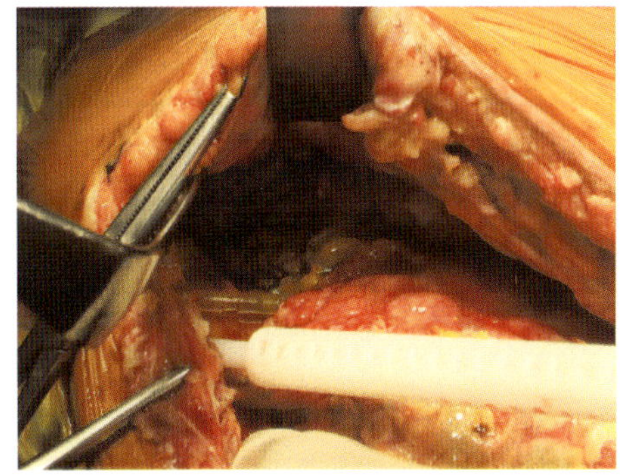

Figure 2: Postoperative day 15. Perforation of donor duodenum appeared to be due to the tip of the intestinal tube penetrating the wall.

anastomosis. The donor portal vein was anastomosed to the recipient's right external iliac vein, and the celiac artery and a Carrel patch extending from the superior mesenteric artery were each anastomosed to the recipient's right external iliac artery. The pancreatic graft was placed inside the abdominal cavity, as it was large relative to the recipient. Since the donor duodenum was distended, an intestinal fistula tube was placed for decompression of the intestinal tract. A 16 Fr Salem sump tube was inserted from the distal part of the ileal Y-limb, and the tip was advanced beyond the anastomosis and fixed inside the donor duodenum.

The total ischemic time was 9 hours and 24 minutes for the pancreas and 10 hours and 54 minutes for the kidney. Blood loss was 370 g.

Postoperative Course. The postoperative course is outlined in Figure 1. The patient had an adequate urine output after transplantation, so dialysis was stopped. Insulin therapy was also discontinued because a decrease of blood glucose was observed. Immunosuppressive therapy was initiated with rabbit antithymocyte globulin (1.5 mg/kg for 4 days), in addition to tacrolimus, mycophenolate mofetil, and steroids. Antithrombotic therapy was commenced on postoperative day 1 with continuous infusion of heparin at 2500 units/day (50 units/kg/day). Warfarin was started on postoperative day 8 and heparin was stopped on postoperative day 11. Valganciclovir was administered to prevent cytomegalovirus (CMV) infection, starting from one week after transplantation. Administration of GFO (a powdered food supplement containing glutamine, fiber, and oligosaccharides suggested to improve intestinal health) was on postoperative day 5. The intestinal tube was allowed to drain spontaneously without negative pressure.

On postoperative day 14, fever (temperature ≥ 38°C) and abdominal pain developed. On postoperative day 15, there were signs of peritoneal irritation. Abdominal CT revealed ascites and free intraperitoneal gas. Generalized peritonitis due to gastrointestinal perforation near the pancreatic graft was diagnosed and emergency laparotomy was performed. The previous surgical wound in the right lower abdomen was reopened. The abdominal cavity contained intestinal fluid, and perforation of the donor duodenum was confirmed (Figure 2). Perforation appeared to be due to the tip of the intestinal tube penetrating the duodenal wall. Partial resection of the duodenal segment including the site of perforation was considered but was judged to be difficult due to severe inflammation and edema of the donor duodenum, as well as the close proximity of the perforation to the anastomotic site. Therefore, the perforation was sutured and the intestinal tube was exchanged for a 9 Fr jejunostomy catheter (3 mm outer diameter) via the same route as the Salem sump tube.

The initial postoperative course was favorable and oral intake was started on day 17 after reoperation, but bowel obstruction developed five days later. It seemed to be caused by adhesions and resolved after decompression with a gastric tube. Oral intake was started again on day 25 following removal of the gastric tube, but fever occurred after six days. Peritonitis was diagnosed two days later and emergency laparotomy was performed via the previous surgical wound (second reoperation). Since there was reperforation of the donor duodenum at the previous perforation site, a 3.5 mm silicon tube (Lilia drain) was inserted through the perforation into the duodenum as a second intestinal tube and was anchored with a purse-string suture.

On day 7 after the second reoperation, peritonitis recurred and another emergency laparotomy was performed via the same surgical wound in the right lower abdomen (third reoperation). Leakage of pancreatic juice was observed from the site where the silicon tube had been inserted into the donor duodenum. This tube was removed and omental patch repair was performed. The intestinal tube was replaced by a new 9 Fr jejunostomy catheter (3 mm outer diameter).

On day 5 after the third reoperation, peritonitis was diagnosed again and yet another emergency laparotomy was performed (fourth reoperation). This time, a midline abdominal incision was made, in addition to reopening the wound in the right lower abdomen. It was found that pancreatic

TABLE 1: Reported cases of donor duodenal perforation after pancreatic transplantation. Pancreatic graft preservation was possible in six patients, including our patient.

Case number	Author	Age	Gender	Complaint	Exocrine drainage	Cause of perforation	Interval from surgery to perforation	Operation
(1)	Gruessner et al. [4]	30	M	Abdominal pain	Enteric	Rejection	27 months	Graft duodenectomy
(2)	Schleibner et al. [5]	33	M	Abdominal pain	Bladder	Simple ulcer	5 months	Direct closure
(3)	Stephanian et al. [6]	32	F	Abdominal pain	Bladder	Cmv duodenitis	18 months	Graft duodenectomy
(4)	Ester et al. [7]	47	F	Hematuria	Bladder	Rejection	1.5 months	Direct closure
(5)	Lee et al. [8]	30	F	Hematuria	Bladder	CMV duodenitis	2 months	Graft pancreatectomy
(6)	Fumimoto et al. [9]	37	F	Abdominal pain	Enteric	Internal hernia	13 months	Graft pancreatectomy
(7)	Miyagi et al. [10]	60	M	Melena	Enteric	Rejection	0.5 months	Graft pancreatectomy
(8)	Yamamoto et al. [11]	45	F	Abdominal pain	Enteric	Avascular necrosis	5 months	Direct closure
(9)	Present case	45	F	Abdominal pain	Enteric	Pressure necrosis	0.5 months	Direct closure

juice was leaking from the edge of the omental patch. The patch was completely removed, and, after extensively peeling off the adhesions around the donor duodenal perforation, it was closed with a simple two-layer suture. Then adhesions were peeled off the terminal ileum and fixed over the sutured duodenal perforation as a small intestinal patch. Damage to the ascending colon, which had probably occurred when adhesions were being removed, was also managed by two-layer suture closure.

GFO was started on day 45 after the fourth reoperation. Around this time, neutropenia and thrombocytopenia developed but resolved after discontinuation of valganciclovir and proton pump inhibitor therapy. On day 69 after the fourth reoperation, a nonfat digested liquid diet was started. Food intake was commenced on day 78, followed by slow transition from a liquid to a solid diet, and central venous nutrition was stopped on day 89. She was discharged on day 121 after the last operation (posttransplantation day 219). At discharge, serum creatinine was 0.61 mg/dL the estimated glomerular filtration rate was 82.1 mL/min/1.73 m^2, urinary protein was negative, C-peptide was 0.53 nmol/L, fasting blood glucose was 116 mg/dL, and HbA1c was 5.0%. The total insulin dose at discharge was 11 units/day (7 units of Novolin R short-acting insulin and 4 units of Apidra ultra-rapid-acting insulin). Two months after discharge, she was readmitted and the intestinal tube was removed uneventfully.

3. Discussion

As of July 2016, our hospital has performed a total of 60 pancreatic transplantations, including 11 from nonbeating heart donors and 49 from brain dead donors. However, this is our first experience of a patient with perforation of the donor duodenum. Our literature search revealed only 8 reported cases worldwide of donor duodenum perforation after pancreatic transplantation (Table 1) [4–11].

In these 9 patients, including our case, perforation occurred from 14 days to 27 months postoperatively. The cause of perforation was rejection in three patients, CMV infection in two patients, and donor duodenal ulcer, intestinal obstruction by an internal hernia, ischemic necrosis at the anastomosis, and compression necrosis due to the tip of an intestinal decompression tube in one patient each. Although we did not perform histopathological examination, rejection was considered unlikely in the present case because function of the transplanted kidney and pancreas was satisfactory. Moreover, CMV prophylaxis was initiated at an early stage, and the CMV antigenemia test and quantitative polymerase chain reaction for CMV-DNA were both negative, so CMV infection was excluded. Ischemic necrosis was also excluded from the macroscopic appearance of the donor duodenum. Accordingly, we concluded that perforation was due to sustained compression of the duodenal wall by the tip of the intestinal tube, which was also suggested by the intraoperative findings. The tube was initially placed away from the duodenal wall, but the donor duodenum may have shortened as edema resolved, allowing the tip of the catheter to compress the duodenal wall and cause perforation. The efficacy of the intestinal tube in pancreas transplant is not established. We opted for the tube insertion because of distention of duodenum but these series of perforation might be avoided without the insertion.

Among the previously reported cases, surgical treatment included simple closure of the perforation in three patients, removal of the donor duodenum in two patients, and total graft removal in three patients. Thus, pancreatic graft preservation was possible in six patients, including our patient. It was reported that 70% of patients who developed intra-abdominal infection after pancreatic transplantation required graft removal [12]. In Japan, the number of brain dead donors is low compared with that in Europe or the United States, so it is desirable to preserve grafts whenever possible. However, patient survival must retain priority, and we should not hesitate to remove the graft if required. In our patient, intestinal perforation occurred in the relatively early postoperative period, and placement of the peritoneal drain and intestinal decompression tube may have prevented the rapid progression of peritonitis. Also, our patient's general condition did not deteriorate despite multiple laparotomies and no other complications developed, which were major factors in allowing successful graft preservation.

4. Conclusion

In the present patient, preservation of the grafted pancreas was achieved by performing laparotomy four times to repair perforation of the donor duodenum causing acute generalized peritonitis, which resulted from the tip of an intestinal tube compressing the duodenal wall after pancreas transplantation. We reported this case because it represents a rare and interesting complication of pancreatic transplantation.

References

[1] H. Egawa, K. Tanabe, N. Fukushima, H. Date, A. Sugitani, and H. Haga, "Current status of organ transplantation in Japan," *American Journal of Transplantation*, vol. 12, no. 3, pp. 523–530, 2012.

[2] C. Troppmann, "Complications after pancreas transplantation," *Current Opinion in Organ Transplantation*, vol. 15, no. 1, pp. 112–118, 2010.

[3] D. S. Nath, A. Gruessner, R. Kandaswamy, R. W. Gruessner, D. E. R. Sutherland, and A. Humar, "Late anastomotic leaks in pancreas transplant recipients—clinical characteristics and predisposing factors," *Clinical Transplantation*, vol. 19, no. 2, pp. 220–224, 2005.

[4] R. W. Gruessner, C. Manivel, D. L. Dunn, and D. E. Sutherland, "Pancreaticoduodenal transplantation with enteric drainage following native total pancreatectomy for chronic pancreatitis: a case report," *Pancreas*, vol. 6, no. 4, pp. 479–488, 1991.

[5] S. Schleibner, J. Theodorakis, W. D. Illner, F. Leitl, D. Abendroth, and W. Land, "Ulcer perforation in the grafted duodenal segment following pancreatic transplantation—a case report," *Transplantation Proceedings*, vol. 24, article 827, 1992.

[6] E. Stephanian, R. W. G. Gruessner, K. L. Brayman et al., "Conversion of exocrine secretions from bladder to enteric drainage in recipients of whole pancreaticoduodenal transplants," *Annals of Surgery*, vol. 216, no. 6, pp. 663–672, 1992.

[7] R. M. Esterl, R. J. Stratta, R. J. Taylor, and S. J. Radio, "Rejection with duodenal rupture after solitary pancreas transplantation: an unusual cause of severe hematuria," *Clinical Transplantation*, vol. 9, no. 3, pp. 155–159, 1995.

[8] H. K. Lee, D. H. Chung, J. Jung et al., "Three cases of pancreas allograft dysfunction," *Journal of Korean Medical Science*, vol. 15, no. 1, pp. 105–110, 2000.

[9] Y. Fumimoto, M. Tanemura, Y. Hoshida, T. Nishida, Y. Sawa, and T. Ito, "Graft duodenal perforation due to internal hernia after simultaneous pancreas-kidney transplantation: report of a case," *Case Reports in Gastroenterology*, vol. 2, no. 2, pp. 244–249, 2008.

[10] S. Miyagi, S. Sekiguchi, N. Kawagishi et al., "Nonmarginal-donor duodenal ulcers caused by rejection after simultaneous pancreas and kidney transplantation: a case report," *Transplantation Proceedings*, vol. 43, no. 9, pp. 3292–3295, 2011.

[11] T. Yamamoto, S. Narumi, M. Okada et al., "Delayed graft duodenal perforation after simultaneous pancreas-kidney transplantation," *Japanese Journal of Gastroenterological Surgery*, vol. 48, no. 11, pp. 929–935, 2015.

[12] R. W. G. Gruessner, D. E. R. Sutherland, C. Troppmann et al., "The surgical risk of pancreas transplantation in the cyclosporine era: an overview," *Journal of the American College of Surgeons*, vol. 185, no. 2, pp. 128–144, 1997.

38

Eculizumab for Thrombotic Microangiopathy Associated with Antibody-Mediated Rejection after ABO-Incompatible Kidney Transplantation

Luca Lanfranco,[1] Melanie Joly,[2] Arnaud Del Bello,[1] Laure Esposito,[1] Noelle Cognard,[2] Peggy Perrin,[2] Bruno Moulin,[2] Nassim Kamar,[1,3,4] and Sophie Caillard[2]

[1]*Department of Nephrology and Organ Transplantation, CHU Rangueil, Toulouse, France*
[2]*Department of Nephrology and Transplantation, University Hospital of Strasbourg, Strasbourg, France*
[3]*Université Paul Sabatier, Toulouse, France*
[4]*INSERM U1043, IFR-BMT, CHU Purpan, Toulouse, France*

Correspondence should be addressed to Nassim Kamar; kamar.n@chu-toulouse.fr

Academic Editor: Ryszard Grenda

Thrombotic microangiopathy is a form of antibody-mediated rejection (ABMR): it is the main complication of ABO-incompatible (ABOi) kidney transplantation (KT). Herein, we report on two cases of ABMR with biological and histological features of thrombotic microangiopathy (TMA) that were treated by eculizumab after ABOi KT. The first patient presented with features of TMA at postoperative day (POD) 13. Because of worsening biological parameters and no recovery of kidney function, despite seven sessions of immunoadsorption, a salvage therapy of eculizumab was started on POD 23. Kidney function slightly improved during the first 4 months after transplantation. Eculizumab was stopped at month 4. However, kidney function worsened progressively, leading to dialysis at month 13 after transplantation. The second patient presented with features of TMA at POD 1. In addition to immunoadsorption therapy, eculizumab was started on POD 6. Kidney function improved. Eculizumab was stopped on POD 64 and immunoadsorption sessions were stopped on POD 102. At the last follow-up (after 9 months), eGFR was at 43 mL/min/1.73 m^2. Our case reports show the beneficial effect of eculizumab to treat ABMR after ABOi KT. However, it should be given early after diagnosing TMA associated with ABMR.

1. Introduction

Mid- and long-term kidney allograft survival rates have been shown to be similar after living-donor ABO-compatible (ABOc) and ABO-incompatible (ABOi) kidney transplantation (KT) [1–3]. In order to ensure successful ABOi KT, the titers of isoagglutinins that are directed against the donor should be decreased: apheresis and rituximab are used to decrease isoagglutinin levels.

Antibody-mediated rejection (ABMR) remains the main complication of ABOi KT. Thrombotic microangiopathy (TMA) is a form of ABMR. It is still a matter of debate whether ABMR is mediated by natural (IgM) or immune (IgG) isoagglutinins. In both cases, ABMR occurs through the activation of the complement system [4]. Eculizumab, a monoclonal anti-C5 antibody that blocks the complement cascade, was used to prevent or treat refractory ABMR after ABOc [5–7] or ABOi KT [8, 9]. Herein, we report on two cases of ABMR with biological and histological features of TMA that were treated with eculizumab after ABOi KT.

2. Case 1

A 64-year-old man (group O) received a first ABOi living unrelated-donor KT for nephroangiosclerosis. The donor was his spouse (group AB). Before, at, and after transplantation, anti-HLA antibodies were assessed by the Luminex SA assay and remained negative. At baseline, anti-A and anti-B isoagglutinin titers that were assessed using hemagglutination

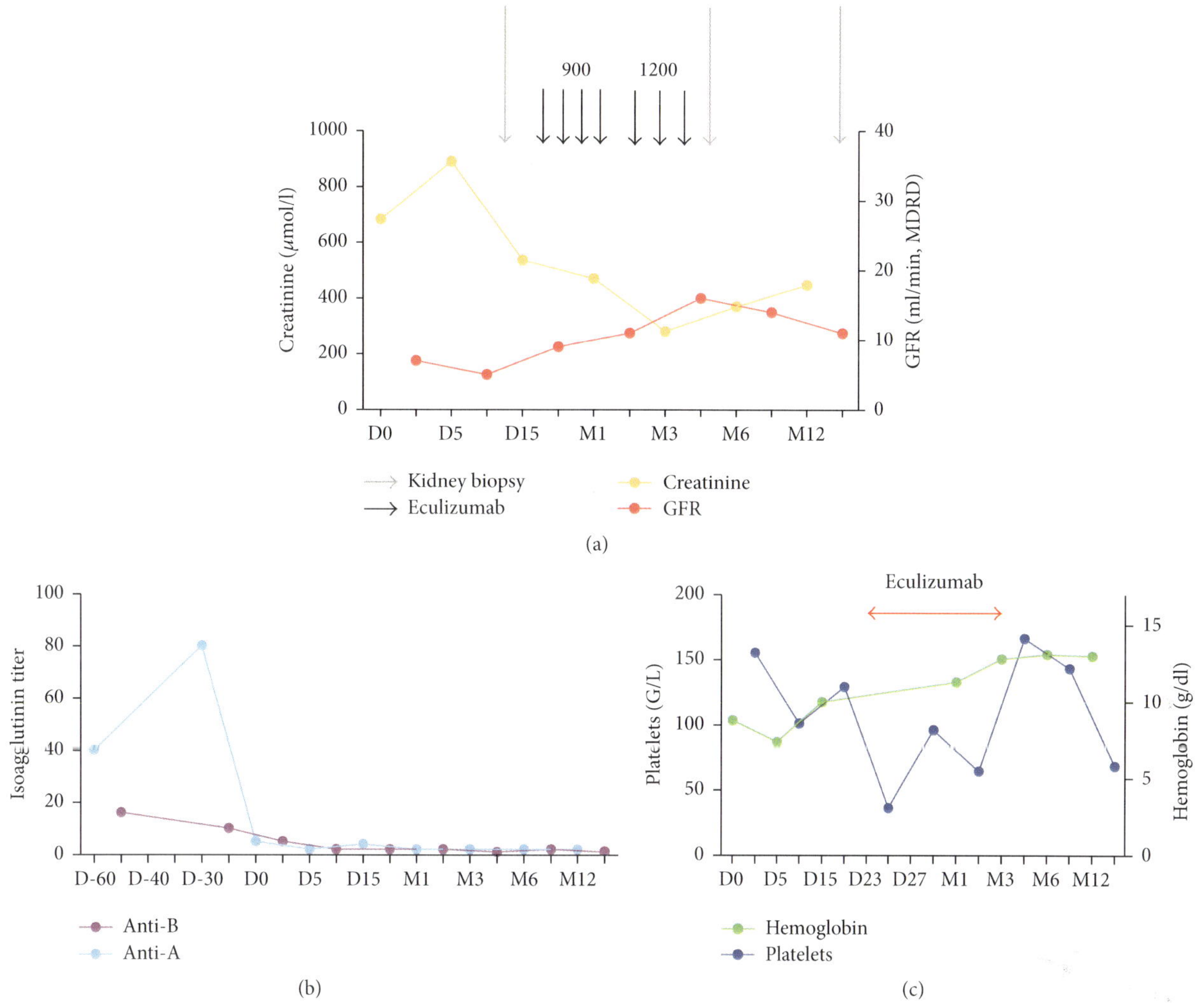

FIGURE 1: Kidney function (a), isoagglutinin titers (b), and hematological parameters (c) in patient 1. Evolution after kidney transplantation.

were 1/80 and 1/10, respectively. The desensitization protocol included eight nonspecific immunoadsorption sessions (Adasorb® reusable columns, Fresenius, Bad Homburg, Germany), two specific-IA sessions (Glycorex® column, Lund, Sweden), and rituximab (375 mg/m^2 given for 30 days before transplantation). At transplantation, both anti-A and anti-B isoagglutinin levels were at 1/5. Basiliximab induction therapy was given on days 0 and 4 (20 mg each). Tacrolimus, mycophenolic acid, and prednisolone were started 12 days before transplantation and were continued thereafter.

At postoperative day (POD) 3, the patient presented with partial kidney allograft venous thrombosis that required surgery, and the graft was reimplanted. Consequently, the patient recovered diuresis, but no graft function. On POD 13, a kidney biopsy was performed and showed the presence of thrombotic microangiopathy without microcirculation inflammation and no features of T-cell mediated rejection. C4d staining was positive. At that time, serum creatinine level was 546 μmol/L (Figure 1). Hemoglobin level was 10.1 g/dL. Schistocyte count was <15‰. Lactate dehydrogenase was 636 IU/L. Platelet count had decreased from 155,000/mm^3 at transplantation to 116,000/mm^3. Tacrolimus trough level was 9.7 ng/mL. Anti-A and anti-B isoagglutinin levels stayed at 1/5. Complement fraction levels were within the normal ranges. No autoimmune disease or phospholipid syndrome was evidenced. Classical viral infections were ruled out. Genetic analysis for the complement pathway ruled out atypical HUS.

We concluded treatment with isoagglutinin-induced ABMR. Hence, we started apheresis using plasma exchanges ($n = 3$) followed by nonspecific IA sessions ($n = 4$). Because of a worsening of platelet count (36,000/mm^3 at day 22) and no recovery of kidney function, a salvage therapy using eculizumab was decided upon. It was started on day 23 at a dose of 900 mg per week for 4 weeks and then 1200 mg every 2 weeks. The platelet count rapidly increased to 96,000/mm^3 (day 29). Hemoglobin level slightly improved and the patient recovered modest kidney function, which permitted dialysis to be stopped at POD 30 (SCr of 460 μmol/L, eGFR CKD Epi 11 mL/min). Kidney function improved during the first 4 months after transplantation and platelet counts returned within the normal range.

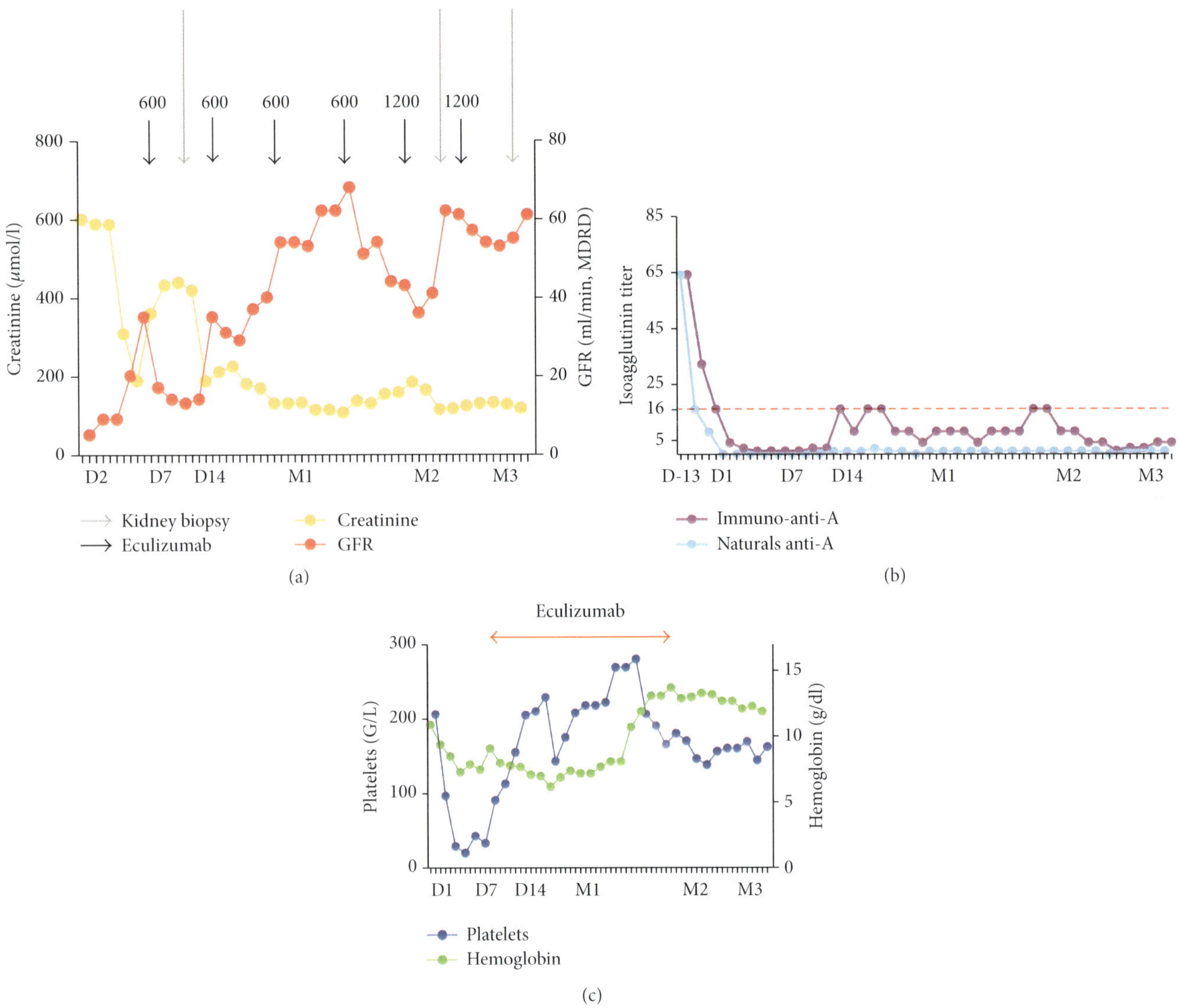

FIGURE 2: Kidney function (a), isoagglutinin titers (b), and hematological parameters (c) in patient 2. Evolution after transplantation.

At month 4, a control kidney biopsy was performed: it revealed no features of cellular or ABMR, but sequelae of the previous TMA episode (t0, i0, g0, v0, ptc0, cg0, cv0, ci2, and ct2). Hence, eculizumab was stopped at month 4. Between months 4 and 12, platelet count remained within the normal range and isoagglutinin levels were unchanged. Conversely, kidney function remained impaired and worsened progressively. At month 13 after transplantation, he started dialysis again.

3. Case 2

A 48-year-old man (group O) received a second ABOi living unrelated-donor KT for IgA nephropathy. The donor was his spouse (group A). No anti-HLA donor specific antibodies (DSA) at or after transplantation were detected. At baseline, natural and immune anti-A isoagglutinins titers were 1/64 each (using hemagglutination). The desensitization protocol included six immunoadsorption sessions (Immunosorba, Fresenius, Bad Homburg, Germany) and rituximab (375 mg/m^2 given 34 days before transplantation). At transplantation, natural and immune anti-A titers were 1/8 and 1/16, respectively. An antithymocyte globulin induction therapy was given from days 0 to 4 (1.3 mg/kg/d). Tacrolimus, mycophenolic acid, and prednisolone were started at 14 days before transplantation and were continued thereafter.

After transplantation, the patient recovered diuresis without a decrease in serum creatinine levels. At POD 1, the patient presented with biological features of TMA, including hemolytic anemia, thrombocytopenia (platelet count at 49,000/mm^3), and no improvement in kidney function (Figure 2). Anti-A level was 1/4. Anti-A-mediated ABMR was suspected and plasmapheresis was initiated: a daily session was given between PODs 1 and 4 and then 3 times weekly until POD 42.

Due to the severity of the clinical and biological presentation, eculizumab was given at a dose of 900 mg on POD

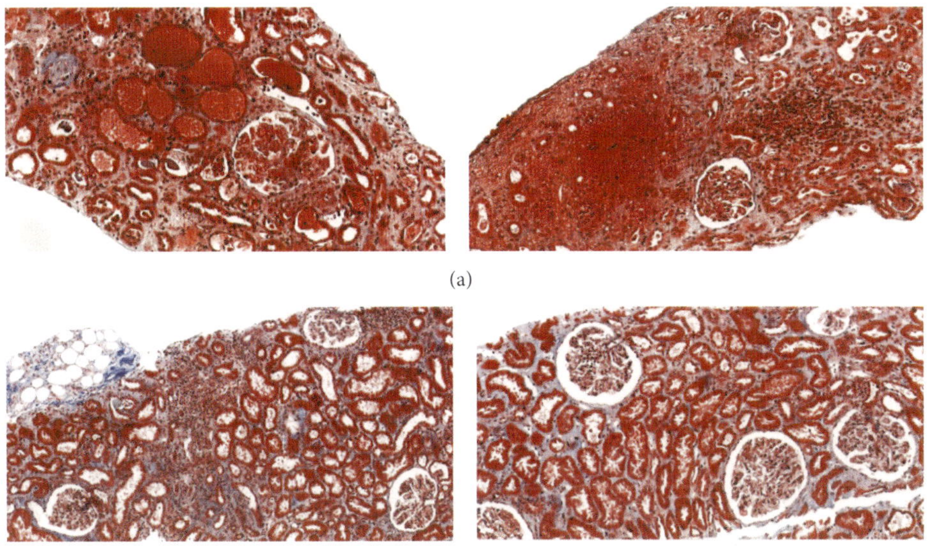

(a)

(b)

FIGURE 3: (a) Kidney allograft biopsy at postoperative day 12 in patient 2: thrombotic microangiopathy lesions, antibody-mediated rejection (t0, i0, g3, and cpt2). (b) Kidney allograft biopsy at postoperative day 54 in patient 2. Lesions of mixed acute cellular and antibody-mediates rejection (i2 i2 ti2 g2 cpt2), IF/TA 1, and no more lesions of thrombotic microangiopathy.

6, 17, 24, and 36 and then of 1200 mg on POD 50 and 64. A first kidney biopsy was done on POD 12 (Figure 3(a)) and revealed thrombotic microangiopathy, glomerulitis (g3), peritubular capillaritis (cpt2), and a peritubular C4d deposition. No histologic sign of acute cellular rejection was seen. Rapidly after initiation of eculizumab, hematological parameters improved, as well as kidney function (Figure 2). Hemodialysis sessions were stopped at POD 16. The patient was discharged at POD 37. At that time, serum creatinine level was at 114 μmol/L (eGFR 62 mL/min/1.73 m^2). During the first month after transplantation, natural isoagglutinin anti-A remained below 1/4 and immune isoagglutinin anti-A increased transiently to 1/16. ADAMTS 13 activity was normal (81%), and genetic analysis for the complement pathway ruled out atypical HUS.

At POD 53, serum creatinine levels increased from 110 to 154 μmol/L, with increasing immuno-anti-A antibody titers, from 1/8 to 1/16, but without biological features of TMA. A second graft biopsy showed an acute mixed rejection (t2 i2 ti2 g2 cpt2) without TMA lesions (Figure 3(b)). Three methylprednisolone pulses were given and immunoabsorption sessions were restarted (2 session/week for 6 weeks). Eculizumab was stopped at POD 64 and immunoadsorption sessions were stopped at POD 102. Kidney function improved. A third graft biopsy was performed on POD 102. It did not reveal any sign of rejection or TMA. At the last follow-up (after 9 months), serum creatinine level was 160 μmol/L (eGFR 43 mL/min/1.73 m^2).

4. Discussion

ABMR is a well-known complication of ABOi kidney transplantation. Most AMR episodes are associated with activation of the complement pathway. ABMR is mediated by the classical pathway cleavage of C3 into C3b and C3a and the downstream formation of the membrane-attack complex, sC5b-9. Eculizumab is a humanized anti-C5 monoclonal antibody that blocks C5b-9 and C5a formation, which prevents the proinflammatory, prothrombotic, and lytic functions of complement [10]. Eculizumab is approved for treatment of paroxysmal nocturnal hemoglobinuria and atypical hemolytic and uremic syndrome (aHUS). Because of its mechanism of action to target the complement pathway, it has been also used in desensitization protocols to prevent ABMR [11, 12]. Although the incidence of ABMR was decreased in patients given eculizumab-based desensitization protocols, compared to those having not received eculizumab [11], at one year, chronic AMR lesions were similar in both groups [12].

Eculizumab has been also used to treat ABMR in ABO-compatible [5–7] and ABOi kidney-transplant patients [8, 9], as well as after ABOi pancreas [8] and heart transplantation [13]. In addition, *in vitro* and *in vivo*, eculizumab was found to inhibit hemolytic reaction after ABO-incompatible red blood-cell transfusion [14, 15].

Biglarnia et al. have reported a case of an intentional ABOi deceased-donor kidney and pancreas transplantation with severe ABMR that occurred at POD 9 during a rebound of isoagglutinins, despite immunoadsorption treatment. The use of two doses of eculizumab (600 mg at PODs 10 and 14) successfully treated the acute episode. At 6 months after transplantation, both kidney and pancreatic functions were normal [8].

Stewart et al. have reported a case of accelerated ABMR that occurred very early after ABOi KT, caused by a rebound in isoagglutinin levels [9]. Biological and histological features of TMA were observed. In the absence of any improvement, despite plasmapheresis, rituximab, intravenous immunoglobulins, and splenectomy, eculizumab was given as a salvage therapy at PODs 8, 10, 12, 14, and 21 [9]. The patient recovered kidney function and had a functional graft at 1 year after transplantation.

Recently, Ikeda et al. have reported two cases of TMA that occurred very early after ABOi kidney transplantation [16]. In both cases, patients had biological and histological features of TMA. Eculizumab was given for 2 and 3 months, respectively, in addition to intravenous immunoglobulins, rituximab, and a few sessions of plasmapheresis (2 and 4 sessions, resp.) [16]. In both cases, biological features of TMA disappeared and kidney function recovered [16].

Similar to the four previous published cases [8, 9, 16], our two patients presented with ABMR and biological features of TMA very early after transplantation. Both were initially treated by apheresis, and eculizumab was added thereafter. Similar to previous published cases [8, 9, 16], in one of the two cases (case 2), a rebound (slight and delayed) in isoagglutinin level was observed. It is important to note that, in the first case, immune isoagglutinin levels were not assessed at that time. In both cases, features of TMA regressed rapidly. The second patient had good kidney function at the last follow-up whereas the first patient had lost his kidney allograft at month 13 after transplantation. This can be explained by the fact that eculizumab was started at POD 23 in the first case, which was much later than for the second patient (POD 6) and the time-periods reported in previous reports [8, 9, 16].

In aHUS, it has been shown that early initiation of eculizumab was associated with greater improvement in kidney function [17]. Finally, it is important to note that eculizumab can fail to prevent [18] and treat ABMR [7], suggesting that there may be other pathways involved in the ABMR mechanisms.

To summarize, we describe the beneficial effect of eculizumab to treat ABMR after ABOi KT. We suggest that eculizumab should be given very early in ABOi KT patients presenting biological and histological features of TMA than can be related to ABMR.

Authors' Contributions

Luca Lanfranco and Melanie Joly equally participated in this study. Luca Lanfranco and Melanie Joly collected the cases and wrote the paper. Arnaud Del Bello, Laure Esposito, Noelle Cognard, and Peggy Perrin participated in the patients' follow-up. Bruno Moulin reviewed the paper. Nassim Kamar and Sophie Caillard designed the study and wrote the paper.

References

[1] N. Kohei, T. Hirai, K. Omoto, H. Ishida, and K. Tanabe, "Chronic antibody-mediated rejection is reduced by targeting B-cell immunity during an introductory period," *American Journal of Transplantation*, vol. 12, no. 2, pp. 469–476, 2012.

[2] G. Opelz, C. Morath, C. Süsal, T. H. Tran, M. Zeier, and B. Döhler, "Three-year outcomes following 1420 ABO-incompatible living-donor kidney transplants performed after ABO antibody reduction: results from 101 centers," *Transplantation*, vol. 99, no. 2, pp. 400–404, 2015.

[3] M. Okumi, D. Toki, T. Nozaki et al., "ABO-Incompatible Living Kidney Transplants: Evolution of Outcomes and Immunosuppressive Management," *American Journal of Transplantation*, vol. 16, no. 3, pp. 886–896, 2016.

[4] O. R. Blume, S. E. Yost, and B. Kaplan, "Antibody-mediated rejection: pathogenesis, prevention, treatment, and outcomes," *Journal of Transplantation*, vol. 2012, Article ID 201754, 7 pages, 2012.

[5] J. E. Locke, C. M. Magro, A. L. Singer et al., "The use of antibody to complement protein C5 for salvage treatment of severe antibody-mediated rejection," *American Journal of Transplantation*, vol. 9, no. 1, pp. 231–235, 2009.

[6] B. J. Orandi, A. A. Zachary, N. N. Dagher et al., "Eculizumab and splenectomy as salvage therapy for severe antibody-mediated rejection after HLA-incompatible kidney transplantation," *Transplantation*, vol. 98, no. 8, pp. 857–863, 2014.

[7] M. Burbach, C. Suberbielle, I. Brochériou et al., "Report of the inefficacy of eculizumab in two cases of severe antibody-mediated rejection of renal grafts," *Transplantation*, vol. 98, no. 10, pp. 1056–1059, 2014.

[8] A.-R. Biglarnia, B. Nilsson, T. Nilsson et al., "Prompt reversal of a severe complement activation by eculizumab in a patient undergoing intentional ABO-incompatible pancreas and kidney transplantation," *Transplant International*, vol. 24, no. 8, pp. e61–e66, 2011.

[9] Z. A. Stewart, T. E. Collins, A. J. Schlueter et al., "Case report: eculizumab rescue of severe accelerated antibody-mediated rejection after ABO-incompatible kidney transplant," *Transplantation Proceedings*, vol. 44, no. 10, pp. 3033–3036, 2012.

[10] V. Frémeaux-Bacchi and C. M. Legendre, "The emerging role of complement inhibitors in transplantation," *Kidney International*, vol. 88, no. 5, pp. 967–973, 2015.

[11] M. D. Stegall, T. Diwan, S. Raghavaiah, L. D. Cornell, J. Burns, and P. G. Dean, "Terminal complement inhibition decreases antibody-mediated rejection in sensitized renal transplant recipients," *American Journal of Transplantation*, vol. 11, no. 11, pp. 2405–2413, 2011.

[12] L. D. Cornell, C. A. Schinstock, M. J. Gandhi, W. K. Kremers, and M. D. Stegall, "Positive crossmatch kidney transplant recipients treated with eculizumab: outcomes beyond 1 year," *American Journal of Transplantation*, vol. 15, no. 5, pp. 1293–1302, 2015.

[13] C. A. Irving, A. R. Gennery, V. Carter et al., "ABO-incompatible cardiac transplantation in pediatric patients with high isohemagglutinin titers," *The Journal of Heart and Lung Transplantation*, vol. 34, no. 8, article no. 5994, pp. 1095–1102, 2015.

[14] C. Weinstock, R. Möhle, C. Dorn et al., "Successful use of eculizumab for treatment of an acute hemolytic reaction after ABO-incompatible red blood cell transfusion," *Transfusion*, vol. 55, no. 3, pp. 605–610, 2015.

[15] C. R. Fata, E. A. Gehrie, and P. P. Young, "Eculizumab inhibits hemolysis in a model of ABO-incompatible red blood cell transfusion," *Transfusion*, vol. 55, no. 7, pp. 1823-1824, 2015.

[16] T. Ikeda, M. Okumi, K. Unagami et al., "Two cases of kidney transplantation-associated thrombotic microangiopathy successfully treated with eculizumab," *Nephrology*, vol. 21, pp. 35–40, 2016.

[17] C. M. Legendre, C. Licht, P. Muus et al., "Terminal complement inhibitor eculizumab in atypical hemolytic-uremic syndrome," *The New England Journal of Medicine*, vol. 368, no. 23, pp. 2169–2181, 2013.

[18] A. Bentall, D. B. Tyan, F. Sequeira et al., "Antibody-mediated rejection despite inhibition of terminal complement," *Transplant International*, vol. 27, no. 12, pp. 1235–1243, 2014.

IVIG Associated Aseptic Meningitis in a Renal Transplant Patient

Tamara Wanigasekera,[1] Rachel J. Grainger,[2] Donal J. Sexton,[1] and Colm Magee[1]

[1] *Transplant, Urology and Nephrology Directorate, Beaumont Hospital, Dublin 9, Ireland*
[2] *Department of Clinical Microbiology, Beaumont Hospital, Dublin 9, Ireland*

Correspondence should be addressed to Tamara Wanigasekera; tamara.wanigasekera@gmail.com

Academic Editor: David Conti

The management of antibody-mediated rejection in renal transplant recipients involves plasmapheresis with IVIG. Aseptic meningitis is a rare adverse effect of IVIG therapy and is a diagnosis of exclusion. We report a case of a renal transplant patient who developed IVIG associated aseptic meningitis in the context of management of antibody-mediated rejection, four years after transplantation.

1. Introduction

IVIG associated meningitis is reported to occur in less than 1% of patients exposed to IVIG [1]. We have identified one prior report of IVIG associated meningitis in a renal transplant patient undergoing treatment of antibody-mediated rejection [2]. It is more frequently reported in the nontransplant setting, for example, the treatment of neuromuscular disorders and of immune deficiency. The initial presentation of IVIG associated meningitis is indistinguishable from infective meningitis.

2. Case Presentation

A 31-year-old male with ESKD secondary to IgA nephropathy received a deceased donor kidney transplant four years prior to presentation. Antibody-mediated rejection (ABMR) was diagnosed on the basis of typical changes on light microscopy (including peritubular capillaritis) and positive staining for C4d staining and the presence in the serum of new donor specific antibodies. The patient was on maintenance immunosuppression consisting of tacrolimus 1.5 mg twice daily, mycophenolate mofetil 750 mg twice daily, and prednisolone 5 mg once daily. He denied noncompliance and had acceptable immunosuppressant drug trough levels.

The patient received 250 mg methylprednisolone daily for three days and underwent five sessions of plasma exchange followed by IVIG (1 g/kg) at a slow rate of 54 ml/hour increasing to 108 ml/hour as per protocol with concomitant IV normal saline and paracetamol, prophylactic cotrimoxazole, and valacyclovir. The total dose received was 90 g. Less than 24 hours after the final dose of IVIG, he presented to emergency services with a severe headache, photophobia, and nuchal rigidity. He had no other neurological symptoms or signs.

Computerized tomography (CT) neuroimaging was noncontributory. Lumbar punctures on days 1 and 2 of admission yielded clear cerebrospinal fluid (CSF) with a polymorphic leukocytosis, elevated protein, and low glucose (Table 1). Gram stain and culture were negative. Serum C-reactive protein and white cell count were normal.

Broad-spectrum empiric antimicrobial therapy was started at presentation. This consisted of high dose intravenous acyclovir, vancomycin, cefotaxime, and amoxicillin.

Microbiological analysis of CSF samples was negative for culture and PCR of typical and atypical bacterial and viral causes of meningitis, as described below.

CSF samples were negative for the following: *Neisseria meningitidis*, *Streptococcus pneumoniae*, *Cryptococcus neoformans*, *Listeria monocytogenes*, cytomegalovirus (CMV),

Table 1: CSF composition.

	Day 1	Day 2
White cell count/mL	3846	1037
Differential	90% polymorphs	79% polymorphs, 16% lymphocytes
Red cell count/mL	50	6
Protein (mg/dL)	139.5	40.0
Glucose (mmol/L)	2.1	3.0

mL = milliliters, mg/dL = milligrams per decilitre, and mmol/L = millimoles per deciliter.

Table 2: Tests of CSF.

Investigation	Result
Gram stain and culture	Negative
Pneumococcal PCR	Negative
Meningococcal PCR	Negative
Listeria monocytogenes PCR	Negative
Acid fast bacilli	Negative
TB culture	Negative
Herpes simplex virus 1&2 PCR	Negative
Varicella zoster virus PCR	Negative
Enterovirus PCR	Negative
Cytomegalovirus PCR	Negative
Cryptococcal antigen	Negative

Table 3: Tests of peripheral blood.

Investigation	Result
Gram stain and culture	Negative
Cryptococcal antigen	Negative
Meningococcal PCR	Negative
Pneumococcal PCR	Negative
Hepatitis C PCR	Negative
Hepatitis B surface antigen Hepatitis B antibodies Hepatitis C antigen HIV1 + 2	Negative

enterovirus, Herpes simplex virus, and Varicella zoster virus as well as acid fast bacilli (Table 2). Serum testing for HIV, hepatitis B, and hepatitis C was also negative (Table 3).

As microbiological tests were negative, initial empirical antimicrobials were discontinued by day seven of admission and the patient was managed supportively with intravenous fluids, analgesia, and antiemetics. IVIG treatment had been completed prior to this presentation and the patient did not require further doses. By day five, the patient was asymptomatic. Four weeks after discharge the patient remained well and was continued on a higher dose of maintenance immunosuppression during this time, with stable graft function.

3. Discussion

As with reported cases of IVIG associated meningitis, this patient's presentation mimicked infective meningitis. Like other reported cases [1–8], he had signs of meningism on examination and had a polymorphic leukocytosis with raised protein on CSF analysis. He also presented within 48 hours of receiving IVIG at a higher doses (1 g/kg) than that used in IVIG replacement in hypogammaglobulinaemia.

When the above case is compared to the prior case of IVIG associated meningitis in a renal transplant patient undergoing treatment of antibody-mediated rejection (Wright et al. [2]) the biochemical picture is similar to differences in clinical presentation.

In the case described by Wright et al. [2] the patient presented with a mild headache, nuchal rigidity, and pyrexia 48 hours after IVIG administration, where the total dose used was higher (120 g). Our patient presented within 24 hours with a severe headache, photophobia, and nuchal rigidity and was afebrile. The main clinical difference was that while our patient had no focal neurological signs, the patient in the case described by Wright et al. developed an abducens nerve palsy on day eight of her admission [2] and took a week later to recover in terms of symptoms. This resolved two weeks later and was postulated to be due to perineuritis [2]. In terms of investigations, both patients had noncontributory imaging and a polymorphonuclear leukocytosis on CSF sampling. In both cases, white cell counts of over 2000 cells/mL, consisting of greater than 70% polymorphs, were found on microscopy. Overall, although both cases were similar in terms of investigation results, our patient received a lower total dose with rapid onset of severe symptoms and swift resolution five days after presentation. This emphasizes the idiosyncratic nature of the IVIG induced drug reaction.

IVIG therapy is used outside the field of transplant medicine in the management of demyelinating disease, autoimmune diseases, and primary and secondary immune deficiency. It is a blood derived product composed of polyclonal human immunoglobulin from up to 15,000 donors. The exact handling of IVIG at the blood brain barrier is incompletely characterised. Murine modeling demonstrates that less than 0.01% crosses the blood brain barrier [9]. The exact mechanism of IVIG associated meningitis is poorly understood and it is thought to be more complex than direct meningeal irritation. Postulated mechanisms include cerebral vasospasm [10], neutrophil activation [10, 11], and hypersensitivity reaction [10]. Neutrophil activation by IVIG has been demonstrated in vivo by antibodies found in IVIG [10] and directly via the FcγRIII neutrophil surface membrane receptor [11]. Cerebral artery vasospasm following IVIG therapy has been demonstrated using transcranial Doppler in small numbers of patients presenting with encephalopathy following IVIG therapy in Guillain-Barre syndrome [12] but may also be a feature of the underlying neurological condition.

There are no established risk factors for anticipating development of IVIG associated aseptic meningitis, although some case reports have observed a background history of migraine [6]. It is common practice to use a slow rate with concurrent IV hydration and antihistamine before medication to minimise the occurrence of adverse effects in IVIG administration.

IVIG is sometimes administered to renal transplant patients in the setting of antibody-mediated rejection. IVIG associated meningitis may initially present in a similar manner to the infusion reaction headache that is commonly observed. It should be a rare diagnosis of exclusion and there are very few reported cases on the renal transplant population. It is important to ensure that typical and atypical organisms are considered when investigating meningitis, especially in the immune-compromised patient. It is a significant complication to be aware of, due to its morbidity and because its presentation mimics the signs and CSF findings of infective meningitis.

References

[1] V. Bharath, K. Eckert, M. Kang, I. H. Chin-Yee, and C. C. Hsia, "Incidence and natural history of intravenous immunoglobulin-induced aseptic meningitis: a retrospective review at a single tertiary care center," *Transfusion*, vol. 55, no. 11, pp. 2597–2605, 2015.

[2] S. E. Wright, Z. H. A. Shaikh, J. A. Castillo-Lugo, and B. Tanriover, "Aseptic meningitis and abducens nerve palsy as a serious side effect of high dose intravenous immunoglobulin used in a patient with renal transplantation," *Transplant Infectious Disease*, vol. 10, no. 4, pp. 294–297, 2008.

[3] N. Veranneman, D. Van Raemdonck, L. Dupont, and G. Verleden, "Repeated, severe headache in a lung transplant patient: a case report," *Acta Clinica Belgica*, vol. 65, no. 4, pp. 269-270, 2010.

[4] Y. Kemmotsu, T. Nakayama, H. Matsuura, and T. Saji, "Clinical characteristics of aseptic meningitis induced by intravenous immunoglobulin in patients with Kawasaki disease," *Pediatric Rheumatology*, vol. 9, article 28, 2011.

[5] A. Chaabane, A. Hamzaoui, K. Aouam et al., "Human intravenous immunoglobulin-induced aseptic meningitis: a case report," *Journal of Clinical Pharmacology*, vol. 52, no. 2, pp. 279–281, 2012.

[6] D. Mullane, L. Williams, A. Merwick et al., "Drug induced aseptic meningitis caused by intravenous immunoglobulin therapy," *Irish Medical Journal*, vol. 105, no. 6, pp. 182-183, 2012.

[7] R. S. Jain, S. Kumar, R. Aggarwal, and J. C. Kookna, "Acute aseptic meningitis due to intravenous immunoglobulin therapy in Guillain-Barre syndrome," *Oxford Medical Case Reports*, vol. 2014, no. 7, pp. 132–134, 2014.

[8] A. Puy-Nunez, M. Dacosta-Balboa, I. Cabo-Lopez et al., "Aseptic meningitis as a complication of immunoglobulin treatment in myasthenia gravis," *Revista De Neurologia*, vol. 62, no. 10, 2016.

[9] I. St-Amour, I. Paré, W. Alata et al., "Brain bioavailability of human intravenous immunoglobulin and its transport through the murine blood-brain barrier," *Journal of Cerebral Blood Flow and Metabolism*, vol. 33, no. 12, pp. 1983–1992, 2013.

[10] S. Jarius, P. Eichhorn, M. H. Albert et al., "Intravenous immunoglobulins contain naturally occurring antibodies that mimic antineutrophil cytoplasmic antibodies and activate neutrophils in a TNFα-dependent and Fc-receptor-independent way," *Blood*, vol. 109, no. 10, pp. 4376–4382, 2007.

[11] S. Higurashi, Y. Machino, E. Suzuki, M. Suzuki, J. Kohroki, and Y. Masuho, "Both the Fab and Fc domains of IgG are essential for ROS emission from TNF-α-primed neutrophils by IVIG," *Biochemical and Biophysical Research Communications*, vol. 417, no. 2, pp. 794–799, 2012.

[12] R. Sztajzel, J. L. Floch-Rohr, and P. Eggimann, "High-dose intravenous immunoglobulin treatment and cerebral vasospasm: a possible mechanism of ischemic encephalopathy?" *European Neurology*, vol. 41, no. 3, pp. 153–158, 1999.

Different Management Options for Transplant Ureteral Obstructions within an Inguinal Hernia

Felix Cheung,[1] Merrit Marion Debartolo,[1]
Leonard Michael Copertino,[2] April Adams Szafran,[1] Chelsea Caron Estrada,[3]
Patrick Gerard Lynch,[4] and Frank Sam Darras[1,3]

[1]*Department of Urology, Stony Brook University Medical Center, Stony Brook, NY 11794, USA*
[2]*Department of Surgery, Stony Brook University Medical Center, Stony Brook, NY 11794, USA*
[3]*Department of Transplant, Stony Brook University Medical Center, Stony Brook, NY 11794, USA*
[4]*Division of Nephrology, Stony Brook University Medical Center, Stony Brook, NY 11794, USA*

Correspondence should be addressed to Felix Cheung; fhkcheung@gmail.com

Academic Editor: Marian Klinger

Ureteral obstruction secondary to an inguinal hernia with transplant ureteral component is an extremely rare entity with only several case reports found in literature. In all previously reported cases, management of the obstruction involved temporary drainage with ureteral stenting or nephrostomy tube placements followed by delayed definitive repair. We present two case reports, here one being the first one managed by immediate definitive repair via ureteral reimplant and herniorrhaphy and a second case by delayed definitive repair after percutaneous nephrostomy tube placement. Both patients continued to do well postoperatively with normalization of renal function on follow-up.

1. Introduction

Transplant ureteral kidney obstruction is not an uncommon occurrence. Different causes of urinary obstruction in kidney transplants may include ischemia to distal ureteral segment, injury, stones, crossing vessels, lymphocele, or ureteral kinking [1]. Ureteral herniation through an inguinal hernia is an extremely rare cause of urinary obstruction, with only several reported cases in literature. Here, we present 2 cases of transplant ureteral herniation and the different approach to management. Both patients continued to do well with normalization of kidney function to baseline after relief of obstruction.

2. Case Report

2.1. Case 1. A 44-year-old obese white male with a history of ESRD secondary to childhood hemolytic-uremic syndrome, with post-DDRT status in 1998, presented with AKI with serum Cr of 3.4 mg/dL from his baseline of 2 mg/dL. He denied any symptoms. Exam was significant for a palpable left inguinal hernia. US revealed moderate to severe hydronephrosis of the transplanted kidney with nonvisualization of the distal ureter, and no bladder abnormalities. Despite IV hydration and adequate bladder emptying, the patient's urine output was marginal and Cr remained elevated at 3.1 mg/dL. A noncontrast CT of the abdomen and pelvis was obtained (Figure 1). A left inguinal hernia was seen to contain the distal transplant ureter with resultant proximal moderate to severe hydronephrosis of the transplant kidney, evident of obstruction.

The patient was taken to the operating room the next day for surgical exploration. A 2 × 3 cm defect between the internal oblique fascia and the shelving edge of the inguinal ligament was exposed, and a highly redundant transplant ureter was reduced (Figure 2). The defect was repaired via preperitoneal approach with nonabsorbent sutures in interrupted fashion. The redundant transplant ureter was

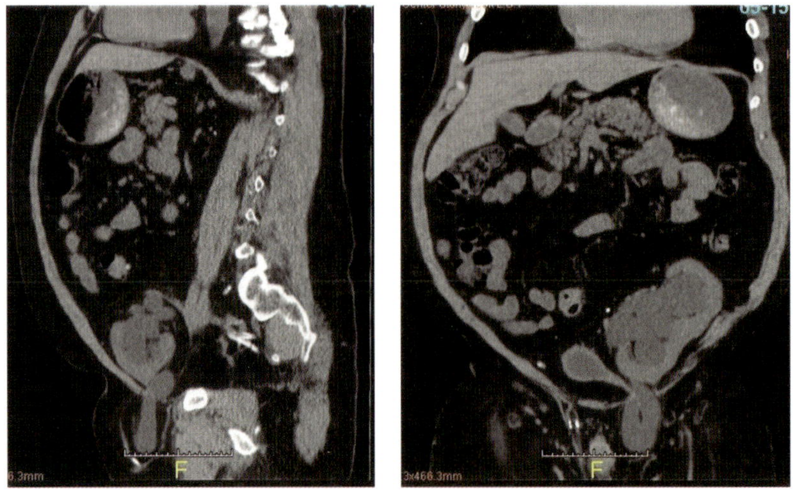

(a) (b)

Figure 1: Noncontrast CT abdomen pelvis in sagittal (a) and coronal (b) views revealing transplant ureter within inguinal hernia resulting in hydroureteronephrosis.

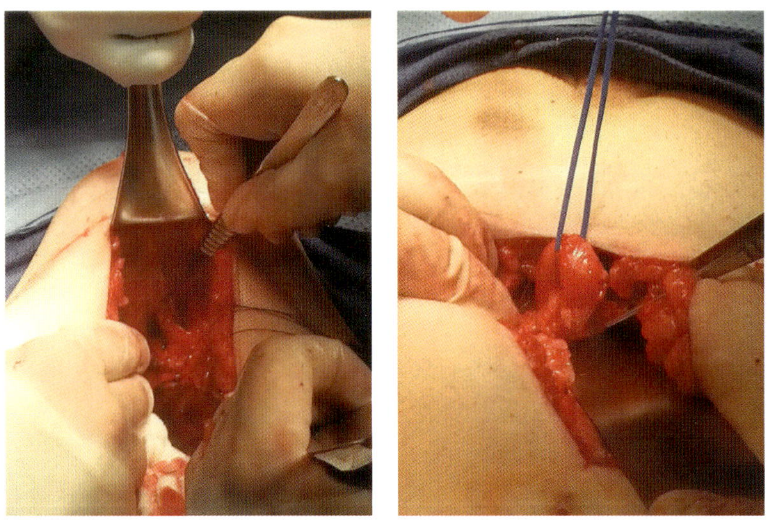

(a) (b)

Figure 2: Hernia defect seen within the preperitoneal space (a); vessel loop around the redundant transplant ureter reduced from the hernia (b).

transected to an appropriate length and reimplanted into the anterior bladder wall over a ureteral stent. The patient tolerated the procedure well without immediate complications. He was discharged on post-op day 2. At two-week follow-up, his Cr had improved to 1.71 mg/dL and remained stable 8 months post-op.

2.2. Case 2. An 88-year-old male with PCKD and ESRD had LRT in 2001. During his hospitalization for pneumonia, he developed AKI with his Cr elevated from 1.5 mg/dL to 2.6 mg/dL. A renal transplant US revealed moderate to severe hydronephrosis with hydroureter; however, the distal portion was not visualized. A CT cystogram was performed which demonstrated vesicoureteral reflux into the collecting system and incarceration of dilated ureter within a right inguinal hernia. The patient was deemed not an ideal surgical candidate in the setting of acute pneumonia. He underwent emergent placement of nephrostomy tube to the transplanted kidney with subsequent improvement of patient's Cr to 1.28 mg/dL. Two months later, he underwent definitive repair of the hernia. A low midline incision was used for exploratory laparotomy and, within the preperitoneal space, the hernia defect was encountered with transplant ureter herniation. The ureter was reduced and herniorrhaphy was performed in preperitoneal fashion. The redundant transplant ureter was revised and reimplanted into the bladder with ureteral stent placement. The existing nephrostomy tube was removed. Postoperatively, the patient's Cr improved to 1.03 mg/dL. He was discharged from hospital on post-op day 7 after normalization of bowel function. At his 4-month follow-up, he continues to do well with normal kidney function (Cr 1.06 mg/dL).

3. Discussion

Common causes of transplant ureteral obstructions include ureteral strictures, malignancy, and calculous disease [1]. Renal transplant hydroureteronephrosis has many etiologies, including ureteral obstruction, reflux, infection, and rejection. Hydronephrosis is usually identified by US while nuclear renal imaging with Lasix can further asses for obstruction. Cystoscopy with ureteral stenting or percutaneous nephrostomy placement can provide the usual first line options to relieve obstruction [1, 2]. In rare instances, inclusion into an inguinal hernia can also cause transplant ureteral obstruction with only three other case reports in literature. Nonetheless, inguinal hernias should be considered in the differential diagnosis in the setting of transplant ureteral obstruction as they represent a common disease process in general and urologic surgical patients and one that urologists and transplant surgeons are able to treat.

Factors that predispose to transplant ureteral obstruction include obesity and redundant ureteral length. Anterior positioning of the transplant ureter in relation to the spermatic cord also is a risk factor [1], although this was not the case for either of our two cases. Regardless of the predisposing influences, ureteroinguinal hernias can be categorized in three different ways depending on their proximity to peritoneum: paraperitoneal (next to peritoneal hernia sac), peritoneal (through peritoneal hernia sac), and extraperitoneal (not associated with a hernia sac altogether) [3]. Concomitant repair of inguinal hernias via a preperitoneal approach during pelvic urologic surgery, particularly with radical retropubic prostatectomy and radical cystoprostatectomy, has been described in the urologic literature [2].

All three prior reports of transplant ureteral obstruction due to inclusion into an inguinal hernia were managed by temporary placement of percutaneous nephrostomy tubes or ureteral stenting prior to delayed definitive surgery as with the scenario presented here in case 2 [1, 4, 5]. However, we also demonstrated that immediate and definitive repair of the ureteral obstruction with herniorrhaphy and ureteral reimplant is a feasible option. This case represents the first report of successful immediate repair of transplant ureteral obstruction. Given our patient's favorable outcome as measured by clinical status, rapid recovery, and Cr improvement, we show that when promptly diagnosed with the appropriate index of suspicion, immediate definitive herniorrhaphy with ureteral reconstruction is a feasible option for selected patients with transplant ureteral obstruction secondary to inclusion into an inguinal hernia.

Abbreviations

AKI: Acute kidney injury
Cr: Creatinine
CT: Computed tomography
DDRT: Deceased donor renal transplantation
ESRD: End stage renal disease
IV: Intravenous
LRT: Living donor related renal transplantation
PCKD: Polycystic kidney disease
US: Ultrasound.

Competing Interests

None of the contributing authors have any conflict of interests, including specific financial interests or relationships and affiliations relevant to the subject matter or materials discussed in the paper.

References

[1] M. S. Ingber, B. J. Girdler, J. F. Moy, M. J. Frikker, and J. B. Hollander, "Inguinal herniation of a transplant ureter: rare cause of obstructive uropathy," *Urology*, vol. 70, no. 6, 2007.

[2] P. N. Schlegel and P. C. Walsh, "The use of the preperitoneal approach for the simultaneous repair of inguinal hernia during surgery on the bladder and prostate," *World Journal of Surgery*, vol. 13, no. 5, pp. 555–559, 1989.

[3] S. Vyas, N. Chabra, S. K. Singh, and N. Khandelwal, "Inguinal herniation of the bladder and ureter: an unusual cause of obstructive uropathy in a transplant kidney," *Saudi Journal of Kidney Diseases and Transplantation*, vol. 25, no. 1, pp. 153–155, 2014.

[4] A. S. Salinas Sánchez, J. Cifuentes Tebar, M. Segura Martín et al., "Obstructive uropathy secondary to ureteral herniation in a pediatric en bloc renal graft," *American Journal of Transplantation*, vol. 5, no. 8, pp. 2074–2077, 2005.

[5] Y. Osman, B. Ali-El-Dein, R. El-Leithy, and A. Shokeir, "Sliding hernia containing the ureter-a rare cause of graft hydroureteronephrosis: a case report," *Transplantation Proceedings*, vol. 36, no. 5, pp. 1402–1404, 2004.

Successful Treatment of Focal Segmental Glomerulosclerosis after Kidney Transplantation with Plasma Exchange and Abatacept in a Patient with Juvenile Rheumatoid Arthritis

Hannelore Sprenger-Mähr,[1,2] Emanuel Zitt,[1,2] Afschin Soleiman,[3] and Karl Lhotta[1,2]

[1]*Department of Nephrology and Dialysis, Academic Teaching Hospital Feldkirch, 6800 Feldkirch, Austria*
[2]*Vorarlberg Institute for Vascular Investigation and Treatment, Academic Teaching Hospital Feldkirch, 6800 Feldkirch, Austria*
[3]*Clinical Pathology and Cytodiagnostics, 6060 Hall in Tirol, Austria*

Correspondence should be addressed to Karl Lhotta; karl.lhotta@lkhf.at

Academic Editor: Ryszard Grenda

Recurrent focal segmental glomerulosclerosis (FSGS) after renal transplantation is difficult to treat. Recently a series of four patients unresponsive to plasma exchange (PE) and rituximab, who were successfully treated with abatacept, has been reported. We present a 26-year-old Caucasian patient who suffered from juvenile rheumatoid arthritis and developed severe proteinuria eleven days after transplantation. An allograft biopsy was suggestive of recurrent focal segmental glomerulosclerosis. He did not respond to PE therapy. A first dose of abatacept produced partial remission. Four weeks later proteinuria again increased and a second biopsy showed progression of disease. After another ineffective course of PE he was given a second dose of abatacept, which was followed by rapid, complete, and sustained resolution of proteinuria. This treatment caused a significant increase in BK and JC viremia. Whether abatacept ameliorated proteinuria via an effect on podocytes or on the patient's primary disease remains speculative.

1. Introduction

Primary focal segmental glomerulosclerosis (FSGS) is a common cause of nephrotic syndrome and leads to end-stage renal disease in approximately 40% of cases. Recurrence after kidney transplantation occurs in 20% to 50% of patients and has been associated with decreased allograft survival [1]. The pathogenesis of primary FSGS is incompletely understood. Recent evidence suggests that immune cell dysfunction and subsequent secretion of a circulating permeability factor and podocyte maladaptation play major roles [2]. Despite ample evidence of the existence of a permeability factor, its clear identification is still lacking. Wei et al. recently provided evidence that soluble urokinase plasminogen activator receptor (suPAR) could be the circulating factor that causes FSGS [3]. Other candidates for the permeability factor are cardiotrophin-like cytokine factor-1 (CLCF-1) [4] and autoantibodies against the costimulatory molecule CD40 [5].

SuPAR probably causes podocyte damage and proteinuria by inducing podocyte B7-1 (CD80) expression, which leads to podocyte migration through inactivation of β1-integrin [3, 6]. This pathophysiological concept provided the framework for a B7-1-targeted therapy in FSGS.

2. Case Presentation

A 26-year-old Caucasian man with end-stage renal disease received kidney transplantation from a deceased donor in October 2013 after having performed chronic peritoneal dialysis and hemodialysis for seven years. He had suffered from juvenile rheumatoid arthritis since early childhood. Because the patient had initially been admitted with end-stage renal disease, his primary renal diagnosis was unknown, but secondary amyloidosis due to rheumatic disease was suspected.

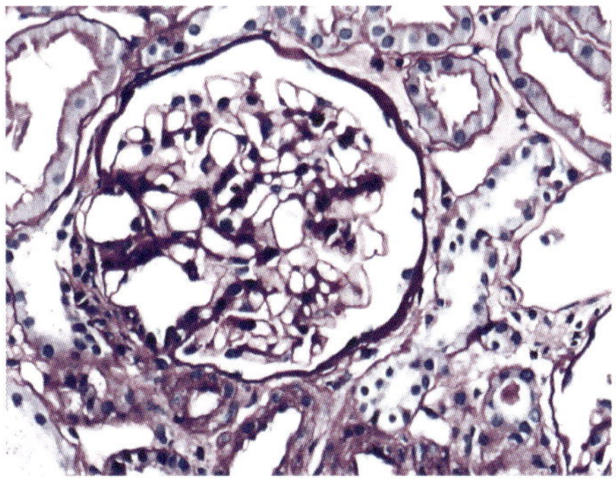

FIGURE 1: Light microscopy of the second biopsy shows mild mesangial matrix expansion and increase in mesangial cell number with focal accentuation (PAS, 200x).

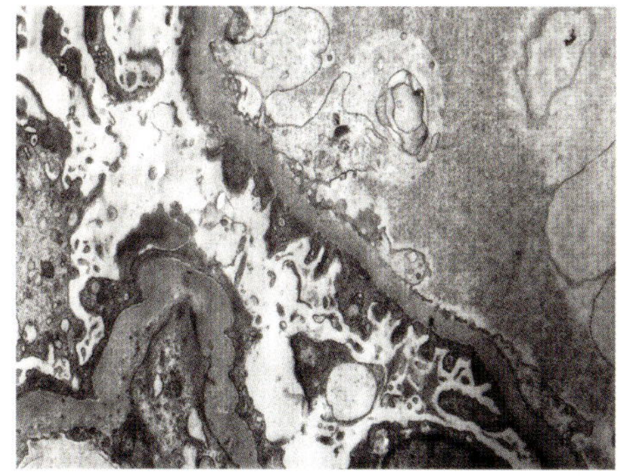

FIGURE 2: Electron microscopy of the renal biopsy reveals partial effacement and flattening of podocyte foot processes. The glomerular basement membrane is normal. No immune complex deposits are detected (4000x).

The patient received induction therapy with basiliximab followed by an immunosuppressive regimen consisting of tacrolimus, mycophenolate mofetil (MMF), and prednisolone. Because of CMV mismatch he also received valganciclovir prophylaxis. He was discharged ten days after transplantation with serum creatinine of 83 μmol/L. On day 11 after transplantation pronounced proteinuria with a protein-creatinine ratio of 3.34 g/g was noted. An allograft biopsy showed ten normal glomeruli with negative immunohistology, and early recurrent primary FSGS was deemed to be the most likely diagnosis. Despite nine PE sessions with exchange of one plasma volume each (5% human albumin as substitution fluid) over a period of three weeks, proteinuria remained significantly elevated after an initial decline from 5.5 g/g to around 3.5 g/g. Treatment with rituximab was not considered a therapeutic option because of severe immunoglobulin deficiency (IgG 370 mg/dL). Instead, after extensive discussion with the patient, a single dose of abatacept 10 mg per kg body weight was given. In order to avoid overimmunosuppression the MMF dose was reduced from 1000 mg to 500 mg daily. Within the next three weeks, proteinuria decreased to 1.5 g/g creatinine but over another three weeks began to rise again until it peaked at 4.5 g/g. The patient's serum creatinine increased to 151 μmol/L. A second allograft biopsy showed progressive disease with diffuse mesangial expansion (Figure 1).

Electron microscopy revealed dystrophic podocytes with flattened foot processes (Figure 2).

The patient was treated with further eight PEs, which reduced proteinuria to around 3.0 g/g creatinine with a tendency to increase. We therefore decided to give a second dose of abatacept. This was followed by a rapid decline in proteinuria to 1.0 g/g and a further decline to 0.15 g/g in the following months. The time course of treatment with PE and abatacept, serum creatinine, and proteinuria is shown in Figure 3.

Two weeks after the second dose of abatacept BK viremia was detected. BK viremia increased to 200.000 copies/mL and JC viremia (6800 copies/mL) was also detected. We discontinued MMF and reduced the tacrolimus dose, aiming for trough levels between 3 and 5 ng/mL, and prednisolone

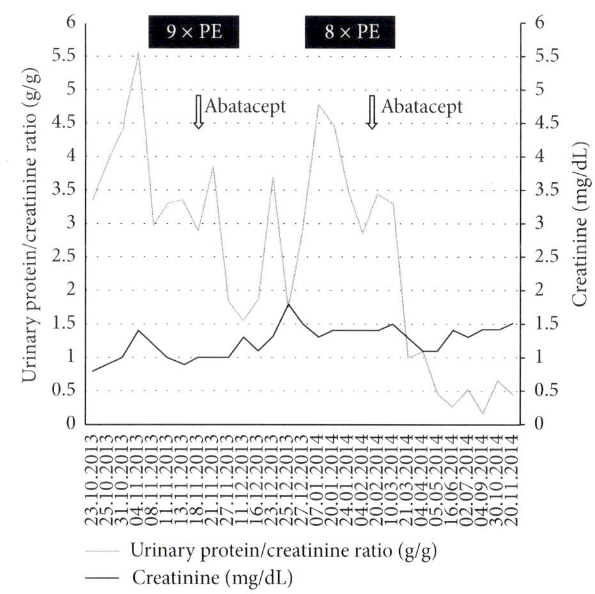

FIGURE 3: Time course of serum creatinine and proteinuria in relation to therapeutic interventions.

to 5 mg daily. JC viremia subsided after five months, whereas mild BK viremia (10.000 copies/mL) persisted. As the patient had negative EBV serology, regular EBV DNA monitoring was performed, which remained negative throughout the disease course. Over the next year, the patient remained in complete remission without proteinuria and with serum creatinine stable at 125 μmol/L.

3. Discussion

Recurrence of primary FSGS after transplantation poses a serious threat to allograft function. Current therapeutic strategies such as high-dose cyclosporine A, cyclophosphamide, PE, and rituximab will induce a remission in only up to 60% of patients [2, 7, 8]. Those patients who do not respond to treatment usually progress to allograft failure. Therefore, a recent report on four patients with refractory recurrent FSGS, who showed a rapid response to abatacept, was highly welcome [9, 10]. Abatacept is a fusion molecule of a modified cytotoxic T lymphocyte-associated antigen 4 (CTLA-4) extracellular domain and a constant-region fragment of human IgG1 [11]. Abatacept and its sister molecule belatacept bind to B7-1 and B7-2 on antigen-presenting cells, thereby blocking T cell activation, and are currently licensed for the treatment of rheumatoid arthritis and the prevention of rejection in kidney transplantation [12–14]. The rationale for the use of abatacept in recurrent FSGS was the observation that B7-1 is expressed de novo on podocytes in proteinuric kidney diseases [6]. B7-1 causes inactivation of β1-integrin via competition between its cytoplasmic tail and talin for binding to β1-integrin [9]. Inactivation of β1-integrin will subsequently cause detachment of foot processes and proteinuria.

The enthusiasm elicited by the first report was rapidly dampened by a letter describing treatment failure of belatacept in five patients with recurrent FSGS [15]. In addition, three further patients, who did not respond to abatacept, were recently reported [16]. This case series also included a patient with minimal change disease, who experienced a marked but only transient reduction of proteinuria after abatacept. Very recently another case series of nine patients with recurrent FSGS after transplantation reported no effect of abatacept or belatacept on proteinuria [17]. It has also been questioned whether podocytes of patients suffering from FSGS or minimal change disease do actually express B7-1, which questions any rationale for B7-1 blockade in proteinuric diseases [17, 18].

Our case includes several interesting aspects. First, the primary renal disease was unknown and the diagnosis of FSGS recurrence came as a surprise. It is possible that there is a link between our patient's renal disease and juvenile rheumatoid arthritis, although such an association has not been described. Abatacept is effective in and approved for the treatment of juvenile rheumatoid arthritis [19]. We therefore cannot rule out that abatacept worked in our patient not by targeting B7-1 on podocytes but by affecting his rheumatic disease. One could imagine that cytokines or other soluble factors produced in rheumatoid arthritis (possibly CLCF-1?) may have been an important cofactor in the pathogenesis of our patient's renal disease and that reduction of these factors by targeting the rheumatic disease may have contributed to remission of proteinuria. Abatacept may also interfere with the effects of CLCF-1 or anti-CD40 autoantibodies and thereby induce remission in FSGS. Another explanation for disease remission would be that abatacept was ineffective and that our patient actually responded, albeit, somehow, delayed, to PE.

It is difficult to know why some patients seem to respond to abatacept while the majority of patients do not. The pathophysiological mechanisms underlying FSGS may be different from case to case, ranging from nonspecific podocyte injury to abnormal immune response (probably in our patient) with production of CLCF-1 or anti-CD40 antibodies and suPAR and up to podocyte expression of molecules including B7-1, B7-2, and CD40.

Following unsuccessful PE therapy, our next choice would have been rituximab.

Our patient's very low serum immunoglobulin levels made us reluctant to prescribe a therapy that might further impair the humoral immune response. We also excluded other treatment options such as high-dose cyclosporine A and steroids or cyclophosphamide because of their potential to cause severe side effects.

Although abatacept's package insert clearly excludes an increased risk for lymphoma in rheumatoid arthritis patients, the situation may be different when it is used in combination with calcineurin inhibitors and MMF. Treatment with belatacept is associated with an increased risk for lymphoma in EBV-negative renal allograft recipients [13]. Our patient had negative EBV serology and therefore belatacept would have been contraindicated. The donor's EBV status was unknown. We discussed our concerns extensively with the patient and decided to monitor EBV DNA regularly. Fortunately, we were unable to detect EBV DNA at any time.

In contrast to previous reports, we found BK virus and JC virus reactivation in our patient following abatacept therapy. To avoid overimmunosuppression we had already halved the MMF dose at initiation of abatacept. Only few data are available on virus replication and virus infection in patients receiving CTLA-4-immunoglobulins. A single-center study compared the incidence of BK virus and JC virus infection in 62 de novo kidney transplant patients, who were enrolled in the BENEFIT studies and received either belatacept or cyclosporine [20]. BK viremia occurred in 4.7% of patients in the belatacept group and in 5% of those in the cyclosporine A group. All five cases of JC virus reactivation were observed in the belatacept group. In our patient JC viremia disappeared and BK viremia decreased significantly after reducing immunosuppression, and the viral infections had no negative effects on the patient's allograft and nervous system. Nevertheless, we feel that the risk of viral infection in kidney transplant recipients treated with abatacept on top of full immunosuppression and plasma exchange is a matter of concern. Careful monitoring and judicious management of immunosuppressive therapy are warranted.

Competing Interests

The authors declare that they have no competing interests.

References

[1] E. M. Briganti, G. R. Russ, J. J. McNeil, R. C. Atkins, and S. J. Chadban, "Risk of renal allograft loss from recurrent glomerulonephritis," *The New England Journal of Medicine*, vol. 347, no. 2, pp. 103–109, 2002.

[2] P. Cravedi, J. B. Kopp, and G. Remuzzi, "Recent progress in the pathophysiology and treatment of FSGS recurrence," *American Journal of Transplantation*, vol. 13, no. 2, pp. 266–274, 2013.

[3] C. Wei, S. El Hindi, J. Li et al., "Circulating urokinase receptor as a cause of focal segmental glomerulosclerosis," *Nature Medicine*, vol. 17, no. 8, pp. 952–960, 2011.

[4] V. J. Savin, M. Sharma, J. Zhou et al., "Renal and hematological effects of CLCF-1, a b-cell-stimulating cytokine of the il-6 family," *Journal of Immunology Research*, vol. 2015, Article ID 714964, 11 pages, 2015.

[5] M. Delville, T. K. Sigdel, C. Wei et al., "A circulating antibody panel for pretransplant prediction of FSGS recurrence after kidney transplantation," *Science Translational Medicine*, vol. 6, no. 256, Article ID 256ra136, 2014.

[6] J. Reiser, G. von Gersdorff, M. Loos et al., "Induction of B7-1 in podocytes is associated with nephrotic syndrome," *The Journal of Clinical Investigation*, vol. 113, no. 10, pp. 1390–1397, 2004.

[7] C. Ponticelli, "Recurrence of focal segmental glomerular sclerosis (FSGS) after renal transplantation," *Nephrology Dialysis Transplantation*, vol. 25, no. 1, pp. 25–31, 2010.

[8] C. E. Araya and V. R. Dharnidharka, "The factors that may predict response to rituximab therapy in recurrent focal segmental glomerulosclerosis: a systematic review," *Journal of Transplantation*, vol. 2011, Article ID 374213, 7 pages, 2011.

[9] C.-C. Yu, A. Fornoni, A. Weins et al., "Abatacept in B7-1-positive proteinuric kidney disease," *The New England Journal of Medicine*, vol. 369, no. 25, pp. 2416–2423, 2013.

[10] B. Haraldsson, "A new era of podocyte-targeted therapy for proteinuric kidney disease," *The New England Journal of Medicine*, vol. 369, no. 25, pp. 2453–2454, 2013.

[11] P. S. Linsley, W. Brady, M. Urnes, L. S. Grosmaire, N. K. Damle, and J. A. Ledbetter, "CTLA-4 is a second receptor for the B cell activation antigen B7," *The Journal of Experimental Medicine*, vol. 174, no. 3, pp. 561–569, 1991.

[12] M. C. Genovese, J.-C. Becker, M. Schiff et al., "Abatacept for rheumatoid arthritis refractory to tumor necrosis factor α inhibition," *The New England Journal of Medicine*, vol. 353, no. 11, pp. 1114–1123, 2005.

[13] F. Vincenti, B. Charpentier, Y. Vanrenterghem et al., "A phase III study of belatacept-based immunosuppression regimens versus cyclosporine in renal transplant recipients (BENEFIT Study)," *American Journal of Transplantation*, vol. 10, no. 3, pp. 535–546, 2010.

[14] R. J. Greenwald, G. J. Freeman, and A. H. Sharpe, "The B7 family revisited," *Annual Review of Immunology*, vol. 23, pp. 515–548, 2005.

[15] N. Alachkar, N. Carter-Monroe, and J. Reiser, "Abatacept in B7-1-positive proteinuric kidney disease," *The New England Journal of Medicine*, vol. 370, no. 13, pp. 1263–1264, 2014.

[16] E. H. Garin, J. Reiser, G. Cara-Fuentes et al., "Case series: CTLA4-IgG1 therapy in minimal change disease and focal segmental glomerulosclerosis," *Pediatric Nephrology*, vol. 30, no. 3, pp. 469–477, 2014.

[17] M. Delville, E. Baye, A. Durrbach et al., "B7-1 blockade does not improve post-transplant nephrotic syndrome caused by recurrent FSGS," *Journal of the American Society of Nephrology*, 2015.

[18] R. Novelli, E. Gagliardini, B. Ruggiero, A. Benigni, and G. Remuzzi, "Any value of podocyte B7-1 as a biomarker in human MCD and FSGS?" *American Journal of Physiology-Renal Physiology*, vol. 310, no. 5, pp. F335–F341, 2016.

[19] N. Ruperto, D. J. Lovell, P. Quartier et al., "Long-term safety and efficacy of abatacept in children with juvenile idiopathic arthritis," *Arthritis and Rheumatism*, vol. 62, no. 6, pp. 1792–1802, 2010.

[20] N. Bassil, L. Rostaing, C. Mengelle et al., "Prospective monitoring of cytomegalovirus, Epstein-Barr virus, BK virus, and JC virus infections on belatacept therapy after a kidney transplant," *Experimental and Clinical Transplantation*, vol. 12, no. 3, pp. 212–219, 2014.

Incidental Eosinophilic Chromophobe Renal Cell Carcinoma in Renal Allograft

Abdullah Alharbi,[1] Maram S. Al Turki,[2] Noura Aloudah,[1,2] and Khaled O. Alsaad[1,2]

[1] *Department of Pathology and Laboratory Medicine, King Abdulaziz Medical City, Riyadh, Saudi Arabia*
[2] *College of Medicine, King Saud bin Abdulaziz University for Health Sciences, Riyadh, Saudi Arabia*

Correspondence should be addressed to Khaled O. Alsaad; khaledalsaad@gmail.com

Academic Editor: David Conti

The incidence of renal cell carcinoma (RCC) in renal allograft in transplant recipients is 0.22–0.25%. De novo clear cell, papillary, and chromophobe RCCs and RCCs with sarcomatoid differentiation originating in renal allograft have been reported. Routine surveillance for graft tumours is not routinely practiced and these tumours are commonly asymptomatic and incidentally discovered. We describe a case of incidental, eosinophilic chromophobe RCC in a 31-year-old, long-term renal transplant male recipient, who presented with acute gastroenteritis 11 years after transplantation. The graft was nonfunctional at the time of presentation. Abdominal ultrasound and computed tomography scan demonstrated 1.8 cm well-defined, round enhancing lesion, confined to the renal allograft and suspicious for malignancy. Pathological examination of graft nephrectomy specimen showed gross, histopathological, and immunohistochemical features of eosinophilic chromophobe RCC. Fifty-five months after surgery, the patient was alive and free of malignancy. To the best of our knowledge, only five chromophobe RCCs originating in a renal allograft were previously described in English literature. We suggest that chromophobe RCC should be considered in the differential diagnosis of renal allograft mass, including eosinophilic tumours, and emphasise the importance of periodic screening of renal allograft in all renal transplant recipients.

1. Introduction

Patients with end stage renal disease (ESRD), particularly those with a history of chronic haemodialysis and subsequent acquired cystic kidney disease, have a high incidence of native kidney epithelial neoplasms [1]. Renal transplantation is the best treatment for patients with ESRD. Due to long-term maintenance immunosuppression therapy, transplant patients have higher incidence for benign and malignant tumours than general population [2], and cancer is a major cause of morbidity and mortality after transplantation [3]. Nonmelanoma skin, genitourinary tract malignancies, and malignant lymphoproliferative diseases are the commonest in kidney transplant recipients [4]. The risk of renal cell carcinoma (RCC) in native kidneys of transplant recipients is approximately 15–30-fold more than general population [5, 6] and the incidence of RCC in native and renal allograft in kidney transplant recipients is 1.1–1.5% and 0.22–0.25%, respectively [7]. Clear cell (conventional) and papillary RCCs are the most common histological tumour types in both native and transplanted kidney [6]. Herein, we describe a rare case of incidental de novo eosinophilic variant of chromophobe RCC (ChRCC) in a renal allograft 11 years after transplantation, discuss the histopathological differential diagnosis, and comment on cancer screening in renal transplant recipients.

2. Case Report

A 31-year-old man underwent living nonrelated kidney transplantation at age of 16 years for ESRD secondary to biopsy-proved immune-complex mediated membranoproliferative glomerulonephritis. The patient was maintained on cyclosporine A, prednisone, and azathioprine immunosuppression regimen. His early posttransplant course was complicated with lymphocele, which was percutaneously

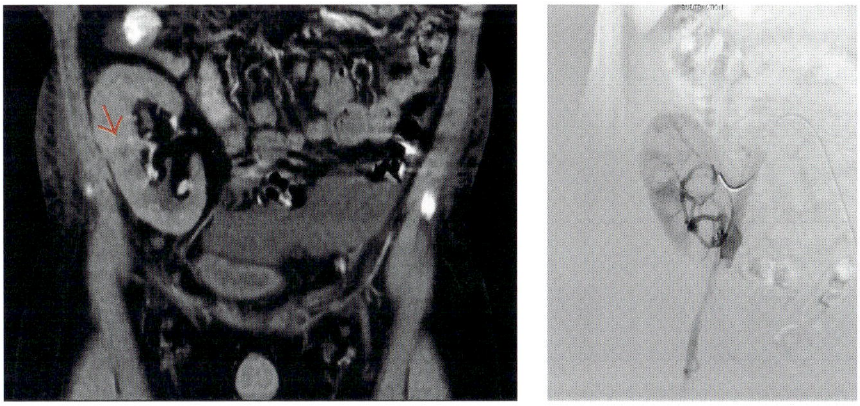

(a) (b)

Figure 1: (a) Computed tomography scan coronal section demonstrates an enhancing, round lesion, suspicious for malignancy in the mid renal zone (arrow). (b) Embolization of the renal artery of the renal allograft was performed before graft nephrectomy.

drained and *pseudomonas aeruginosa* urinary tract infection, which was treated by meropenem. The patient was noncompliant with his immunosuppression therapy and the clinical and radiological follow-up was not optimal due to patient's poor compliance. He experienced multiple episodes of acute cellular graft rejection, which resulted in severe transplant glomerulopathy, global glomerulosclerosis, severe interstitial fibrosis, and tubular atrophy and severe chronic allograft arteriopathy. Radiological studies during the follow-up period showed no evidence of tumour neither in native kidneys nor in renal allograft. Haemodialysis was resumed 11 years after transplantation due to failed renal allograft. Four weeks after resuming haemodialysis, the patient presented to the hospital emergency with a history of watery diarrhea, vomiting, and fever associated with rigor and mild diffuse abdominal pain for 3 days. In addition, he reported an episode of gross haematuria. The patient's vital signs were as follows: body temperature 37.9°C, respiratory rate 20/min, heart rate 101/min, and blood pressure 138/93 mmHg. His oxygen saturation was 100% on room air. Physical examination revealed mild generalised abdominal and graft tenderness. The rest of the physical examination was unremarkable. Urine analysis showed white blood cells (WBC) 7/HPF, red blood cells (RBC) 1/HPF, and protein 600 mg/dl. Laboratory tests showed haemoglobin level of 143 g/l, white blood cell count 3.9×10^9/L, platelet 150×10^9/L, normal electrolytes, blood urea nitrogen 6.2 mmol/L, and serum creatinine 801 μmol/L. Abdominal ultrasonography (US) demonstrated 14.3 cm renal allograft with well-defined, round lesion at the mid zone of the kidney, measuring 1.8 cm in maximum dimension, highly suspicious for malignancy. Both native kidneys were atrophic with no evidence of cystic changes or focal lesion. Abdominal computed tomography (CT) scan showed 1.8 cm enhancing lesion in the middle third of renal allograft (Figure 1(a)). The patient was diagnosed with acute gastroenteritis and mass suspicious for malignancy in the renal allograft. He was treated with cefazolin and gentamycin, which resolved the gastroenteritis. Later, the patient was admitted electively and underwent embolization of the renal artery of the renal allograft (Figure 1(b)) and graft nephrectomy.

Table 1: Primary antibodies used for IHC, their clone, dilution, and source.

Antibody	Clone	Dilution	Source
Pan CK	AE1/AE3	1/100	Cell Marque, CA, USA
CK8/18	TSIFB5	RTU	Ventana, AZ, USA
CK7	OV-TL12/30	1:50	Cell Marque
EMA	E29	1:50	Cell Marque
E-Cadherin	NCH-38	1:50	Cell Marque
RCC	SPM314	1:20	Dako, Denmark
Vimentin	V9	1:300	Dako
CD10	56C6	RTU	Ventana
CD117 (C-KIT)	YR145	1:400	Cell Marque

CK, cytokeratin; RTU, Ready to Use; EMA, epithelial membrane antigen; RCC, renal cell carcinoma.

Gross examination of the graft nephrectomy specimen showed well-defined, solitary, round, mahogany corticomedullary tumour in the mid zone of the renal allograft, measuring 1.6 cm in maximum dimension. No tumour central scar, haemorrhage, or necrosis was seen. The tumour was confined to the kidney and showed no extracapsular extension. Sections from the tumour were fixed in 10% buffered formalin, paraffin-embedded, sectioned at 5 μm, mounted on coated glass-slides, and stained by routine haematoxylin and eosin stain (H&E). A panel of diagnostic immunohistochemical (IHC) stains was performed (Table 1). All immunoassays were performed according to the manufacturer's guidelines, using automated platform (Ventana Benchmark XT, Tucson, AZ, USA) and heat antigen retrieval by ultracell condition solution PH 8.4. Ultraview universal DAB detection kit was used for reaction visualization. Proper positive and negative controls were utilized for all IHC stains.

Histopathological examination showed well-circumscribed eosinophilic variant of ChRCC. The tumour consisted of medium to large, round, and polygonal neoplastic cells that

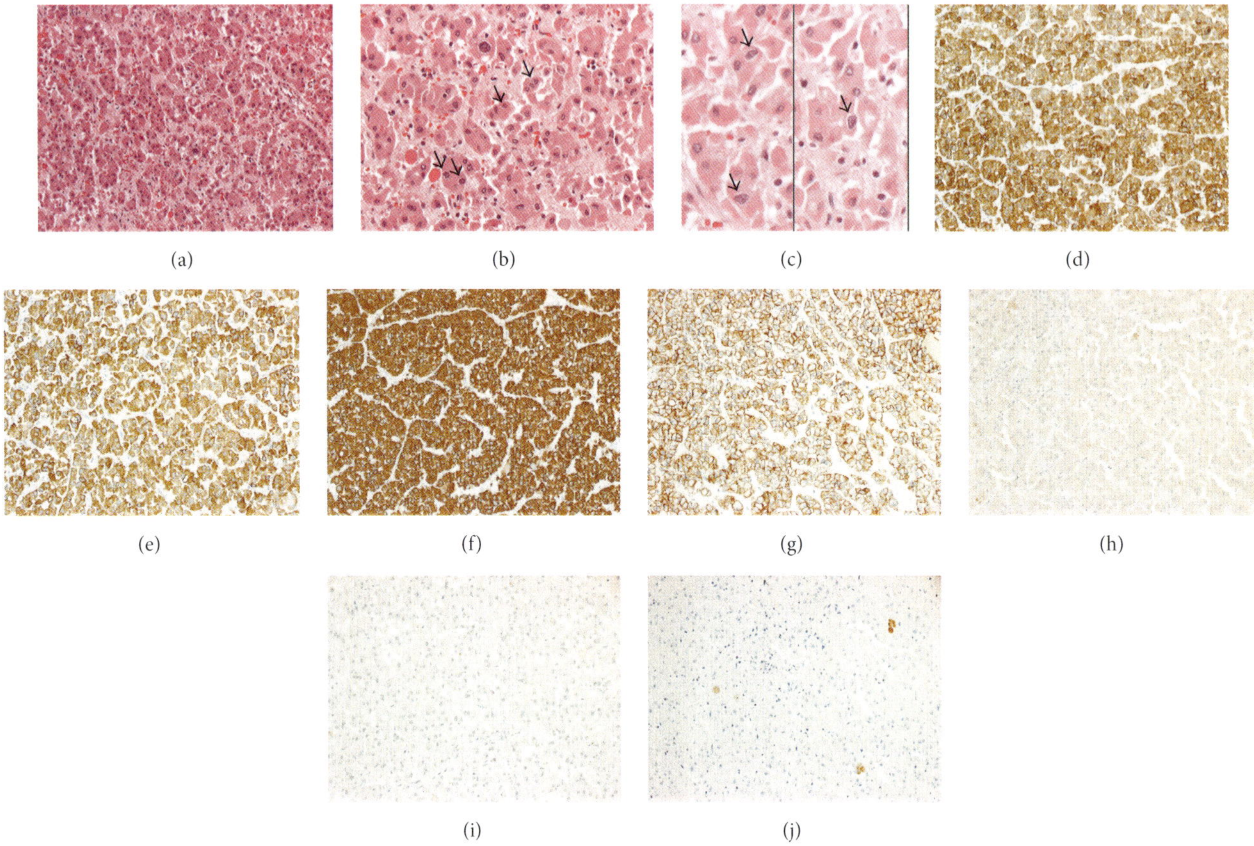

FIGURE 2: (a) Histopathological examination of the renal allograft tumour showed eosinophilic chromophobe renal cell carcinoma. The tumour consisted of medium to large round and polygonal neoplastic cells arranged in variably sized nests and cords and poorly formed acini [H&E ×200]. (b) Tumour cells exhibited hyperchromatic nuclei, irregular "raisinoid" nuclear membranes (arrows) and voluminous, and dense eosinophilic cytoplasm [H&E ×400]. (c) Tumour cells "raisinoid," wrinkled nuclear membranes, and perinuclear cytoplasmic clearing (arrows) [H&E ×600]. Immunophenotypically, the tumour cells exhibited positive immune reaction to pancytokeratin (CK) (d), low-molecular weight CK (e), CK7 (diffuse and strong staining, (f)), and E-cadherin (g), while staining for renal cell carcinoma (h), CD10 (i), and CD117 (j) antibodies was negative [(d–j) ×200].

exhibited mild degree of nuclear pleomorphism and arranged predominantly in variably sized nests, cords, and poorly formed acini and had hyperchromatic nuclei, indistinct nucleoli, irregular "raisinoid" or round nuclear cell membranes, abundant amount of dense eosinophilic cytoplasm, and poorly defined cell membranes (Figures 2(a)–2(c)). Scattered binucleated cells and occasional neoplastic cells with pale cytoplasm and perinuclear cytoplasmic clearing were present (Figure 2(c)). Mitotic activity was inconspicuous. No papillary growth pattern, foamy histiocytes, psammoma bodies, or background of extensive network of thin-walled "chicken-wire" vasculature was identified and no tumour necrosis was seen. There was no sarcomatoid differentiation. Lymphovascular invasion was not identified. Immunohistochemically, the neoplastic cells exhibited diffuse positive cytoplasmic staining for pancytokeratin (CK), low-molecular weight CK (CK8/18), CK7, and epithelial membrane antigen (EMA), and membranous staining for E-cadherin (Figures 2(d)–2(g)), while IHC staining for vimentin, CD10, CD117, and renal cell carcinoma (RCC) marker was negative (Figures 2(h)–2(j)). The remaining kidney showed severe segmental and global glomerular sclerosis, severe interstitial fibrosis and tubular atrophy, severe, widespread arteriolar hyalinosis, and severe chronic allograft arteriopathy.

The patient had an uneventful postoperative clinical course. On follow-up, the patient remains clinically stable on haemodialysis and without clinical or radiological evidence of locoregional recurrence or distant metastasis at 55 months after graft nephrectomy.

3. Discussion

Renal cell carcinoma of the native kidneys affects 1–3% of all renal transplant recipients with 5.6 years' estimated median interval time between renal transplantation and the occurrence of RCC [8]. In renal allograft, de novo RCC is rare and RCCs transmitted from donor represent only 0.02% to 0.2% of cases [9]. In a retrospective analysis, Leveridge et al. [6] reported 45 RCCs in 3,568 recipients who had renal transplant over a period of 43 years; 39 patients had RCC

in the native kidney, while 8 were diagnosed with RCC in renal allograft. The majority of renal allograft tumours are diagnosed incidentally when a biopsy or radiological investigations are performed for other clinical indications [10]. The interval between transplantation and allograft tumour diagnosis ranges between 2 and 258 months (mean 56); early detected tumours most likely represent donor-derived tumours [11, 12]. In our patient, the chromophobe RCC was incidentally discovered in renal allograft 11 years after transplantation by a diagnostic workup for acute gastroenteritis and presumed to be a de novo disease. Unfortunately no genetic analysis or leukocytes antigen typing to further confirm the recipient origin of the tumour was performed.

Various histological types of renal allograft de novo RCC were reported. In most reported series of cases, papillary RCC was the most common type, followed by clear cell (conventional) RCC [6, 13]. De novo ChRCC in renal allograft is extremely rare and only five cases were found in the English literature, one in paediatric age group and the remaining ones in adults [7, 14–17]. Table 2 summarizes the clinicopathological features of reported renal allografts ChRCC.

Chromophobe RCC is uncommon distinct type of RCC that is derived from the intercalated cells in the collecting ducts and accounts of approximately 5% of all native renal neoplasms. Morphologically it is classified into two main variants: classical and eosinophilic [18]. The classical variant is the most common and characterised by alveoli and/or trabeculae of large, polygonal neoplastic cells with voluminous, pale, flocculent, reticulated cytoplasm, irregular nuclear membrane, perinuclear cytoplasmic clearing, and prominent cell membrane. The classical network of delicate, anastomosing capillaries in the background is not a usual feature of ChRCC. The eosinophilic variant of CRCC is very rare and exhibits similar nuclear features encountered in classical CRCC; however, the neoplastic cells tend to be arranged in more solid growth pattern and have dense eosinophilic, slightly granular, abundant cytoplasm and visible to indistinct cell membrane [19]. All previously reported ChRCC in renal allografts were classical variant [7, 14–17]. To the best of our knowledge, the current case represents the first eosinophilic ChRCC in renal allograft, which expands the spectrum of histomorphology of renal allograft RCC.

The histopathological differential diagnosis of eosinophilic ChRCC includes eosinophilic variant of conventional RCC, oncocytoma, and hybrid oncocytic/chromophobe tumour/renal cell carcinoma (HOCT). The latter two entities can be very difficult to distinguish even for an experienced urological pathologist. Several histological, histochemical, and immunohistochemical features distinguish ChRCC from other mimicking entities. In the current case the absence of typical tumour vascular component and the immunophenotypical features of the tumour easily excluded eosinophilic variant of conventional RCC, and the presence of readily identified irregular, raisinoid nuclear contour and cytoplasmic perinuclear clearing and strong diffuse immunohistochemical positivity for CK7 favour ChRCC over oncocytoma (CK7 tends to be negative or only focally positive in oncocytoma). Hybrid oncocytoma/chromophobe tumour/renal cell carcinoma is rare kidney tumour, which can be associated with renal oncocytosis and Birt-Hogg-Dube syndrome; rare sporadic HOCT were also described. These tumours exhibit histopathological features of both renal oncocytoma and ChRCC and can be extremely difficult to classify [20]. Although some neoplastic cells with round nuclear contour were seen in our case, noticeable numbers of cells with raisinoid nuclear membrane and the strong diffuse cytoplasmic (rather than focal or peripherally enhanced positivity) made us lean toward the diagnosis of eosinophilic variant of ChRCC over HOCT [21]. It is worth mentioning that overreliance on CK7 as main discriminator between eosinophilic variant of ChRCC and HOCT is not recommended as cases with strong diffuse IHC reaction can be also encountered in HOCT and cases demonstrating classic cytological features of ChRCC can be negative [22]. Thus, favoured diagnosis is a subjective matter and ultimately depends on the conventional light microscopic examination of H&E stained slides in many cases. Molecular genetics techniques such as fluorescence in situ hybridization (FISH) demonstrating variable monosomy for chromosome 1, 2, 6, 10, 13, 17, 21, or Y can be very valuable in diagnosing and help in distinguishing ChRCC from other mimickers, particularly oncocytoma, which shows no chromosomal loss. However an overlapping numerical chromosomal changes with HOCT are well documented as these tumours can exhibit mono- and polysomies of chromosomes 1, 2, 6, 9, 10, 13, 17, 21, and 22 [21]. Unfortunately molecular genetics studies were not performed on our case.

In general, ChRCC tends to be low-grade and has better prognosis compared to conventional (clear) RCC with a mortality rate < 10% [19]. Large tumour size and presence of tumour necrosis and sarcomatoid differentiation are associated with worse prognosis. Our patient had well-circumscribed tumour that was confined to the renal allograft and showed no evidence of necrosis or sarcomatoid change.

Renal cell carcinoma can be silent and has insidious biological behavior, which result in a large tumour size. Similar to the current case, all reported ChRCC were discovered incidentally by radiological investigations for other clinical indications [7, 14] or as part of routine checkup or surveillance [15, 16]. This highlights the importance of the clinical relevance of radiological graft screening in kidney transplant recipients, which allow early detection of the tumour, provide wider range of treatment options, and result in excellent clinical outcome. Ploussard et al. [15] follow up a cohort of 2396 renal transplant recipients by annual US and reported 17 RCC arising in renal allograft, of which all were staged T1N0M0 and only one patient had a tumour > 4 cm.

Renal allograft tumours can be treated by different treatment modalities that include graft nephrectomy, nephron-sparing surgery, cryoablation, and radiofrequency ablation [23]. Allograft nephrectomy is indicated in tumours larger than 4 cm, in tumours located in the mid zone of the graft, in a recurrent disease, or in tumours arising in a nonfunctional graft. Nephron-sparing surgery or other nephron-sparing therapeutic options should be considered in small tumours with low-risk of local recurrence, especially in functioning

TABLE 2: Clinicopathological features of reported chromophobe renal cell carcinoma in renal allograft.

Reference	Age at RCC diagnosis (yr)/sex	Primary kidney disease	Interval before RCC diagnosis (yr)	Treatment	Tumour location	Tumour size (cm) & histological variant	Clinical follow-up
Greco et al. [14], 2005	13.5/M	Juvenile nephronophthisis	5	Graft nephrectomy	Near the hilum	2.1, classical	N/A
Ploussard et al. [15], 2012†	58/M	Polycystic kidney	8	Graft nephrectomy	Upper pole	0.5, classical	Alive, NED at 96 mo
Ajabnoor et al. [16], 2014	52/F	N/A	15	Graft nephrectomy	Mid renal	8, classical	N/A
Troxell and Higgins [17], 2016	27/M	N/A	9	Partial graft nephrectomy	Unknown	3.5, classical	Graft failed at 5 yr; NED at 6 yr, died of unrelated cause
Althaf et al. [7], 2016	20/F	Unknown	5	Graft nephrectomy	Renal pelvis	3.5, classical	N/A
Current case	31/M	IC-MPGN	11	Graft nephrectomy	Mid renal	1.6, eosinophilic	Alive, NED at 55 mo

†Chromophobe RCC was combined with papillary RCC measuring 4 cm and conventional (clear) cell RCC measuring 0.5 cm. RCC, renal cell carcinoma; yr, year; cm, centimeter; N/A, not available; NED, no evidence of disease; mo, months; IC-MPGN, immune-complex mediated membranoproliferative glomerulonephritis.

43

Immune Complex Mediated Glomerulonephritis with Acute Thrombotic Microangiopathy following Newly Detected Hepatitis B Virus Infection in a Kidney Transplant Recipient

Tracey Salter,[1] Hannah Burton,[1] Sam Douthwaite,[2] William Newsholme,[3] Catherine Horsfield,[4] and Rachel Hilton[1]

[1] *Departments of Nephrology and Transplantation, Guy's and St Thomas' NHS Foundation Trust, London, UK*
[2] *Department of Virology, Guy's and St Thomas' NHS Foundation Trust, London, UK*
[3] *Department of Infectious Diseases, Guy's and St Thomas' NHS Foundation Trust, London, UK*
[4] *Department of Histopathology, Guy's and St Thomas' NHS Foundation Trust, London, UK*

Correspondence should be addressed to Tracey Salter; traceysalter@doctors.org.uk

Academic Editor: David Conti

Hepatitis B virus (HBV) presents a risk to patients and staff in renal units. To minimise viral transmission, there are international and UK guidelines recommending HBV immunisation for patients commencing renal replacement therapy (RRT) and HBV surveillance in kidney transplant recipients. We report the case of a 56-year-old male who was immunised against HBV before starting haemodialysis. He received a deceased donor kidney transplant three years later, at which time there was no evidence of HBV infection. After a further six years he developed an acute kidney injury; allograft biopsy revealed an acute thrombotic microangiopathy (TMA) with glomerulitis, peritubular capillaritis, and C4d staining. Due to a "full house" immunoprofile, tests including virological screening were undertaken, which revealed acute HBV infection. Entecavir treatment resulted in an improvement in viral load and kidney function. HBV genotyping demonstrated a vaccine escape mutant, suggesting "past resolved" infection that reactivated with immunosuppression, though posttransplant acquisition cannot be excluded. This is the first reported case of acute HBV infection associated with immune complex mediated glomerulonephritis and TMA. Furthermore, it highlights the importance of HBV surveillance in kidney transplant recipients, which although addressed by UK guidelines is not currently practiced in all UK units.

1. Introduction

Blood borne virus (BBV) infection presents a risk to both patients and staff in renal centres, with HBV historically associated with outbreaks in haemodialysis units. Globally there exist numerous clinical practice guidelines (CPG) which aim to minimise viral transmission. International CPG recommend that patients who require RRT should be immunised against HBV [1, 2]. There is specific guidance for HBV surveillance in patients receiving regular hospital haemodialysis; those deemed to have achieved protective immunity (anti-hepatitis B surface antibody [anti-HBs] >10 mIU/mL) need to only be tested for hepatitis B surface antigen (HBsAg) annually [1, 2]. In addition, there is international [3] and UK [4] guidance addressing HBV surveillance in kidney transplant recipients.

TMA is characterised by microangiopathic haemolytic anaemia, thrombocytopenia associated with hyaline thrombi, and varying degrees of end organ failure. Numerous and varied causes are recognised, including viral infection [5]. However, there are no reports of TMA in association with acute HBV infection. Here we describe the case of a kidney transplant recipient who developed TMA synchronous to newly detected HBV infection in the absence of other likely causes.

renal allograft [15]. In our case, the renal allograft tumour was surgically treated by graft nephrectomy because the graft was nonfunctional and because of anatomical location of the tumour.

In summary, ChRCC is extremely rare in renal allograft. We described a case of incidentally discovered, de novo eosinophilic variant of ChRCC, originating in a nonfunctional renal allograft 11 years after transplantation, which was treated by graft nephrectomy. This is the first case of eosinophilic ChRCC, which expands the spectrum of morphological variants of renal allograft RCC. Early detection of renal allograft tumours by annual radiological screening should be implemented regardless of the graft functionality throughout recipient's lifetime.

Authors' Contributions

Dr. A. Alharbi performed gross examination of the graft nephrectomy specimen and participated in histopathological analysis and writing the manuscript. Miss M. S. Al Turki performed literature review and obtained histopathological images. Dr. N. Aloudah performed diagnostic histopathological analysis of the pathology specimen. Dr. K. O. Alsaad performed diagnostic histopathological analysis of the pathology specimen and wrote the manuscript.

References

[1] I. Ishikawa, Y. Saito, Z. Onouchi et al., "Development of acquired cystic disease and adenocarcinoma of the kidney in glomerulonephritic chronic hemodialysis patients," *Clinical Nephrology*, vol. 14, no. 1, pp. 1–6, 1980.

[2] N. A. Muruve and D. A. Shoskes, "Genitourinary malignancies in solid organ transplant recipients," *Transplantation*, vol. 80, no. 6, pp. 709–716, 2005.

[3] A. C. W. Chapman Jr and G. Wong, "Cancer in the transplant recipient," *Cold Spring Harb Perspect Med*, vol. 3, no. 7, Article ID a015677, Jul 2013.

[4] R. Saleeb, H. Faragalla, G. M. Yousef, R. J. Stewart, and C. Streutker, "Malignancies in a renal transplant population: the St. Michael's Hospital experience," *Urology Annals*, vol. 8, no. 2, pp. 163–167, 2016.

[5] B. L. Kasiske, J. J. Snyder, D. T. Gilbertson, and C. Wang, "Cancer after kidney transplantation in the united states," *The American Journal of Transplantation*, vol. 4, no. 6, pp. 905–913, 2004.

[6] M. Leveridge, M. Musquera, A. Evans et al., "Renal cell carcinoma in the native and allograft kidneys of renal transplant recipients," *Journal of Urology*, vol. 186, no. 1, pp. 219–223, 2011.

[7] M. M. A. Althaf, M. S. Al-Sunaid, M. S. A. Abdelsalam et al., "Chromophobe renal cell carcinoma occurring in the renal allograft of a transplant recipient presenting with weight loss," *Saudi journal of kidney diseases and transplantation : an official publication of the Saudi Center for Organ Transplantation, Saudi Arabia*, vol. 27, no. 1, pp. 139–143, 2016.

[8] T. Klatte, C. Seitz, M. Waldert et al., "Features and outcomes of renal cell carcinoma of native kidneys in renal transplant recipients," *BJU International*, vol. 105, no. 9, pp. 1260–1265, 2010.

[9] S. Yaich, N. El'Aoud, S. Zaghdane et al., "Primary adenocarcinoma in a kidney allograft: a case report and review of the literature," *Transplantation Proceedings*, vol. 43, no. 2, pp. 660–662, 2011.

[10] G. Zavos, J. Kakisis, J. Bokos, P. Pappas, J. Boletis, and A. Kostakis, "De novo renal cell carcinoma in a kidney allograft 13 years after transplantation: a case report and review of the literature," *Urologia Internationalis*, vol. 78, no. 3, pp. 283–285, 2007.

[11] I. Penn, "Primary kidney tumors before and after renal transplantation," *Transplantation*, vol. 59, no. 4, pp. 480–485, 1995.

[12] K. I. Park, H. Inoue, Y. Arai, T. Yoshiki, and T. Tomoyoshi, "Enucleation of renal cell carcinoma in an allograft kidney 21 years after transplantation," *British Journal of Urology*, vol. 80, no. 2, pp. 339-340, 1997.

[13] F. Cornelis, X. Buy, M. André et al., "De novo renal tumors arising in kidney transplants: midterm outcome after percutaneous thermal ablation," *Radiology*, vol. 260, no. 3, pp. 900–907, 2011.

[14] A. J. Greco, J. H. Baluarte, K. E. C. Meyers et al., "Chromophobe renal cell carcinoma in a pediatric living-related kidney transplant recipient," *American Journal of Kidney Diseases*, vol. 45, no. 6, pp. e105–e108, 2005.

[15] G. Ploussard, D. Chambade, P. Meria et al., "Biopsy-confirmed de novo renal cell carcinoma (RCC) in renal grafts: A single-centre management experience in a 2396 recipient cohort," *BJU International*, vol. 109, no. 2, pp. 195–199, 2012.

[16] R. Ajabnoor, E. Al-Sisi, G. Zafer, and J. Al-Maghrabi, "Chromophobe renal cell carcinoma in renal allograft: Case report," *Life Science Journal*, vol. 11, no. 7, pp. 9–14, 2014.

[17] M. L. Troxell and J. P. Higgins, "Renal cell carcinoma in kidney allografts: histologic types, including biphasic papillary carcinoma," *Human Pathology*, vol. 57, pp. 28–36, 2016.

[18] J. J. Hsieh, M. P. Purdue, S. Signoretti et al., "Renal cell carcinoma," *Nature Reviews Disease Primers*, vol. 3, Article ID 17009, 2017.

[19] V. Podduturi, C. J. Yourshaw, and H. Zhang, "Eosinophilic variant of chromophobe renal cell carcinoma," in *Proceedings of the Bayl Univ Med Cent*, vol. 28, pp. 57-58.

[20] N. B. Delongchamps, L. Galmiche, D. Eiss et al., "Hybrid tumour 'oncocytoma-chromophobe renal cell carcinoma' of the kidney: A report of seven sporadic cases," *BJU International*, vol. 103, no. 10, pp. 1381–1384, 2009.

[21] F. Petersson, Z. Gatalica, and P. Grossmann, "Sporadic hybrid oncocytic/chromophobe tumor of the kidney: a clinicopathologic, histomorphologic, immunohistochemical, ultrastructural, and molecular cytogenetic study of 14 cases," *Virchows Archiv*, vol. 456, no. 4, pp. 355–365, 2010.

[22] O. N. Kryvenko, M. Jorda, P. Argani, and J. I. Epstein, "Diagnostic Approach to Eosinophilic Renal Neoplasms," *Archives of Pathology and Laboratory Medicine*, vol. 138, no. 11, pp. 1531–1541, 2014.

[23] S. M. Baughman, W. J. Sexton, C. W. Glanton, N. C. Dalrymple, and J. T. Bishoff, "Computerized tomography guided radio frequency ablation of a renal cell carcinoma within a renal allograft," *The Journal of Urology*, vol. 172, no. 4, pp. 1262-1263, 2004.

2. Case Report

A fifty-six-year-old Arab male developed end stage kidney disease (ESKD) in association with hypertension and type 2 diabetes mellitus and commenced unit haemodialysis. At the time his serology tested negative for HBsAg and HBV core antibody (cAb). In accordance with UK guidance he received a full course of vaccination against HBV infection, receiving HBVaxPro 10 μg at 0, 1, and 6 months; subsequent anti-HBs titre following completion of immunisation was 965 mIU/mL. He was therefore deemed to have acquired protective immunity and was scheduled for annual monitoring of anti-HBs levels, with a booster indicated for any level <100 mIU/mL. One year after immunisation the anti-HBs level was 155 mIU/mL, suggesting that protective immunity had been maintained and that no booster was required.

Three years after starting dialysis he received a donation after cardiac death (DCD) deceased donor kidney transplant. At the time he remained HBsAg and cAb negative. Induction immunosuppression comprised basiliximab and methylprednisolone. Maintenance immunosuppression was ciclosporin (target level 200–300 μg/L), mycophenolate mofetil 500 mg four times daily, and corticosteroids. The postoperative course was complicated by delayed graft function and T cell-mediated rejection requiring treatment with pulsed methylprednisolone and antithymocyte globulin (ATG) (Figure 1(a)). Cytomegalovirus (CMV) viraemia was detected and treated with valganciclovir. Thereafter his kidney function improved to a baseline serum creatinine of 130 μmol/L. Maintenance immunosuppression comprised twice-daily tacrolimus with levels maintained between 7 and 12 μg/L, mycophenolate mofetil 500 mg twice daily, and prednisolone 5 mg daily.

Over the next five years his allograft function remained stable. Two immunosuppression-related issues arose: *Escherichia coli* sepsis secondary to cellulitis and a pyogenic granuloma of his thumb. In line with current practice at our renal unit, anti-HBs levels were not checked and no boosters were administered after transplant.

Six years after transplantation he presented to his local hospital nonspecifically unwell, and was found to have acute kidney injury (AKI) with a rise in creatinine from a baseline of 100 μmol/L to almost 350 μmol/L. He was transferred to this hospital for further management (Figure 1(b)).

Allograft biopsy revealed TMA with glomerulitis (g3), mild peritubular capillaritis (ptc1), and acute tubular injury, together with C4d staining (C4d2) (Figure 2). This was attributed to antibody-mediated rejection, although no donor-specific antibody was detected in peripheral blood, and he commenced treatment with pulsed intravenous methylprednisolone (3x 500 mg), plasma exchange (4-litre exchanges), and intravenous immunoglobulin (400 mg/kg). Serum creatinine remained significantly raised at 255 μmol/L (Figure 1(b)).

As a possible cause for TMA, tacrolimus was stopped. Immunosuppression then comprised mycophenolate mofetil 500 mg twice daily and prednisolone 5 mg daily.

The biopsy was further examined, and, in light of the extent of the glomerular thrombotic process and endothelial hypercellularity, a native immunoperoxidase panel was performed. This revealed a "full house" immunoprofile (IgA++, IgG++, IgM++, C3++, and C1q++) within the glomeruli, with deposition in the mesangial matrix and also at subendothelial loci (Figure 2), consistent with an immune complex mediated glomerulonephritis. This finding triggered both virological and lupus screening.

Initial HBV testing revealed the following: HBsAg detected; hepatitis B e antigen detected; hepatitis B e antibody not detected; hepatitis B core IgM not detected; HBV viral load (Roche) HBV DNA log value 8.15. Serology was negative for the following: CMV, BK virus, Epstein-Barr virus, HIV, hepatitis C virus, delta virus, and parvovirus. Lupus and antiphospholipid screening tests were negative, as was *E. coli* 0157 serology. All previous tests for HBsAg had been negative, most recently at the time of transplantation.

Liver function tests, including markers of synthetic function, were normal. He commenced treatment with Entecavir and completed ten plasma exchanges for ongoing TMA with thrombocytopenia.

The source of his HBV infection was sought. He denied any risk factors. His immediate contacts all screened negative for HBV infection. The allograft donor was HBsAg and cAb negative. Hepatitis B genotyping showed a vaccine escape mutant. One possibility is that the HBV cAb result at the time of starting dialysis was a false negative (commercial assays for the detection of HBV cAb can show marked variability in detecting cAb in comparative studies). He could thus have had resolved HBV infection prior to transplantation which later reactivated, with HBV sAb driving viral mutation. Another possibility is new acquisition of mutated HBV, against which the vaccine-induced sAb was not protective. Revisiting his history revealed that he had travelled to Mecca in the months prior to his presentation with AKI; it is possible that HBV could have been acquired during ritual head-shaving.

A repeat allograft biopsy was performed after two weeks of Entecavir treatment. This showed resolution of the TMA, but with residual immune complex mediated glomerulonephritis.

After one month of Entecavir treatment the HBV viral load had dropped from a log value of 8.15 to a log value of 4.65; the creatinine had fallen from 250 μmol/L to 211 μmol/L; the haemoglobin had risen, and the platelet count had normalised. Tacrolimus was not restarted. Two weeks later, both the HBV viral load and serum creatinine had further improved to 24884 IU/mL and 171 μmol/L, respectively. Several months later, transplant function remains stable at this new baseline and HBV viral load continues to fall.

We hypothesise that the acute allograft dysfunction was secondary to an infection associated (HBV) immune complex mediated glomerulonephritis. Our patient developed acute HBV despite successful HBV vaccination before transplant.

3. Discussion

It is widely accepted that patients receiving RRT should be vaccinated against HBV, ideally well in advance of ESKD.

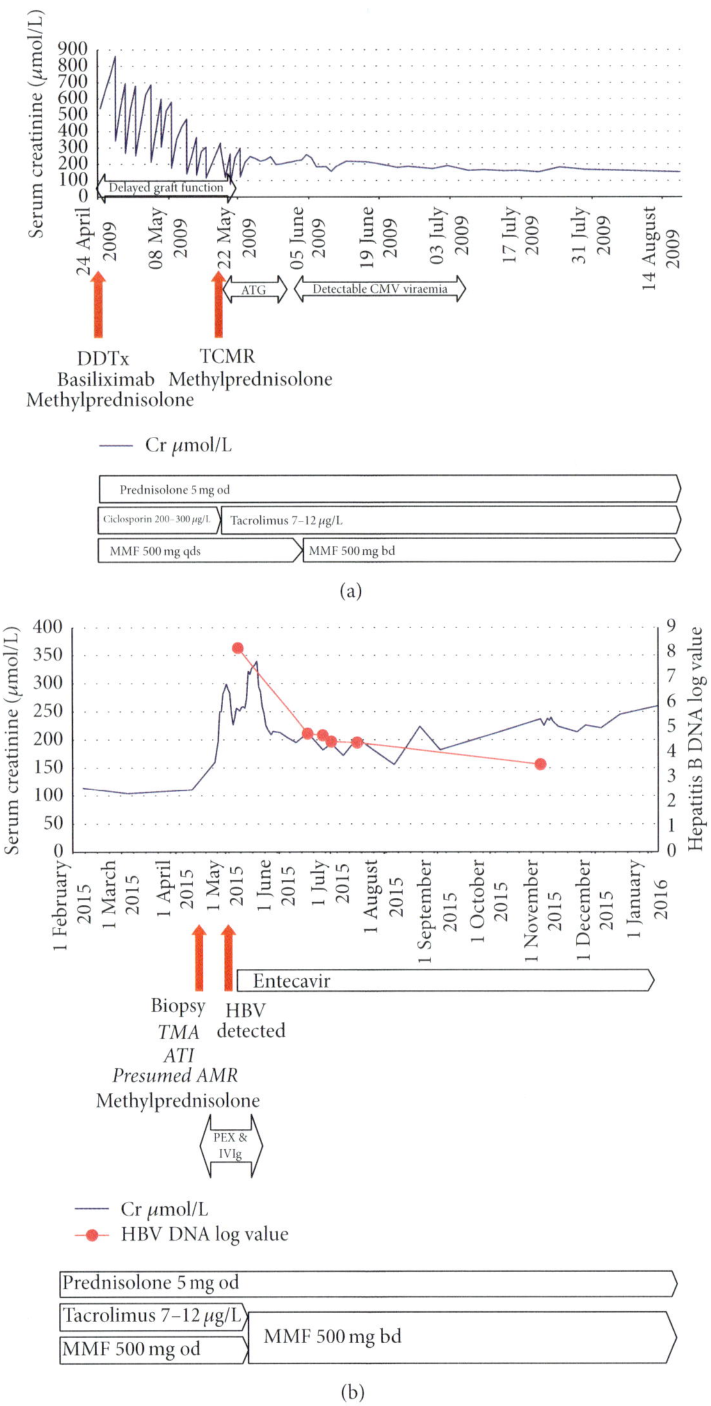

Figure 1: (a) Events following transplantation. (b) Events following his presentation with AKI.

Anti-HBs levels should be checked annually and boosted as indicated [2, 6, 7].

The importance of preventing HBV infection among solid organ transplant candidates and recipients is twofold; immunosuppressed individuals are more susceptible to infection with HBV and if infected with HBV are more likely to develop chronic HBV infection. Furthermore, a transplant candidate may be offered an organ from a HBsAg-negative, HBcAb-positive ("core-positive") donor, so there is additional benefit to completing HBV immunisation before transplantation [8].

If a kidney transplant recipient has not been vaccinated against HBV prior to transplantation then current best practice is to vaccinate between 2 and 6 months after transplant, thereby avoiding the risk that high dose immunosuppression may blunt the vaccine response [9]. The response

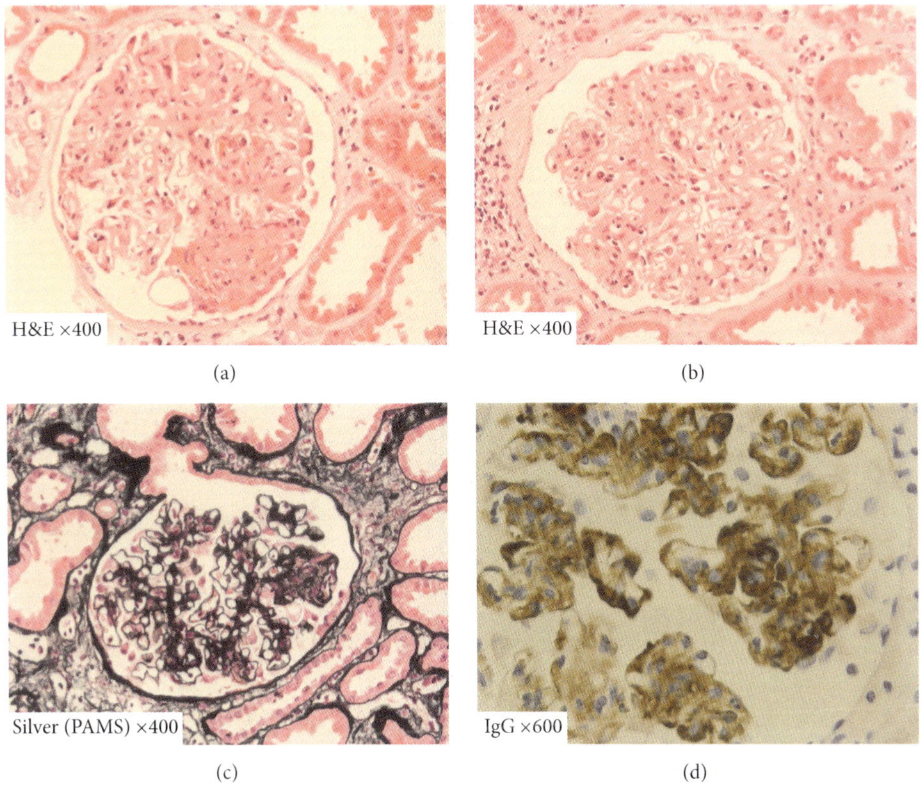

FIGURE 2: (a) Acute thrombotic occlusion of capillary loops, with segmental endocapillary hypercellularity due to inflammation, with endothelial cell swelling, and with fragmented red blood cells. (b) Mild increase in mesangial cells and moderate expansion of the mesangial matrix. Occasional inflammatory cells in capillary loops. (c) Segmental endocapillary hypercellularity with endothelial cell swelling due to inflammatory cells. (d) Positive staining for immunoglobulin G in the matrix and along glomerular capillary walls. Staining for immunoglobulins A and M and C3 and C1q was also positive.

to HBV vaccine administration after transplantation varies greatly, with response rates ranging between 17 and 89% [10–12]. Unfortunately, HBsAb levels decline more rapidly in immunosuppressed patients, even in those who develop protective levels [10, 13], and booster doses produce blunted responses [10]. These results underscore the value of pretransplant immunisation, ideally prior to the onset of advanced kidney failure.

The need for hepatitis B vaccination boosters is controversial and practice varies from country to country. There have however been reports of clinically significant HBV infection in previously immunised dialysis patients in whom production of HBsAb was no longer measurable [1].

It is widely accepted that annual measurement of HBsAb levels inform the use of booster doses of hepatitis B vaccine for dialysis patients. The European Consensus Group on hepatitis B immunity have expanded this recommendation to include patients with impaired immune function [14].

KDIGO [3] and the UK Renal Association [4] recommend HBV vaccination for kidney transplant recipients ideally before transplant, with an antibody check 6–12 weeks after the vaccination course. Annual antibody level checks before and after transplantation are recommended, with a booster to be given if the antibody level drops below 10 mIU/mL.

Our case demonstrates that HBV can cause clinically significant disease after transplantation, even when a patient has been vaccinated against HBV before transplantation with apparently protective response. This case is an illustrative example of the possible benefits of following the current International and UK Renal Association guidance.

This case is also notable for the association between acute HBV infection and biopsy-proven TMA with immune complex mediated glomerulonephritis causing acute allograft dysfunction. HBV infection is associated with a range of kidney diseases, most commonly membranous nephropathy and mesangiocapillary glomerulonephritis. However, an association or even causative role for HBV in TMA and immune complex mediated glomerulonephritis has not previously been reported.

Competing Interests

The authors declare that there is no conflict of interests regarding the publication of this paper.

References

[1] CDC, "Recommendations for preventing transmission of infections among chronic hemodialysis patients," *Morbidity and*

Mortality Weekly Report: Recommendations and Reports, vol. 50, pp. 1–43, 2001.

[2] Renal Association Guidelines, http://www.renal.org/guidelines/modules/blood-borne-virus-infection#S5.

[3] http://kdigo.org/clinical_practice_guidelines/pdf/TxpGL_publVersion.pdf.

[4] Clinical Practice Guidelines, *Post-Operative Care of the Kidney Transplant Recipient*, Guideline 8.1.2, UK Renal Association, 5th edition, 2011.

[5] R. L. Da Silva, "Viral-associated thrombotic microangiopathies," *Hematology/Oncology and Stem Cell Therapy*, vol. 4, no. 2, pp. 51–59, 2011.

[6] A. F. Charest, A. Grand'Maison, J. McDougall, and M. B. Goldstein, "Evolution of naturally acquired hepatitis B immunity in the long-term hemodialysis population," *American Journal of Kidney Diseases*, vol. 42, no. 6, pp. 1193–1199, 2003.

[7] I. Tsouchnikas, E. Dounousi, K. Xanthopoulou, S. Papakonstantinou, V. Thomoglou, and D. Tsakiris, "Loss of hepatitis B immunity in hemodialysis patients acquired either naturally or after vaccination," *Clinical Nephrology*, vol. 68, no. 4, pp. 228–234, 2007.

[8] R. T. Chung, S. Feng, and F. L. Delmonico, "Approach to the management of allograft recipients following the detection of hepatitis B virus in the prospective organ donor," *American Journal of Transplantation*, vol. 1, no. 2, pp. 185–191, 2001.

[9] L. G. Rubin, M. J. Levin, P. Ljungman et al., "2013 IDSA clinical practice guideline for vaccination of the immunocompromised host," *Clinical Infectious Diseases*, vol. 58, no. 3, pp. e44–e100, 2014.

[10] C. Loinaz, J. R. de Juanes, E. Moreno Gonzalez et al., "Hepatitis B vaccination results in 140 liver transplant recipients," *Hepatogastroenterology*, vol. 44, no. 13, pp. 235–238, 1997.

[11] S.-H. Chang, K.-S. Suh, N.-J. Yi et al., "Active immunization against de novo hepatitis B virus infection in pediatric patients after liver transplantation," *Hepatology*, vol. 37, no. 6, pp. 1329–1334, 2003.

[12] B. Serrano, J.-M. Bayas, L. Bruni, and C. Díez, "Solid organ transplantation and response to vaccination," *Vaccine*, vol. 25, no. 42, pp. 7331–7338, 2007.

[13] P. J. Grob, U. Binswanger, K. Zaruba et al., "Immunogenicity of a hepatitis B subunit vaccine in hemodialysis and in renal transplant recipients," *Antiviral Research*, vol. 3, no. 1, pp. 43–52, 1983.

[14] European Consensus Group on Hepatitis B Immunity, "Are booster immunisations needed for lifelong hepatitis B immunity?" *The Lancet*, vol. 355, pp. 561–565, 2000.

Urinary Obstruction of Transplanted Kidney Caused by Uterine Adenomyosis and 2-Year Posthysterectomy Psoas Abscess in Conjunction with Transplanted Kidney

Yuta Takezawa, Yoshifumi Kadono, Takahiro Nohara, and Atsushi Mizokami

Department of Urology, Kanazawa University Hospital, 13-1 Takara-machi, Kanazawa, Japan

Correspondence should be addressed to Yoshifumi Kadono; yskadono@yahoo.co.jp

Academic Editor: David Conti

Urinary obstruction of the transplanted kidney caused by uterine leiomyoma is an extremely rare condition. To the best of our knowledge, there are only two reports in English literature. Psoas abscess secondary to renal graft pyelonephritis is also uncommon. We present this unusual case and its treatment course. A 43-year-old female presented with renal dysfunction. She was started on peritoneal dialysis from the age of 26 years and received kidney transplantation from her mother (living donor) at the age of 27 years. Computed tomography (CT) revealed right hydronephrosis and a large uterine mass compressing the distal ureter of the transplanted kidney. After a simple total hysterectomy, her renal function improved. Two years following the hysterectomy, she experienced painful urination, fever, right abdominal pain, and right lower limb pain. CT and T2-weighed magnetic resonance imaging of her pelvis demonstrated right psoas abscess in conjunction with transplanted kidney. She was treated with broad-spectrum antibiotics alone, which resulted in a good response. Urinary obstruction of the transplanted kidney caused by uterine leiomyoma is an extremely rare condition. Psoas abscess secondary to transplanted kidney pyelonephritis is also rare. We should keep these rare diseases in mind when treating such cases.

1. Introduction

Ureteral obstruction and urinary leak represent the most frequent urological complications after renal transplantation [1]. The incidence of transplant ureteric obstruction is 2%–5% among all transplants, and most of these occur within the first 4 months after surgery [1, 2]. The most common cause of urinary obstruction is ureteric stenosis because of the surgical technique used; other causes include edema, ischemia, necrosis of the ureter, intraluminal blood clot, lymphocele, and hematoma [2]. Urinary obstruction of the transplanted kidney caused by uterine leiomyoma is an extremely rare condition. To the best of our knowledge, there are only two reports in the English literature [2, 3]. There is one report of an ovarian tumor causing urinary obstruction [4]. Furthermore, the present case also suffered from psoas abscess secondary to graft pyelonephritis 2 years after the operation. Psoas abscess is also a rare condition, but it is now diagnosed and reported more frequently because of the increased use of computed tomography (CT) scans [5]. However, psoas abscess secondary to renal graft pyelonephritis is extremely uncommon. We present this unusual case and its treatment course.

2. Case Report

A 43-year-old female who received kidney transplantation from a living donor presented with renal dysfunction. Her history revealed purpura nephritis, which was diagnosed at the age of 2 years and culminated in end-stage renal disease at the age of 26 years. She was started on peritoneal dialysis from the age of 26 years, and she received kidney transplantation from her mother (living donor) at the age of 27 years. Her renal dysfunction steadily progressed from the age of 42 years, and she was referred to our department to investigate the cause of the renal dysfunction. She was given cyclosporine, azathioprine, and prednisolone. Physical examination was normal. Blood pressure was 152/95 mmHg, heart rate was 90 beats/min, body temperature was 36.7°C,

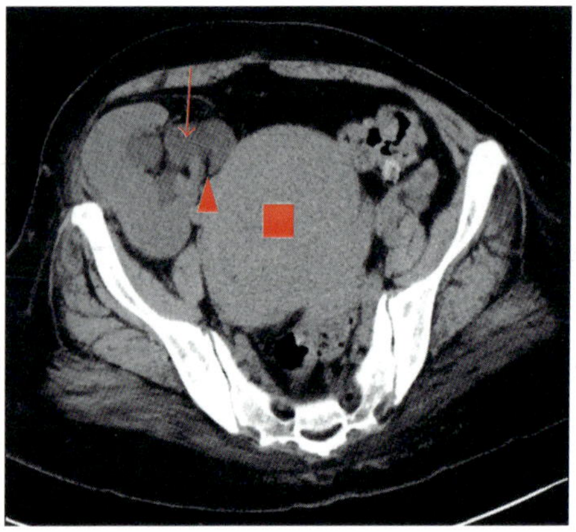

Figure 1: Plain computed tomography. A large uterine tumor (red square) compressed the distal ureter of the transplanted kidney (red arrowhead), causing hydronephrosis (red arrow).

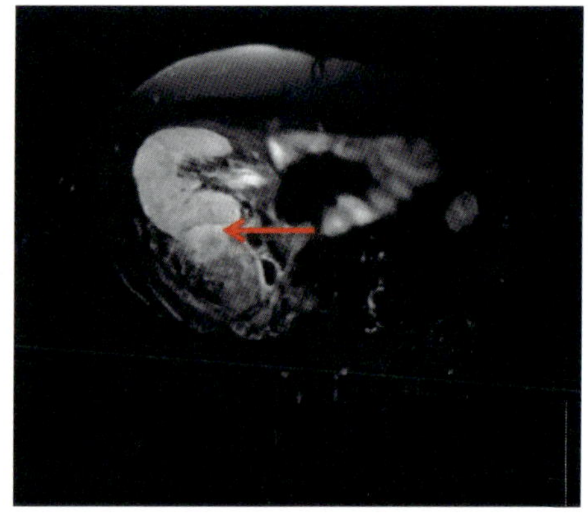

Figure 2: Contrasted T2-weighted magnetic resonance imaging. Right psoas abscess was in conjunction with the transplanted kidney. Ring-enhancement lesion was exhibited on magnetic resonance imaging (red arrow).

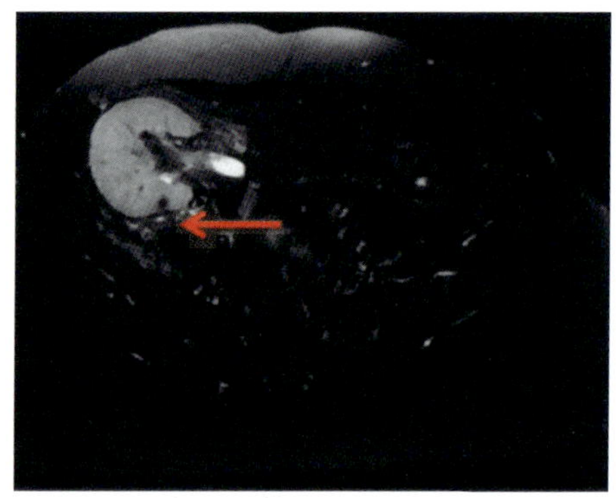

Figure 3: Contrast T2-weighted magnetic resonance imaging. After the patient was given antibiotics, right psoas abscess ameliorated within 2 months (red arrow).

and Body Mass Index (BMI) was 29.8. On laboratory examination, she had anemia (Hb, 6.6 g/dl), her serum creatinine (Cr) level was 1.88 mg/dl, and her urine was clear. CT revealed a large uterine mass compressing the distal ureter of the transplanted kidney and causing hydronephrosis (Figure 1).

First, a 5 Fr ureteral stent was retrogradely placed in the transplanted ureter. However, a percutaneous nephrostomy was needed because the serum Cr levels and hydronephrosis of the transplanted kidney did not improve. Serum Cr and hydronephrosis immediately improved after the nephrostomy, but it was necessary to perform a simple hysterectomy to remove the nephrostomy tube. The hysterectomy was performed a month later, and the pathological diagnosis was uterine adenomyosis.

Two years after the hysterectomy, she experienced painful urination, fever, right abdominal pain, and right lower limb pain. Physical examination revealed right abdominal tenderness on the transplanted kidney. Her blood pressure was 120/85 mmHg, heart rate was 110 beats/min, and body temperature was 38.5°C. Her white blood cell count was $1.32 \times 10^4/\mu l$, C-reactive protein level was 14.4 mg/dl, and serum Cr level was 2.73 mg/dl. Urinalysis revealed pyuria. T2-weighed magnetic resonance imaging (MRI) of her pelvis demonstrated right psoas abscess in conjunction with the transplanted kidney (Figure 2). Immediately, broad-spectrum antibiotics were administered. β-Streptococcus was isolated from the urine culture. The blood bacterial culture was negative. Her fever and abdominal pain were quickly alleviated, and T2-weighed MRI after 2 months revealed abscess improvement (Figure 3). Immunosuppressive agent was not changed during the entire treatment course. No relapses have occurred after the completion of treatment.

3. Discussion

The most common cause of urinary obstruction is ureteric stenosis because of the surgical technique used; other causes include edema, ischemia, necrosis of the ureter, intraluminal blood clot, lymphocele, and hematoma [2]. Two reports of the extremely rare urinary obstruction of the transplanted kidney caused by uterine leiomyoma were found in the English literature [2, 3]. However, a clinician must consider this rare condition, which could be fatal for patients with a transplanted kidney, when making an early treatment plan. In the present case, the patient underwent ureteral stent placement, which was ineffective because of the severe ureteral stenosis, and a percutaneous nephrostomy was needed. A simple hysterectomy was then performed. Previously, two reported cases of urinary obstruction caused by uterine tumor also involved a simple total hysterectomy [2, 3]. We should keep this option in mind to improve and maintain the transplanted kidney function. If the diagnosis was possible before transplantation, the patient may need to have performed preoperative enucleation or hysterectomy.

Psoas abscess secondary to renal graft pyelonephritis is also uncommon [5–7]. Intravenous drug use, human immunodeficiency virus, and Acquired Immune Deficiency Syndrome (AIDS) are emerging as common risk factors for the development of primary psoas abscesses [8]. A previous report stated that Crohn's disease is the most common cause of secondary psoas abscess in the western world [9]. In the present case, the patient was diagnosed with a psoas abscess secondary to the pyelonephritis of the transplanted kidney. The patient underwent a simple total hysterectomy, but the postoperative status was not related to the cause of psoas abscess because it occurred 2 years after the hysterectomy. The urine culture revealed β-streptococcus, while the blood bacterial culture was negative. *S. aureus* is implicated in most cases with primary psoas abscess. Other causative organisms include *Streptococcus* sp., *Escherichia coli*, *Mycobacterium tuberculosis*, *Mycoplasma pneumonia*, *Proteus*, *Pasteurella*, and *Bacteroides* spp. [5, 6]. In our case, the pathogens of the psoas abscess were not identified; however, it was considered to be a secondary event leading to pyelonephritis by reasons of the positive urine bacterial culture, the negative blood bacterial culture, and the adjacent position of infected transplanted kidney and psoas abscess. Yacoub et al. reported that psoas abscess should initially be nonsurgically treated with antibiotics, with or without percutaneous drainage. The administration of antibiotics alone for abscesses smaller than 3 cm in the largest diameter and percutaneous drainage for those larger than 3 cm could be recommended. Surgical drainage is a rare treatment option [5]. In our case, the diameter of the abscess was smaller than 3 cm; therefore, the administration of broad-spectrum antibiotics without drainage was selected as the first-line treatment and was greatly effective. We need to carefully consider the treatment plan, taking into account the patient's systematic condition and abscess size.

4. Conclusions

Urinary obstruction of the transplanted kidney caused by uterine leiomyoma is an extremely rare condition. Psoas abscess secondary to transplanted kidney pyelonephritis is also rare. We should keep these rare diseases in mind when treating such cases.

Abbreviations

AIDS: Acquired Immune Deficiency Syndrome
BMI: Body Mass Index
Cr: Creatinine
CT: Computed tomography
MRI: Magnetic resonance imaging.

Competing Interests

The authors of this paper have no conflict of interests to disclose.

References

[1] M. Harza, C. Baston, A. Preda et al., "Impact of ureteral stenting on urological complications after kidney transplantation surgery: a single-center experience," *Transplantation Proceedings*, vol. 46, no. 10, pp. 3459–3462, 2014.

[2] M. Abate, N. K. Wadhwa, and E. P. Nord, "Uterine leiomyoma causing urinary obstruction of the transplanted kidney," *Clinical Nephrology*, vol. 73, no. 4, pp. 314–317, 2010.

[3] T. Hara, M. Tsuchida, K. Takai, S. Takiguchi, and K. Naito, "Ureteral obstruction in a transplanted kidney secondary to a subserous myoma uteri [2]," *Transplantation*, vol. 75, no. 11, pp. 1915–1916, 2003.

[4] J. E. Bernie and M. Hart, "Ureteral obstruction in a transplant kidney caused by an ovarian tumor," *Transplantation*, vol. 71, no. 3, pp. 485–486, 2001.

[5] W. N. Yacoub, H. J. Sohn, S. Chan et al., "Psoas abscess rarely requires surgical intervention," *American Journal of Surgery*, vol. 196, no. 2, pp. 223–227, 2008.

[6] A. S. Badurdeen, P. N. Rajakrishna, H. M. Herath, A. W. Wazil, and N. Nanayakkara, "Bilateral psoas abscess in a renal transplant patient.," *The Ceylon Medical Journal*, vol. 57, no. 4, pp. 175–176, 2012.

[7] N. Ozgur, N. Seyahi, U. Sili et al., "Candidal psoas abscess following persistent pyuria in a renal transplant recipient," *International Urology and Nephrology*, vol. 46, no. 1, pp. 269–273, 2014.

[8] R. O. Santaella, E. K. Fishman, P. A. Lipsett, R. E. Condon, and M. D. Allo, "Primary vs secondary iliopsoas abscess: presentation, microbiology, and treatment," *Archives of Surgery*, vol. 130, no. 12, pp. 1309–1313, 1995.

[9] S. N. Agrawal, A. J. Dwivedi, and M. Khan, "Primary psoas abscess," *Digestive Diseases and Sciences*, vol. 47, no. 9, pp. 2103–2105, 2002.

Collecting Duct Carcinoma of the Native Kidney in a Renal Transplant Recipient

Ian Zheng,[1] Mahmoud Alameddine,[1] Yaohong Tan,[2] Zhobin Moghadamyeghaneh,[1,3] Joshua S. Jue,[1] Ali Yusufali,[1] Ahmed Farag,[1,4] and Gaetano Ciancio[1]

[1]*Department of Surgery, Division of Transplantation, Miami Transplant Institute, University of Miami Miller School of Medicine, Miami, FL 33136, USA*
[2]*Department of Pathology, University of Miami Miller School of Medicine, Miami, FL 33136, USA*
[3]*Department of Surgery, University of California, San Francisco, CA 94143, USA*
[4]*Department of Surgery, Zagazig University School of Medicine, Zagazig, Egypt*

Correspondence should be addressed to Mahmoud Alameddine; dralameddine@hotmail.com

Academic Editor: Mahmoud Sadeghi

Collecting duct carcinoma (CDC) is a rare and aggressive form of renal cell carcinoma (RCC) arising from the epithelium of Bellini's duct. It presents earlier in life and has a poorer prognosis than the clear-cell type. Historically, immunosuppressed renal transplant patients are more likely to develop malignancies than the general population. We report a case of CDC of the native kidney in a 59-year-old man who initially underwent kidney transplantation five years before the time of presentation. To our knowledge, CDC in the setting of renal transplant and long-term immunosuppression has not been previously described.

1. Introduction

Renal cell carcinoma (RCC) accounts for 2% to 3% of all adult malignancies [1]. The most common type of RCC is a clear cell, followed by papillary and chromophobe [2]. Collecting Duct Carcinoma (CDC) is a rare form of RCC that arises from the epithelium of Bellini ducts, located in the distal collecting duct of the renal medulla. It comprises about 1% of all RCC cases [3] and presents earlier in life and at a more advanced stage. CDC behaves more aggressively and is often unresponsive to conventional therapies [4]. Due to its rarity, definitive treatment for advanced and/or metastatic CDC has not been established.

In kidney transplant recipients, the estimated incidence of RCC is fivefold higher than in the general population [5]. An immunosuppressed status, deficient immune surveillance of malignant cells [6, 7], and reduced protection against oncogenic viruses [8, 9] may all contribute to the increased risk of cancer in transplant patients. The RCC subtypes of postrenal transplant patients include clear-cell carcinomas, chromophobe, and papillary carcinomas [10, 11]; however, CDC has not been previously reported in this setting.

The goal of this study is to report a novel case of postrenal transplant CDC in the native kidney that was complicated by distant metastases and to improve understanding of clinical and pathological characteristics. Treatment options for this disease in transplant patients will also be discussed.

2. Case Report

A 59-year-old male presented to the emergency department complaining of a 3-day history of suprapubic pain and macroscopic hematuria. The patient denied fever or dysuria. His physical examination was unremarkable, except suprapubic tenderness to palpation. Past medical history was consistent with smoking (30 pack-years, stopped 10 years prior to presentation), morbid obesity (135 Kg), hypertension for 7 years, diabetes mellitus for 15 years, hepatitis C virus (diagnosed during the pretransplant evaluation), and end-stage renal disease (on hemodialysis for 3 years). He received

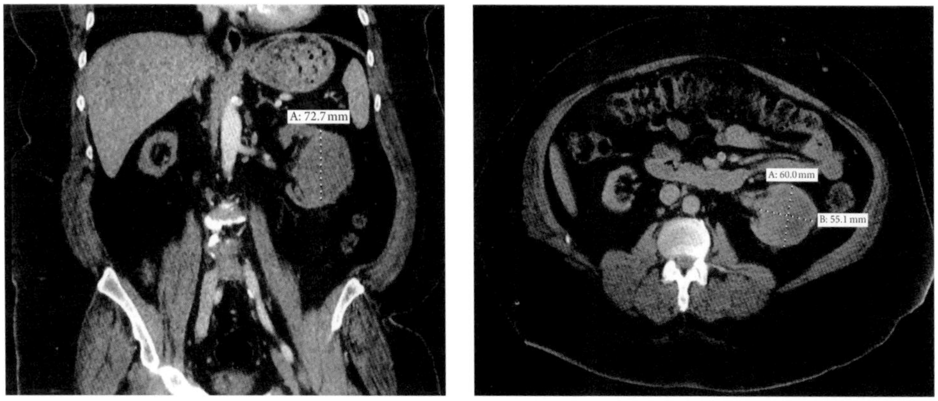

(a) (b)

FIGURE 1: Coronal (a) and transverse (b) views of abdominal computed tomography demonstrate 7.27 × 6.00 × 5.50 cm heterogeneous mass in the left native kidney. Both kidneys show signs of atrophy.

a kidney transplant from a deceased donor five years before the time of presentation. The donor was a 17-year-old male with no evidence of malignancy who died from a head injury. As part of the patient's pretransplant workup, an abdominal ultrasound revealed no kidney masses, but a liver biopsy showed stage 2 cirrhosis. The patient received induction immunosuppression both during and after the transplant that included thymoglobulin (1 mg/kg) and methyl prednisolone (500 mg Intravenous) for three daily doses and basiliximab (20 mg) for two daily doses. He was maintained on steroid-free immunosuppressant therapy consisting of low-dose tacrolimus (12-hour trough level: 6–8 ng/ml) and enteric coated mycophenolate sodium.

In the emergency department, an abdominal ultrasound showed a normal appearing kidney allograft; however, the native kidneys were not properly visualized. For better assessment of the urinary tract, a computerized tomography scan (CT) was ordered. A suspicious heterogeneous mass was noted within the left native kidney that measured 6.0 × 5.5 × 7.3 cm in anteroposterior, transverse, and craniocaudal dimensions (Figure 1). Those findings were confirmed by MRI of the abdomen, raising the possibility of renal malignancy. No distant metastasis was identified. Consequently, hand-assisted laparoscopic radical nephrectomy was performed a few days later.

Gross examination of the kidney revealed an ill-defined gray tan solid mass present in the middle lower pole of the left kidney, measuring 7.5 × 6.5 × 5.0 cm. The tumor extended into the renal sinus and perinephric adipose tissue with metastasis to a regional lymph node. Histologic examination demonstrated widely infiltrative high-grade adenocarcinoma with variable architectural patterns. Some areas showed solid tumor nests (Figure 2(a)), while another showed linear and single cell infiltration with prominent desmoplasia (Figure 2(b)). The tumor cells had marked nuclear pleomorphism, high nuclear : cytoplasmic (N : C) ratio, and prominent nucleoli (Figure 2(c)). Mitosis was brisk and the Fuhrman nuclear grade was 4 (ISUP/WHO Grade 4) [12]. The criteria for grade 4 include extreme nuclear pleomorphism and/or sarcomatoid and/or rhabdoid differentiation. In this case, sarcomatoid or rhabdoid component was not found; however, extreme nuclear pleomorphism was identified and characterized the specimen as a grade 4. Immunohistochemistry revealed that the tumor cells retained INI-1. The specimen was also positive for Pax8 and CK7 and negative for GATA3 and p63. Based on these morphologic and pathologic features, a diagnosis of collecting duct carcinoma was rendered. The American Joint Committee on Cancer (AJCC) pathology staging was pT3aN1M0.

The morphologic differential diagnosis included medullary carcinoma and urothelial carcinoma (UC). Medullary carcinoma is usually seen in patients with sickle cell trait, with a different history and patient age. Retention of INI-1 unequivocally ruled out medullary carcinoma. High-grade UC may also have similar morphology, although the absence of p63 and Gata-3 is inconsistent with high-grade UC.

Consequently, his immunosuppression regimen was modified to include sirolimus instead of mycophenolate sodium, as well as the addition of low-dose tacrolimus and oral prednisone. The patient was kept on close metastatic surveillance. Six months later, multiple bilateral pulmonary and bone metastases were noted on follow-up imaging. Cancer progression was confirmed pathologically by CT guided biopsy of the lesions. He was subsequently started on a tyrosine kinase inhibitor (TKI) in the form of sunitinib 37.5 mg daily for 4 weeks on and 2 weeks off as a first-line therapy while his immunosuppression regimen was adjusted to include tacrolimus and everolimus (0.75 mg twice daily). At that time, his kidney function was optimum (serum creatinine 0.6 mg/dl). Palliative radiation therapy was required to control his bone pain. Later, sunitinib was stopped after the development of drug toxicity, which included altered mental status, urinary tract infection, fatigue, anemia, leukopenia, thrombocytopenia, and diarrhea. However, the allograft function remained stable with a serum creatinine of 0.8 mg/dl. Follow-up imaging demonstrated worsening metastatic disease, so palliative care was established.

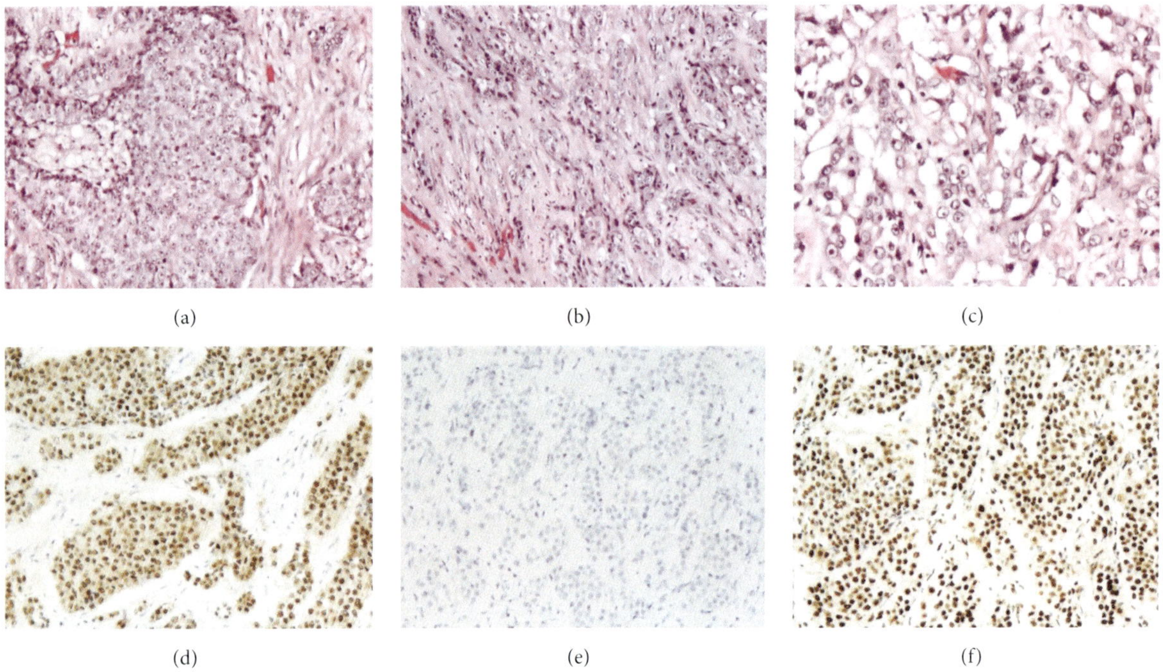

Figure 2: Histologic and immunophenotypic features of collecting duct carcinoma. (a) Tumor cells form solid sheets (20x). (b) Linear and single cell infiltration (20x). (c) Prominent large nucleoli (40x). (d) Positive for PAX8, consistent with renal origin. (e) Negative for GATA-3, ruled out urothelial origin. (f) INI-1 retained, ruled out medullary carcinoma.

3. Description of Hand-Assisted Laparoscopic Radical Nephrectomy

After induction with general anesthesia and preparation of the surgical field, the patient was placed in a right semidecubitus position. Since the patient was morbidly obese with a huge truncal circumference, we performed the hand port at the left pararectal line (8 cm) to gain closer access to the left kidney. A Gelport with a 10 mm trocar was first placed into the abdominal cavity through the left pararectal incision. Under direct visualization, one 5 mm port was placed at the level of the ribcage at the midclavicular line, while the other was placed 3 cm superomedially to the iliac crest. The colon was initially reflected medially to the level of the aorta. The ureter was identified, released from its attachments, and divided. Using the electrothermal bipolar tissue sealing grasper, the upper pole was separated from the adrenal gland. In the approach to the renal hilum, the renal artery and vein were dissected and controlled by the vascular stapler. After the kidney and the tumor had been freed from surrounding attachments, the specimen was removed through the hand port. No complications were encountered, with an estimated blood loss of 200 mL and a total operative time of 3 hours.

4. Discussion

CDC is a rare pathologic type of RCC that behaves more aggressively and presents more often with metastatic disease than the clear-cell RCC. Early diagnosis is uncommon but most important to improve the prognosis of CDC patients. Diagnosis of CDC is often based on histopathological findings. The clinical symptoms of CDC are often nonspecific, including hematuria, flank pain, a palpable abdominal mass, or distant metastasis [13]. Typical CT findings include an inner medullary location, renal sinus involvement, infiltrative growth that can reach the cortex, heterogeneous and weak enhancement, and a cystic component [13]. Microscopic findings can be quite varied and may present with a variety of growth patterns, including tubular, papillary, microcystic papillary, pseudopapillary, cribriform, and solid patterns [14]. Nuclear atypia is often prominent and atypical mitotic figures are usually present [14]. In the center of the tumor, desmoplastic stromal reaction and infiltration with inflammatory cells can be observed. Histochemical analysis characteristically reveals low and high molecular weight cytokeratins, *Ulex europaeus* agglutinin 1, vimentin, and peanut lectin [14, 15].

Our patient presented with hematuria and CT findings of a large heterogenous mass that extended into the renal sinus, a common presentation for CDC. Microscopically, the patient's tumor showed features that ruled in CDC, including high-grade cytologic features with desmoplastic stroma and focal gland formation. A positive immunohistochemical stain for cytokeratins is characteristic for CDC and ultimately clinched the diagnosis.

The largest analysis of CDC addressing the survival and the demographic factors was done by Pepek et al. using the Surveillance, Epidemiology, and End Results (SEER) database. This study found that the 3-year relative survival rate for the localized, regional, and distant disease was 93%,

45%, and 6%, respectively [16]. Additionally, no significant difference was seen in disease presentation and relative survival based on race and sex [16].

Clinical research has been predominantly focused on clear-cell RCC rather than non-clear-cell due to the scarcity of non-clear-cell histology. In the majority of patients with CDC, surgery is the primary treatment. In more advanced cases, some studies have shown that patients respond to chemotherapy with gemcitabine and cisplatin (GC) [17, 18]. In a multicenter, prospective study that administered GC as first-line therapy, 23 CDC patients had a response rate of 26% and an overall survival of 10.5 months [19]. Targeted therapy, such as sunitinib, sorafenib, temsirolimus, and everolimus, has also been used with moderate success [20–22]. However, due to high rates of metastasis and local recurrence, nephrectomy and chemotherapy have not been found to effectively control aggressive forms of this disease [23]. About 2/3 of patients with CDC die within two years of its detection [14]. Since CDC frequently metastasizes and often presents with a poor prognosis, early detection and diagnosis are crucial.

Kidney transplant patients are at an increased risk of developing various types of malignancies. Renal transplant recipients are 3-4 times more likely to develop a malignancy, most notably integumentary and lymphoproliferative diseases, compared to patients on dialysis (transplant waiting list) [10]. Wong and Chapman also reported a small chance of transmission of cancer from the donors to the recipients [24]. This increased incidence of tumors also includes de novo malignancies, which are more aggressive and incur an increased mortality in transplant recipients compared to the general population [25]. For renal cancers, Kasiske et al. reported the incidence of RCC to be 15 times higher in the native kidney of patients after renal transplantation than in the general population and 39% higher than those on the kidney transplant waiting list [26]. According to Klatte and Marberger, the risk of RCC is increased in men, patients with acquired cystic kidney disease, African-Americans, recipients aged 65 years or older, donors aged 50 years or older, longer pretransplant dialysis time, and microscopic hematuria [27]. Renal cancer also occurs more often in the native kidneys (90%) than the graft kidney (10%) [28]. In another study, RCC of the native kidney in the context of a renal transplant was found to have an incidence within 0.35%–3.9%, with histologies consisting primarily of clear-cell carcinoma and papillary renal cell carcinoma [10]. Rare cancer subtypes of the native kidney postkidney transplant, such as collecting duct carcinoma, have not been described in the literature.

The increased incidence of malignancy in kidney transplant patients is complicated by the necessity of immunosuppressant therapy to prevent rejection of the renal allograft. Many studies have shown that prolonged immunosuppression plays a fundamental role in cancer occurrence. This is thought to do with impaired identification of tumors cells, diminished antiviral defense, and direct oncogenic effects of the drugs [29]. The typical maintenance immunosuppressive therapy for renal transplant recipients consists of a calcineurin inhibitor (CNI), an antimetabolite, and prednisone [30]. Growing evidence suggests that CNI (cyclosporine and tacrolimus) promote neoplastic changes due to the production of several cytokines that regulate tumor growth and metastasis [31].

A study by Javaid et al. indicated that sirolimus may be an alternative for both anticancer and antirejection effects [32]. Sirolimus is an orally administered inhibitor of mechanistic Target of Rapamycin (mTOR) that inhibits the production of interleukin-2 (IL-2). IL-2 is thought to enhance tumor regression and promote the immune response to neoplastic changes. The use of sirolimus has been associated with lower rates of squamous cell carcinoma of the skin and other malignancies in kidney transplant recipients [33, 34].

In the setting of RCC, everolimus, another inhibitor of mTOR, has shown better progression-free survival compared to placebo in patients whose disease had progressed on treatment with a TKI [35]. Since the duration and dose of immunosuppressant may be a contributing factor to the increased risks of malignancy, further studies are needed to find the optimal regimen for transplant recipients with malignancies. Our patient received a combined regimen consisting of sunitinib and everolimus. Nevertheless, drug toxicity from combining a TKI and mTOR inhibitor is a concerning issue. The results of a phase 1 study by Kanesvaran et al. [36] demonstrated that combination therapy with sunitinib and everolimus in the treatment of metastatic RCC was poorly tolerated. Despite lower everolimus doses used in kidney transplant patients, an exacerbated risk for drug toxicity still exists that adds to the deleterious effect of CNI. Several studies investigated the side effects of combining a TKI with an mTOR inhibitor. These trials used the combinations of sorafenib plus everolimus [37], sunitinib plus temsirolimus [38], and sunitinib plus everolimus [39]. Most of these studies were prematurely terminated due to significant toxicity that included thrombocytopenia, infection, hemorrhage, and gastrointestinal toxicity. Extra consideration should be given to the patient's renal function because of the deleterious effect of the targeted anticancer therapy on the kidney, especially in the setting of kidney transplantation [40].

Unfortunately, the prognosis for CDC patients is poor with all immunosuppressive agents. A previous study by Pickhardt found that less than 1/3 of patients survive more than two years [41]. This histology is commonly associated with metastases to the retroperitoneal lymph nodes, bones, lungs, and adrenal glands [20]. There is even a case with metastases to the heart, in a case report by Voss et al. [42], who recommended investigation with MRI in all patients with CDC and cardiac symptoms. Despite its typically aggressive behavior, cases without direct invasion or metastases have been described. In a case report by Hu et al., an early diagnosis of CDC was made after a presentation of right flank pain [23]. The tumor was locally resected, with no recurrence after ten months, suggesting that CDC may be very manageable if detected in an early stage. With posttransplant patients being at an increased risk of malignancy [10, 26], some authors have advocated for annual ultrasonography of native kidneys in transplant patients [11]. This may be especially beneficial in patients with congenital cystic disease, acquired cystic disease, or even a single cyst in native kidneys [28]. Further studies are needed to evaluate the risk of CDC with the use of immunosuppressive therapy.

In conclusion, CDC is a rare and aggressive disease that may present with gross hematuria. A full evaluation of the urinary tract, including the native kidneys, is essential in transplant patients presenting with gross hematuria. Modification of immunosuppression should be considered as part of the treatment for CDC. Routine evaluation of native kidneys for malignancy is advised for early detection of CDC in post-kidney-transplant patients. Further investigation is needed to determine the high-risk group for CDC patients who would benefit from the screening programs.

Authors' Contributions

Ian Zheng and Mahmoud Alameddine have contributed equally to this work.

References

[1] R. Siegel, D. Naishadham, and A. Jemal, "Cancer statistics, 2013," *CA Cancer Journal for Clinicians*, vol. 63, no. 1, pp. 11–30, 2013.

[2] F.-M. Deng and J. Melamed, "Histologic variants of renal cell carcinoma: does tumor type influence outcome?" *Urologic Clinics of North America*, vol. 39, no. 2, pp. 119–132, 2012.

[3] F. Algaba, H. Akaza, A. López-Beltrán et al., "Current pathology keys of renal cell carcinoma," *European Urology*, vol. 60, no. 4, pp. 634–643, 2011.

[4] N. Tokuda, S. Naito, O. Matsuzaki, Y. Nagashima, S. Ozono, and T. Igarashi, "Collecting duct (Bellini duct) renal cell carcinoma: a nationwide survey in Japan," *The Journal of Urology*, vol. 176, no. 1, pp. 40–43, 2006.

[5] S. Karami, E. L. Yanik, L. E. Moore et al., "Risk of renal cell carcinoma among kidney transplant recipients in the united states," *American Journal of Transplantation*, vol. 16, no. 12, pp. 3479–3489, 2016.

[6] F. M. Burnet, "Immunological aspects of malignant disease.," *Lancet*, vol. 1, no. 7501, pp. 1171–1174, 1967.

[7] D. Keast, "Immunosurveillance and cancer," *The Lancet*, vol. 296, no. 7675, pp. 710–712, 1970.

[8] A. C. Allison, L. D. Berman, and R. H. Levey, "Increased tumour induction by adenovirus type 12 in thymectomized mice and mice treated with anti-lymphocyte serum [39]," *Nature*, vol. 215, no. 5097, pp. 185–187, 1967.

[9] L. W. Law, R. C. Ting, and A. C. Allison, "Effects of antilymphocyte serum on induction of tumours and leukaemia by murine sarcoma virus," *Nature*, vol. 220, no. 5167, pp. 611-612, 1968.

[10] A. Jakes, P. Jani, M. Menon et al., "Renal squamous cell carcinoma of a native kidney after renal transplant: a case report," *Transplantation Proceedings*, vol. 48, no. 1, pp. 259–261, 2016.

[11] L. E. Ianhez, M. Lucon, W. C. Nahas et al., " Renal cell carcinoma in renal transplant patients," *Urology*, vol. 69, no. 3, pp. 462–464, 2007.

[12] B. Delahunt, J. C. Cheville, G. Martignoni et al., "The international society of urological pathology (ISUP) grading system for renal cell carcinoma and other prognostic parameters," *American Journal of Surgical Pathology*, vol. 37, no. 10, pp. 1490–1504, 2013.

[13] A. K. Mishra, R. Manikandan, L. N. Dorairajan, J. K. Mittal, and J. S. Rekha, "Bellini duct carcinoma: a rare entity," *Journal of Clinical and Diagnostic Research*, vol. 10, no. 10, 2016.

[14] N. Kuroda, M. Toi, M. Hiroi, and H. Enzan, "Review of collecting duct carcinoma with focus on clinical and pathobiological aspects," *Histology and Histopathology*, vol. 17, no. 4, pp. 1329–1334, 20023.

[15] H. J. Rumpelt, S. Störkel, R. Moll, T. Schärfe, and W. Thoenes, "Bellini duct carcinoma: further evidence for this rare variant of renal cell carcinoma," *Histopathology*, vol. 18, no. 2, pp. 115–122, 1991.

[16] J. Pepek, P. Johnstone, and A. Jani, "Influence of demographic factors on outcome of collecting duct carcinoma: a surveillance, epidemiology, and end results (SEER) database analysis," *Clinical Genitourinary Cancer*, vol. 7, no. 2, pp. E24–E27, 2009.

[17] M. Peyromaure, N. Thiounn, F. Scotté, A. Vieillefond, B. Debré, and S. Oudard, "Collecting duct carcinoma of the kidney: a clinicopathological study of 9 cases," *Journal of Urology*, vol. 170, no. 4, pp. 1138–1140, 2003.

[18] S. Dason, C. Allard, A. Sheridan-Jonah et al., "Management of renal collecting duct carcinoma: a systematic review and the McMaster experience," *Current Oncology*, vol. 20, no. 3, pp. e233–e232, 2013.

[19] S. Oudard, E. Banu, A. Vieillefond et al., "Prospective multicenter phase ii study of gemcitabine plus platinum salt for metastatic collecting duct carcinoma: results of a GETUG (Groupe d'Etudes des Tumeurs Uro-Génitales) study," *Journal of Urology*, vol. 177, no. 5, pp. 1698–1702, 2007.

[20] R.-N. Zhao, L.-H. Nie, R. Gong et al., "Active targeted therapy for metastatic collecting duct carcinoma of the kidney: a case report and review of the literature," *International Urology and Nephrology*, vol. 45, no. 4, pp. 1017–1021, 2013.

[21] N. M. Tannir, E. Plimack, C. Ng et al., "A phase 2 trial of sunitinib in patients with advanced non-clear cell renal cell carcinoma," *European Urology*, vol. 62, no. 6, pp. 1013–1019, 2012.

[22] J. Ansari, A. Fatima, S. Chaudhri, R. I. Bhatt, M. Wallace, and N. D. James, "Sorafenib induces therapeutic response in a patient with metastatic collecting duct carcinoma of kidney," *Onkologie*, vol. 32, no. 1-2, pp. 44–46, 2009.

[23] Y. Hu, H. Zhou, G. Wang, Z. Song, C. Zhao, and Y. Wang, "Collecting duct carcinoma of the kidney: a case report," *Oncology Letters*, vol. 9, no. 6, pp. 2902–2904, 2015.

[24] G. Wong and J. R. Chapman, "Cancers after renal transplantation," *Transplantation Reviews*, vol. 22, no. 2, pp. 141–149, 2008.

[25] I. Doycheva, S. Amer, and K. D. Watt, "De novo malignancies after transplantation: risk and surveillance strategies," *Medical Clinics of North America*, vol. 100, no. 3, pp. 551–567, 2016.

[26] B. L. Kasiske, J. J. Snyder, D. T. Gilbertson, and C. Wang, "Cancer after kidney transplantation in the United States," *The American Journal of Transplantation*, vol. 4, no. 6, pp. 905–913, 2004.

[27] T. Klatte and M. Marberger, "Renal cell carcinoma of native kidneys in renal transplant patients," *Current Opinion in Urology*, vol. 21, no. 5, pp. 376–379, 2011.

[28] G. M. Frasca, S. Sandrini, L. Cosmai et al., "Renal cancer in kidney transplanted patients," *Journal of Nephrology*, vol. 28, no. 6, pp. 659–668, 2015.

[29] S. Domhan, M. Zeier, and A. Abdollahi, "Immunosuppressive therapy and post-transplant malignancy," *Nephrology Dialysis Transplantation*, vol. 24, no. 4, pp. 1097–1103, 2009.

[30] W. Wong, J.-P. Venetz, N. Tolkoff-Rubin, and M. Pascual, "2005 Immunosuppressive strategies in kidney transplantation: which role for the calcineurin inhibitors?" *Transplantation*, vol. 80, no. 3, pp. 289–296, 2005.

[31] M. Guba, C. Graeb, K.-W. Jauch, and E. K. Geissler, "Pro- and anti-cancer effects of immunosuppressive agents used in organ transplantation," *Transplantation*, vol. 77, no. 12, pp. 1777–1782, 2004.

[32] M. M. Javaid, S. Chowdhury, A. Henderson, and J. Olsburgh, "Advanced native kidney renal cell carcinoma in renal transplant recipients: role of sirolimus as dual anti-cancer and anti-rejection agent," *Clinical Nephrology*, vol. 79, no. 2, pp. 154–160, 2013.

[33] J. Alberu, M. D. Pascoe, J. M. Campistol et al., "Lower malignancy rates in renal allograft recipients converted to sirolimus-based, calcineurin inhibitor-free immunotherapy: 24-month results from the CONVERT trial," *Transplantation*, vol. 92, no. 3, pp. 303–310, 2011.

[34] J. M. Campistol, J. Eris, R. Oberbauer et al., "Sirolimus therapy after early cyclosporine withdrawal reduces the risk for cancer in adult renal transplantation," *Journal of the American Society of Nephrology*, vol. 17, no. 2, pp. 581–589, 2006.

[35] R. J. Motzer, B. Escudier, S. Oudard et al., "Efficacy of everolimus in advanced renal cell carcinoma: a double-blind, randomised, placebo-controlled phase III trial," *The Lancet*, vol. 372, no. 9637, pp. 449–456, 2008.

[36] R. Kanesvaran, K. Watt, J. D. Turnbull, A. J. Armstrong, M. C. Wolkowiez, and D. J. George, "A single-arm phase 1b study of everolimus and sunitinib in patients with advanced renal cell carcinoma," *Clinical Genitourinary Cancer*, vol. 13, no. 4, pp. 319–327, 2015.

[37] T. Ikezoe, C. Nishioka, T. Tasaka et al., "The antitumor effects of sunitinib (formerly SU11248) against a variety of human hematologic malignancies: enhancement of growth inhibition via inhibition of mammalian target of rapamcycin signaling," *Molecular Cancer Therapeutics*, vol. 5, no. 10, pp. 2522–2530, 2006.

[38] P. H. Patel, P. L. Senico, R. E. Curiel, and R. J. Motzer, "Phase i study combining treatment with temsirolimus and sunitinib malate in patients with advanced renal cell carcinoma," *Clinical Genitourinary Cancer*, vol. 7, no. 1, pp. 24–27, 2009.

[39] A. M. Molina, D. R. Feldman, M. H. Voss et al., "Phase 1 trial of everolimus plus sunitinib in patients with metastatic renal cell carcinoma," *Cancer*, vol. 118, no. 7, pp. 1868–1876, 2012.

[40] C. Porta, L. Cosmai, M. Gallieni, P. Pedrazzoli, and F. Malberti, "Renal effects of targeted anticancer therapies," *Nature Reviews Nephrology*, vol. 11, no. 6, pp. 354–370, 2015.

[41] P. J. Pickhardt, "Collecting duct carcinoma arising in a solitary kidney: imaging findings," *Clinical Imaging*, vol. 23, no. 2, pp. 115–118, 1999.

[42] J. N. Voss, N. M. Nkwam, T. A. McCulloch, and G. S. Mann, "Collecting duct carcinoma with cardiac metastases: a case report & literature review," *Urology Case Reports*, vol. 5, pp. 27–30, 2016.

Reconstruction of a Damaged Lower Polar Artery for Kidney Transplantation Using Tubularised Donor Aorta

A. J. Vicéns-Morton, C. Callaghan, and J. Olsburgh

Guy's and St Thomas NHS Foundation Trust, Renal Department, London, UK

Correspondence should be addressed to A. J. Vicéns-Morton; ajvm81@yahoo.com

Academic Editor: Ryszard Grenda

Introduction. Live donors, extended donor criteria, and the maximum usage of organs with anatomical variants are some of the mechanisms used to increase the number of organs available. *Case.* We present the case of a kidney transplant, in which the organ had an iatrogenic injury to a lower pole arterial branch during retrieval. The donor was a 35-year-old male (DCD, Maastricht III). The right kidney was accepted; it had three veins in a single cava patch and three renal arteries, the main artery with aorta patch that is 8 cm long. A small lower pole artery was sectioned during retrieval surgery at approximately 1 cm from its origin as well as a third small mid-lower pole artery. The lower pole damaged artery was reconstructed using tubularised aorta patch to a total length of 5 cm. No additional donor vessels had been sent. After construction of the tubulised aorta, E-E anastomosis to the damaged polar artery was done with interrupted 7-0 Prolene sutures. *Conclusion.* While the waiting list for a kidney continues to rise and we continue to have organ shortness, vascular retrieval injury should not be an absolute contraindication for transplant.

1. Introduction

Kidney transplantation is the gold standard renal replacement therapy for patients suffering from end-stage renal disease (ESRD); it is more cost effective than haemodialysis and provides a better quality of life [1]. With the advance of medicine and the increased life expectancy, the demand for organs has increased globally.

Many novel techniques and protocols have been introduced in order to increase the number of organs available. Live donors were responsible for 31,5% of kidney transplants in the UK last year (according to NHS-BT, 2972 kidneys were transplanted; 937 were from a live donor). Also, the use of "extended donor criteria" and the maximum usage of organs with anatomical and/or vascular variants are mechanisms used to increase the number of organs available, although this makes great demands on the transplant surgeons.

We present the case of a kidney transplant, in which the organ had an iatrogenic injury to a lower pole arterial branch occurring during retrieval. Reconstruction was performed using donor's tubularised aortic patch and the recipient has had a satisfactory outcome. To the best of our knowledge, this is the first case report of this technique.

2. Case

The donor was a 35-year-old male, Maastricht category III, who died after cardiac arrest (DCD) due to intracranial haemorrhage secondary to trauma. The right kidney was sent to another centre first and declined due to vascular damage. It then went through the fast-track scheme and was accepted by our team at Guy's Hospital. Once we had the kidney, the initial evaluation showed a right kidney, with three veins in a single cava patch, three renal arteries, the main artery with aorta patch that is 8 cm long, a small lower pole artery, which was sectioned during retrieval surgery at approximately 1 cm from its origin, and a third small mid-lower pole artery. The ureter had bifid renal pelvis.

During bench surgery the kidney was well perfused well with Soltran solution. From the three veins in the single cava patch, it was decided to ligate the posterior branch in order to allow the single patch to be more mobile. The small mid-lower pole artery was already damaged and was deemed unreconstructable and was therefore tied off. The main artery was left with a 1 cm aortic patch. The lower pole damaged artery was reconstructed using tubularised aorta patch to a total length of 5 cm. No additional donor vessels had been sent.

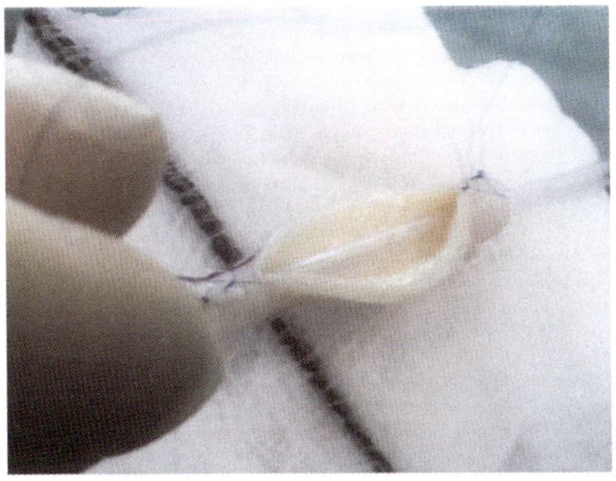

Figure 1: Aortic patch over Nelaton 8 ch catheter.

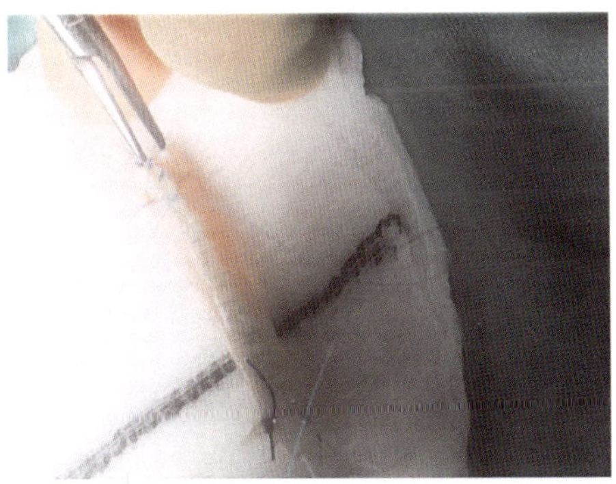

Figure 2: Aortic patch over Nelaton 8 ch catheter.

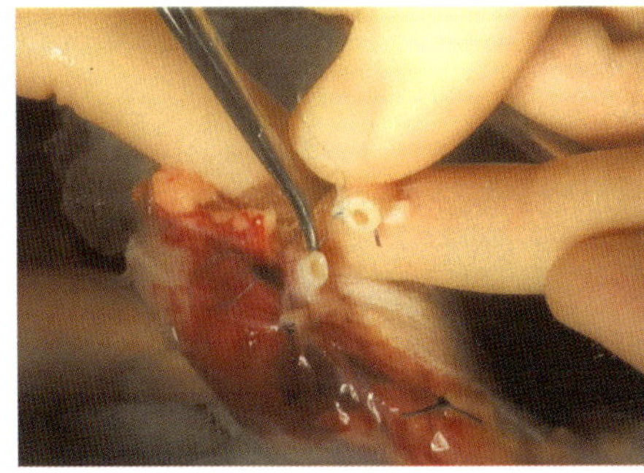

Figure 3: Start of the E-E anastomosis between tubulised aortic patch and polar renal artery.

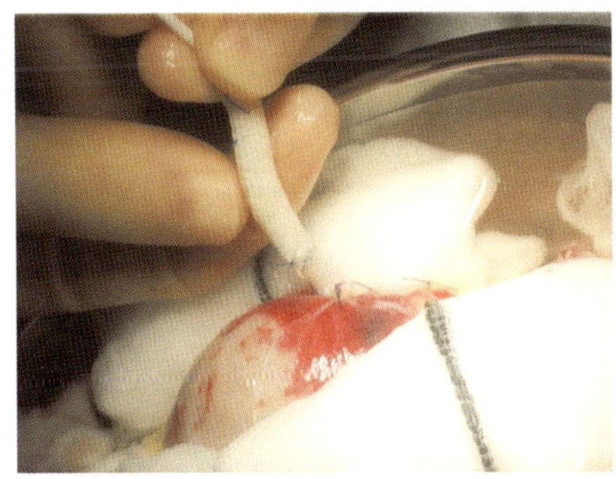

Figure 4: Completed E-E anastomosis between tubulised aortic patch and polar renal artery.

Although the inferior epigastric artery is sometimes preferred for this kind of reconstruction, in this case, it would probably have been too small for the reconstruction; also, the availability of a long and healthy aortic patch and the fact that during benching we did not know the status of the recipient vessels made us decide to take this approach.

The reconstruction was carried out with an aorta patch that is 5 cm in length that was part of the main artery patch of the organ. Using an 8 ch Nelaton bladder catheter as a mold a 5 cm long aorta segment was tubularised using 3 7-0 Prolene interrupted stiches in the distal area to avoid stenosis and Prolene 7-0 continuous suture in the rest of the patch to minimize bleeding risk. After construction of the tubulised aorta, E-E anastomosis to the damaged polar artery was done with interrupted 7-0 Prolene (Figures 1–4 showing steps of the vascular reconstruction).

The recipient was 68-year-old male, with past medical history of ESRD secondary to IgA nephropathy on peritoneal dialysis and no other medical issues nor surgical procedures. After a detailed discussion with the patient, regarding the benefits and the risks due to the surgery and donors/organ characteristics, the patient was happy to proceed and signed the consent.

Transplant surgery was performed in the right iliac fossa with an extraperitoneal approach to the iliac vessels. The common cava patch was anastomosed to the recipient's external iliac vein. The main artery was anastomosed to the common iliac artery. Finally the reconstructed artery with the tubulised patch anastomosed the external iliac artery. After completion of all three vascular anastomoses the kidney was reperfused (Figures 5, 6, and 7). The ureter was anastomosed to the bladder over a double J stent. A Robinson drain was left and wound was closed. The cold ischemic time was 27 hours and 15 minutes and warm ischemic time was 75 min.

There were no immediate postoperative complications. The first ultrasound was performed two hours after finishing the surgery in the recovery ward, showing good perfusion of the kidney.

After 48 hours a second ultrasound was performed. The presence of a superficial haematoma within the subcutaneous tissues and slightly reduced perfusion within the interpolar region was reported; otherwise appearance of the transplant kidney was satisfactory.

Haemoglobin fell from 11.2 (preoperatively) to 6.4 gr/dl. A decision to transfuse two units of blood cells and a relook surgery was reached. There was subcutaneous and perigraft haematoma and no active bleeding. The three vascular anastomoses were identified, both arteries, main and reconstructed, had good thrill, and the vein was soft and had good outflow. A new drain was left at the surgical site and wound closure was performed.

Three days later, the ultrasound was repeated showing that the right iliac fossa transplant kidney had normal cortical thickness and appearance. There was no pelvicalyceal dilatation. The previously demonstrated superficial collection was no longer present. There was satisfactory global vascularity. The sampled interlobular and arcuate vessels demonstrate

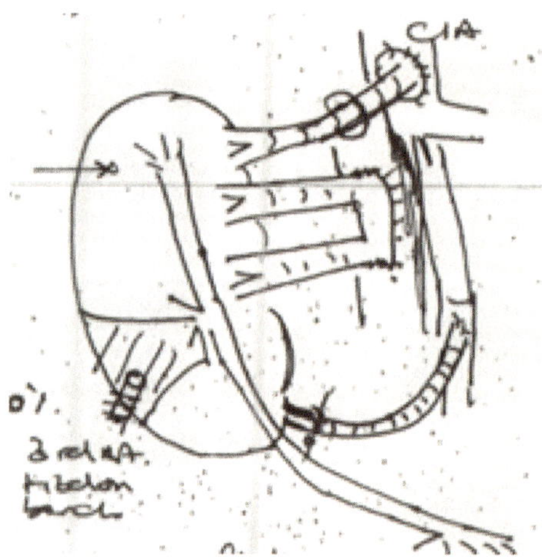

Figure 5: Drawing of the transplant showing ischemic area and all three vascular anastomoses.

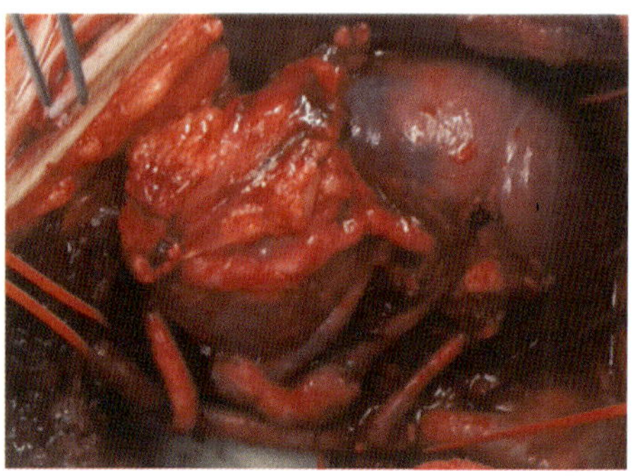

Figure 6: Kidney after reperfusion, all three vascular anastomoses.

normal flow with resistive indices between 0.65 and 0.8. The two renal arteries and veins had normal spectral waveforms, with a final impression of normal appearances of right iliac fossa transplant kidney.

Ureteric stent was removed at week 4 after transplant. Three months after transplantation the patient was stable and had no dialysis requirements with creatinine of 187.

3. Discussion

Donor kidneys with damaged vessels are often declined when offered for transplantation because of increased risk of thrombosis, bleeding, or compromised renal function. The use of these organs represents a technical challenge to the transplant surgeons [2].

The retrieval technique has a definitive impact on the final outcome after transplantation. During harvesting of the kidneys all the structures should be carefully identified. Renal arteries should be preserved and explanted with a common aortic patch when possible. Polar arteries may originate far away from the main renal artery, for example, common iliac artery. If a common patch is impossible to preserve, patches for each artery should be obtained. All the arteries and veins as well as existing patches must be dissected from

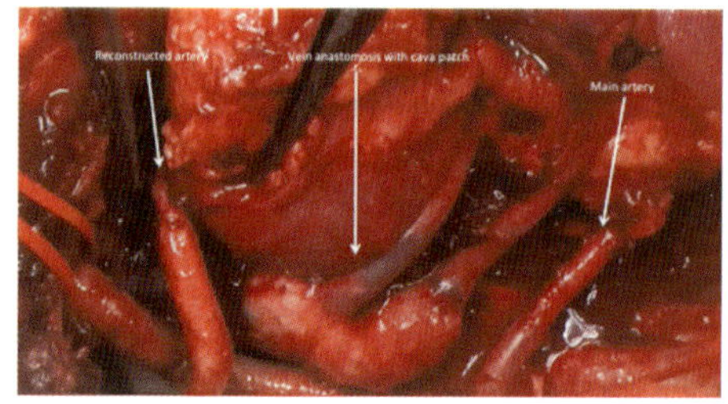

Figure 7: Close look at all three vascular anastomoses after reperfusion.

perivascular tissue. Cannulation of every single artery and perfusion should be performed ex vivo immediately [1].

Some of the problems that can be found in the organs are arteriosclerosis, renal artery stenosis, and intimal desquamation requiring shortening of the renal artery. Generally patches with severe arteriosclerosis and intimal lesions should be removed [1].

The presence of vascular anomalies, disease of the vessels, or iatrogenic injury to the vasculature during organ procurement may necessitate reconstruction of these vessels ex vivo prior to transplantation to salvage these allografts for transplant [3].

Some of the techniques most frequently used for reconstructing vessels include end-to-side (E-S) anastomosis of a branch vessel to the main artery, anastomosis of a branch vessel to the aortic patch, side-to-side (S-S) anastomosis of two aortic patches, anastomosing two renal arteries together to form a single stem, end-to-end (E-E) anastomosis of the main renal artery to a donor arterial graft, E-E anastomosis of the main renal artery to a synthetic graft, and anastomosis of a polar artery to the inferior epigastric artery of the recipient [3].

Reconstruction of the donor renal artery is associated with higher rates of arterial complications postoperatively [3]. Ex vivo reconstruction of the artery is a significant risk factor for the development of arterial thrombosis and arterial stenosis postoperatively [4]. The renal artery stenosis, the most frequent vascular complication after renal transplant and vascular reconstruction, increases this risk [3].

The 5-year graft survival for kidneys with reconstructed renal arteries was 84.3% in deceased donor renal transplantations (86.1% without arterial reconstruction) [5].

The gold standard for evaluation of the perfusion after renal transplantation is colour duplex sonography. The method is cost effective and suitable to detect vascular problems [6]. Further imaging diagnostic tools include angiography and renal scintigraphy. When doubts persist, a second surgical look should be indicated [1].

4. Conclusion

While the waiting list for a kidney continues to rise and we continue to have organ shortness, vascular retrieval injury should not be an absolute contraindication for transplantation. There are many different options and techniques available in order to repair vascular damage. We describe a new technique using the aortic patch. Which technique to use will depend on the vascular defect we are dealing with and the availability of extra vessels sent by the retrieval team.

References

[1] J. H. Beckmann, S. Jackobs, and J. Klempnauer, "Arterial reconstruction in kidney transplantation," *Transplantationsmedizin: Organ der Deutschen Transplantationsgesellschaft*, vol. 20, no. 1, pp. 2–7, 2008.

[2] M. H. Kamel, A. A. Thomas, P. Mohan, and D. P. Hickey, "Renal vessel reconstruction in kidney transplantation using a polytetrafluoroethylene (PTFE) vascular graft," *Nephrology Dialysis Transplantation* , vol. 22, no. 4, pp. 1030–1032, 2007.

[3] L. C. McLoughlin, N. F. Davis, C. M. Dowling et al., "Ex vivo reconstruction of the donor renal artery in renal transplantation: A case-control study," *Transplant International*, vol. 5, pp. 458–466, 2014.

[4] T. Bessede, S. Droupy, Y. Hammoudi et al., "Surgical prevention and management of vascular complications of kidney transplantation," *Transplant International*, vol. 25, no. 9, pp. 994–1001, 2012.

[5] M. Duran, "Vascular Challenges in Renal Transplantation," *Annals of Transplantation*, vol. 19, pp. 464–471, 2014.

[6] J. Radermacher, M. Mengel, S. Ellis et al., "The renal arterial resistance index and renal allograft survival," *The New England Journal of Medicine*, vol. 349, no. 2, pp. 115–124, 2003.

47

Immune Reconstitution Inflammatory Syndrome Occurring in a Kidney Transplant Patient with Extrapulmonary Tuberculosis

Jose Iglesias,[1,2] Kandria Jumil Ledesma,[3] Paul J. Couto,[3] and Jessie Liu[4]

[1] *Department of Nephrology, Jersey Shore University Medical Center, Neptune, NJ 07753, USA*
[2] *Rowan University School of Osteopathic Medicine, Stratford, NJ 08084, USA*
[3] *American University of Antigua College of Medicine, Coolidge, Antigua and Barbuda*
[4] *Ocean Renal Associates, 210 Jack Martin Boulevard, Brick, NJ 08724, USA*

Correspondence should be addressed to Jose Iglesias; jiglesias23@gmail.com

Academic Editor: Binnaz Handan Ozdemir

Tuberculosis (TB) occurring in solid organ transplantation (SOT) is associated with significant morbidity and mortality usually due to delays in diagnosis, drug toxicity encountered with antimycobacterial therapy, and drug-drug interactions. TB in SOT patients may mimic other infectious and noninfectious posttransplant complications such as posttransplant lymphoproliferative disorder (PTLD) and systemic cytomegalovirus infection. Immune reconstitution inflammatory syndrome (IRIS) is a host response resulting in paradoxical worsening of an infectious disease which occurs after the employment of effective therapy and reversal of an immunosuppressed state. We describe the development of immune reconstitution inflammatory syndrome (IRIS), a unique complication occurring during the treatment of extrapulmonary tuberculosis occurring after transplant which resulted from decreasing immunosuppression in a patient who received Alemtuzumab induction therapy. Although (IRIS) has been originally described in HIV/AIDS patients receiving highly active antiretroviral therapy (HAART), solid organ transplant recipients with diagnosed or occult TB whose immune system may undergo immune reconstitution during their posttransplant course represent a new high risk group.

1. Introduction

SOT recipients have a high risk of developing TB during the posttransplant period usually due to reactivation of latent infection [1, 2]. Extrapulmonary and disseminated TB is a common presentation and poses diagnostic challenges and delays in diagnosis [3–5]. Treatment of TB in patients who have received SOT poses many therapeutic dilemmas due to drug interactions and drug toxicity [6, 7]. IRIS is a recognized complication of HIV/AIDS patients with TB undergoing HAART [8–10]. IRIS has recently been described with increasing frequency in solid organ transplant recipients who are undergoing treatment for TB and other opportunistic infections who have necessarily had to have their immunosuppression curtailed [9, 10]. Although IRIS has been increasingly reported in SOT recipients, this entity may still remain unrecognized. Underrecognition of IRIS in these patients may lead to extensive testing, unnecessary changes in therapy, and decreases in immunosuppression. We present an illustrative case of IRIS during treatment of nonpulmonary TB in the setting of Alemtuzumab induction therapy occurring 3 months after renal transplantation.

2. Case Report

A 32-year-old Asian woman received a successful two-antigen mismatched deceased donor renal transplant. She underwent Alemtuzumab and Methylprednisone induction. The immediate posttransplant course was uncomplicated. She was discharged with a nadir serum creatinine of 0.9 mg/dL. Immunosuppression consisted of Mycophenolic acid delayed release (MMF) 720 mg twice daily

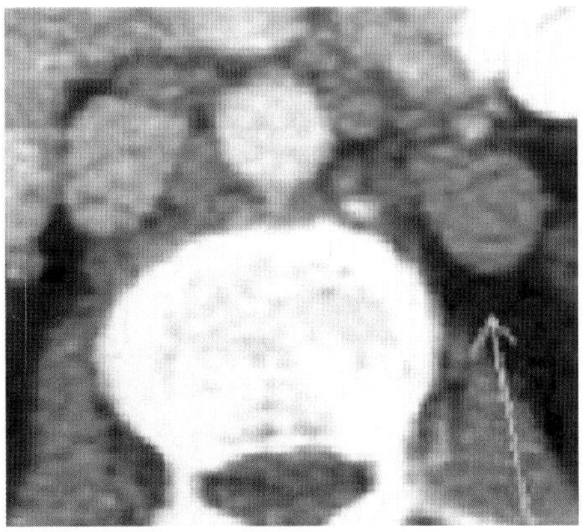

FIGURE 1: CT scan revealing para-aortic lymphadenopathy.

and Tacrolimus therapy (target trough 9–12 ng/mL). Three months after transplant the patient developed elevated liver enzymes associated with fever of 102°F. Initial blood cultures, CMV, parvovirus B-19 and EBV by quantitative polymerase chain reaction were negative. Computed tomographic imaging studies (CT) revealed periaortic lymphadenopathy (Figure 1). Liver biopsy revealed noncaseating granulomas and no evidence of posttransplant lymphoproliferative disorder (Figure 2(a)). Para-aortic lymph node biopsy revealed acid fast bacilli which were confirmed to be Mycobacterium tuberculosis (MTB) by nucleic acid amplification test and culture (Figure 2(b)). Review of pretransplant records revealed that the patient developed a 5 mm induration on tuberculin skin testing. Based on a history of prior administration of the BCG vaccine and a completely normal radiograph of the chest, the decision to forego Isoniazid prophylaxis against latent TB was made. Treatment was begun with Isoniazid 300 mg daily, Rifampin 450 mg daily, Ethambutol 800 mg daily, and Pyrazinamide 1000 mg daily. Her immunosuppression was reduced to maintain target Tacrolimus trough levels of 6 ng/mL and MMF was decreased to 180 mg twice daily. Resolution of symptoms occurred after initiation of therapy and reduction of immunosuppression. Five months after initiation of therapy the patient developed fever, weight loss, back pain, and weakness. CT scan demonstrated multiple lobulated peripherally enhancing fluid collections within the iliopsoas muscles as well as within the left hepatic lobe, most suggestive of abscesses (Figure 3). Empirical intravenous Ampicillin/Sulbactam was initiated at 3.1 grams every 8 hours. She underwent drainage of fluid collections, and gram stain, and cultures were obtained. Gram stain and acid fast stain of fluid revealed multiple neutrophils and no organisms. Fluid cultures revealed no growth of bacteria or MTB. The diagnosis of IRIS was established, corticosteroids were not administered, and the patient was maintained on two-drug anti-TB therapy consisting of Rifampin and Isoniazid. During the course of therapy, she was rehospitalized for fever of unknown origin.

Fever, abdominal pain, and fullness slowly resolved over the course of therapy. Repeat CT imaging of the abdomen revealed resolving iliopsoas fluid collections (Figure 4). After 4 months of 4-drug regimen, the patient was continued on Rifampin and Isoniazid. The patient finished one year of antituberculosis therapy and has remained symptom-free with a functioning allograft. This patient received lymphocyte depleting induction with Alemtuzumab and her immunosuppression was reduced after the diagnosis of active TB. As IRIS may occur in the setting of treatment for TB and immune reconstitution, the time course of her illness and her total lymphocyte count are displayed (Figure 5).

3. Discussion

SOT recipients have a high risk of developing TB during the posttransplant period usually due to reactivation of latent infection [1, 2, 4]. MTB infection in SOT can result in extremely high mortality rates and high rates of organ rejection [1, 3, 4, 7]. Extrapulmonary and disseminated TB may occur in up to 12–50% of posttransplant TB cases and is particularly challenging as it may mimic other infectious and noninfectious complications observed in the posttransplant course such as PTLD and systemic opportunistic fungal and viral infections [3–5, 7]. Drug toxicity and drug interactions are important issues to consider in SOT recipients undergoing antimycobacterial therapy [1, 4, 6, 7].

Rifampin induces hepatic and intestinal CYP3A4 resulting in protracted difficulty in maintaining therapeutic drug levels of calcineurin inhibitors (CNI), inhibitors of the mammalian target of Rapamycin (MTOR), and corticosteroids [11, 12]. Rifampin also induces intestinal, renal, and hepatic enzymes involved in the conversion of MMF into the active mycophenolic acid (MPA) resulting in marked decrease in active drug [13]. Acute rejection may occur and IRIS may develop as immunosuppression is decreased by clinicians and as concurrent drug-drug interactions occur [1, 2, 4, 9]. Thus, in the clinical setting of transplantation, treatment of TB can result in rejection rates and allograft loss in 33% of cases [1, 2, 4, 7].

IRIS can be described as a pathological hyperinflammatory host response when reversal of either pathogen or iatrogenic immunosuppression occurs resulting in paradoxical worsening of disease during effective antimicrobial therapy [9]. IRIS has been reported commonly in the HIV/AIDS population with MTB receiving HAART [9, 10]. In SOT, IRIS has been reported in recipients undergoing treatment for mycotic infections, BK polyoma nephropathy, and systemic cytomegalovirus (CMV) [9]. IRIS has recently been described with increasing frequency in SOT recipients who are undergoing treatment for TB and other opportunistic infections who have necessarily had to have their immunosuppression curtailed [9, 10, 14]. Review of the literature documenting IRIS in SOT has revealed 3 case reports and 1 retrospective study documenting 9 cases, which include 6 liver, 4 kidney, 1 heart, and 1 heart lung transplant [10, 14–16].

In SOT undergoing treatment for active TB, IRIS usually occurs within 3 months [10]. Risk factors appear to be liver transplantation, use of Rifampin, CMV infection, and the presence of extrapulmonary TB [10]. Although IRIS has been increasingly reported in solid organ transplant recipients, this entity may still remain unrecognized.

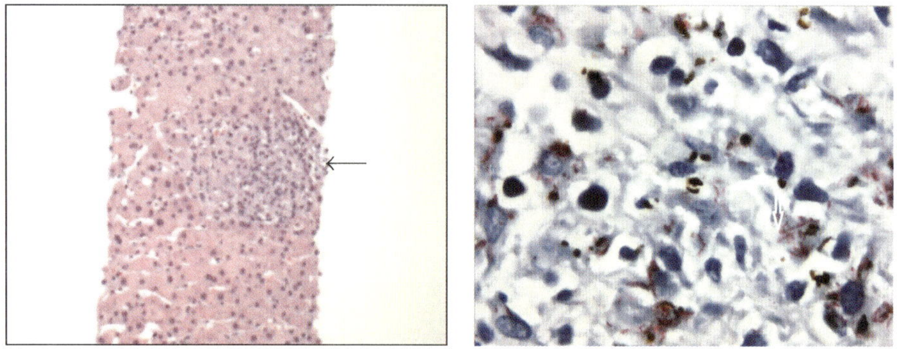

(a) (b)

Figure 2: (a) Liver biopsy with Hematoxylin and Eosin stain demonstrating a noncaseating granuloma. (b) Para-aortic lymph node biopsy with Acid fast stain demonstrating the presence of multiple acid fast bacilli.

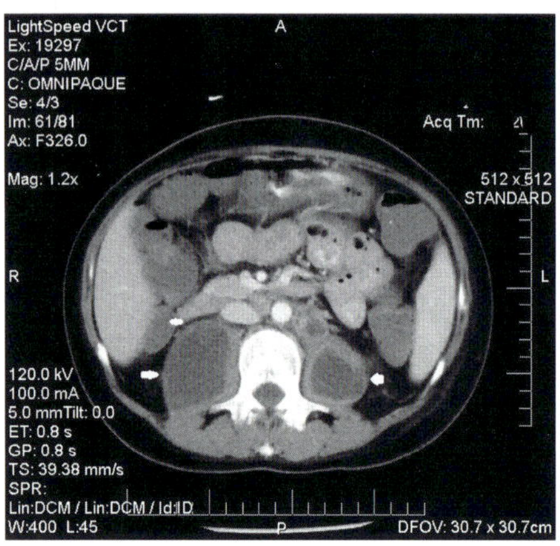

Figure 3: Abdominal CT scan demonstrating large hypodense iliopsoas fluid collections (white arrows).

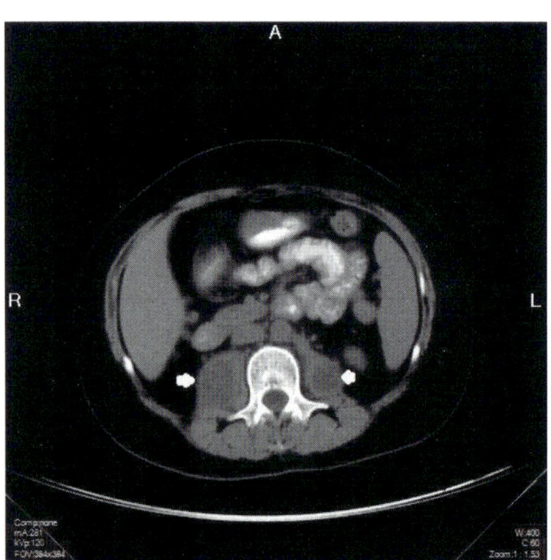

Figure 4: Abdominal CT scan demonstrating resolving iliopsoas fluid collections.

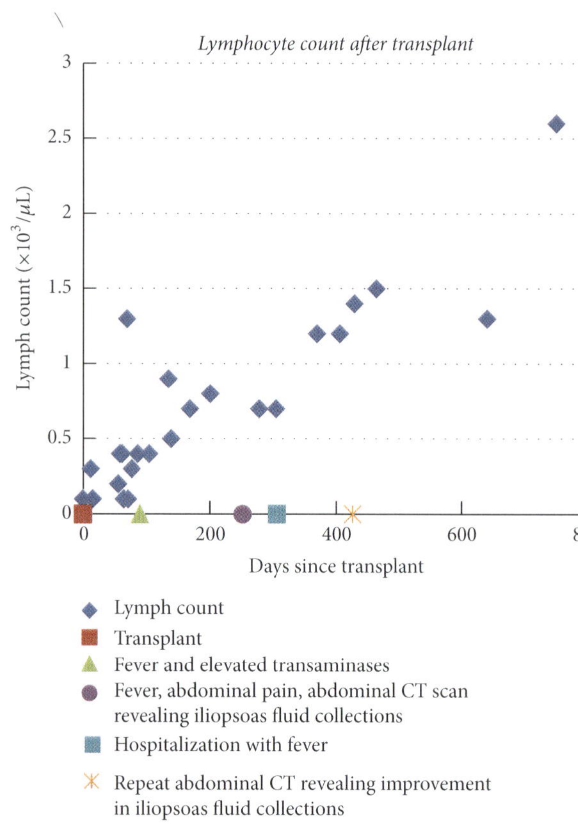

Figure 5: Timeline of clinical events and total lymphocyte count (diamond) from the time of transplant (red square), onset of elevated transaminases and fever (triangle), development of fever and abdominal masses (circle), rehospitalization with fever (blue square), and clinical improvement (star).

Although a working paradigm of the pathophysiology of IRIS occurring in the posttransplant setting has not been established, current evidence suggests an imbalance between pathogen directed host inflammatory (Th1, Th17) and anti-inflammatory (Th-2, Tregs) effector cells resulting in hyperinflammatory response to a pathogen with ensuing tissue damage [9]. Both MTB infection and immunosuppressive therapy have effects on T cell repertoire resulting in polarization towards a Th2 cell response [9, 10, 17]. TB infection results in the modulation of the immune response by increasing the generation of Cd4 Th2 subtypes and Treg cells [9, 17, 18]. In the clinical setting of transplantation the polarization of Cd4 cells into Th1 and Th17 subtypes mediates allograft rejection [9]. Conversely, increases in Tregs and polarization towards Cd4 Th2 cells lead to degrees of tolerance. Calcineurin inhibitors (CNI), mycophenolate (MMF), corticosteroids, and MTOR inhibitors decrease Th1 and Th2 generation [9, 19]. Furthermore, corticosteroids increase Th2 and Treg generation [9, 19]. MTOR inhibitors result in decrease in Th1, Th2, and Th17 cells while increasing generation of Tregs [9, 19, 20]. Induction therapy with the lymphocyte depleting antibody Alemtuzumab and antithymocytic globulins results in decreases in Th1 and TH17 Tcell repertoire and preferential increases in Treg cells during the proliferation and recovery period that occurs after T cell depletion [19, 21].

It is important to also consider epidemiological data involving TB to further examine high risk population subgroups within which our patient resides. According to the Centers for Disease Control and Prevention (CDC), one-third of the world's population is infected with TB [22]. In 2015, the TB incidence rate per 100,000 persons has remained relatively stable at approximately 3.0 since 2013 [22]. Alternative data collected from 1993 to 2006 found that almost one-fifth of US tuberculosis cases are extrapulmonary in nature [23]. There is an especially high incidence of TB in the United States in Asian patients. According to a report on tuberculosis trends conducted by the CDC, compared to non-Hispanic Caucasians, the TB incidence rate among the Asian population was 28.5 times greater, at 18.2 cases per 100,000 persons, the highest among all racial groups [24]. With respect to patients with chronic renal failure on hemodialysis, there is also a high prevalence of latent TB infection. Population-based cohort studies have designated relative risks of TB ranging from 3.4 to 25.3 in dialysis patients compared with the general population [25]. The use of the anti-CD52 monoclonal antibody, Alemtuzumab, has also been linked to the development of various opportunistic infections, including TB. In a Hong Kong study, researchers recommended TB prophylaxis in those who are administered Alemtuzumab after 7 out of 27 immunosuppressed patients developed TB, 3 of which were extrapulmonary [26]. However, it must be noted that the large variety of potential infections with Alemtuzumab therapy makes it difficult to have universal prophylaxis strategies and rather requires vigilant surveillance and awareness by the treating physician [27]. This is true not only for those treated with Alemtuzumab, but for all high risk population subgroups.

4. Conclusion

Immune Reconstitution Inflammatory Syndrome (IRIS) has primarily been studied in the context of HIV/AIDS-associated paradoxical exacerbation of infection symptoms after recovery of an immunosuppressed state. Although there have been increasing reports of IRIS occurring in the setting of SOT and infections with MTB and a variety of opportunistic infections, we believe that IRIS is an underrecognized complication in this high risk group. This report demonstrates the difficulties encountered when IRIS develops in a SOT recipient during the management of extrapulmonary MTB infection by reduction in immunosuppression and institution of appropriate antimycobacterial therapy. It is possible that decreasing immunosuppression may have further exacerbated the development of IRIS in this patient. The potential for the development of IRIS in SOT with MTB may have an impact on treatment strategies for physicians managing transplant immunosuppression. Clinicians should therefore be cognizant of the potential of IRIS not only in HIV/AIDS cases but also in solid organ transplant patients. Caution should be used in decreasing immunosuppression in SOT patients undergoing treatment for MTB. Developing greater awareness among treatment providers about the paradoxical nature of IRIS is essential for the safe and proper management of patients that have undergone therapeutic immunosuppression for transplantation. What is clear is that further investigation into IRIS associated with solid organ transplantation must be completed to develop not only our understanding but also appropriate treatment protocol for this complex phenomenon.

Authors' Contributions

All authors contributed equally to writing the case report, reviewing literature, and arranging graphics.

References

[1] J. M. Aguado, J. A. Herrero, J. Gavaldá et al., "Clinical presentation and outcome of tuberculosis in kidney, liver, and heart transplant recipients in Spain," *Transplantation*, vol. 63, no. 9, pp. 1278–1286, 1997.

[2] N. Singh and D. L. Paterson, "Mycobacterium tuberculosis infection in solid-organ transplant recipients: impact and implications for management," *Clinical Infectious Diseases*, vol. 27, no. 5, pp. 1266–1277, 1998.

[3] J. Torre-Cisneros, A. Doblas, J. M. Aguado et al., "Tuberculosis after solid-organ transplant: incidence, risk factors, and clinical characteristics in the resitra (spanish network of infection in transplantation) cohort," *Clinical Infectious Diseases*, vol. 48, no. 12, pp. 1657–1665, 2009.

[4] P. Muñoz, C. Rodríguez, and E. Bouza, "*Mycobacterium tuberculosis* infection in recipients of solid organ transplants," *Clinical Infectious Diseases*, vol. 40, no. 4, pp. 581–587, 2005.

[5] J.-E. C. Holty and R. R. Sista, "*Mycobacterium tuberculosis* infection in transplant recipients: early diagnosis and treatment of resistant tuberculosis," *Current Opinion in Organ Transplantation*, vol. 14, no. 6, pp. 613–618, 2009.

[6] J. Aguado, J. Torre-Cisneros, J. Fortun et al., "Tuberculosis in solid-organ transplant recipients: consensus statement of the Group for the Study of Infection in transplant recipients (GESITRA) of the Spanish society of infectious diseases and

clinical microbiology," *Clinical Infectious Diseases*, vol. 48, no. 9, pp. 1276–1284, 2009.

[7] J.-E. C. Holty, M. K. Gould, L. Meinke, E. B. Keeffe, and S. J. Ruoss, "Tuberculosis in liver transplant recipients: a systematic review and meta-analysis of individual patient data," *Liver Transplantation*, vol. 15, no. 8, pp. 894–906, 2009.

[8] V. C. C. Cheng, P. L. Ho, R. A. Lee et al., "Clinical spectrum of paradoxical deterioration during antituberculosis therapy in non-HIV-infected patients," *European Journal of Clinical Microbiology and Infectious Diseases*, vol. 21, no. 11, pp. 803–809, 2002.

[9] H.-Y. Sun and N. Singh, "Opportunistic infection-associated immune reconstitution syndrome in transplant recipients," *Clinical Infectious Diseases*, vol. 53, no. 2, pp. 168–176, 2011.

[10] H.-Y. Sun, P. Munoz, J. Torre-Cisneros et al., "Mycobacterium tuberculosis—associated immune reconstitution syndrome in solid-organ transplant recipients," *Transplantation*, vol. 95, no. 9, pp. 1173–1181, 2013.

[11] B. T. Ngo, M. Pascoe, and D. Khan, "Drug interaction between rifampicin and sirolimus in transplant patients," *Saudi Journal of Kidney Diseases and Transplantation*, vol. 22, no. 1, pp. 112–115, 2011.

[12] A. M. Baciewicz, C. R. Chrisman, C. K. Finch, and T. H. Self, "Update on rifampin, rifabutin, and rifapentine drug interactions," *Current Medical Research and Opinion*, vol. 29, no. 1, pp. 1–12, 2013.

[13] D. R. J. Kuypers, G. Verleden, M. Naesens, and Y. Vanrenterghem, "Drug interaction between mycophenolate mofetil and rifampin: possible induction of uridine diphosphate-glucuronosyltransferase," *Clinical Pharmacology and Therapeutics*, vol. 78, no. 1, pp. 81–88, 2005.

[14] S. Place, C. Knoop, M. Remmelink et al., "Paradoxical worsening of tuberculosis in a heart-lung transplant recipient," *Transplant Infectious Disease*, vol. 9, no. 3, pp. 219–224, 2007.

[15] T. Asano, H. Kawamoto, J. Asakuma, T. Tanimoto, H. Kobayashi, and M. Hayakawa, "Paradoxical worsening of tuberculosis after anti-TB therapy in a kidney transplant recipient," *Transplantation Proceedings*, vol. 32, no. 7, pp. 1960–1962, 2000.

[16] A. Mohapatra, G. Basu, I. Sen et al., "Tuberculosis in a renal allograft recipient presenting with intussusception," *Indian Journal of Nephrology*, vol. 22, no. 1, pp. 52–56, 2012.

[17] X. Chen, B. Zhou, M. Li et al., "$CD4^+CD25^+FoxP3^+$ regulatory T cells suppress *Mycobacterium tuberculosis* immunity in patients with active disease," *Clinical Immunology*, vol. 123, no. 1, pp. 50–59, 2007.

[18] K. M. Quinn, R. S. McHugh, F. J. Rich et al., "Inactivation of CD4+CD25+ regulatory T cells during early mycobacterial infection increases cytokine production but does not affect pathogen load," *Immunology and Cell Biology*, vol. 84, no. 5, pp. 467–474, 2006.

[19] A. Demirkiran, T. K. Hendrikx, C. C. Baan, and L. J. W. Van Der Laan, "Impact of immunosuppressive drugs on CD4+ CD25+FOXP3+ regulatory T cells: does in vitro evidence translate to the clinical setting?" *Transplantation*, vol. 85, no. 6, pp. 783–789, 2008.

[20] J. Arias-Diaz, J. A. Ildefonso, J. J. Muñoz, A. Zapata, and E. Jiménez, "Both tacrolimus and sirolimus decrease Th1/Th2 ratio, and increase regulatory T lymphocytes in the liver after ischemia/reperfusion," *Laboratory Investigation*, vol. 89, no. 4, pp. 433–445, 2009.

[21] E. Havari, M. J. Turner, J. Campos-Rivera et al., "Impact of alemtuzumab treatment on the survival and function of human regulatory T cells in vitro," *Immunology*, vol. 141, no. 1, pp. 123–131, 2014.

[22] *Center for Disease Control and Prevention: Tuberculosis (TB) Data and Statistics*, CDC, 2016, https://www.cdc.gov/tb/statistics/.

[23] H. M. Peto, R. H. Pratt, T. A. Harrington, P. A. LoBue, and L. R. Armstrong, "Epidemiology of extrapulmonary tuberculosis in the United States, 1993–2006," *Clinical Infectious Diseases*, vol. 49, no. 9, pp. 1350–1357, 2009.

[24] C. Scott, H. L. Kirking, C. Jeffries, S. F. Price, and R. Pratt, "Tuberculosis trends—United States, 2014," *Morbidity and Mortality Weekly Report*, vol. 64, no. 10, pp. 265–269, 2015.

[25] C. C. Dobler, S. P. McDonald, and G. B. Marks, "Risk of tuberculosis in dialysis patients: a nationwide cohort study," *PLoS ONE*, vol. 6, no. 12, Article ID e29563, 2011.

[26] W.-Y. Au, A. Y. H. Leung, E. W. C. Tse, W. W. W. Cheung, T. W. H. Shek, and Y.-L. Kwong, "High incidence of tuberculosis after alemtuzumab treatment in Hong Kong Chinese patients," *Leukemia Research*, vol. 32, no. 4, pp. 547–551, 2008.

[27] S. I. Martin, F. M. Marty, K. Fiumara, S. P. Treon, J. G. Gribben, and L. R. Baden, "Infectious complications associated with alemtuzumab use for lymphoproliferative disorders," *Clinical Infectious Diseases*, vol. 43, no. 1, pp. 16–24, 2006.

48

Brincidofovir Use after Foscarnet Crystal Nephropathy in a Kidney Transplant Recipient with Multiresistant Cytomegalovirus Infection

Romain Vial,[1,2] Christine Zandotti,[3] Sophie Alain,[4] Alexandre Decourt,[1,2] Noémie Jourde-Chiche,[1,2] Raj Purgus,[1] Charleric Bornet,[5] Laurent Daniel,[2,6] Valérie Moal,[1,2] and Tristan Legris[1]

[1]*Centre de Néphrologie et Transplantation Rénale, Hôpital Conception, Assistance Publique-Hôpitaux de Marseille, Marseille, France*
[2]*Aix-Marseille University, Marseille, France*
[3]*Fédération de Bactériologie-Virologie-Hygiène, Hôpital Timone, Assistance Publique-Hôpitaux de Marseille, Marseille, France*
[4]*Laboratoire de Bactériologie-Virologie-Hygiène, Centre Hospitalier Universitaire, Limoges, France*
[5]*Pharmacie Hospitalière, Hôpital Conception, Assistance Publique-Hôpitaux de Marseille, Marseille, France*
[6]*Laboratoire d'Anatomie Pathologique, Hôpital Timone, Assistance Publique-Hôpitaux de Marseille, Marseille, France*

Correspondence should be addressed to Tristan Legris; tristan.legris@ap-hm.fr

Academic Editor: Frieder Keller

Background. Cytomegalovirus (CMV) antiviral drug resistance constitutes an increasing challenge in transplantation. Foscarnet is usually proposed when resistance for ganciclovir is suspected, but its use is limited by its nephrotoxicity. *Case Presentation.* We report a case of multiresistant CMV disease in a kidney transplant recipient. Foscarnet was prescribed after ganciclovir treatment failure in a patient with two mutations in the UL97 viral gene. Foscarnet induced biopsy-proven kidney crystal precipitation that resulted in severe acute transplant failure and nephrotic syndrome. Despite a large decrease in immunosuppression, CMV disease was not controlled and a salvage therapy with Brincidofovir (BCV), which is an oral lipid conjugate of cidofovir with limited nephrotoxicity, was attempted. Clinical and virological remission was observed after a 21-day course of BCV, despite mild and reversible liver toxicity. However, a new relapse could not be effectively cured by BCV due to a new mutation in the UL54 gene, which is known to confer resistance to cidofovir. A new course of foscarnet finally resulted in prolonged CMV remission. Herein, we present a review of foscarnet nephropathy cases in solid-organ transplanted patients. *Conclusions.* This unique case highlights the potential benefit of BCV use during resistant CMV infection, although mutations in the UL54 gene may limit its therapeutic efficacy. These findings need to be confirmed in clinical trials.

1. Introduction

Human cytomegalovirus (CMV) infections represent a major clinical issue after solid-organ transplantation, especially when the donor's serological status is positive and the recipient is seronegative (D+/R−) [1]. Despite improvement in diagnosis, prevention, and treatment strategies [2–4], concerns related to antiviral drug resistance (ADR) constitute an increasing challenge for the transplant physician. ADR was tested in a retrospective French cohort study of D+/R− kidney transplant recipients up to one year after transplant if the viremia increased during antiviral therapy. ADR was observed in 16% of the 80 patients who were treated preemptively versus 3% of the 32 patients who received 3 months of valganciclovir-based prophylaxis ($p = 0.05$) [5]. Other risk factors for ADR include the type of transplant (highest risk for lung and kidney-pancreas recipients), D+/R− serostatus, delay in commencement of prophylaxis, high peak blood viral load ($>10^5$ copies/ml), increased duration of antiviral exposure, and suboptimal drug concentration [6]. Intravenous ganciclovir (GCV) or oral valganciclovir (vGCV) is recommended as the first-line treatments for CMV disease within the transplant population [2]. Other drugs, such as foscarnet (FOS) and cidofovir (CDV), are typically proposed as second-line therapies when ADR is suspected. However, FOS and CDV cause significant nephrotoxicity, and FOS also induces electrolyte abnormalities. Brincidofovir (BCV), which is a new orally bioavailable lipid acyclic nucleoside phosphonate that is converted intracellularly into CDV diphosphate, has limited renal toxicity [7]. Here, we report a case of BCV use in the setting of FOS nephrotoxicity in a transplant recipient with CMV ADR.

2. Case Presentation

A 42-year-old woman with stage 5D chronic kidney disease related to MYH9-related disease received her first kidney transplant from a familial living donor. Repeated anti-HLA antibody blood testing was negative, despite previous blood transfusions and pregnancies. The A, B, DR, and DQ HLA mismatches were 0/1/1/1, respectively. The CMV serostatus was D+/R−. Her immunosuppressive regimen consisted of an induction with antithymocyte globulins and a maintenance regimen with ciclosporin A, azathioprine, and steroids. She also received cotrimoxazole and vGCV prophylaxis for 6 months (900 mg/d). With the exception of two deep venous thrombosis episodes, the first seven months after transplantation was unremarkable with good transplant function (serum creatinine level = 100 μmol/L). One month after vGCV discontinuation on day (D) 222 after graft, she was admitted for a fever of 38.2°C and epigastric pain without diarrhea. Her biological tests revealed a severe lymphocytopenia (150/mm^3). Her serum creatinine level was 122 μmol/L. The blood and urine cultures and liver and pancreatic tests were unremarkable, whereas her pp65 antigenemia was strongly positive (600 positive cells/200000 polymorphonuclear leukocytes (PC)). The chest X-ray and fundus examination did not suggest pulmonary or retinal CMV involvement. An upper gastrointestinal endoscopy revealed gastritis with a positive CMV polymerase chain reaction (PCR). Due to the diagnosis of possible CMV gastrointestinal disease [4], a first intravenous GCV treatment (10 mg/kg/d) was started together with a decrease in immunosuppression (half azathioprine dose), resulting in a slow but sustained decrease in the CMV antigenemia. Two months of GCV was needed to obtain viral clearance defined by two consecutive weekly negative antigenemia results.

One week after GCV discontinuation on D288, she was readmitted for fever recurrence and abdominal pain and a relapse of CMV disease was observed (antigenemia = 20 PC). No retinitis was found again. As digestive symptoms were similar to recent primary CMV infection, no new upper endoscopy was performed. A new GCV-based treatment (10 mg/kg/day) was started. No clinical or biological improvement was noted after two weeks of treatment (antigenemia = 115 PC) despite azathioprine withdrawal. Genotypic testing for ADR in the UL97 kinase gene revealed two common mutations (A594V and L595S) associated with moderate viral resistance for GCV [13] and no mutation in the UL54 DNA polymerase gene. The kidney graft function was stable (serum creatinine level = 100 μmol/L). Thus, a second-line treatment with intravenous FOS (180 mg/kg/d) was initiated at D306. A fast decrease in the CMV viral load was observed that allowed FOS weaning at D320. A second relapse of CMV infection (same symptoms, antigenemia = 25 PC, blood quantitative CMV PCR = 351000 DNA copies/mL) at D329 led us to restart FOS at the same dose. Unfortunately, 6 days after this new FOS course a severe acute graft failure was noted (serum creatinine level = 450 μmol/L, blood ciclosporin trough level = 200 ng/mL) that was associated with an acute nephrotic syndrome (urinary protein creatinine ratio = 4.5 g/g and serum albumin = 2.6 g/dL). A transplant biopsy showed diffuse tubular necrosis and tubular and intraglomerular crystal deposits that obstructed capillaries and were suggestive of FOS nephropathy. No sign of acute rejection or CMV transplant infection was noted on the biopsy (Figure 1). At that time, the CMV antigenemia had become negative, blood CMV PCR was weak (1381 copies/mL), and FOS was stopped, which allowed a partial reversal of the glomerulopathy and transplant failure (serum creatinine level = 150 μmol/L and proteinuria = 1 g/d).

However, at D341 a third CMV relapse occurred (antigenemia = 78 PC, PCR = 141000 copies/mL). Because the FOS toxicity was recent, we decided to begin a double-dose of GCV therapy [14] together with intravenous immunoglobulins (2 infusions of 0.3 g/kg/d at a 10-day interval) and a decrease in the ciclosporin target trough level (100 ng/mL). One month later, persistent low-grade symptoms and mild but positive CMV antigenemia (5–15 PC) reflected the failure of this regimen. A second genotypic testing for ADR revealed the same L595S mutation in the UL97 gene without mutation in the UL54 gene. To avoid new FOS toxicity, oral BCV was introduced (100 mg orally twice a week) at D376 for 21 days with good results on clinical and viral parameters (negative antigenemia and blood PCR after 17 days). A mild isolated cytolysis (alanine and aspartate aminotransferase (ALT and AST) = 137 and 104 IU/L, respectively) and moderate epigastric pain were observed during therapy. Liver ultrasonography was normal. The liver enzymes returned to normal levels and the abdominal pain disappeared after BCV discontinuation. Nevertheless, at D412 a 4th relapse was observed (antigenemia = 16 PC, blood PCR = 95700 copies/mL) and was again treated with BCV for 15 days (200 mg/week). After 15 days of BCV, persistent diarrhea and abdominal pain indicated a new upper gastrointestinal endoscopy together with a colonoscopy. CMV PCR biopsies of stomach and large bowel were positive (3380 and 3020 copies/mL, respectively). Blood CMV antigenemia and PCR were 9 PC and 38200 copies/mL, respectively, after 15 days of BCV. A new mild and isolated cytolysis (ALT = 143, ASAT = 155 IU/L) appearing at the same time led us to definitely stop BCV. Liver enzymes returned to normal levels after BCV discontinuation. No liver biopsy was performed. A third genotypic ADR test, performed at the end of the second course of BCV, revealed a novel F412L mutation in the UL54 DNA polymerase gene that was associated with moderate resistance for GCV and CDV but not FOS [15]. Before reinitiating FOS, a new transplant biopsy

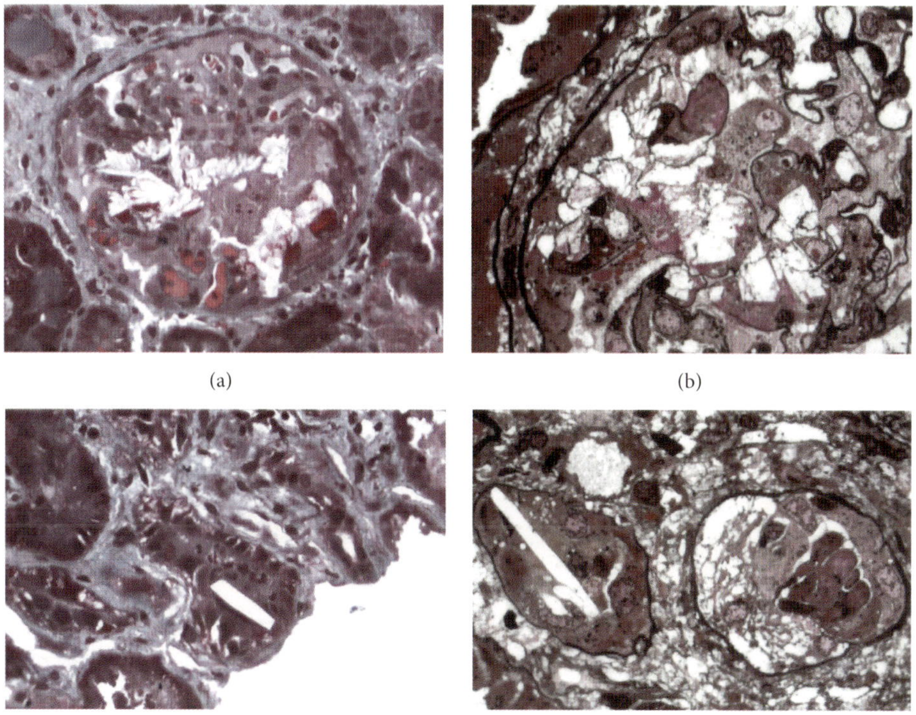

(a) (b) (c) (d)

FIGURE 1: Foscarnet nephropathy in the kidney transplant. (a) Masson's trichrome staining (×200) showed intraglomerular crystalline precipitation obstructing the capillaries and crushing the mesangium together with fibrinoid thrombi. (b) Jones methenamine silver staining (×400) also revealed FOS crystals within the glomerular capillaries. (c) Masson's trichrome staining (×200) showed crystals that resembled short sticks with angular edges in the tubular lumen. (d) Jones methenamine silver staining (×400) also revealed FOS crystals within the tubular lumen.

was performed at D441 (serum creatinine = 150 μmol/L and proteinuria = 1 g/g). Seven of the 25 glomeruli were sclerotic. Interstitial fibrosis and tubular atrophy were mild without crystals, rejection, or CMV signs. A new two-month course of intravenous FOS (50 mg/kg/d, dose tailored to decreased glomerular filtration rate) was necessary to achieve a complete resolution of CMV infection (negative antigenemia and PCR) without any new FOS nephropathy. Figure 2 describes the course of the CMV disease together with the course of immunosuppression and blood lymphocyte counts.

Currently, the patient's overall condition is normal 6 months after the final treatment, without secondary CMV prophylaxis. Repeated CMV antigenemia tests have been negative, and the graft function remains stable (mean creatinine = 130 μmol/L, proteinuria = 0.6 g/g, without anti-HLA antibodies).

3. Discussion

To our knowledge, we report the first published case of refractory CMV infection treated with BCV in a kidney transplant recipient. BCV (formerly CMX001) is a lipid conjugate of CDV and is highly active in vitro against various double-stranded DNA viruses, such as adenoviruses, herpesviruses, human papillomaviruses, polyomaviruses (including BK virus), and orthopoxviruses [7]. BCV can inhibit the UL54 CMV DNA polymerase when it is converted intracellularly into CDV. Interestingly, BCV's in vitro activity is increased by 422-fold compared to CDV [16], probably due to its more efficient cellular uptake facilitated by the lipid chain. In contrast to CDV, which is actively secreted from the blood into kidney proximal tubule cells by organic anion transporters (OAT), BCV is not a substrate of OAT1 and thus has a lower risk of nephrotoxicity.

A phase 2 study of BCV involved 230 CMV-seropositive allogeneic hematopoietic cell transplant (HCT) recipients who were randomized to receive BCV or a placebo to prevent CMV events. The incidence of CMV events was significantly lower among patients who received BCV at a dose of 100 mg twice weekly than among those who received the placebo. Diarrhea, vomiting, and abdominal pain were the most common adverse effects in the group that received this dose. No increased risk of nephrotoxicity was observed [17]. However, in the recent phase 3 SUPPRESS trial, despite an antiviral effect seen at the end of the on-treatment period at week 14 following HCT (with patients who received BCV experiencing fewer clinically significant CMV infections than patients in the placebo group (24 percent versus 38 percent, $p = 0.002$)), the primary endpoint of prevention of significant CMV infection at week 24 was not reached (data reported at the 2016 BMT Tandem Meetings). These clinical results

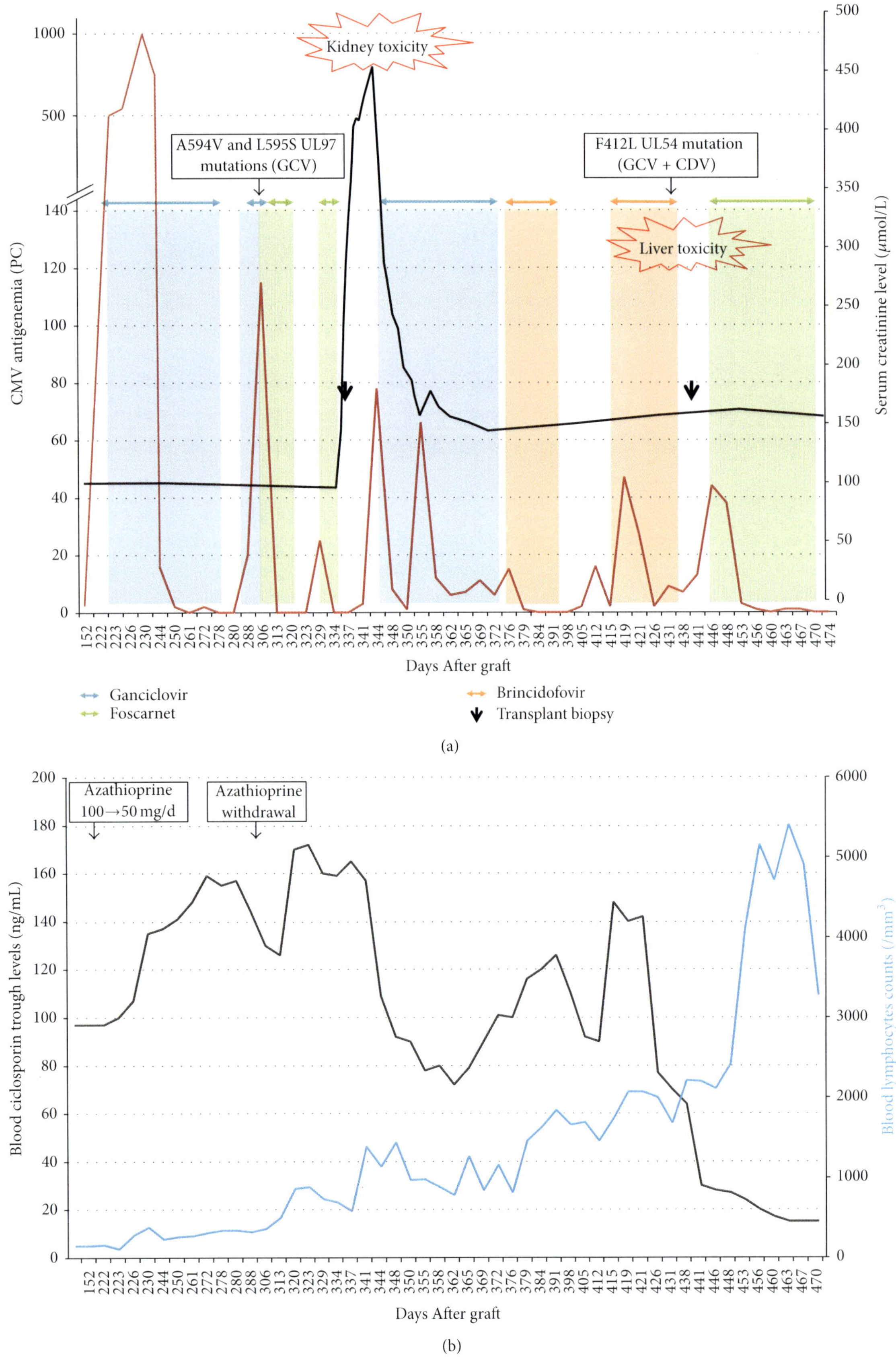

Figure 2: Course of multiresistant CMV disease. (a) Evolution of CMV antigenemia (red line) and kidney transplant function (serum creatinine level, blue line) together with antiviral therapies and genotypic mutations. PC: positive cells/200000 polymorphonuclear leukocytes. GCV: ganciclovir. CDV: cidofovir. (b) Evolution of blood ciclosporin levels (black line) and lymphocytes counts (blue line).

TABLE 1: Summary of cases of biopsy-proven foscarnet nephropathy during CMV infection in solid organ transplantation.

Reference	Type of transplant	Indication of FOS	Time to nephropathy after FOS initiation	Peak serum creatinine	Proteinuria	Biopsy results	Outcome
[8, 9]	Kidney D+/R−	CMV syndrome Persistent high CMV viremia after 65 days of GCV	30 days (single treatment)	387 μmol/L	7 g/d	Birefringent crystal precipitation surrounded by macrophages in glomeruli and tubules. Fibrinoid thrombi. Black crystals with Von Kossa's reaction.	FOS withdrawn after 27 days. Seven months after FOS nephropathy: creatinine level at 158 μmol/L, proteinuria at 2 g/d. Second transplant biopsy: moderate interstitial fibrosis and tubular atrophy with sclerosis of half glomeruli, no crystal, and positive in situ CMV PCR.
[10]	Lung D−/R+	CMV bronchiolitis M460I mutation in the UL97 gene	35 days (second treatment; first treatment of 4 weeks)	475 μmol/L	NR	Autopsy: birefringent short crystals with angular edges in glomeruli (with rupture of capillaries and Bowman's capsule) and in tubules with tubular necrosis and granulomas.	No FOS withdrawal. Death 5.5 months after CMV disease (mild acute rejection, chronic lung rejection). Crystals found in lungs, esophagus, kidney, epicardium, pericardium, and tricuspid valve at autopsy.
[11]	Kidney D−/R+	Asymptomatic reactivation of GCV resistant strain despite prophylactic valganciclovir	21 days (single treatment)	Anuria, hemodialysis	NR	Crystals in tubules and in one-third of glomeruli with rupture of the basement membrane, tubular necrosis, and macrophages.	Multiorgan (kidney, pancreas, and myocardium) damage due to FOS crystal precipitation. Pancreatitis and myocarditis resolved. Graft loss and dialysis therapy continued.
[12]	Kidney D+/R−	CMV hepatitis and retinitis A594V mutation in the UL97 gene	After 14 days (single treatment)	157 μmol/L	NR	Birefringent crystals in the tubular lumens. Black crystals with Von Kossa's reaction.	FOS withdrawal. Ten months after FOS nephropathy: creatinine level at 112 μmol/L. Second transplant biopsy: disappearance of crystal deposition.
PR	Kidney D+/R−	CMV gastritis A594V and L595S mutations in the UL97 gene	6 days (second treatment; first treatment of 14 days)	450 μmol/L	4.5 g/g of creatininuria	Crystals in glomeruli and tubules.	FOS withdrawal followed by Brincidofovir. Second biopsy: disappearance of crystals, sclerosis of one-third glomeruli, mild interstitial fibrosis, and tubular atrophy. Third treatment with FOS: resolution of CMV disease. One year after FOS nephropathy: creatinine level at 130 μmol/L, proteinuria at 0.6 g/g.

CMV, cytomegalovirus; FOS, foscarnet; GCV, ganciclovir; NR, not reported; PCR, polymerase chain reaction; PR, present report.

in a population at risk for kidney injuries together with the in vitro findings mentioned above prompted us to try BCV in our difficult case of GCV resistance and previous FOS nephrotoxicity. Since our personal experience, BCV use has been recently reported in other case studies as a potential curative treatment involving severe resistant dsDNA viral infections (CMV, HSV, and VZV) in HCT recipients and immunocompromised cancer patients [18–21].

In our report, BCV treatment resulted initially in a remission of CMV disease but was marked by abdominal pain, diarrhea, and ALT elevation. Liver metabolism has been proposed to be the most likely major route of elimination for BCV [7]. Mild dose-dependent ALT elevations were observed in 10 to 40% of stem-cell recipients [17]. The known metabolic pathway of BCV, the course of our clinical case, the typical damage, and the rechallenging situation are clearly enough to confirm a BCV induced liver damage, even if mild and likely dose-dependent. However, it was difficult to distinguish between side effect of BCV and gastrointestinal CMV infection itself, regarding abdominal pain and diarrhea.

Similar to CDV, CMV resistance to BCV only involves UL54 DNA polymerase mutations and not UL97 mutations [15]. In the phase 2 trial mentioned above, no known resistance-associated mutations were detected in the BCV arms. Two mutations (M827I and R1052C) in the UL54 gene were found in a small number of subjects without decreased susceptibility to BCV, CDV, GCV, or FOS [22]. Our case and another case in a lung transplant recipient treated with BCV [23] illustrated that BCV could be associated with the A987G and F412L UL94 mutations known to confer ADR to CDV.

Thus, BCV could constitute an antiviral alternative in cases with UL97 mutations when FOS is contraindicated or in cases of FOS nephrotoxicity. Foscarnet nephropathy was initially described in the 1980s as a frequent complication in AIDS patients undergoing treatment for CMV infection [24]. In vivo trisodium foscarnet crystals mixed with sodium calcium salt were first identified by infrared microscopy in the glomerular capillary lumens and tubules of AIDS patients [25]. Importantly, isotonic saline infusion of 1.5 to 2.5 liters per day was demonstrated to reduce this renal toxicity by increasing FOS clearance and constituted the best preventive strategy [24]. Nonetheless, renal failure is possible with FOS despite appropriate hydration. Cases of biopsy-proven FOS crystal precipitation in the transplantation field are relatively scarce and are summarized in Table 1. With the exception of one lung recipient, all patients were kidney transplant recipients. FOS nephropathy does not seem to appear during the first days of therapy but rather after several weeks of treatment. Glomerular crystallization seems to be associated with worse acute kidney injury than isolated tubular crystallization [12]. At worst, FOS nephropathy led to kidney graft loss. Interestingly, FOS precipitation was also observed in the lungs, heart, pancreas, and gastrointestinal tract in two patients with severe systemic crystal dissemination [10, 11].

In conclusion, BCV appeared to be useful in this complicated case of CMV resistance. Although CMV became also resistant to BCV and some mild toxicity occurred, the length of BCV course allowed FOS nephropathy to recover, which facilitated repeated use of FOS, ultimate clearance of the virus, and preserved transplant function. A clinical trial of BCV to manage resistant CMV disease is needed.

Competing Interests

The authors declare that there is no conflict of interests regarding the publication of this paper.

Acknowledgments

The authors thank Chimerix Inc. (Durham, NC, USA) for the generous delivery of Brincidofovir for compassionate use. Brincidofovir was delivered after temporary permission (Autorisation Temporaire d'Utilisation, ATU) was received from the French Agence Nationale de Securité du Médicament et des Produits de Santé (ANSM).

References

[1] E. Beam and R. R. Razonable, "Cytomegalovirus in solid organ transplantation: epidemiology, prevention, and treatment," *Current Infectious Disease Reports*, vol. 14, no. 6, pp. 633–641, 2012.

[2] C. N. Kotton, D. Kumar, A. M. Caliendo et al., "Updated international consensus guidelines on the management of cytomegalovirus in solid-organ transplantation," *Transplantation*, vol. 96, no. 4, pp. 333–360, 2013.

[3] R. R. Razonable and A. Humar, "Cytomegalovirus in solid organ transplantation," *American Journal of Transplantation*, vol. 13, no. s4, pp. 93–106, 2013.

[4] P. Ljungman, M. Boeckh, H. H. Hirsch et al., "Definitions of cytomegalovirus infection and disease in transplant patients for use in clinical trials," *Clinical Infectious Diseases*, vol. 64, no. 1, pp. 87–91, 2017.

[5] L. Couzi, S. Helou, T. Bachelet et al., "High incidence of anticytomegalovirus drug resistance among D+R− kidney transplant recipients receiving preemptive therapy," *American Journal of Transplantation*, vol. 12, no. 1, pp. 202–209, 2012.

[6] A. K. Le Page, M. M. Jager, J. M. Iwasenko, G. M. Scott, S. Alain, and W. D. Rawlinson, "Clinical aspects of cytomegalovirus antiviral resistance in solid organ transplant recipients," *Clinical Infectious Diseases*, vol. 56, no. 7, pp. 1018–1029, 2013.

[7] R. Lanier, L. Trost, T. Tippin et al., "Development of CMX001 for the treatment of poxvirus infections," *Viruses*, vol. 2, no. 12, pp. 2740–2762, 2010.

[8] E. Justrabo, G. Zanetta, L. Martin et al., "Irreversible glomerular lesions induced by crystal precipitation in a renal transplant after foscarnet therapy for cytomegalovirus infection," *Histopathology*, vol. 34, no. 4, pp. 365–369, 1999.

[9] G. Zanetta, L. Maurice-Estepa, C. Mousson et al., "Foscarnet-induced crystalline glomerulonephritis with nephrotic syndrome and acute renal failure after kidney transplantation," *Transplantation*, vol. 67, no. 10, pp. 1376–1378, 1999.

[10] V. Tischler, M. M. Schuurmans, A. Boehler, and A. Gaspert, "Crystal precipitation and granulomatous inflammation in multiple organs after foscarnet therapy in a lung transplant

recipient," *The Journal of Heart and Lung Transplantation*, vol. 31, no. 9, pp. 1037–1040, 2012.

[11] C. Philipponnet, P.-A. Michel, M. Daudon, I. Brocheriou, and J.-J. Boffa, "Intravascular foscarnet crystal precipitation causing multiorgan failure," *American Journal of Kidney Diseases*, vol. 65, no. 1, pp. 152–155, 2014.

[12] D. Iwami, Y. Ogawa, H. Fujita et al., "Successful treatment with foscarnet for ganciclovir-resistant cytomegalovirus infection in a kidney transplant recipient: a case report," *Nephrology*, vol. 21, no. S1, pp. 63–66, 2016.

[13] N. S. Lurain and S. Chou, "Antiviral drug resistance of human cytomegalovirus," *Clinical Microbiology Reviews*, vol. 23, no. 4, pp. 689–712, 2010.

[14] P. West, M. Schmiedeskamp, H. Neeley, J. Oberholzer, E. Benedetti, and B. Kaplan, "Use of high-dose ganciclovir for a resistant cytomegalovirus infection due to UL97 mutation," *Transplant Infectious Disease*, vol. 10, no. 2, pp. 129–132, 2008.

[15] S. Chou, "Phenotypic diversity of cytomegalovirus DNA polymerase gene variants observed after antiviral therapy," *Journal of Clinical Virology*, vol. 50, no. 4, pp. 287–291, 2011.

[16] S. L. Williams-Aziz, C. B. Hartline, E. A. Harden et al., "Comparative activities of lipid esters of cidofovir and cyclic cidofovir against replication of herpesviruses in vitro," *Antimicrobial Agents and Chemotherapy*, vol. 49, no. 9, pp. 3724–3733, 2005.

[17] F. M. Marty, D. J. Winston, S. D. Rowley et al., "CMX001 to prevent cytomegalovirus disease in hematopoietic-cell transplantation," *New England Journal of Medicine*, vol. 369, no. 13, pp. 1227–1236, 2013.

[18] D. El-Haddad, F. El Chaer, J. Vanichanan et al., "Brincidofovir (CMX-001) for refractory and resistant CMV and HSV infections in immunocompromised cancer patients: a single-center experience," *Antiviral Research*, vol. 134, pp. 58–62, 2016.

[19] J. F. Camargo, M. I. Morris, L. M. Abbo et al., "The use of brincidofovir for the treatment of mixed dsDNA viral infection," *Journal of Clinical Virology*, vol. 83, pp. 1–4, 2016.

[20] K. M. Mullane, C. Nuss, J. Ridgeway et al., "Brincidofovir treatment of acyclovir-resistant disseminated varicella zoster virus infection in an immunocompromised host," *Transplant Infectious Disease*, vol. 18, no. 5, pp. 785–790, 2016.

[21] S. Voigt, J. Hofmann, A. Edelmann, A. Sauerbrei, and J. Kühl, "Brincidofovir clearance of acyclovir-resistant herpes simplex virus-1 and adenovirus infection after stem cell transplantation," *Transplant Infectious Disease*, vol. 18, no. 5, pp. 791–794, 2016.

[22] E. Randall Lanier, S. Foster, T. Brundage et al., "Analysis of mutations in the gene encoding cytomegalovirus DNA polymerase in a phase 2 clinical trial of brincidofovir prophylaxis," *Journal of Infectious Diseases*, vol. 214, no. 1, pp. 32–35, 2016.

[23] D. R. Kaul, S. Stoelben, E. Cober et al., "First report of successful treatment of multidrug-resistant cytomegalovirus disease with the novel anti-CMV compound AIC246," *American Journal of Transplantation*, vol. 11, no. 5, pp. 1079–1084, 2011.

[24] G. Deray, F. Martinez, C. Katlama et al., "Foscarnet nephrotoxicity: mechanism, incidence and prevention," *American Journal of Nephrology*, vol. 9, no. 4, pp. 316–321, 1989.

[25] L. Maurice-Estepa, M. Daudon, C. Katlama et al., "Identification of crystals in kidneys of AIDS patients treated with foscarnet," *American Journal of Kidney Diseases*, vol. 32, no. 3, pp. 392–400, 1998.

Massive Ascites in a Renal Transplant Patient after Laparoscopic Fenestration of a Lymphocele

Shohei Kawaguchi,[1] Takahiro Nohara,[2] Takashi Shima,[1] Satoko Matsuyama,[2] Chikako Nose,[3] Junya Yamahana,[3] Yoshifumi Kadono,[2] Chikashi Seto,[1] Masahiko Kawabata,[3] and Atsushi Mizokami[2]

[1]*Department of Urology, Toyama Prefectural Central Hospital, Toyama, Japan*
[2]*Department of Integrative Cancer Therapy and Urology, Kanazawa University Graduate School of Medical Science, Kanazawa, Japan*
[3]*Department of Internal Medicine, Toyama Prefectural Central Hospital, Toyama, Japan*

Correspondence should be addressed to Shohei Kawaguchi; shohei_k2001@yahoo.co.jp

Academic Editor: Marian Klinger

Retroperitoneal lymphocele is a common complication of renal transplantation. Here, we report the case of a 67-year-old woman with massive ascites after fenestration surgery for a lymphocele that developed following renal transplantation. She had been on continuous ambulatory peritoneal dialysis for 9 years. Living donor renal transplantation was performed and an intrapelvic lymphocele subsequently developed. The lymphocele did not resolve after aspiration therapy; therefore, laparoscopic fenestration was performed. Although the lymphocele disappeared, massive ascites appeared in its stead. Half a year later, the ascites was surgically punctured, which then gradually resolved and disappeared 6 weeks later. Aspiration therapy should be considered in patients on long-term peritoneal dialysis, although laparoscopic fenestration is safe and effective.

1. Introduction

Retroperitoneal lymphocele is a common complication after renal transplantation. The incidence rate of lymphocele after renal transplantation is 1%–26% [1]. The lymphocele is usually small, asymptomatic, and incidentally diagnosed during routine ultrasonography. However, symptomatic lymphoceles may affect graft function and thus require treatment. The treatment options for lymphoceles occurring after renal transplantation include simple aspiration, sclerotherapy, and drain placement. Laparoscopic and open peritoneal fenestration surgeries are more invasive options. Previous studies found that laparoscopic fenestration is a safe, effective, and possible first-line treatment for larger, symptomatic lymphoceles when there is a high risk for graft dysfunction [2, 3].

To the best of our knowledge, this is the first report of massive ascites developing in a renal transplant patient after peritoneal fenestration surgery for a symptomatic lymphocele.

2. Case Presentation

A 67-year-old woman who had been on continuous ambulatory peritoneal dialysis (CAPD) for 9 years received a living donor renal transplant. There was no history of peritonitis during CAPD. Graft function was good and her serum creatinine level was 0.9 mg/dL 5 days after the transplantation. The patient received combination immunosuppressive therapy with methylprednisolone, tacrolimus, mycophenolate mofetil, and basiliximab.

Perirenal fluid collection, detected 8 days after transplantation during routine ultrasonography, increased on a daily basis. On day 14, simple aspiration was performed as lower abdominal pressure was increasing. The creatinine level of the drainage was equivalent to that of the serum. After aspiration, fluid immediately reaccumulated in the perirenal space (Figure 1(a)). On day 32, laparoscopic surgery to fenestrate the lymphocele into the peritoneal cavity was performed by introducing a ~5 cm incision in the peritoneum. The septa of the lymphocele were then removed.

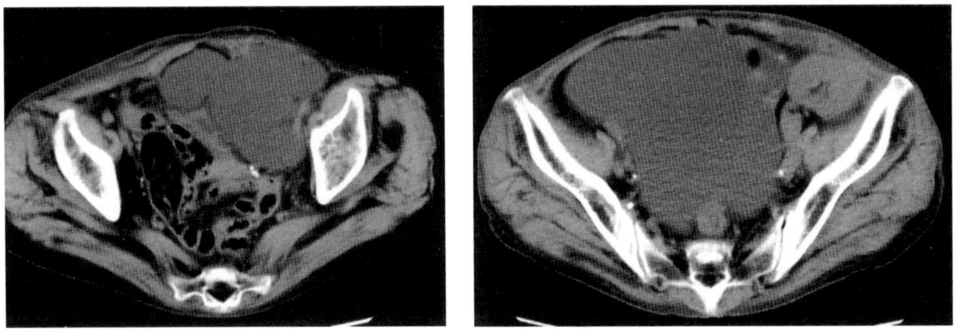

(a) (b)

FIGURE 1: The lymphocele developed from around the graft to the front of the bladder after transplantation (a). The ascites developed and increased after fenestration surgery (b).

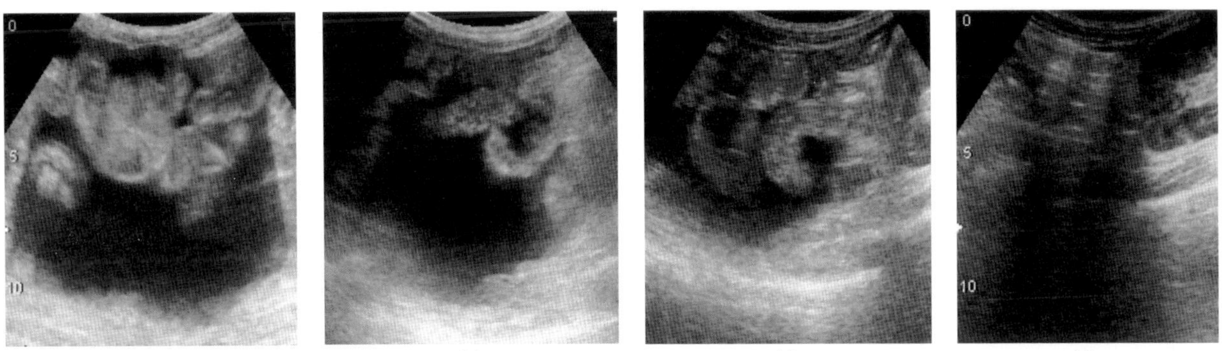

(a) (b) (c) (d)

FIGURE 2: Lower abdominal ultrasonography. (a) Before percutaneous abdominal puncture; (b) 2 weeks after abdominal puncture; (c) 4 weeks after abdominal puncture; and (d) 6 weeks after abdominal puncture (ascites completely resolved).

Three days after fenestration, the lymphocele had almost completely resolved. However, ascites was detected with ultrasonography 5 days after fenestration, which gradually increased. On day 79, abdominal computed tomography was performed because of intense abdominal fullness (Figure 1(b)). Massive ascites was detected and a diagnostic puncture was performed. Laboratory analysis of the fluid revealed the following characteristics: specific gravity (1.017), total protein concentration (2.8 g/dL), Rivalta reaction (negative), and ratio of ascites to serum lactate dehydrogenase (0.5). Culture and cytodiagnosis of the ascites and a T-Spot tuberculosis assay were all negative. The patient was followed up as an outpatient because the ascites was transudative and not cancerous or tuberculous.

On day 163 after fenestration, the patient presented to the outpatient clinic with prominent abdominal fullness. A percutaneous abdominal puncture was performed and 2 L of ascitic fluid was aspirated. Two weeks after aspiration, the ascites significantly decreased and the abdominal fullness was resolving. The ascites continued to decrease and disappeared 6 weeks after aspiration (Figure 2). There was no recurrence after 2.5 years of follow-up.

3. Discussion

Lymphocele after renal transplantation results from transection of the lymphatic vessels accompanying the external iliac vessels during transplantation surgery and subsequent lymph accumulation in a nonepithelized retroperitoneal cavity. Dissection around the external iliac vessels is necessary to perform vascular anastomoses. However, extensive dissection is a risk factor for lymphocele formation [4]. Limited dissection and careful ligation of iliac lymphatic vessels decrease the incidence rate of lymphoceles [5].

Management of lymphocele after renal transplantation is variable. Aspiration therapy is performed to reduce leakage of lymphatic fluid, and fenestration surgery is performed to allow the peritoneum to absorb the fluid. Laparoscopic surgery to fenestrate the lymphocele into the peritoneal cavity is preferred because the rate of recurrence (8%) is lower than that with open surgery (16%) and aspiration therapy (59%) [1].

Long-term CAPD can lead to structural changes in the peritoneal membrane, such as loss of mesothelial cells, thickening of the submesothelial zone, and alterations of blood vessel walls [6]. Functional transport abnormalities of the peritoneal membrane, such as loss of ultrafiltration, occur subsequent to these structural changes [7].

In the present case, we performed laparoscopic fenestration after simple aspiration. Although the lymphocele disappeared, a large quantity of ascites developed. Nine years of CAPD may have produced structural changes in and loss of function of the peritoneal membrane. A massive amount of lymph fluid then leaked from around the external iliac vessels and accumulated in the peritoneal cavity without absorption. A percutaneous abdominal puncture was performed 5 months after fenestration, and the ascites subsequently decreased and disappeared 6 weeks after aspiration. The resolution of the ascites may have been caused by the decrease in lymph fluid leakage due to long-term high abdominal pressure.

Laparoscopic fenestration is a safe and effective first-line treatment for symptomatic lymphocele occurring after renal transplantation. However, aspiration therapy, such as percutaneous catheter drainage with or without sclerotherapy, should be considered for patients with peritoneal function that is impaired by long-term peritoneal dialysis.

Competing Interests

The authors declare that they have no competing interests.

Acknowledgments

The authors would like to thank Enago (https://www.enago.jp/) for the English language review.

References

[1] A. Lucewicz, G. Wong, V. W. T. Lam et al., "Management of primary symptomatic lymphocele after kidney transplantation: a systematic review," *Transplantation*, vol. 92, no. 6, pp. 663–673, 2011.

[2] H. S. Lee, D. J. Joo, K. H. Huh et al., "Laparoscopic fenestration versus percutaneous catheter drainage for lymphocele treatment after kidney transplantation," *Transplantation Proceedings*, vol. 45, no. 4, pp. 1667–1670, 2013.

[3] F. Ulrich, S. Niedzwiecki, P. Fikatas et al., "Symptomatic lymphoceles after kidney transplantation—multivariate analysis of risk factors and outcome after laparoscopic fenestration," *Clinical Transplantation*, vol. 24, no. 2, pp. 273–280, 2010.

[4] E. Zagdoun, M. Ficheux, T. Lobbedez et al., "Complicated lymphoceles after kidney transplantation," *Transplantation Proceedings*, vol. 42, no. 10, pp. 4322–4325, 2010.

[5] O. Øyen, V. Siwach, P.-D. Line et al., "Improvement of post-transplant lymphocele treatment in the laparoscopic era," *Transplant International*, vol. 15, no. 8, pp. 406–410, 2002.

[6] I. Savidaki, D. Karavias, F. Sotsiou et al., "Histologic change of peritoneal membrane in relation to adequacy of dialysis in continuous ambulatory peritoneal dialysis patients," *Peritoneal Dialysis International*, vol. 23, no. 2, pp. S26–S30, 2003.

[7] R. T. Krediet, "The peritoneal membrane in chronic peritoneal dialysis," *Kidney International*, vol. 55, no. 1, pp. 341–356, 1999.

50

Successful Use of Ectopic Pelvic Kidney for Living Related Donation Technical Aspects

R. C. Minnee,[1] H. J. A. N. Kimenai,[1] J. van de Wetering,[2] and J. N. M. Ijzermans[1]

[1] *Department of Surgery, Division of HPB & Transplant Surgery, Erasmus University Medical Center (Erasmus MC), Rotterdam, Netherlands*
[2] *Department of Nephrology, Erasmus University Medical Center (Erasmus MC), Rotterdam, Netherlands*

Correspondence should be addressed to R. C. Minnee; rcminnee@hotmail.com

Academic Editor: David Conti

Ectopic pelvic kidneys can provide an additional source of organs for transplantation. They are often excluded from donation in living donation programs mainly due to aberrant vascular and urinary anatomies. We present a donor with an ectopic left kidney, who successfully donated his kidney. The use of ectopic pelvic kidney for living kidney transplantation is a highly demanding surgical procedure but after extensive preoperative investigation in high volume centers with surgical expertise in vascular reconstruction and access surgery, ectopic pelvic kidneys should not be a contraindication for donation and should be considered as a viable option.

1. Introduction

Live donor kidney transplantation is the optimal method of renal replacement therapy for most patients with end stage renal disease in terms of short- and long-term results [1]. Shortage of available donor kidneys compels us to expand the supply of living donor kidneys. Essentially, the donor kidney must be anatomically and functionally suitable for transplantation, and the donor must be in good medical and psychological health and left with a good renal function from the remaining kidney.

The use of ectopic pelvic kidneys can provide an additional source of organs for transplantation.

Ectopic pelvic kidney is a relatively rare congenital anomaly in which the kidney fails to ascend to its lumbar position during embryonic development. The incidence of pelvic kidneys is reported as 1 in 1000 autopsies; only routine ultrasound screening in children revealed a lower incidence of 1 in 5000 [2, 3]. The location of an ectopic kidney can be pelvic, lumbar, abdominal, and thoracic or crossed fused. Ectopic pelvic kidney slightly occurs more on the left side with predominance in male subjects. Due to malrotation, the ectopic pelvic kidney might have a flattened, discoid shape. This incomplete rotation leads to an undeveloped renal pelvis with a variety of congenital anatomies such as a shorter ureter, defective ureteral drainage, and multiple renal arteries and renal veins. Ectopic pelvic kidneys are often excluded from donation in living donation programs mainly due to these aberrant vascular and urinary anatomies resulting in only a few successful case reports [4–15]. We advocate the use of these kidneys for transplantation in high volume transplant centers and present a successful living-unrelated kidney transplantation of an ectopic pelvic kidney; in addition, we present a review of the literature to focus on the technical aspects.

2. Case Report

The donor was a 43-year-old man donating a kidney to his wife. In the past, he underwent arthroscopic meniscus repair on his left knee and micro discectomy of a herniated nucleus pulposus. He did not use any medication and reported no allergies. During workup, an ectopic left kidney and a normally placed right kidney were found. Physical examination was normal with a BMI of 25.7. Blood and urine examination revealed no abnormalities. His measured creatinine clearance was 123 mL/min. The computed tomography (CT) angiogram performed showed 1 artery, 1 vein, and 1 ureter of the left

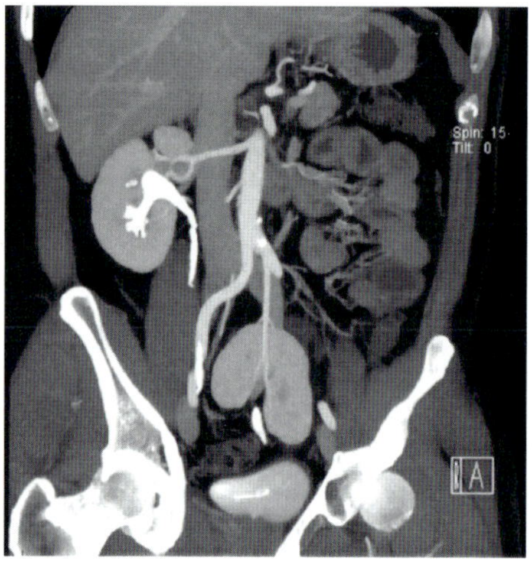

Figure 1: CT scan with coronal image of ectopic left pelvic kidney showing the middle polar artery.

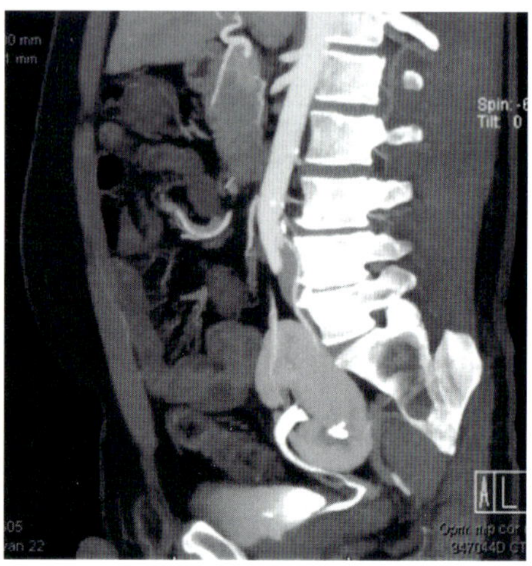

Figure 2: CT scan with sagittal image of ectopic left pelvic kidney showing the upper and middle polar artery.

kidney (Figures 1 and 2). The ectopic left kidney had a relative function of 40% in conventional technetium-99m (Tc-99m) mercaptoacetyltriglycine (MAG3) scan. During the renal transplant multidisciplinary meeting, it was recommended to select the left kidney for donation.

A left open donor nephrectomy was performed through a Gibson incision. The donor kidney had additional blood vessels undetected on CT scan. There were an additional upper polar artery and an additional middle polar artery (Figure 3). On the bench, an end-to-side anastomosis was made between the middle polar artery and the main renal artery with Prolene 7.0 (Figure 4).

The recipient was the donor's 43-year-old wife with end stage renal failure secondary to tubulointerstitial nephritis. The donor kidney was placed in the right iliac fossa. The renal vein was anastomosed to the common iliac vein, whereas the reconstructed renal artery was anastomosed end to side to the external iliac artery and the upper polar artery to the common iliac artery. The anastomosis time for all anastomoses was

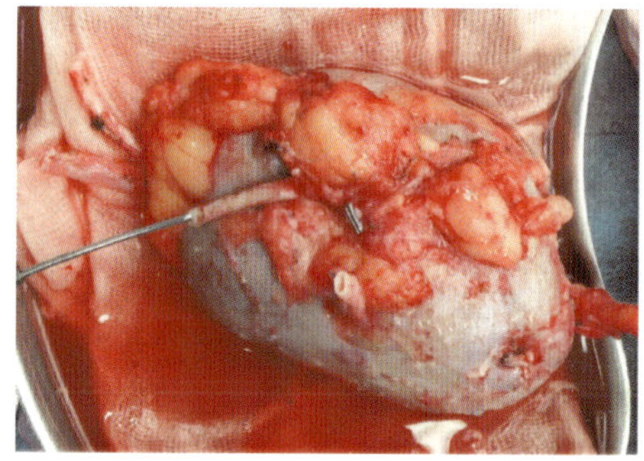

Figure 3: Left pelvic kidney with additional upper polar artery and an additional middle polar artery before reconstruction.

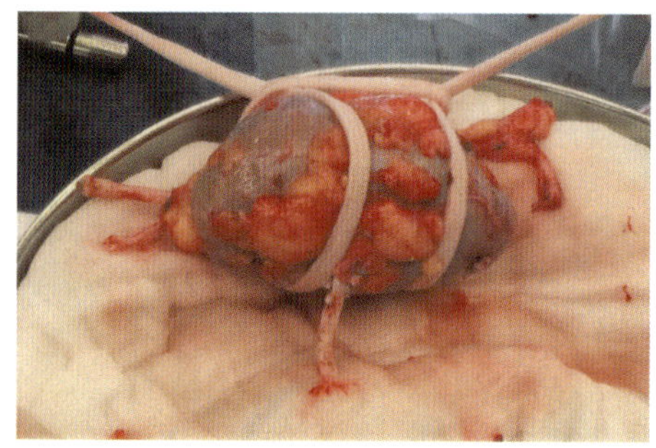

Figure 4: After end-to-side reconstruction of the middle polar artery and main renal artery.

32 minutes. The method used to establish urinary continuity was extravesical ureteroneocystostomy and closure of the abdominal wall in layers. The ureteroneocystostomy was stented with an externally draining 8-French catheter for 9 days. According to local protocol, a standard dose of 12.000 U heparin daily was given during the first 5 days due to the arterial reconstruction. The postoperative course of the donor and the patient was uneventful.

3. Discussion

The use of an ectopic kidney for transplantation in a living transplant program has been only reported in thirteen patients (Table 1) [4–15]. In all cases, extensive investigation of live donors was carried out. The majority of ectopic kidneys had multiple renal vessels especially renal arteries (77%). However, despite comprehensive investigation in 4 cases (29%) (including our case), discrepancy was found between the preoperative imaging and operative findings [4, 11, 14]. In all 4 cases, additional renal veins and/or arteries were visualized. So, even after extensive preoperative imaging, a cautious approach should be undertaken during the donor nephrectomy for the existence of additional vascular structures.

Several studies reported clinicoradiological discrepancies between preoperative CT renal angiography and operative findings ranging from 5% to 15% [16–18]. Retrospectively, Johnson et al. could not identify 3 of the 12 discrepancies between CT angiographic and operative findings on image review [16]. This reveals an effect of experience on reporting

TABLE 1

Author	Number of patients	Donor-recipient relationship	Kidney	Number of arteries*	Number of veins*	Number of ureters*	Number of arteries#	Number of veins#	Number of ureters#	Discrepancy imaging versus surgery
Kim 1973	1	Sister to brother	Left	1	1	1	1	1	1	N
Spanos 1976	2	Mother to son	Right	3	1	1	3	1	1	N
		Brother to brother	Right	2	1	1	2	1	1	N
Bacharach 1984	1	Brother to brother	Right	2	1	1	3	1	1	Y
Luke 2003	1	Uncle to niece	Left	2	2	1	2	2	1	N
Grogan 2004	1	Son to mother	Right	1	1	1	1	1	1	N
Boughey 2004	1	Father to son	Right	3	1	1	3	2	1	Y
Li 2006	1	Unrelated	Right	3	3	1	3	3	1	N
Papanikolaou 2007	1	Mother to son	Left	1	1	1	1	1	1	N
Goldsmith 2009	1	Father to son	Left	2	1	1	3	2	1	Y
He 2012	1	Wife to husband	Left	2	2	1	2	2	1	N
Yaich 2014	1	Son to father	Left	3	1	1	3	1	1	N
Siemens 2015	1	Father to son	Left	2	1	1	2	1	1	N

*Number of arteries/veins and ureters on preoperative imaging; #number of arteries/veins and ureters during explantation.

TABLE 2

Author	Number of patients	AT	Vascular reconstruction	Vascular reconstruction	Postoperative course	Graft function
Kim 1973	1	N/A	N	—	Uneventful	Immediate
Spanos 1976	2	N/A	N	2 arteries ETS, smallest on internal iliac artery	Uneventful	Immediate
		N/A	N	No reconstruction, smallest artery ligated	Uneventful	Immediate
Bacharach 1984	1	N/A	Y	2 arteries STS, smallest artery ligated	Uneventful	Immediate
Luke 2003	1	32 min	Y	2 arteries STS, 2 renal veins ETS	Uneventful	Immediate
Grogan 2004	1	N/A	N	—	Uneventful	Immediate
Boughey 2004	1	N/A	Y	2 arteries STS, 2 renal veins ETS	Uneventful	Immediate
Li 2006	1	N/A	Y	2 arteries STS, smallest on internal iliac artery, 3 renal veins reconstructed with vein interponate	Uneventful	Immediate
Papanikolaou 2007	1	N/A	N	—	Uneventful	Immediate
Goldsmith 2009	1	50 min	Y	2 arteries ETS, 1 artery ETE on epigastric artery with vein interponate, 2 renal veins ETS	Uneventful	Immediate
He 2012	1	45 min	N	1 artery ETS, 1 artery ETE on internal iliac artery, 2 renal veins ETS	Uneventful, 6 weeks later lymphocele followed by surgery	Immediate
Yaich 2014	1	N/A	N	1 artery ETS, 2 small arteries ligated	Uneventful	Immediate
Siemens 2015	1	N/A	N	2 arteries ETS	Acute vascular rejection	2 HD sessions

N/A: not applicable; ETS: end-to-site anastomosis; STS: side-to-side anastomosis; ETE: end-to-end anastomosis; AT: anastomosis time.

accuracy and greater awareness of potential reporting pitfalls, which was the case in our report.

All kidney grafts showed immediate graft function except in one case requiring two hemodialysis sessions (Table 2). All arterial and venous reconstructions were flawless, showing that reconstruction of multiple renal vessels in ectopic pelvic kidneys is feasible for transplantation [4, 11, 13–15].

Ureteral duplication occurs in approximately 0.8% of the general population and the incidence of duplicated ureters in ectopic pelvic kidney is unknown [19]. Approximately 50% of ectopic kidneys have a hydronephrosis. Half of these cases are due to obstruction of the ureteropelvic or the ureterovesical junction (70% and 30%, resp.), 25% from reflux grade III or greater, and 25% from the malrotation alone [20]. Despite all aberrant urinary anatomies described in the literature, all transplanted ectopic pelvic kidneys reported in the literature had a normal single ureter and urinary collecting system. When the ureter is very short, ureteroureterostomy or pyelovesicostomy is an alternative option.

Laparoscopic donor nephrectomy has been performed in 2 cases [8, 12]. Key points for laparoscopic donor nephrectomy are careful interpretation of the preoperative imaging and use of a Endo Retract™ articulating fan retractor to increase the working space [12].

Hence, these donors should have extensive investigations of the renal vasculature and anatomy variation using computed tomography angiography or magnetic resonance angiography. Intravenous pyelography can also be performed to detect urinary tract abnormality and, additionally, nuclear renography is necessary to assess the renal function of each kidney.

The main limitation in all the case reports is the presence of publication bias. Only successful transplantations are most likely reported and published.

The use of ectopic pelvic kidney for living kidney transplantation is a highly demanding surgical procedure but nonetheless a feasible one. After extensive preoperative investigation in high volume centers with surgical expertise in vascular reconstruction and access surgery, ectopic pelvic kidneys should not be a contraindication for donation and should be considered as a viable option. Since the presence of an ectopic pelvic kidney is a relatively common condition, it must be noted that the use of these kidneys may expand the donor pool in experienced hands.

References

[1] C. L. Davis and F. L. Delmonico, "Living-donor kidney transplantation: A review of the current practices for the live donor," *Journal of the American Society of Nephrology*, vol. 16, no. 7, pp. 2098–2110, 2005.

[2] S. P. Dretler, C. Olsson, and R. C. Pfister, "The anatomic, radiologic and clinical characteristics of the pelvic kidney: an analysis of 86 cases," *Journal of Urology*, vol. 105, no. 5, pp. 623–627, 1971.

[3] C. P. Sheih et al., "Renal abnormalities in schoolchildren," *Pediatrics*, vol. 84, no. 6, pp. 1086–1090, 1989.

[4] M. D. Bacharach and N. L. Tilney, "Use of an ectopic pelvic donor kidney for transplantation," *Transplantation Proceedings*, vol. 16, no. 6, pp. 1663–1665, 1984.

[5] E. L. Grogan, W. A. Nylander, and D. Shaffer, "Living-related transplantation of an ectopic pelvic kidney [3]," *Transplantation*, vol. 77, no. 6, p. 953, 2004.

[6] C. H. Kim and O. Fjeldborg, "Transplantation of pelvic kidney: A case report," *Scandinavian Journal of Urology and Nephrology*, vol. 7, no. 2-3, pp. 236–238, 1973.

[7] V. Papanikolaou, D. Giakoustidis, N. Antoniadis, N. Ouzounidis, D. Takoudas, and A. Antoniadis, "Living-related transplantation of an ectopic pelvic kidney," *International Journal of Urology*, vol. 14, no. 4, pp. 357–359, 2007.

[8] T. A. Siemens et al., "Pelvic kidney for living transplantation: case report and review of the literature," *Jornal Brasileiro de Nefrologia*, vol. 37, no. 3, pp. 418–421, 2015.

[9] P. K. Spanos, R. Weil, R. L. Simmons, and J. S. Najarian, "Successful transplantation of ectopic kidneys from living related donors," *The American Journal of Surgery*, vol. 131, no. 3, pp. 360–362, 1976.

[10] S. Yaich et al., "Use of a pelvic kidney for living transplantation," *Saudi Journal of Kidney Diseases and Transplantation*, vol. 25, no. 2, pp. 408-409, 2014.

[11] J. C. Boughey, O. E. Emovon, F. Afzal et al., "Living donor transplantation of a pelvic kidney," *Clinical Transplantation*, vol. 18, no. 3, pp. 336–338, 2004.

[12] B. He and A. Mitchell, "Laparoscopic donor nephrectomy for ectopic kidney," *Transplantation Proceedings*, vol. 44, no. 10, pp. 3051–3054, 2012.

[13] J. Li, S. Nadalin, A. Paul et al., "The symptomatic pelvic kidney: A new source of organs for living donor kidney transplantation?" *Transplantation*, vol. 82, no. 9, pp. 1241-1242, 2006.

[14] P. J. Goldsmith, M. Marco, Z. Hussain, C. Newstead, J. P. A. Lodge, and N. Ahmad, "Kidney Transplantation Using the Inferior Epigastric Vessels for Multiple Anastomoses from a Pelvic Kidney," *Journal of the American College of Surgeons*, vol. 209, no. 1, p. -e3, 2009.

[15] P. P. W. Luke, V. C. McAlister, A. M. Jevnikar et al., "Use of a pelvic kidney for living transplantation: Case report and review of the literature," *American Journal of Transplantation*, vol. 3, no. 2, pp. 235–238, 2003.

[16] J. E. Johnson, E. J. Loveday, L. J. Archer, P. Lear, and M. J. Thornton, "Preoperative evaluation of live renal donors using multislice CT angiography," *Clinical Radiology*, vol. 60, no. 7, pp. 771–777, 2005.

[17] J. F. Platt, J. H. Ellis, M. Korobkin, and K. Reige, "Helical CT evaluation of potential kidney donors: Findings in 154 subjects," *American Journal of Roentgenology*, vol. 169, no. 5, pp. 1325–1330, 1997.

[18] J. J. Del Pizzo, G. N. Sklar, J. W. You-Cheong, B. Levin, T. Krebs, and S. C. Jacobs, "Helical computerized tomography arteriography for evaluation of live renal donors undergoing laparoscopic nephrectomy," *Journal of Urology*, vol. 162, no. 1, pp. 31–34, 1999.

[19] J. T. J. Privett, W. D. Jeans, and J. Roylance, "The incidence and importance of renal duplication," *Clinical Radiology*, vol. 27, no. 4, pp. 521–530, 1976.

[20] C. J. Shapiro E, "Anomalies of the upper urinary tract," in *Campbell-Walsh Urology*, pp. 3123–3160, Elsevier, 2011.

51

Spontaneous Renal Allograft Rupture Caused by Acute Tubular Necrosis

Deepak Shankar Ray and Sharmila Thukral

Rabindranath Tagore International Institute of Cardiac Sciences, Narayana Health Hospitals, 124 EM Bypass, Mukundapur, Kolkata, India

Correspondence should be addressed to Sharmila Thukral; sharmilathukral@gmail.com

Academic Editor: Henkie P. Tan

Renal allograft rupture (RAR) is a rare but lethal complication of renal transplantation. It potentially threatens graft and patient survival. RAR is frequently associated with acute rejection, but other causes like renal vein thrombosis and acute tubular necrosis have also been observed. Most commonly a graft nephrectomy is required, but graft repair can also be attempted in selected cases to salvage the graft. Herein, we describe a rare case of spontaneous renal allograft rupture in the early posttransplant period due to acute tubular necrosis. A 42-year-old male, living donor renal allograft recipient, experienced RAR on the sixth posttransplant day. Surgical exploration showed two lacerations of 10 cm and 5 cm length at the upper and mid pole of the kidney. Histologically, the graft demonstrated acute tubular injury; no features of humoral or cellular rejection were identified. The successful management of this complication resulted in the salvage of the patient and the graft. This case demonstrates that early diagnosis and prompt treatment of a life-threatening RAR can salvage the graft.

1. Introduction

Spontaneous renal allograft rupture is a rare yet potentially life-threatening complication of renal transplantation. It is associated with a high incidence of graft loss [1]

The consequences are fatal in 6% of the cases and graft loss is the outcome in another 53% [2]

Most of these cases are immunologically mediated and caused by acute rejection. Acute tubular necrosis is only rarely responsible for this complication [3, 4].

With improvements in the immunosuppressive regimens, the incidence of this complication has decreased. Recognition and prompt management of allograft rupture are important because of its likely devastating outcomes. Usually, graft nephrectomy is necessary in these cases, but conservative surgical intervention has also been tried successfully.

We report an unusual case of a renal allograft recipient who developed a spontaneous RAR. The rupture was secondary to a relatively uncommon cause, acute tubular necrosis. The graft was successfully salvaged by surgical repair.

This case emphasises that the transplant team must be aware of this fatal complication and the current management strategies.

2. Case History

A 42-year-old gentleman, suffering from End-Stage Renal Disease (ESRD) secondary to vesicoureteral reflux (VUR). VUR was detected at the age of four years. He developed progressive proteinuria 12 years later followed by slowly progressive decline of renal function culminating in ESRD and was started on hemodialysis in Jan 2010. He underwent a live spousal blood group compatible renal transplant on 19th Feb 2010. The graft was lost to chronic allograft nephropathy in 2015 and second live donor renal transplant was planned. Donor was 33-year-old male, altruistic with HLA mismatch 3/6, ABO compatible, and CDC cross-match negative. Optical internal urethrotomy was done one day prior to transplant as he had urethral stricture diagnosed by micturating cystourethrogram. Induction was done with antithymocyte globulin in the dose of 3 mg/kg and triple

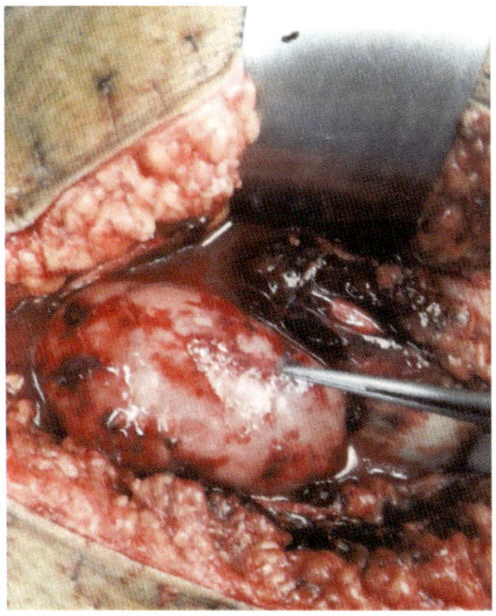

FIGURE 1: Two ruptures, 10 cm and 5 cm one at upper pole and one at midportion, respectively.

immunosuppression was given with tacrolimus, mycophenolate mofetil, and prednisolone. The second transplant was done on 20th April 2016. Donor nephrectomy was done laparoscopically, the warm ischaemia time being 10 minutes. There was no injury to the renal vein or artery during donor nephrectomy. After anastomosis of the renal vein to the external iliac vein, there was avulsion at the venous anastomotic site. There was no thrombosis or stenosis of the vein and no heparin was required intraoperatively.

Venous avulsion was repaired with 6.0 Prolene immediately, after which the arterial and venous blood flows were normal. The recipient was hemodynamically stable in the intraoperative and immediate posttransplant period. Immediate postoperative graft function was poor.

In the next six postoperative days, his urine output remained around 2–4 liters/day. His serum creatinine came down very slowly from 9.97 mg/dL to 8.37 mg/dL by the fifth posttransplant day. Drain fluid decreased from 190 ml/day to 80 ml/day by the fifth posttransplant day. Hemoglobin remained stable, and no significant perigraft collection was seen on sonography. In view of poor allograft function, a renal biopsy was planned on sixth postoperative day, but his drain volume suddenly increased on that day and a frank hemorrhagic collection of 1 liter was drained within half an hour. The patient complained of severe abdominal pain and the urine output dropped. The graft became swollen and tender.

Aggressive resuscitation was started and the patient was immediately reexplored in the operation theatre. A hematoma with large amount of blood clots was evacuated. There were two ruptures in the transplant kidney, 10 cm and 5 cm, one at upper pole and one at midportion, respectively, along the convex border (Figure 1). There was no leak at the anastomotic site and no other source of bleeding was found. The coagulation profile of the patient was normal. Ruptures were repaired with 3-0 Prolene hemolock and reinforced by TACOSIL.

An allograft biopsy was done in the operating room.

The patient was shifted to transplant unit and the patient was given two sessions of plasmapheresis followed by 5 gm of IVIG on the first and second posttransplant day, while awaiting the graft biopsy report.

The donor specific antibodies were negative by flow cytometry. Histopathology showed normocellular and uniform glomeruli. There were no capillary wall thickening and no fibrin thrombi or necrosis. Tubules showed vacuolation and degeneration and necrosis of epithelial cells. There was severe acute tubular necrosis. There was no tubulitis. There were no interstitial infiltration, fibrosis, and endarteritis. C4d stain was negative in the peritubular capillaries and glomerular capillaries.

In Figures 2(a) and 2(b) the patient improved symptomatically; drain volume came down to less than 50 ml by the sixteenth posttransplant day. It also became mainly serous collection and the drain was removed after 8 days.

His graft function improved significantly and he was discharged after 10 days of repair of the rupture with good urine output and a serum creatinine of 1.9 mg/dl (Figure 3).

3. Discussion

Renal allograft rupture is defined as a superficial or deep tear of the renal capsule as well as renal parenchyma [5].

It was first reported in 1968 by Murray et al. [6].

The prevalence of RAR ranges from 0.3% to 9.6% with a mean of 3.4% [7].

It typically occurs within three weeks after transplantation [4].

The most frequent cause of RAR is acute graft rejection. It is the main predisposing factor in 60–80% of the cases [8].

Other factors contributing to RAR include ischaemic acute kidney injury, acute tubular necrosis, damaged hilar lymphatic channels, renal vein thrombosis, ureteral obstruction with subsequent hydronephrosis, renal biopsy, trauma, nephrostomy tubes, and development of renal cell cancer [4, 5, 9–11].

The pathogenetic mechanism of RAR is not fully understood. Cortical and capsular ischaemia resulting from interstitial oedema and cellular inflammatory cell infiltration, in the setting of acute rejection, is considered the major cause of RAR by exerting capsular tension, tearing, and rupture. This may occur even many years after transplantation [12].

Interstitial oedema was found in 85% cases and major ischaemic damage in 15%. Graft biopsy is the etiological factor in 15% and hydronephrosis in 4%.

Hemodialysis with heparin is the possible factor in 46% cases [13]. Clinically, RAR is most commonly characterised by sudden onset of abdominal pain, graft tenderness, and swelling, and decreased haematocrit with hemorrhagic shock. It is generally associated with oliguria or anuria, sometimes with gross hematuria, fever, and bleeding from incision. Clinical diagnosis may be confirmed by ultrasound or CT scan [7]. Immediate ultrasound evaluation can confirm the diagnosis with 87% sensitivity and 100% specificity [14].

The management of RAR is urgent exploratory operation to control the bleeding, perform nephrectomy if indicated, and evacuate the hematoma to reduce the possibility of secondary infection.

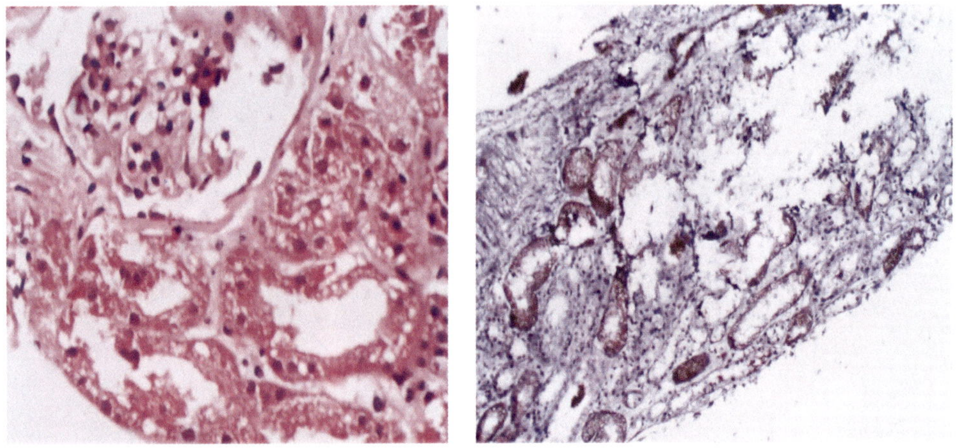

(a) H&E stain (40x) showing ATN, no inflammatory cell infiltration, tubulitis, or peritubular capillaritis noted

(b) C4D is negative

FIGURE 2

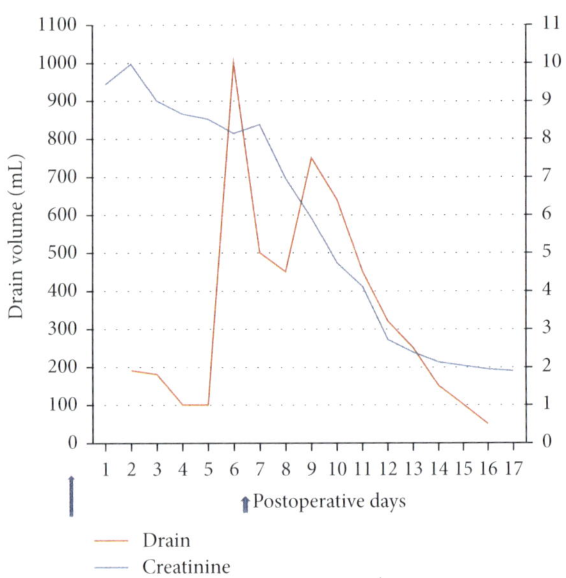

FIGURE 3: Time course of events.

Early reports of conservative management of RAR showed poor results with less than 30% success rates. The high rate of graft nephrectomies was due to the failure to control bleeding and inability to reverse rejection, postoperative multiorgan failure, and uncontrollable coagulopathy. Over the past two decades, improvements in the surgical techniques have significantly reduced the transplant related mortality and morbidity. Current literature demonstrate that the ruptured grafts can be salvaged with a success rate as high as 80%. Recurrent rupture occurs in only 5% patients [15].

With salvage rates between 40 and 100% and variable long-term complications and performance of the repaired graft, it is worth trying to salvage spontaneously ruptured grafts. Only in those patients whose hemodynamic status cannot be stabilised by appropriate aggressive hemodynamic support, graft nephrectomy should be considered as a definite treatment [1, 8, 9].

4. Conclusion

RAR is still encountered in clinical practice. In spite of advances in immunosuppression, most of the cases are due to acute rejection. Acute tubular necrosis is an uncommon cause of RAR. The life-threatening nature of this complication mandates early recognition and treatment. Although transplant nephrectomy is a definite treatment, with advances in the surgical techniques, attempts can be made to salvage the graft when hemorrhage can be controlled and RAR does not compromise survival of the patient.

References

[1] F. Gomez-Veiga, V. Chantada-Abal, J. Garcia-Buitron, and M. Gonzalez-Martin, "Spontaneous rupture of transplanted kidney. Experience with 500 transplants," *Arch Esp Urol*, vol. 46, pp. 295–302, 1993.

[2] J. A. Van Der Viliet, G. Kootstra, A. M. Tegzess et al., "Management of rupture in allograft kidney," *The Netherlands Journal of Surgery*, vol. 32, no. 2, pp. 45–48, 1980.

[3] B. W. Hochleitner, R. Kafka, B. Spechtenhauser et al., "Renal allograft rupture is associated with rejection or acute tubular necrosis, but not with renal vein thrombosis," *Nephrology Dialysis Transplantation*, vol. 16, no. 1, pp. 124–127, 2001.

[4] P. Szenohradszky, G. Smehák, and E. Szederkényi, "Renal allograft rupture: a clinicopathologic study of 37 nephrectomy cases in a series of 628 consecutive renal transplants," *Transplantation Proceedings*, vol. 31, no. 5, pp. 2107–2111, 1999.

[5] H. Shahrokh, H. Rasouli, M. A. Zargar, K. Karimi, and K. Zargar, "Spontaneous kidney allograft rupture," *Transplantation Proceedings*, vol. 37, no. 7, pp. 3079-3080, 2005.

[6] J. E. Murray, R. E. Wilson, N. L. Tilney et al., "Five years' experience in renal transplantation with immunosuppressive drugs: survival, function, complications, and the role of lymphocyte depletion by thoracic duct fistula," *Annals of Surgery*, vol. 168, no. 3, pp. 416–435, 1968.

[7] G. J. Azar, A. A. Zarifian, G. D. Frentz, R. J. Jesi, and E. E. Ethredge, "Renal allogrsft rupture: a clinical review," *Clinical Transplantation*, vol. 9, pp. 71–73, 1995.

[8] D. Heimbach, W. D. Miersch, H. Buszello, G. Schoeneich, and H. U. Klehr, "Is the transplant-preserving management of renal allograft rupture justified?" *British Journal of Urology*, vol. 75, no. 6, pp. 729–732, 1995.

[9] M. D. Garcia Sanchez de la Nieta, A. I. Sánchez-Fructuoso, R. Alcázar et al., "Higher graft salvage rate in renal allograft rupture associated with acute tubular necular," *Transplantation Proceedings*, vol. 36, no. 10, pp. 3016–3018, 2004.

[10] N. Busi, E. Capocasale, and M. P. Mazzoni, "Spontaneous renal allograft rupture without acute rejection," *Acta Bio-Medica*, vol. 75, pp. 131–133, 2004.

[11] G. Fernandez-Juarez, J. Pascual, F. J. Burgos et al., "Late rupture of the renal graft: not always graft rejection," *Nephrology Dialysis Transplantation*, vol. 13, no. 2, pp. 496–498, 1998.

[12] S. Askandarani, N. Aloudah, H. Al Enazi, K. O. Alsaad, and A. Altamimi, "Late renal allograft rupture associated with cessation of immunosuppression following graft failure," *Case Reports in Transplantation*, vol. 2011, Article ID 512893, 5 pages, 2011.

[13] M. Goldman, L. De Pauw, P. Kinnaert, P. Vereerstraeten, J. Van Geertruyden, and C. Toussaint, "Renal allograft rupture: possible causes and results of surgical conservative management," *Transplantation*, vol. 32, no. 2, pp. 153–155, 1981.

[14] H. Oesterwitz, V. Strobelt, G. May, and R. Horlbeck, "Spontaneous kidney transplant rupture- effect of immunosuppressive therapy on incidence of rupture: a clinical review," *Z Urol Nephrol*, vol. 83, no. 4, pp. 157–163, 1990.

[15] W. P. Homan, J. S. Cheigh, S. J. Kim et al., "Renal allograft fracture: clinicopathological study of 21 cases," *Annals of Surgery*, vol. 186, no. 6, pp. 700–703, 1977.

52

Primary Cytomegalovirus Infection Causing Guillain-Barré Syndrome in a Living Renal Allograft Recipient

Massini Merzkani, Ezra Israel, and Mala Sachdeva

Division of Kidney Diseases and Hypertension, North Shore University Hospital and Long Island Jewish Medical Center, Hofstra Northwell School of Medicine, Great Neck, NY, USA

Correspondence should be addressed to Mala Sachdeva; msachdeva@northwell.edu

Academic Editor: David Conti

Guillain-Barré Syndrome (GBS) is a common acute autoimmune polyneuropathy in adults. There have been few reported cases of Guillain-Barré Syndrome associated with active cytomegalovirus (CMV) infection in renal transplant recipients. Here we present a case of active CMV viremia inducing Guillain-Barré Syndrome in a renal transplant recipient. We discuss the treatment regimen utilized. Furthermore, we performed a review of the literature and discuss the cases of CMV induced GBS in renal transplant recipients.

1. Introduction

In solid organ transplantation, neurologic complications are not uncommon. Guillain-Barré Syndrome (GBS), also called acute inflammatory demyelinating polyneuropathy, is a common form of acute neuropathy in adults. Worldwide, its incidence is 1.3 per 100,000 population [1]. GBS carries a high incidence in bone marrow transplant recipients [2]. In kidney transplant recipients, GBS has been a rare occurrence and optimal treatment in this population has not yet been defined. On the contrary, CMV in kidney transplantation is not uncommon. Long-term CMV infection in a renal transplant recipient increases the risk for allograft failure and mortality [3]. The first case of Guillain-Barré Syndrome occurring in association with cytomegalovirus (CMV) infection was first reported in a renal transplant recipient in 1970 [4]. Second case was reported by Bale et al. 1980 of an active CMV infection inducing Guillain-Barré Syndrome [5]. There have been approximately a total of eleven cases that had this association worldwide in renal transplant recipients.

Optimal treatment for Guillain-Barré Syndrome in the immunosuppressed kidney transplant recipient is still unknown. Here we report a case of CMV induced GBS in a living unrelated renal transplant recipient who was treated with good clinical response with the combination of oral valganciclovir, plasma exchange, and intravenous immunoglobulins (IVIG).

2. Case

This is a 47-year-old Caucasian male with a history significant for a living unrelated renal transplant two years prior to presentation and recent acute cytomegalovirus (CMV) infection. He presented with a two-day history of worsening, ascending lower extremity weakness, numbness, and tingling. The weakness had worsened rapidly to the point where he had difficulty ambulating and imbalance. Seven days prior to presentation, he had first presented with fever, chills, myalgias, and headache of one-week duration. Work-up at that time revealed acute CMV infection and he was started on oral valganciclovir at treatment doses. On review of systems, the patient complained of mild shortness of breath that worsened on exertion. He denied fever, chills, nausea, vomiting, diarrhea, lightheadedness, cough, lower extremity edema, or any changes in his urine output. He denied any recent travel, sick contacts, recent history of insect bites, or vaccinations.

His past medical history was significant for hypertension, dyslipidemia, asthma, and a distant history of melanoma. The etiology of his end stage kidney disease was biopsy proven focal segmental glomerulosclerosis presumed to be secondary to anabolic steroid use. He had a living unrelated kidney transplant two years prior to presentation. Induction was with steroids and basiliximab. His posttransplant course was complicated by biopsy proven BK Virus Nephropathy one year after transplant for which he was successfully treated with reduction in immunosuppression and intravenous immunoglobulin. At the time of transplantation, the donor was CMV positive, and the recipient was CMV negative. He received prophylaxis with valganciclovir for CMV more than one year. His current immunosuppression regimen consisted of prednisone 5 mg daily, tacrolimus 1.5 mg every twelve hours, and mycophenolate mofetil 500 mg every twelve hours.

On physical examination, the patient appeared anxious but was awake, alert, and oriented to person, place, and time. Vital signs included a blood pressure of 137/98 mmHg, pulse rate of 81/min, temperature of 97 degrees Fahrenheit, respiratory rate of 16 breaths/min, and a pulse oximetry of one hundred percent on room air. Physical examination was significant for a neurological examination, which demonstrated decreased motor strength in proximal and distal muscles in both upper and lower limbs (grades 3/5 and 2/5, resp.). He had absent deep tendon reflexes in his lower extremities. His gait could not be assessed due to lower extremity weakness and inability to ambulate. Two days before, his neurological exam was noncontributory except for decreased temperature sensation in his hands and feet.

Laboratory data from one week prior to presentation included mild thrombocytopenia, mild increase in liver transaminases, and a stable creatinine. Diagnosis of acute CMV infection was made based on a positive serum CMV IgM titer of 149 au/ml (normal < 30 au/ml), negative CMV IgG, and CMV PCR with 4800 copies/ml. Lumbar puncture and other serologic work-ups were negative. MRI of the brain done revealed no acute changes. Due to a diagnosis of acute CMV infection, he was started on oral valganciclovir. Laboratory data at this presentation included white blood cell count 5.9 k/microliter; hemoglobin 16.8 grams/deciliter; platelets 312 k/microliter; sodium 139 mmol/liter; potassium 3.6 mmol/liter; chloride 105 mmol/liter; bicarbonate 23 mmol/liter; blood urea nitrogen 17 mg/dl; and creatinine 1.28 mg/dl (at baseline). Urine heavy metal screen was negative for arsenic, cadmium, mercury, or lead. HIV, HTLV I/II, HBV, HCV, HSV, EBV, and HHV-6 PCR analyses were all negative. Lumbar puncture showed cerebrospinal fluid protein at 63 mg/dL, glucose of 68 mg/dL, cell count of 1, and albumin of 52.7 mg/dL. CMV PCR was positive in the CSF. Serum CMV PCR was 4000 copies/mL.

Based on positive serum and cerebrospinal fluid CMV PCR, the typical albuminocytologic dissociation of CSF analysis, and progressive neurological manifestations, a diagnosis of CMV associated Guillain-Barré Syndrome was made.

The patient was on an immunosuppression regimen that consisted of prednisone 5 mg daily, tacrolimus 1.5 mg every twelve hours, and mycophenolate mofetil 500 mg every twelve hours. The mycophenolate mofetil was discontinued, and the Prograf dosage was reduced to target FK506 troughs of 5–7. In addition to reduction in immunosuppression, the patient received eleven treatments of plasma exchange over a course of two weeks (each exchange consisted of two plasma volumes each with albumin as the replacement) and a total of 1 g/kg body weight of intravenous immunoglobulin (IVIG) in two divided doses. He was continued on valganciclovir 900 mg orally two times a day. After 72 hours, the patient began to improve with increased motor strength and improved negative inspiratory flow and vital capacity measurements. Every successive plasma exchange treatment seemed to subjectively show a favorable response to his motor recovery and muscle strength. After a two-week hospitalization, the patient regained his ability to ambulate and he was subsequently discharged on oral valganciclovir. He was continued on treatment doses of valganciclovir at 900 mg orally two times a day as an outpatient. His serum CMV PCR was negative after two weeks of treatment. One month later, the patient returned with lower extremity weakness and was readmitted for a presumed relapse. At this time, his CMV PCR was still negative. The patient was then treated with a total of 7 plasma exchanges. He regained his motor strength once again after initiation of plasma exchange and subjectively reported progressive improvement with each treatment. The patient had no adverse reactions to the IVIG or to the plasmapheresis. He has been in remission after treatment. His renal function has remained stable through all of this.

3. Discussion

Guillain-Barré Syndrome has rarely been reported in the kidney transplant recipient. When clinical findings occur, it is usually preceded by either viral or bacterial infections that can be active during clinical presentation. Common pathogens that have been associated with GBS are *Campylobacter jejuni*, cytomegalovirus, Epstein-Barr virus, and *Mycoplasma pneumonia* [1]. Since CMV is common in the renal transplant recipient, it still remains unclear why GBS has not been reported more frequently in this population. Whether there is true underreporting of this association or whether there is some protective effect from the immunosuppression for GBS needs to be further elucidated. In the general population, morbidity and mortality with GBS are high with approximately 20% requiring artificial ventilation, 15–30% being left with severe disability and residual deficits, and about 5–10% requiring long-term use of a mechanical ventilator [13, 14]. Mortality can occur in 4–10% [15, 16]. In a transplant recipient, the course can be more severe; however, it is unpredictable. Thus, once clinically suspected, there should be prompt initiation of treatment to prevent further sequela.

The initial diagnosis of Guillain-Barré Syndrome is usually based upon the clinical presentation. The symptoms of GBS include ascending numbness, paresthesias, pain, or weakness in the limbs. GBS often can progress to ascending symmetric muscle weakness that can vary from mild difficulty with ambulation to nearly complete paralysis of all extremities, facial, and respiratory muscles [17]. Sensory involvement is common, but not as severe.

On physical examination, patients typically have motor weakness with absent or decreased deep tendon reflexes. Most patients usually have a lumbar puncture performed which can show increased cerebrospinal fluid (CSF) protein and usually have a normal CSF white blood cell count. Nerve conduction studies can confirm the diagnosis [17]. The presented patient showed typical clinical features and laboratory testing consistent with GBS. In addition, in his case there was a clear precedent acute CMV infection. See Table 1.

TABLE 1: Summary of cases with cytomegalovirus infection associated with Guillain-Barre Syndrome in renal transplant recipients.

Cases	Location	Age of recipient	Gender of recipient	Type of kidney transplant	CMV serostatus recipient/donor	CMV prophylaxis	Time after transplant when CMV infection developed	Immunosuppression regimen	Induction	Antiviral medication used for treatment	IVIG dose used for treatment	Use of plasma	Outcome
Drachman et al. 1970 [4]	US	28	Male	Cadaveric	NS/ NS	NS	5 months	Prednisone, azathioprine	None	No	No	No	Full recovery
Bale et al., 1980 [5]	USA	40	Male	Living	NS/ NS	NS	3 months	Prednisone and 3 days of radiation	NS	No	No	No	NS
Donaghy et al., 1989 [6]	UK	48	Male	Cadaveric	D+/R−	NS	7 weeks	Steroids, azathioprine, cyclosporine	NS	NS	NS	NS	NS
De Maar et al. 1999 [7]	Netherlands	58	Male	Cadaveric	D+/R−	NS	3 months	Cyclosporine, mycophenolate, prednisolone	None	Ganciclovir at a dose of 5 mg/kg every 12 h for 21 days	5 doses	No	Full recovery
El Sabrout et al. 2001 [8]	Texas	44	Male	Cadaveric	D+/R−	2-week preemptive course of ganciclovir followed by 3 months of oral acyclovir	2 years, 2 months	Mycophenolate mofetil, received for acute rejection of OKT3	NS	Steroids, no improvement	No	No	Partial recovery
El Sabrout et al. 2001 [8]	USA	47	Male	Cadaveric	D+/R−	NS	~7 years	Unknown, received for acute rejection of OKT3	NS	IV ganciclovir 5 mg/kg × 14 days	6 doses	No	Full recovery
Keithi-Reddy et al. 2007 [9]	India	48	Male	Cadaveric	D−/R−	NS	3 months post	Prednisolone, cyclosporine, mycophenolate mofetil	NS	IV ganciclovir 5 mg/kg every 12 hours for 21 days	5 doses	No	Full recovery
Alvarez et al. 2010 [10]	Spain	62	Male	Unknown	NS	NS	2.5 months	Steroids, tacrolimus, mycophenolate mofetil	NS	IV ganciclovir	5 doses	No	Full recovery
Alvarez et al. 2010 [10]	Spain	22	Female	Cadaveric	D+/R−	NS	5 weeks	Steroids, tacrolimus, mycophenolate mofetil	NS	IV ganciclovir	5 doses	4 cycles of plasmapheresis	Full recovery
Papasotiriou et al. 2013 [11]	Greece	28	NA	Cadaveric	D+/R−	IV ganciclovirfor 2 weeks, then 3 months with valganciclovir	190 days	Prednisone, tacrolimus, mycophenolate mofetil	Basiliximab, solumedrol	IV ganciclovir for 21 days. Then valacyclovir after 21 days. After 2 weeks, foscarnet	No IV IG	No	Had a relapse, then full recovery
Shaban et al. 2016 [12]	USA	62	Female	Cadaveric	D+/R−	Valganciclovir for 6 months	7 months	Tacrolimus and prednisone	Basiliximab and steroids	IV ganciclovir for 21 days	6 doses	No	Full recovery

NS = not specified, D = donor, and R = recipient.

In the reported renal transplant recipients, most of the cases occurred in middle aged, males and the majority of the cases occurred within the first six months after transplantation, likely a reflection of net immunosuppression and opportunistic infection susceptibility at this time. Induction therapy was unknown for the majority, but most of the cases were on triple-drug regimen for their transplant which consisted of prednisone, a calcineurin inhibitor, and an antimetabolite.

Initial therapy in the nontransplant GBS patient is geared toward acute management of the ill patient. Usage of intravenous immunoglobulin (IVIG) or plasma exchange has shown to reduce time to recovery and still remain the most effective strategy to treat GBS [15, 17].

Treatment with intravenous immune globulin has been shown to be at least as effective as plasma exchange alone [15]. IVIG can be given at a dose of 0.4 g/kg bodyweight daily for five consecutive days [17]. Of the 11 cases reported in the literature in renal transplant recipients, six cases received IVIG. The plasma exchange regimen frequently consists of 5 plasma volume exchanges over a two-week period [17]. Interestingly, of the cases reported only one received plasma exchange. In solid organ transplantation for active CMV disease, it is common practice to decrease immunosuppression. This consists of reduction in prednisone, targeting a lower calcineurin inhibitor trough level, and decreasing the dosage of the antimetabolite. Addition of an antiviral medication is important to decrease active viral replication and decrease long-term outcomes.

Regarding general standard CMV prophylaxis in the renal transplant recipients, recipients are generally received prophylaxis for three to six months depending on the donor and recipient CMV status at the time of transplant. In one study, prophylaxis with valganciclovir 900 mg PO once a day for 200 days in kidney transplant recipients who are CMV mismatch donor positive and recipient negative showed a decrease in late CMV disease [18]. Regarding CMV acute infection, treatment depends on the severity of the disease and could include ganciclovir intravenously if the infection is severe or oral valganciclovir (900 mg twice a day) if the disease is mild [19]. Our patient received a total of one year of prophylaxis at the discretion of the physician due to his susceptibility to developing other opportunistic infections, such as BK Virus after transplant, and concern that he was being over immunosuppressed. However, to the authors surprise, the patient developed CMV even after receiving one year of prophylaxis when he did not seem to be over immunosuppressed.

In our literature review, the majority of the cases (seven out of the 11) reported with Guillain-Barré received treatment with intravenous ganciclovir for 14 to 21 days and there was improvement in most of the cases with recovery of neurological status. Our patient received oral treatment doses of antiviral therapy and did well. In patients who have recurrent CMV disease or fail to respond after adequate therapy genotypic testing should be a consideration. Other alternative therapies for CMV resistant strains could include foscarnet or cidofovir [19].

4. Conclusion

GBS presenting after CMV infection is not widely reported in a renal transplant recipient. Due to its debilitating nature, clinicians must be mindful of the presenting signs and symptoms as the diagnosis of GBS warrants rapid and timely initiation of therapy. Exact treatment is still unknown. In the cases thus reported, an antiviral medication (oral or intravenous) in combination with plasma exchange, IVIG, or both has been utilized. Our case is the first case with success using oral antiviral medications in combination with IVIg and plasma exchange. Because plasma exchange in patients with GBS has been shown to improve muscle strength early on and reduce the need for mechanical ventilation, we decided to treat our patient with this, which was atypical for other case reports [20]. Our patient showed daily improvement with every successive plasma exchange. In addition, after the short relapse, the patient responded very well to another short course of plasma exchange. In addition to decreasing the level of immunosuppression, we suggest using a combination of antiviral medication, plasma exchange, and IVIG in the treatment of CMV induced Guillain-Barre Syndrome in the renal transplant recipient.

References

[1] S. Kuwabara, "Guillain-Barré syndrome," *Drugs*, vol. 64, no. 6, pp. 597–610, 2004.

[2] C. Ponticelli and M. R. Campise, "Neurological complications in kidney transplant recipients," *Journal of Nephrology*, vol. 18, no. 5, pp. 521–528, 2005.

[3] S. K. Arthurs, A. J. Eid, R. A. Pedersen et al., "Delayed-onset primary cytomegalovirus disease and the risk of allograft failure and mortality after kidney transplantation," *Clinical Infectious Diseases*, vol. 46, no. 6, pp. 840–846, 2008.

[4] D. A. Drachman, P. Y. Paterson, B. S. Berlin, and J. Roguska, "Immunosuppression and the Guillain-Barré Syndrome," *JAMA Neurology*, vol. 23, no. 5, pp. 385–393, 1970.

[5] J. F. Bale, L. C. Bloomer, and P. F. Bray, "Guillain-Barrélike Polyneuropathy After Renal Transplant: Possible Association with Cytomegalovirus Infection," *JAMA Neurology*, vol. 37, no. 12, p. 784, 1980.

[6] M. Donaghy, J. A. Gray, W. Squier et al., "Recurrent guillain-barré syndrome after multiple exposures to cytomegalovirus," *American Journal of Medicine*, vol. 87, no. C, pp. 339–341, 1989.

[7] E. F. De Maar, D. M. Kas-Deelen, A. E. J. De Jager, H. The, A. M. Tegzess, and W. J. Van Son, "Inflammatory demyelinating polyneuropathy in a kidney transplant patient with cytomegalovirus infection," *Nephrology Dialysis Transplantation* , vol. 14, no. 9, pp. 2228–2230, 1999.

[8] R. A. El Sabrout, B. Radovancevic, V. Ankoma-Sey, and C. T. van Buren, "Guillain-Barré syndrome after solid organ transplantation," *Transplantation*, vol. 71, no. 9, pp. 1311–1316, 2001.

[9] S. R. R. Keithi-Reddy, R. M. Chakravarthi, S. M. Hussaini, R. R. Venkatapuram, and J. M. K. Murthy, "Cytomegalovirus disease with Guillain-Barré syndrome in a cadaver renal allograft

recipient: Cause or coincidence," *International Urology and Nephrology*, vol. 39, no. 3, pp. 967–970, 2007.

[10] T. G. Alvarez, A. García Herrera, A. Mazuecos Blanca, and C. Lancho Novillo, "Guillain-barré syndrome in kidney transplant," *Nefrología*, vol. 30, no. 2, pp. 260-261, 2010.

[11] M. Papasotiriou, E. Papachristou, M. Marangos et al., "Cytomegalovirus polyradiculopathy of late onset in a young renal transplant recipient," *Clinical Nephrology*, vol. 80, no. 1, pp. 75–78, 2013.

[12] E. Shaban, "Lateonset cytomegalovirus infection complicated by Guillain–Barre syndrome in a kidney transplant recipient: case report and review of the literature," *Infection*, vol. 44, no. 2, pp. 255–258, 2016.

[13] A. F. Hahn, "Guillain-Barre syndrome," *The Lancet*, vol. 352, no. 9128, pp. 635–641, 1998.

[14] J. T. Kissel, D. R. Cornblath, and J. R. Mendell, "Guillain-Barre Syndrome," in *Diagnosis and Management of Peripheral Nerve Disorders*, Oxford University Press, New York, NY, USA, 2001.

[15] F. G. van der Meche and P. I. Schmitz, "A randomized trial comparing intravenous immune globulin and plasma exchange in Guillain-Barré syndrome. Dutch Guillain-Barré Study Group," *The New England Journal of Medicine*, vol. 326, no. 17, pp. 1123–1129, 1992.

[16] Y. A. Rajabally and A. Uncini, "Outcome and its predictors in Guillaine-Barré syndrome," *Journal of Neurology, Neurosurgery & Psychiatry*, vol. 83, no. 7, pp. 711–718, 2012.

[17] P. A. van Doorn, L. Ruts, and B. C. Jacobs, "Clinical features, pathogenesis, and treatment of Guillain-Barré syndrome," *The Lancet Neurology*, vol. 7, no. 10, pp. 939–950, 2008.

[18] A. Humar, Y. Lebranchu, F. Vincenti et al., "The efficacy and safety of 200 days valganciclovir cytomegalovirus prophylaxis in high-risk kidney transplant recipients," *American Journal of Transplantation*, vol. 10, no. 5, pp. 1228–1237, 2010.

[19] R. R. Razonable and A. Humar, "Cytomegalovirus in solid organ transplantation," *American Journal of Transplantation*, vol. 13, no. s4, pp. 93–106, 2013.

[20] J. C. Raphael, C. Chastang, J.-P. Jais, and D. Brunel, "Efficiency of plasma exchange in Guillain-Barré syndrome: Role of replacement fluids," *Annals of Neurology*, vol. 22, no. 6, pp. 753–761, 1987.

53

Renal Transplantation with Simultaneous Aortoiliac Reconstruction Using a Polytetrafluoroethylene Vascular Graft for Severe Atherosclerosis

Go Anan,[1] Koji Nanmoku,[2] Masaki Shimbo,[1] Masahiko Nagahama,[3] Takaaki Kimura,[2] Yasunaru Sakuma,[2] Fumiyasu Endo,[1] Yasuhiro Komatsu,[3] Kazunori Hattori,[1] and Takashi Yagisawa[2]

[1]*Department of Urology, St. Luke's International Hospital, Tokyo, Japan*
[2]*Surgical Branch, Institute of Kidney Diseases, Jichi Medical University Hospital, Shimotsuke, Japan*
[3]*Division of Nephrology, Department of Medicine, St. Luke's International Hospital, Tokyo, Japan*

Correspondence should be addressed to Go Anan; goanan@tohoku-mpu.ac.jp

A ademic Editor: Ryszard Grenda

Studies on aortoiliac reconstruction for severe atherosclerosis with renal transplantation are limited. Here, we report a rare experience of the simultaneous reconstruction of the external iliac artery caused by severe atherosclerosis with polytetrafluoroethylene vascular graft and renal transplantation in a 55-year-old female; she was unable to undergo standard renal artery anastomosis to the right external iliac artery because of severe atherosclerosis, which would result in complete occlusion. Next, we directly anastomosed the donor renal artery to the polytetrafluoroethylene graft. After transplantation, delayed graft function occurred; therefore, the patient had to undergo hemodialysis. On day 7 after transplantation, her creatine level started to decrease. She was discharged from the hospital on the 14th day after transplantation. After 1 month, her serum creatinine level reduced to 1.12 mg/dL. After 3 years of transplantation, her serum creatinine level was 1.2 mg/dL. The simultaneous implantation of the polytetrafluoroethylene graft and renal transplantation was feasible as well as safe, with no infectious complications and stable renal function noted on long time follow-up. Although our case was rare, it emphasizes the need for transplant surgeons to gain surgical skills for vascular surgery using vascular grafts.

1. Introduction

Atherosclerosis of the iliac arteries occurs frequently in patients with end-stage renal disease who are awaiting renal transplants [1]. Several renal transplant candidates present with iliac artery atherosclerosis; this increases the technical difficulty of the procedure. As reported previously, 0.7%–3.6% of the recipients underwent aortoiliac reconstruction before, during, and after renal transplantation [2–8]. The indications for renal transplantation in these cases were controversial because of the difficulty associated with vascular dissection and the risk of infection. In addition, the vascular reconstruction timing remains controversial in both simultaneous and staged renal transplantation [2]. Here, we report a case of renal transplantation, wherein, owing to the emergency nature of the case, aortoiliac reconstruction was performed with the simultaneous implantation of a vascular graft.

2. Case Presentation

The patient was a 55-year-old woman with end-stage renal disease of unknown cause who had been undergoing hemodialysis for the past 4 years before receiving a living-related renal transplant from her husband in September 2014. Before the transplantation, the recipient's computed tomography (CT) scan revealed moderate to severe atherosclerosis of the bilateral iliac arteries. Also, the donor's CT revealed two left renal arteries. For blood type-compatible and donor-specific antibody-positive recipients, desensitization was performed before transplantation with three sessions of double filtration plasmapheresis or plasma exchange and two doses

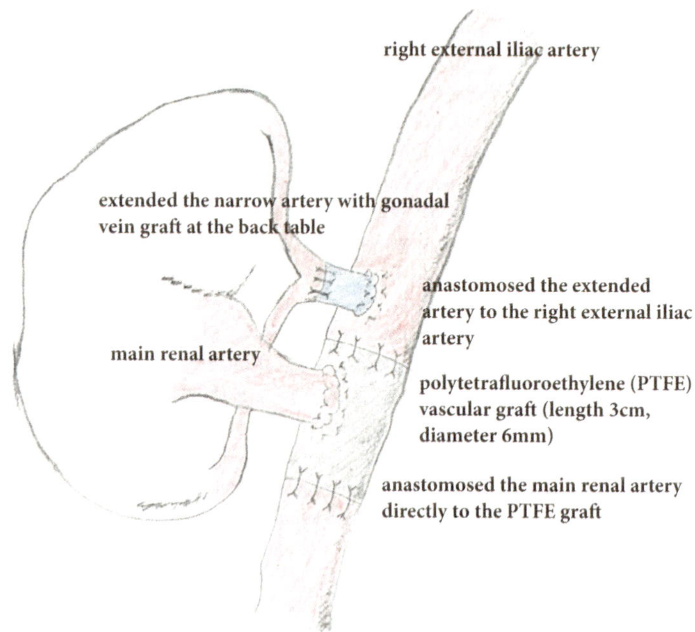

Figure 1: An illustration of aortoiliac reconstruction using polytetrafluoroethylene vascular graft.

of rituximab (100 mg). Immunosuppressive agents included triple immunosuppressive therapy with extended-release tacrolimus, mycophenolate mofetil, and methylprednisolone. Briefly, the transplant bed was made in the right iliac fossa. At the back table, there were two donor renal arteries, namely, the main artery and one narrow artery. Because the length of the narrow artery was short, it had to be extended using the donor's gonadal vein graft with end-to-end anastomosis using a 6-0 monofilament at the back table. Usually when there are two donor renal arteries, we connect the two arteries conjointly or side-to-end at the back table. However, as the length of one artery was short and the distance between the two arteries was large to connect, we thought that connecting the two arteries will enable anastomotic stenosis. Therefore, we decided to intracorporeally anastomose each renal artery to the iliac artery. The transplanted renal vein was anastomosed to the right external iliac vein side-to-end using a 5-0 monofilament with continuous sutures. First, considering the position of the two arteries, we decided to anastomose the extended artery to the right external iliac artery side-to-end using a 6-0 monofilament with continuous sutures. Second, before anastomosing the main artery to the iliac artery, we punched out the external iliac artery using an aorta punch; however, the cavity in the artery was narrow. Firstly, we performed endarterectomy to create sufficient space for anastomosis with the renal artery. However, we could not make a sufficient cavity to ensure adequate blood flow. Therefore, we decided to reconstruct the external artery using a polytetrafluoroethylene (PTFE) vascular graft to achieve adequate blood flow. We were unable to undertake the standard renal artery anastomosis to the right external iliac artery owing to severe atherosclerosis, which would result in complete occlusion. After reconstructing the external artery with the PTFE vascular graft (length, 3 cm; diameter, 6 mm),

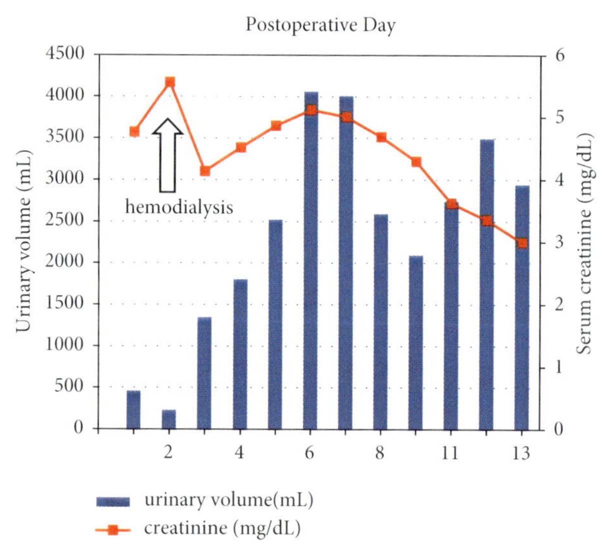

Figure 2: The clinical course of urinary volume and renal function.

the transplanted main renal artery was anastomosed directly to the PTFE graft side-to-end using a 5-0 monofilament with continuous sutures (Figure 1). The surgical procedure lasted for 9 h and 14 min; the total ischemic time was 3 h and 20 min, and we could not confirm the first urine during the operation. The total bleeding volume was 450 mL; the same volume was transfused during the transplantation.

After transplantation, delayed graft function occurred, for which the patient had to undergo hemodialysis session on the third day after transplantation. Seven days after the transplantation, her serum creatinine level started to decrease (Figure 2). The patient was discharged from the hospital on the 14th day after transplantation. Her serum creatinine level had reduced to 3.01 mg/dL on the day of discharge. Furthermore, after 1 month of discharge, her serum creatinine level reduced even further to 1.12 mg/dL. Presently, after 3 years of transplantation, her serum creatinine level is stable (1.2 mg/dL). She showed no sign of arterial graft infection after the renal transplantation. As she received an internalized antiplatelet agent before the transplantation because of coronary disease, internal resumption was resumed from seven days after transplantation to date.

3. Discussion

The number of renal transplant candidates with extended indications, such as older age and advanced atherosclerosis, is currently increasing [1, 2]. This has increased the number of cases that are difficult to treat using vascular anastomosis. However, studies on aortoiliac reconstruction with renal transplantation are limited. In transplant recipients with iliac artery atherosclerosis, it is possible to perform additional vascular procedures simultaneously, before performing transplantation in selected cases [2–8]. In the simultaneous aortoiliac reconstruction group, perioperative surgical complications, such as bleeding and infection, have been noted. No perioperative mortality was related to the additional vascular procedure [2]. Moreover, simultaneous aortoiliac reconstruction was not associated with increased risk of delayed graft function or with a longer hospital stay [2]. However, in our case, delayed graft function occurred, necessitating the need for hemodialysis. Contrarily, another study on 11 patients reported simultaneous aortoiliac reconstruction, wherein two grafts were lost because of bleeding from the anastomotic site and primary nonfunction resulting from prolonged warm ischemia [3]. No infectious complications of the vascular graft were noticed during the 4 years in all 11 renal recipients [3]. Contrarily, one recipient died because of prosthetic graft infection secondary to a urinary tract fistula [4].

Considering the advantages and disadvantages, we have summarized the differences in the vascular procedures before or during transplantation [2–8]. Several advantages were noted in simultaneous transplantation with vascular reconstruction. First, no technical difficulties in the dissection caused by reoperation were noticed. Second, the hospitalization time and cost are reduced as compared with those of separate operations. Third, general anesthesia is required only once; thus, risks caused by anesthesia are decreased. There were also several disadvantages. First, the operation procedure was complex and difficult to perform. Second, there was an inherent risk of prosthesis infection in immunosuppressed patients. Third, there was a risk of graft function because of the long ischemic time and extra procedure.

At our institution, up to two renal arteries are usually selected in the left kidney as donors to secure a long renal vein. In the case of two renal arteries, we normally connect the two arteries conjointly or side-to-end at the back table. Therefore, we selected the left kidney as the donor in this case. It is notable that the increased use of kidneys with multiple renal arteries does not affect any clinical outcome of the recipient besides total ischemia time [9].

In our case, the patient showed no symptoms of vascular disorders. At our institution, we do not usually perform enhanced CT scan and vascular 3D reconstruction before transplantation. Thus, we could not predict severe arteriosclerosis of the external iliac artery from nonenhanced CT scan in this case. In mild arteriosclerosis cases, we normally perform endarterectomy to make sufficient space for successful anastomosis with the renal artery. If severe arteriosclerosis of the iliac artery is predicted before transplantation, we consider anastomosis to the iliac artery on the contralateral side and the common iliac artery. During the transplantation, we could not make sufficient space to anastomose the renal artery after endarterectomy; therefore, we finally decided to reconstruct the external artery using the PTFE vascular graft. We successfully performed the simultaneous implantation of PTFE graft with stable renal function and no infectious complications. From our experience, we noted some important points for successful aortoiliac reconstruction performed simultaneously with renal transplantation. First, surgeons should always be prepared for sudden vascular reconstruction. Renal transplant surgeons should continuously gain and enhance their skills in performing anastomosing prosthesis. Second, to avoid prosthesis infection, it is important to ensure hemostasis and prevent urinary and lymph fistulas.

4. Conclusion

The simultaneous implantation of the PTFE graft with renal transplantation because of severe atherosclerosis is feasible and safe, because stable renal function and no infectious complications were noted in our patient.

References

[1] K. Nanmoku, Y. Watarai, S. Narumi et al., "Surgical techniques and procedures for kidney transplant recipients with severe atherosclerosis," *Experimental and Clinical Transplantation*, vol. 15, no. 6, pp. 594–601, 2017.

[2] D. J. Han, Y. H. Kim, Y. S. Chung et al., "Effects of simultaneous Iliac artery angioplasty on graft and patient survival after living-donor kidney transplantation," *Transplantation*, vol. 97, no. 8, pp. 826–831, 2014.

[3] A. Özçelik, J. Treckmann, A. Paul et al., "Results of kidney transplantation with simultaneous implantation of vascular graft," *Transplantation Proceedings*, vol. 39, no. 2, pp. 509-510, 2007.

[4] P. Gouny, B. Lenot, B. Decaix et al., "Aortoiliac surgery and kidney transplantation," *Annals of Vascular Surgery*, vol. 5, no. 1, pp. 26–31, 1991.

[5] D. Patrono, R. Verhelst, A. Buemi et al., "Renal allograft implantation on prosthetic vascular grafts: short- and long-term results," *World Journal of Surgery*, vol. 37, no. 7, pp. 1727–1734, 2013.

[6] I. Matia, M. Adamec, M. Varga, L. Janousek, K. Lipar, and O. Viklicky, "Aortoiliac reconstruction with allograft and kidney transplantation as a one-stage procedure: long term results," *European Journal of Vascular and Endovascular Surgery*, vol. 35, no. 3, pp. 353–357, 2008.

[7] M. Tsivian, F. Neri, B. Nardo et al., "Aortoiliac surgery concomitant with kidney transplantation: a single center experience," *Clinical Transplantation*, vol. 23, no. 2, pp. 164–167, 2009.

[8] Z. Galazka, T. Grochowiecki, T. Jakimowicz, M. Kowalczewski, and J. Szmidt, "Is severe atherosclerosis in the aortoiliac region a contraindication for kidney transplantation?" *Transplantation Proceedings*, vol. 43, no. 8, pp. 2908–2910, 2011.

[9] K. Nanmoku, A. Kurosawa, T. Kubo et al., "Selection criteria for kidney laterality in retroperitoneoscopic living donor nephrectomy and the usefulness of pretransplant intervention," *Transplantation Proceedings*, vol. 49, no. 5, pp. 924–929, 2017.

54

Fatal Donor-Derived Carbapenem-Resistant *Klebsiella pneumoniae* Infection in a Combined Kidney-Pancreas Transplantation

Giovanni Varotti,[1] Ferdinando Dodi,[2] Anna Marchese,[3] Alessia Terulla,[1] Massimo Bertocchi,[1] and Iris Fontana[1]

[1]*Kidney Transplant Unit, IRCCS San Martino University Hospital, IST National Institute for Cancer Research, Genoa, Italy*
[2]*Department of Infectious Disease, IRCCS San Martino University Hospital, IST National Institute for Cancer Research, Genoa, Italy*
[3]*Department of Microbiology, IRCCS San Martino University Hospital, IST National Institute for Cancer Research, Genoa, Italy*

Correspondence should be addressed to Giovanni Varotti; gvarotti@hotmail.com

Academic Editor: Graeme Forrest

Carbapenem-resistant *Klebsiella pneumoniae* (CR-KP) infections in solid organ transplant recipients are associated with high morbidity and mortality. We report a case of a fatal donor-derived CR-KP infection in a combined kidney-pancreas transplant. Given the short interval of time between donor hospitalization and organ procurement, information concerning the donor CR-KP positivity arrived only 72 hours after transplant. Based on this experience, we believe that knowledge of the donor's CR-KP status should be mandatory before procurement and, if positive, pancreas donation should be contraindicated.

1. Introduction

First described in 2001 concerning an isolate collected in a North Carolina Hospital in 1996, CR-KP infections have spread rapidly worldwide, becoming a serious healthcare problem associated with increased cost and length of stay as well as worse patient outcomes [1, 2]. Its impact can be particularly devastating in solid organ transplant recipients, as they are a very high-risk population because of either their immunosuppressed status or their prolonged hospitalization [3, 4].

Moreover, given their stay in intensive care units under mechanical ventilation and their severe illness requiring vasopressor support, deceased multiorgan donors are also another high-risk category for CR-KP transmission, leading potentially to donor-derived infection of recipients [5].

Unfortunately, definitive information concerning the donor's cultures may be still unknown during the times of procurement and implantation, resulting in an indefinite risk for donor-derived CR-KP transmission.

2. Case Report

We report the case of a 37-year-old diabetic female, who underwent a combined kidney-pancreas transplant in our centre in April 2014.

Donor was a 26-year-old male who remained in ICU for only 18 hours before procurement and was considered a "standard" risk for infections.

Simultaneous pancreas and left kidney transplant was performed by first placing the pancreatic graft in the right lower intraperitoneal cavity, with vascularization on the recipient's right common iliac axis and a duodenoenterostomy for the exocrine drainage. Then a standard kidney transplant was performed placing the graft in the left iliac fossa.

Intravenous (IV) amoxicillin doses were continued for 48 hours as perioperative antibiotic prophylaxis.

On POD 3, the donor's sputum, bronchoalveolar lavage cultures, and the rectal swab were positive for carbapenem-resistant *Klebsiella pneumoniae* (CR-KP), susceptible only to colistin (MIC = 2 mg/L); the donor's blood cultures were negative. Combined IV preemptive antibiotic therapy with colistin (loading dose: 9.000.000 IU, maintenance dose: 2.000.000 IU/BID), meropenem (dose: 2 gr./BID), and tigecycline (loading dose: 100 mg, maintenance dose: 50 mg/BID) was started.

Four days later, the recipient's blood cultures revealed a CR-KP infection and a picture of peritonitis required an urgent relaparotomy which showed an enteric leak from duodenoileal anastomosis with surrounding necrotic tissue, which imposed the removal of the pancreatic graft.

Evidence of CR-KP was confirmed in the intraoperative swabs collected from the duodenal graft.

Comparison of all the donor's isolates to the recipient's blood isolate by pulsed-field gel electrophoresis [1] revealed an identical profile, confirming the donor-derived infection. The identifications of the KPC-3 gene were achieved by PCR and sequencing using primers and conditions previously described [6]. Genomic DNA was prepared, digested with *Xba*I (New England Biolabs Inc., MA, USA) and subjected to PFGE with the CHEF DRII device (Bio-Rad, Milan, Italy). All isolates exhibited the same PFGE macrorestriction profile, confirming the donor-derived infections.

Antibiotic was continued for six weeks, until cultures tested negative; on POD 70, the patient was discharged with normal kidney function, remaining colonized for CR-KP by positive rectal swab.

One month later, the patient was readmitted for a pseudoaneurysm of the right common iliac artery with surrounding liquid collection, found to be CR-KP positive and colistin resistant (MIC = 3 mg/L, EUCAST confirmed). Patient underwent right iliac replacement with heterologous homograft which was then infected by CR-KP requiring a subsequent silver graft substitution. Triple IV antibiotic therapy with ertapenem (500 mg/daily), meropenem (2 g/BID), and tigecycline (loading dose: 100 mg, maintenance dose: 50 mg/BID) was reintroduced but the iliac wound cultures remained CR-KP positive, subsequently developing a picture of sepsis. In the following weeks, the patient's condition progressively worsened and, unfortunately, she died as a result of multiorgan failure 195 days after transplant.

3. Discussion

There is very little data on this argument and, to the best of our knowledge, this is the first case reporting a donor-derived CR-KP infection in a kidney-pancreas transplant recipient. In the 15 published cases of donor-derived CR-KP infection in solid organ transplant (5 kidneys, 5 livers, 3 lungs, 1 combined liver-kidney, and 1 heart), 13 had an uneventful outcome while 2 recipients died (one after receiving a lung from an asymptomatic carrier of CR-KP in the respiratory tract and one after receiving a kidney from a donor with CR-KP urine infection) [3–5, 7, 8]. These initial experiences suggest that, in well-defined conditions and following a strict follow-up, organs from colonized CR-KP donors may be considered for transplantation, avoiding their use when the donor's blood cultures were positive or when the organ is directly involved in CR-KP infection, such as lungs in the case of the airway infection or kidneys in urinary tract isolation [7, 8].

However, our experience revealed peculiar aspects of pancreas donation. In a colonized subject, the CR-KP bacteria remain silent and mainly at the level of the gastrointestinal tract; in this setting, in the event of a pancreas transplant in which the graft necessarily includes a duodenal tract, there could be a high potential risk of direct bacterial transmission from the duodenal graft to the recipient.

In our case, the intraoperative swab collected proved the presence of CR-KP bacteria in the explanted duodenal graft. However, we cannot state that the CR-KP infection was directly responsible for the duodenal-ileal anastomotic leak but it was certainly one of the main causes of the sequence of unfavourable events which led to the patient's death. As a result of this experience, we believe that pancreas donation should also be contraindicated in the event of colonized CR-KP donors.

Given the short time interval between donor hospitalization and organ procurement (<24 hours), we learnt of the positivity of the rectal swab only three days after transplant. We believe it would be crucial to receive this information before harvesting, to optimize the organ allocation process. These reasons highlight the importance of prompt interinstitutional information sharing among the donor's hospital doctors, local organ coordination centre, and transplant teams. Moreover, we believe that in selected cases, such as ours, the use of faster diagnostic assays such as real-time PCR [9, 10] should be encouraged for rapid CR-KP detection.

Abbreviations

CR-KP: Carbapenem-resistant *Klebsiella pneumoniae*
ICU: Intensive care units.

Competing Interests

The authors declare that there is no conflict of interests regarding the publication of this paper.

References

[1] L. S. Munoz-Price, L. Poirel, R. A. Bonomo et al., "Clinical epidemiology of the global expansion of *Klebsiella pneumoniae* carbapenemases," *The Lancet Infectious Diseases*, vol. 13, no. 9, pp. 785–796, 2013.

[2] J. A. Fishman and P. A. Grossi, "Donor-derived infection-the challenge for transplant safety," *Nature Reviews Nephrology*, vol. 10, no. 11, pp. 663–672, 2014.

[3] E. Goldberg, J. Bishara, S. Lev, P. Singer, and J. Cohen, "Organ transplantation from a donor colonized with a multidrug-resistant organism: a case report," *Transplant Infectious Disease*, vol. 14, no. 3, pp. 296–299, 2012.

[4] A. Mularoni, A. Bertani, G. Vizzini et al., "Outcome of transplantation using organs from donors infected or colonized with carbapenem-resistant gram-negative bacteria," *American Journal of Transplantation*, vol. 15, no. 10, pp. 2674–2682, 2015.

[5] J. Bishara, E. Goldberg, S. Lev, P. Singer, T. Ashkenazi, and J. Cohen, "The utilization of solid organs for transplantation in the setting of infection with multidrug-resistant organisms: an expert opinion," *Clinical Transplantation*, vol. 26, no. 6, pp. 811–815, 2012.

[6] A. Marchese, E. Coppo, R. Barbieri, and E. Debbia, "Emergence of KPC-2 carbapenemase-producing *Klebsiella pneumoniae* strains and spread of an isolate of sequence type 258 in the neuro-rehabilitation Unit of an Italian hospital," *Journal of Chemotherapy*, vol. 22, no. 3, pp. 212–214, 2010.

[7] E. J. Ariza-Heredia, R. Patel, E. A. Blumberg et al., "Outcomes of transplantation using organs from a donor infected with *Klebsiella pneumoniae* carbapenemase (KPC)-producing *K. pneumoniae*," *Transplant Infectious Disease*, vol. 14, no. 3, pp. 229–236, 2012.

[8] T. Giani, V. Conte, S. Mandalà et al., "Cross-infection of solid organ transplant recipients by a multidrug-resistant *Klebsiella pneumoniae* isolate producing the OXA-48 carbapenemase, likely derived from a multiorgan donor," *Journal of Clinical Microbiology*, vol. 52, no. 7, pp. 2702–2705, 2014.

[9] M. Hindiyeh, G. Smollen, Z. Grossman et al., "Rapid detection of *blaKPC* carbapenemase genes by real-time PCR," *Journal of Clinical Microbiology*, vol. 46, no. 9, pp. 2879–2883, 2008.

[10] J. M. Cole, A. N. Schuetz, C. E. Hill, and F. S. Nolte, "Development and evaluation of a real-time PCR assay for detection of *Klebsiella pneumoniae* carbapenemase genes," *Journal of Clinical Microbiology*, vol. 47, no. 2, pp. 322–326, 2009.

55

Successful Renal Transplantation between Identical Twins with Very Brief Immunosuppression

Idris Yakubu[1], **Abdolreza Haririan**[2], **Stephen Bartlett**[2] **and Tracy Sparkes**[1]

[1] *Pharmacy, University of Maryland Medical Center, Baltimore, MD, USA*
[2] *University of Maryland School of Medicine, Baltimore, MD, USA*

Correspondence should be addressed to Idris Yakubu; idrisyakubu90@gmail.com

Academic Editor: Ryszard Grenda

Renal transplantation between monozygous identical twins provides an opportunity to utilize minimal immunosuppression to maintain stable allograft function, thereby alleviating the toxicities of immunosuppressive therapy. Despite monozygosity, there is a possibility of discordant protein presentation in identical twins that could trigger alloimmune response and lead to graft injury. Therefore, the optimal immunosuppression regimen in this patient population is unknown, and the safety of immunosuppression withdrawal remains controversial. Herein, we describe two patients who underwent successful renal transplantation from monozygotic identical twin donors. Monozygosity was determined using short tandem repeat (STR) analysis. All immunosuppression was successfully discontinued at 2 days and 3 weeks, respectively, after transplantation. Both patients are alive with functioning renal grafts at 1 year and 5 years after transplant, respectively. These two cases suggest that immunosuppression can be withdrawn safely and rapidly in select monozygous identical twin renal transplant recipients.

1. Introduction

Although advances in immunosuppression have led to improvement in short-term renal transplant graft outcomes, the vast majority of transplant recipients must remain on immunosuppressive medications for the lifetime of their allografts in order to prevent rejection. Due to the effects of immunosuppression, transplant patients are vulnerable to infection and malignancy. Additionally, immunosuppressive drugs increase the risk of posttransplant metabolic complications such as diabetes, hypertension, hyperlipidemia, and obesity, which are important risk factors for cardiovascular diseases—the leading cause of death in renal transplant recipients [1–5]. Living related kidney transplantation between identical twins provides a unique opportunity to further optimize patient and graft outcomes, given the low risk of allograft rejection. This low immunological risk also confers an opportunity to minimize or withdraw immunosuppression, thereby reducing or altogether avoiding the toxicities associated with immunosuppressive medications [6, 7].

This concept was demonstrated by the first successful kidney transplant that was performed over 6 decades ago by Dr. Joseph E. Murray at the Peter Bent Brigham Hospital in Boston. The recipient was a 24-year-old male who developed renal failure from glomerulonephritis and received a kidney transplant from his monozygotic identical twin brother. No immunosuppression was utilized, due to lack of availability. The recipient had a functioning graft for 9 years after transplant until he expired due to a myocardial infarction [7]. Since the discovery of pharmacological immunosuppression in the early 1960s and advances in understanding of the immunological mechanisms involved in rejection, various immunosuppression strategies have been used in this patient population [7–13]. When utilized, the appropriate choice of or the optimal dosing of the immunosuppressive agent(s) required remains unclear. Growing knowledge of the possibility of genetic differences between identical twins has further contributed to a variety of opinions on the optimal approach for these patients. Herein, we describe two cases of kidney transplantation between identical twins where

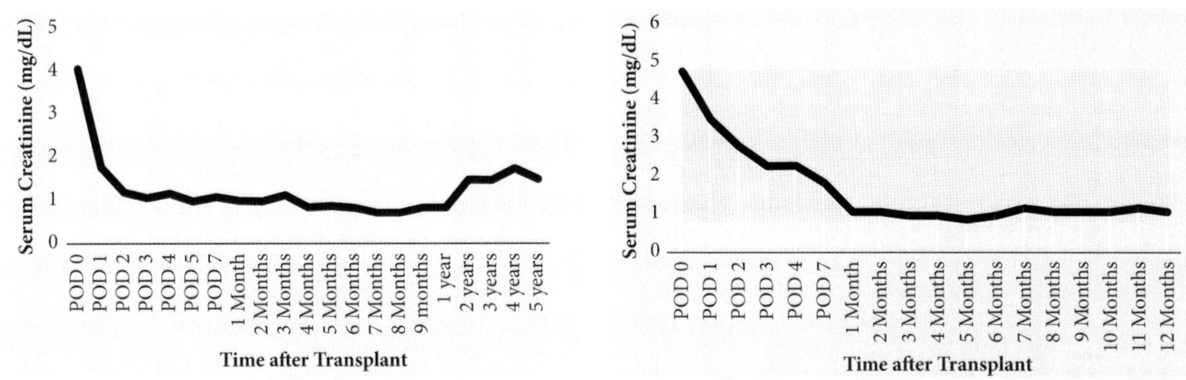

(a) Serum creatinine trend after transplantation

(b) Serum creatinine trend after transplantation

Figure 1

immunosuppression was safely and rapidly withdrawn after transplant, despite the presence of donor specific antibody in one patient.

2. Case Presentation

2.1. Patient 1. A 60-year-old Caucasian female with a history of ESRD secondary to hypertension and type 1 diabetes mellitus received a living related renal transplant from her HLA identical twin sister. At the time of transplant, monozygosity had yet to be determined. Therefore, she received a 3-day course of steroids, consisting of methylprednisolone 500 mg intraoperatively, followed by 250 mg and 125 mg on postoperative days (POD) 1 and 2, respectively. She also received maintenance immunosuppression of tacrolimus with a target trough level of 6 ng/mL and mycophenolic acid (Myfortic®) 360 mg twice daily. Postoperatively, blood samples from the donor and recipient were sent for short tandem repeat (STR) analysis in order to determine monozygosity. Given the use of maintenance immunosuppression, opportunistic infection prophylaxis was provided with oral sulfamethoxazole-trimethoprim 400-80 mg daily for *Pneumocystis jirovecii* pneumonia, fungal prophylaxis with oral clotrimazole 10 mg four times daily and cytomegalovirus (CMV) prophylaxis with valganciclovir 900 mg daily. She experienced immediate graft function and was discharged with no complications on postoperative day (POD) 5 with a serum creatinine (SCr) of approximately 1.0 mg/dL. The STR analysis occurred one week after transplant and demonstrated allelic identity at all 16 loci tested, consistent with monozygosity. Therefore, the transplant team decided to discontinue maintenance immunosuppression. Tacrolimus was stopped 12 days after transplant, and mycophenolate was stopped one week later. Infection prophylaxis was also discontinued once maintenance immunosuppression was stopped. She continues to have stable graft function at 5 years after transplant, with a baseline SCr of approximately 1.5 mg/dL (Figure 1(a)). She has experienced several episodes of mild acute kidney injury, which were attributed to her poorly controlled diabetes mellitus. She underwent a protocol allograft biopsy at 3 months after transplant, which showed no significant interstitial fibrosis and tubular atrophy, minimal arterial sclerosis, and mild arteriolar hyalinosis, with no evidence of acute allograft rejection. At 17 months after transplant, she underwent a second biopsy due to an elevation in SCr. The second biopsy showed mild tubular injury, without evidence of allograft rejection. No interventions were indicated based on the results of the 2 allograft biopsies, beside attempts to optimize her glycemic control. She has had no infectious or neoplastic complications from short-term immunosuppression.

2.2. Patient 2. A 71-year-old Caucasian female received a living related renal transplant from her identical twin sister. She developed ESRD due to chronic cystitis related to ureteral obstruction. Prior to transplantation, she made normal amounts of urine and had been on hemodialysis for 6 months. Her past surgical history included an ileal loop conduit urinary diversion and ileostomy drainage bag placement. Given the recipient's structural bladder anomaly, a ureteral anastomosis was made to the small bowel over a 6-French 30 cm double-J stent which extended from the renal pelvis out to the ileal conduit. Prior to transplant, monozygosity was confirmed via an STR analysis, which revealed that she was identical to her sister in all 16 polymorphic gene loci that were evaluated. Additionally, she was found to be a six-antigen match on HLA typing and had a negative anti-human globulin (AHG) crossmatch. Interestingly, a class II donor specific antibody (DSA) to DPB1∗05:01/DPA1∗02:02 with a mean fluorescence intensity (MFI) of 1,359 was identified four months prior to transplant. The antibody screening was repeated 10 days prior to transplant and revealed an MFI of 1,458. Based on the confirmation of monozygosity, the transplant team proceeded with transplantation without maintenance immunosuppression. She received a 3-day steroid taper course consisting of methylprednisolone 500 mg intraoperatively, followed by 250 mg and 125 mg intravenously on POD 1 and 2, respectively. She did not receive antibody induction therapy or further maintenance immunosuppression beyond the corticosteroids. Due to rapid immunosuppression withdrawal, she did not receive prophylaxis against opportunistic infections. She experienced immediate graft function, although her SCr was initially slow to decline (Figure 1(b)). Her hospital course was uncomplicated, and she was discharged home on POD 4 with a SCr of 2.3 mg/dL. She experienced a urinary tract infection (UTI) approximately 1 month after transplant, which resolved after ureteral stent removal and treatment with a 7-day course of oral ciprofloxacin. At 1 year after transplant, she continues to have excellent graft function with a baseline serum creatinine of 1.0 ng/mL (Figure 1(b)). A protocol kidney biopsy was attempted approximately 3 months after transplant, which however could not be performed due to lack of a clear window. Repeat posttransplant surveillance DSA screening with high resolution typing at the time of the attempted biopsy revealed persistence of Class II DPB1∗05:01/DPA1∗02:02 antibody, with a stable MFI of 1,030. She remains free from long-term complications due to brief immunosuppression, including infections, malignancy, or metabolic complications.

3. Discussion

The optimal immunosuppressive agent, magnitude, and duration of immunosuppression after monozygotic twin kidney transplantation remain controversial [9–13]. While our center's approach to date has been to rapidly minimize immunosuppression, this is not necessarily the approach followed elsewhere. In a study of 120 identical twin renal transplant recipients in the United States (US) and 12 recipients in the United Kingdom (UK), 68% and 33% of patients, respectively, were discharged on some form of immunosuppression, with steroids being the most commonly used agent in both groups [11]. At various follow-up time points, fewer patients were on each immunosuppressive agent. This suggests that, in some patients, immunosuppression was only given for a short period of time after transplantation. However, the timeframe of discontinuation of immunosuppression was not reported, and it is unclear if all cases were truly monozygotic identical twins. In the US cohort, although the 5-year graft survival rate among those who received immunosuppression was numerically better compared to those who did not, the difference was not statistically significant (93.9% versus 84.0%, $p = 0.12$) [11]. Additionally, in an Organ Procurement Transplant Network (OPTN) database study, Krishnan et al. evaluated the use of immunosuppressive agents at discharge and 6 months and 1, 2, and 3 years after transplant in identical twin kidney transplant recipients. The authors found that 71% and 34% of patients were on some form of immunosuppression at time of discharge and 1 year, respectively. Of those patients receiving immunosuppression at discharge, 59% were maintained on immunosuppression beyond 6 months after transplant and 33% of patients were on some form of immunosuppression therapy at 3 years after transplant. Patient and graft survival rates were similar from the time of transplant up to five years between those who received immunosuppression at discharge and those who did not ($p =$ 0.98 and 0.54, respectively). After 5 years, patients who had received immunosuppression at discharge had worse patient survival rates, compared to those who did not ($p \leq 0.04$), likely due to both short and long-term complications from immunosuppression. Renal function at 6 months onwards was superior in those not receiving immunosuppression ($p \leq 0.007$). The average serum creatinine at 3 years after transplant was 1.46 ± 0.96 in patients receiving immunosuppression, compared to 1.13 ± 0.21 in those not on immunosuppression ($p = 0.003$). This difference in renal function was attributed to calcineurin inhibitor induced nephrotoxicity in patients receiving immunosuppression. The authors concluded that immunosuppression minimization in monozygotic twin transplantation may allow for better graft function and recommended the use of perioperative high dose steroids to minimize the potential for immune system activation from surgical tissue damage, followed by a rapid steroid taper to avoid the consequences of chronic immunosuppression [12].

The optimal method of determining monozygosity is unclear. A variety of methods have been used to identify monozygosity, including HLA typing, blood typing, chorionicity, evaluation of placenta after birth, deoxyribonucleic acid (DNA) finger printing, and reciprocal skin grafting [7, 14]. These methods have several limitations and are prone to misinterpretations. Standard HLA typing which is commonly used to determine zygosity may not accurately diagnose monozygosity, as 25% of dizygotic twins can be identical in all HLA loci [15, 16]. STR analysis has been shown to provide a greater sensitivity and precision in identifying differences between identical twins [17, 18]. Furthermore, advances in immunology and biology have shown that monozygous twins may not be completely identical as previously believed. Several mechanisms for differences, including postzygotic genetic changes, antenatal environmental effects, and postnatal environmental experiences have been postulated. These differences could lead to minor antigen presentation and trigger an alloimmune response against the transplanted organ [19, 20]. However, the possibility of antibody formation against donor HLA antigens in monozygous identical twins has not been reported in the literature. Our second patient was reported to have a class II antibody with borderline MFI, according to the threshold value used in our laboratory for detection of DSA. We are not certain if this was a false positive finding due to the limitations of MFI or the technique. One could postulate that the finding of antibody in this patient was possibly due to somatic genetic mutations in the donor that led to abnormal protein presentation and triggered antibody formation in the recipient.

In our center's twin transplant experience, the patients received a short course of steroids to decrease innate immune response resulting from ischemia-reperfusion injury, which has been shown to increase the risk of graft rejection [21, 22]. Previous studies have shown that the presence of preformed anti-HLA antibodies directed against a donor's class II antigens confers a high risk of humoral rejection [23, 24]. However, this does not necessarily correlate with an increased risk of rejection and graft loss in renal transplant recipients [25, 26]. Despite the presence of pretransplant DSA in patient 2, we decided not to use chronic immunosuppression, given her low antibody titers in the setting of a negative flow crossmatch and the results of HLA typing and STR. Therefore, we opted for minimum perioperative immunosuppression to prevent potential immunologic response to ischemia-reperfusion injury with close posttransplant surveillance and monitoring. Based on these experiences, our center performs STR analysis ahead of time in cases of identical twin transplants, to avoid unnecessary immunosuppression.

Previous published cases on identical twin transplantation have mostly been limited to a younger adult population with an average age of 30 years. Younger recipient age has been demonstrated to confer an increased risk of rejection after transplantation, due to a more robust immune response. Consequently, most transplant centers tend to favor more intense immunosuppression strategies in the younger transplant population [27]. The advanced age (>60 years old) of both patients provided an added opportunity to allow minimum immunosuppression utilization. Elderly patients have a less competent immune system, which reduces their risk of rejection after transplantation and contributes to a greater vulnerability to the toxicities of immunosuppressive therapy, including an increased risk of infections and death [28, 29].

In conclusion, these cases demonstrate that immunosuppression can be safely withdrawn in monozygotic identical twin transplant recipients. The consideration for immunosuppression withdrawal or minimization in this patient population needs to be individualized, and several important factors need to be considered, including confirmation of true monozygosity by means of reliable methods and analysis of the risk versus benefit of immunosuppression, including the likelihood of primary disease recurrence. We recommend the use of steroids perioperatively to prevent rejection resulting from activation of innate immune response due to ischemic reperfusion injury, along with close posttransplant monitoring.

Abbreviations

ESRD: End stage renal disease
STR: Short tandem repeat
HLA: Human leukocyte antigen
CKD: Chronic kidney disease
AHG: Anti-human globulin
DSA: Donor specific antibody
MFI: Mean fluorescence intensity
IV: Intravenously
POD: Postoperative day
UTI: Urinary tract infection
US: United States
UK: United Kingdom
OPTN: Organ Procurement and Transplantation Network.

References

[1] A. Lindholm, D. Albrechtsen, L. Frödin, G. Tufveson, N. H. Persson, and G. Lundgren, "Ischemic heart disease—major cause of death and graft loss after renal transplantation in scandinavia," *Transplantation*, vol. 60, no. 5, pp. 451–457, 1995.

[2] K. Sato, F. Tadokoro, K. Ishida et al., "Causes of death after renal transplantation: A long-term follow-up study," *Transplantation Proceedings*, vol. 26, pp. 2017-2018, 1994.

[3] A. O. Ojo, J. A. Hanson, R. A. Wolfe, A. B. Leichtman, L. Y. Agodoa, and F. K. Port, "Long-term survival in renal transplant recipients with graft function," *Kidney International*, vol. 57, no. 1, pp. 307–313, 2000.

[4] J. D. Briggs, "Causes of death after renal transplantation," *Nephrology Dialysis Transplantation* , vol. 16, no. 8, pp. 1545–1549, 2001.

[5] A. E. El-Agroudy, M. A. Bakr, A. B. S. El-Dein, and M. A. Ghoneim, "Death with functioning graft in living donor kidney transplantation: Analysis of risk factors," *American Journal of Nephrology*, vol. 23, no. 3, pp. 186–193, 2003.

[6] I. I. N. Doxiadis, J. M. A. Smits, G. M. T. Schreuder et al., "Association between specific HLA combinations and probability of kidney allograft loss: the taboo concept," *The Lancet*, vol. 348, no. 9031, pp. 850–853, 1996.

[7] J. P. Merrill, J. E. Murray, J. H. Harrison, and W. R. Guild, "Successful homotransplantation of the human kidney between identical twins," *Journal of the American Medical Association*, vol. 160, no. 4, pp. 277–282, 1956.

[8] N. L. Tilney, "Renal transplantation between identical twins: A review," *World Journal of Surgery*, vol. 10, no. 3, pp. 381–388, 1986.

[9] A. Hauch, J. Heneghan, M. Killackey et al., "Living-related kidney transplant in two sets of HLA-identical twins," *Journal of Surgery and Transplantation Science*, vol. 1, no. 1, article 1003, 2013.

[10] M. Gumprich, G. Woeste, K. Kohlhaw, J. T. Epplen, and W. O. Bechstein, "Living related kidney transplantation between identical twins," *Transplantation Proceedings*, vol. 34, no. 6, pp. 2205-2206, 2002.

[11] N. Kessaris, D. Mukherjee, P. Chandak, and N. Mamode, "Renal transplantation in identical twins in United States and United Kingdom," *Transplantation*, vol. 86, no. 11, pp. 1572–1577, 2008.

[12] N. Krishnan, P. M. Buchanan, N. Dzebisashvili, H. Xiao, M. A. Schnitzler, and D. C. Brennan, "Monozygotic transplantation: Concerns and opportunities," *American Journal of Transplantation*, vol. 8, no. 11, pp. 2343–2351, 2008.

[13] K. K. Yong, E. Y. Hye, H. K. Su et al., "Long-term follow-up of three identical twin transplant recipients without maintenance immunosuppressive therapy," *Nephrology*, vol. 13, no. 5, pp. 447-448, 2008.

[14] D. M. St. Clair, J. B. St. Clair, C. P. Swainson, F. Bamforth, and G. A. Machin, "Twin zygosity testing for medical purposes," *American Journal of Medical Genetics*, vol. 77, no. 5, pp. 412–414, 1998.

[15] E. Day, P. K. Kearns, C. J. Taylor, and J. A. Bradley, "Transplantation between monozygotic twins: How identical are they?" *Transplantation*, vol. 98, no. 5, pp. 485–489, 2014.

[16] P. Gringras and W. Chen, "Mechanisms for differences in monozygous twins," *Early Human Development*, vol. 64, no. 2, pp. 105–117, 2001.

[17] C. H. Tzeng, J. Y. Lyou, Y. R. Chen et al., "Polymerase chain reaction-amplified short tandem repeat analysis for single parentage testing in Taiwan," *Journal of Genetics and Molecular Biology*, vol. 11, pp. 93–98, 2000.

[18] M.-J. Yang, C.-H. Tzeng, J.-Y. Tseng, and C.-Y. Huang, "Determination of twin zygosity using a commercially available STR analysis of 15 unlinked loci and the gender-determining marker amelogenin - A preliminary report," *Human Reproduction*, vol. 21, no. 8, pp. 2175–2179, 2006.

[19] G. Machin, "Non-identical monozygotic twins, intermediate twin types, zygosity testing, and the non-random nature of monozygotic twinning: A review," *American Journal of Medical Genetics Part C: Seminars in Medical Genetics*, vol. 151, no. 2, pp. 110–127, 2009.

[20] G. W. Montgomery, G. Zhu, J. J. Hottenga et al., "HLA and genomwide allele sharing in dizygotic twins," *The American Journal of Human Genetics*, vol. 79, article 1052, 2006.

[21] P. Boros and J. S. Bromberg, "New cellular and molecular immune pathways in ischemia/reperfusion injury," *American Journal of Transplantation*, vol. 6, no. 4, pp. 652–658, 2006.

[22] A. Siedlecki, W. Irish, and D. C. Brennan, "Delayed graft function in the kidney transplant," *American Journal of Transplantation*, vol. 11, no. 11, pp. 2279–2296, 2011.

[23] H. S. Pollinger, M. D. Stegall, J. M. Gloor et al., "Kidney transplantation in patients with antibodies against donor HLA class II," *American Journal of Transplantation*, vol. 7, no. 4, pp. 857–863, 2007.

[24] Q. Mao, P. I. Terasaki, J. Cai et al., "Extremely high association between appearance of HLA antibodies and failure of kidney grafts in a five-year longitudinal study," *American Journal of Transplantation*, vol. 7, no. 4, pp. 864–871, 2007.

[25] M. A. Mujtaba, W. Goggins, A. Lobashevsky et al., "The strength of donor-specific antibody is a more reliable predictor of antibody-mediated rejection than flow cytometry crossmatch analysis in desensitized kidney recipients," *Clinical Transplantation*, vol. 25, no. 1, pp. E96–E102, 2011.

[26] J. M. Gloor, J. L. Winters, L. D. Cornell et al., "Baseline donor-specific antibody levels and outcomes in positive crossmatch kidney transplantation," *American Journal of Transplantation*, vol. 10, no. 3, pp. 582–589, 2010.

[27] A. Rana, B. Murthy, Z. Pallister et al., "Profiling risk for acute rejection in kidney transplantation: recipient age is a robust risk factor," *Journal of Nephrology*, vol. 30, no. 6, pp. 859–868, 2017.

[28] B. A. Bradley, "Rejection and recipient age," *Transplant Immunology*, vol. 10, no. 2-3, pp. 125–132, 2002.

[29] D. Weiskopf, B. Weinberger, and B. Grubeck-Loebenstein, "The aging of the immune system," *Transplant International*, vol. 22, no. 11, pp. 1041–1050, 2009.

Permissions

All chapters in this book were first published in CRT, by Hindawi Publishing Corporation; hereby published with permission under the Creative Commons Attribution License or equivalent. Every chapter published in this book has been scrutinized by our experts. Their significance has been extensively debated. The topics covered herein carry significant findings which will fuel the growth of the discipline. They may even be implemented as practical applications or may be referred to as a beginning point for another development.

The contributors of this book come from diverse backgrounds, making this book a truly international effort. This book will bring forth new frontiers with its revolutionizing research information and detailed analysis of the nascent developments around the world.

We would like to thank all the contributing authors for lending their expertise to make the book truly unique. They have played a crucial role in the development of this book. Without their invaluable contributions this book wouldn't have been possible. They have made vital efforts to compile up to date information on the varied aspects of this subject to make this book a valuable addition to the collection of many professionals and students.

This book was conceptualized with the vision of imparting up-to-date information and advanced data in this field. To ensure the same, a matchless editorial board was set up. Every individual on the board went through rigorous rounds of assessment to prove their worth. After which they invested a large part of their time researching and compiling the most relevant data for our readers.

The editorial board has been involved in producing this book since its inception. They have spent rigorous hours researching and exploring the diverse topics which have resulted in the successful publishing of this book. They have passed on their knowledge of decades through this book. To expedite this challenging task, the publisher supported the team at every step. A small team of assistant editors was also appointed to further simplify the editing procedure and attain best results for the readers.

Apart from the editorial board, the designing team has also invested a significant amount of their time in understanding the subject and creating the most relevant covers. They scrutinized every image to scout for the most suitable representation of the subject and create an appropriate cover for the book.

The publishing team has been an ardent support to the editorial, designing and production team. Their endless efforts to recruit the best for this project, has resulted in the accomplishment of this book. They are a veteran in the field of academics and their pool of knowledge is as vast as their experience in printing. Their expertise and guidance has proved useful at every step. Their uncompromising quality standards have made this book an exceptional effort. Their encouragement from time to time has been an inspiration for everyone.

The publisher and the editorial board hope that this book will prove to be a valuable piece of knowledge for researchers, students, practitioners and scholars across the globe.

List of Contributors

Julie Belliere, Arnaud Del Bello, Laure Esposito and Isabelle Cardeau Desangles
Department of Nephrology and Organ Transplantation, CHU Rangueil, TSA 50032, 31059 Toulouse Cedex 9, France

Céline Guilbeau-Frugier and Caroline Capuani
Université Paul Sabatier, 31062 Toulouse, France
Department of Pathology, CHU Rangueil, 31059 Toulouse, France

Lionel Rostaing and Nassim Kamar
Department of Nephrology and Organ Transplantation, CHU Rangueil, TSA 50032, 31059 Toulouse Cedex 9, France
Université Paul Sabatier, 31062 Toulouse, France
INSERM U1043, IFR-BMT, CHU Purpan, 31059 Toulouse, France

L. Friedrich, F. Barbey, M. Pascual and J.-P. Venetz
Centre de Transplantation d'Organes, Centre Hospitalier Universitaire Vaudois, Avenue du Bugnon 46,
1011 Lausanne, Switzerland

Vivek B. Kute, Himanshu V. Patel, Manoj R. Gumber, Pankaj R. Shah and Hargovind L. Trivedi
Department of Nephrology and Clinical Transplantation, Institute of Kidney Diseases and Research Center, Dr. H. L. Trivedi Institute of Transplantation Sciences (IKDRC-ITS), Civil Hospital Campus, Asarwa, Ahmedabad, Gujarat 380016, India

Aruna V. Vanikar
Department of Pathology, Laboratory Medicine, Transfusion Services and Immunohematology, IKDRC-ITS, Ahmedabad, India

Pranjal R.Modi
Department of Urology and Transplantation, IKDRC-ITS, Ahmedabad, India

Kazuro Kikkawa, Takahito Wakamiya, Hiroki Kusumoto, Nagahide Matsumura, Yasuo Kohjimoto and Isao Hara
Department of Urology, Wakayama Medical University, 811-1 Kimiidera, Wakayama 641-0012, Japan

C. Estrada, H. Suh and E. P. Nord
Division of Nephrology, Department of Medicine, School of Medicine, State University of New York at Stony Brook, HSC T-16 Rm 080, Stony Brook, NY 11794, USA

A. G. Desai
Division of Pulmonology, Department of Medicine, School of Medicine, State University of New York at Stony Brook, Stony Brook, NY 11794, USA

L. M. Chirch
Division of Infectious Diseases, Department of Medicine, School of Medicine, State University of New York at Stony Brook, Stony Brook, NY 11794, USA

R. Seidman
Department of Pathology, School of Medicine, State University of New York at Stony Brook, Stony Brook, NY 11794, USA

F. Darras
Transplantation Services, School of Medicine, State University of New York at Stony Brook, Stony Brook, NY 11794, USA

Michael V. Holmes and Rachel Hilton
Directorate of Nephrology, Transplantation and Urology, Guy's Hospital, Guy's and St Thomas' NHS Foundation Trust, London SE1 9RT, UK

Ranjababu Kulasegaram
Department of HIV and Genitourinary Medicine, Guy's and St Thomas' NHS Foundation Trust, London SE19RT, UK

Sebastian B. Lucas
Department of Histopathology, Guy's and St Thomas' NHS Foundation Trust, London SE19RT, UK

Terry Wong
Department of Gastroenterology, Guy's and St Thomas' NHS Foundation Trust, London SE19RT, UK

Yingchun Wang, Wei Li and Ping L. Zhang
Department of Anatomic and Clinical Pathology, Beaumont Health System, Royal Oak, MI 48073, USA

Mona Doshi
Division of Nephrology, Wayne State University School of Medicine, Detroit, MI 48201, USA

Salman Khan
Dallas Nephrology Associates, Dallas, TX 75204, USA

M. Tozzi
Vascular Surgery, Insubria University, Circolo University Teaching Hospital, Via Guicciardini 9, 21100 Varese, Italy

B. Molteni, M. Franchin, G. Ietto, G. Soldini, V. Bertocchi and G. Carcano
Department of Organ Transplant, Insubria University, Circolo University Teaching Hospital, Via Guicciardini 9, 21100 Varese, Italy

Joanna C. Masters
Skaggs School of Pharmacy and Pharmaceutical Sciences, University of California, San Diego, La Jolla, CA 92093, USA

Mita M. Shah
University of California, San Diego Medical Center, Center for Transplantation, La Jolla, CA 92037, USA
University of California, San Diego Medical Center, Department of Medicine, Division of Nephrology and Hypertension, San Diego, CA 92103, USA'

Ashley A. Feist
University of California, San Diego Medical Center, Center for Transplantation, La Jolla, CA 92037, USA

Catherine Quinlan, Atif Awan and Denis Gill
Paediatric Renal Transplant Centre, The Children's University Hospital, Temple Street, Dublin 1, Ireland

Mary Waldron
Our Lady's Children's Hospital, Crumlin, Dublin 12, Ireland

Dilly Little, David Hickey and Peter Conlon
Renal Transplant Unit, Beaumont Hospital, Dublin 9, Ireland

Mary Keogan
National Histocompatibility and Immunogenetics Services for Solid Organ Transplantation, Beaumont Hospital, Dublin 9, Ireland

Vital Hevia, Victoria Gómez, Sara Álvarez, Víctor Díez Nicolás, Carmen Gómez del Cañizo, Andrea Orosa and F. J. Burgos Revilla
Department of Urology, Hospital Ramón y Cajal, Ctra. Colmenar km 9, 100, 28034 Madrid, Spain
Cristina Galeano Álvarez
Department of Nephrology, Hospital Ramón y Cajal, Ctra. Colmenar km 9, 100, 28034 Madrid, Spain

Michael Sosin and Matthew Cooper
Medstar Georgetown Transplant Institute, Georgetown University Hospital, 3800 Reservoir Road, NW, Main Hospital Building, Second Floor, Washington, DC 20007, USA

Wuya Lumeh
Georgetown University School of Medicine, Medical Dental Building, 3900 Reservoir Road, NW, Washington, DC 20057, USA

Zhanyong Bing and John E. Tomaszewski
Department of Pathology and Laboratory Medicine, Hospital of the University of Pennsylvania, 3400 Spruce Street, Philadelphia, PA 19104, USA

Mahesh Eswarappa, P. Vijay Varma, Rakesh Madhyastha, Sujeeth Reddy, M. S. Gireesh and K. C. Gurudev
Department of Nephrology, M. S. Ramaiah Medical College and Teaching Hospital, MSR Nagar, MSRIT Post, Bangalore, Karnataka 560054, India

Vijaya V. Mysorekar
Department of Pathology, M. S. Ramaiah Medical College and Teaching Hospital, MSR Nagar, MSRIT Post, Bangalore, Karnataka 560054, India

Beena Hemanth
Department of Microbiology, M. S. Ramaiah Medical College and Teaching Hospital, MSR Nagar, MSRIT Post, Bangalore, Karnataka 560054, India

Sumayah Askandarani
Division of Nephrology, Department of Medicine, King Abdulaziz Medical City, Riyadh 11426, Saudi Arabia

Noura Aloudah and Hanan Al Enazi
Department of Pathology and Laboratory Medicine, King Abdulaziz Medical City, Riyadh 11426, Saudi Arabia

Khaled O. Alsaad
Department of Pathology and Laboratory Medicine, King Abdulaziz Medical City, Riyadh 11426, Saudi Arabia
King Abdullah International Medical Research Centre and College of Medicine, King Saud bin Abdulaziz University for Health Sciences, King Abdulaziz Medical City, Riyadh 11426, Saudi Arabia

Abdulrahman Altamimi
Department of Hepatobiliary Sciences and Liver Transplantation, King Abdulaziz Medical City, Riyadh 11426, Saudi Arabia

Dean Markić, Maksim Valenčić, Anton Maričić, Kristian Krpina, Dražen Rahelić, Juraj Ahel and Nino Rubinić
Department of Urology, University Hospital Rijeka, 51000 Rijeka, Croatia

Lidija Orlić and Sanjin Rački
Department of Nephrology and Dialysis, University Hospital Rijeka, 51000 Rijeka, Croatia

Matteo Tozzi
Vascular Surgery, Department of Surgery and Center for Research on Organ Transplantation, Insubria University School of Medicine, Circolo University Hospital, 21100 Varese, Italy

Luigi Boni, Gabriele Soldini and Marco Franchin
General Surgery 1, Department of Surgery and Center for Research on Organ Transplantation, Insubria University School of Medicine, Circolo University Hospital, 21100 Varese, Italy

Gabriele Piffaretti
Vascular Surgery, Department of Surgery and Morphological Sciences, Insubria University School of Medicine, Circolo University Hospital, Via Guicciardini 9, 21100 Varese, Italy

Rachael Leek, Erika Aldag, Iram Nadeem and Vikraman Gunabushanam
Department of Abdominal Transplant, Aurora St. Luke's Medical Center, Milwaukee, WI, USA

Ajay Sahajpal
Department of Abdominal Transplant, Aurora St. Luke's Medical Center, Milwaukee, WI, USA
University of Wisconsin School of Medicine and Public Health, Madison, WI 53726, USA

David J. Kramer
University of Wisconsin School of Medicine and Public Health, Madison, WI 53726, USA
Department of Critical Care, Aurora St. Luke's Medical Center, Milwaukee, WI, USA

Thomas J.Walsh
Weill Cornell Medicine, Cornell University and New York Presbyterian Hospital, New York, NY, USA

G. Schlaf, E. Schabel and W. Altermann
Tissue Typing Laboratory (GHATT), University Hospital Halle/Saale, Magdeburger Straße 16, 06112 Halle, Germany

B. Pollok-Kopp
Department of Transfusion Medicine, University Hospital Göttingen, Robert-Koch-Straße 40, 37075 Göttingen, Germany

Dilip Samarapungavan, Krishna Pothugunta, Gampala Reddy, Leslie Rocher, Francis Dumler, Vandad Raofi, Steven Cohn and Alan Koffron
Division of Nephrology and Transplantation, William-Beaumont Hospital, Royal Oak, MI 48037, USA

Ravi Parasuraman
Division of Nephrology and Transplantation, William-Beaumont Hospital, Royal Oak, MI 48037, USA
Kidney Transplant Outreach Program, William-Beaumont Hospital, Royal Oak, MI 48037, USA
Oakland University, William Beaumont School of Medicine, Royal Oak, MI 48037, USA

Ping L. Zhang
Division of Renal Pathology, William-Beaumont Hospital, Royal Oak, MI 48037, USA

Dilip Samarapungavan, Leslie Rocher and Alan Koffron
Division of Transplantation and Department of Pathology, Royal Oak, MI 48703, USA

Ravi Parasuraman
Division of Transplantation and Department of Pathology, Royal Oak, MI 48703, USA
Oakland University William Beaumont School of Medicine, William Beaumont Hospital, Royal Oak, MI 48703, USA

Ping L. Zhang
Beaumont Health System, Royal Oak, MI 48703, USA

Masataka Banshodani, Hideki Kawanishi, Seiji Marubayashi, Sadanori Shintaku, Misaki Moriishi and Shinichiro Tsuchiya
Department of Artificial Organs, Akane-Foundation, Tsuchiya General Hospital, 3-30 Nakajimacho, Naka-ku, Hiroshima 730-8655, Japan

Fumio Shimamoto
Department of Pathology, Faculty of Human Culture and Science, Prefectural University of Hiroshima, 1-1-71 Ujina-Higashi, Minami-ku, Hiroshima 734-8558, Japan

Kiyohiko Dohi
Department of Surgery, Akane-Foundation, Tsuchiya GeneralHospital, 3-30 Nakajimacho, Naka-ku, Hiroshima 730-8655, Japan

Hideki Ohdan
Department of Gastroenterological and Transplant Surgery, Applied Life Sciences, Institution of Biomedical and Health Sciences, Hiroshima University, 1-2-3 Kasumi, Minami-ku, Hiroshima 734-8551, Japan

Morgan S. Martin and Alison A. Smith
Department of Surgery, Tulane University School of Medicine, New Orleans, LA, USA

Monica Lobo
Department of Pathology, Tulane University, School of Medicine, New Orleans, LA, USA

Anil S. Paramesh
Tulane University School of Medicine, Tulane Abdominal Transplant Institute, New Orleans, LA, USA

Srey Ram Kuy
Division of Vascular Surgery, Department of Surgery, Medical College of Wisconsin, 9200WWisconsin Avenue, Milwaukee, WI 53226, USA

Chun He
Department of Pathology, Medical College of Wisconsin, Milwaukee, WI, USA

David C. Cronin II
Division of Transplantation, Department of Surgery, Medical College of Wisconsin, Milwaukee, WI, USA

Hugo Bonatti
Department of Surgery, Vanderbilt University Medical Center, Nashville, TN, USA
Meritus Surgical Specialists, Hagerstown, MD, USA

Naureen Iqbal
Department of Surgery, Vanderbilt University Medical Center, Nashville, TN, USA
Geisinger, Wilkes-Barre, PA, USA

Catherine Kling
Department of Surgery, Vanderbilt University Medical Center, Nashville, TN, USA
Surgery, University of Washington, Seattle, WA, USA

Willie Melvin
Department of Surgery, Vanderbilt University Medical Center, Nashville, TN, USA
Stone Crest Medical Center Clinic, Smyrna, TN, USA

James Broome
Department of Surgery, Vanderbilt University Medical Center, Nashville, TN, USA
St.Thomas Endocrine Surgical Specialists, Nashville, TN, USA

Pradeep V. Kadambi and Ann K. Gamilla-Crudo
University of Texas Medical Branch, 301 University Boulevard, Galveston, TX 77555, USA

Mohammad Almiani, Michelle A. Josephson and W. James Chon
University of Chicago, 5841 S Maryland Avenue, MC 5100, Chicago, IL 60637, US

Emma J. Griffin
University of Glasgow Medical School, Glasgow G12 8QQ, UK

Peter C. Thomson, Marc Clancy and Conal Daly
Renal Unit, Western Infirmary, Dumbarton Road, Glasgow G11 6NT, UK

David Kipgen
Department of Pathology, Southern General Hospital, Glasgow G51 4TF, UK

Bruna Natacha Leite Costa, Constantino Fernández Rivera, Maria Calvo Rodríguez, Andrés López Muñiz, Tamara Ferreiro Hermida and Ángel Alonso Hernández
Department of Nephrology, Xerencia de Xestión Integrada A Coruña, A Coruña, Spain

Felipe Sacristán Lista, Pilar Iglesias Díaz and Teresa Hermida Romero
Department of Pathological Anatomy, Xerencia de Xestión Integrada A Coruña, A Coruña, Spain

Makoto Ryosaka, Kazuya Omoto, Taiji Nozaki, Kazuhiko Yoshida, Yugo Sawada, Hajime Hirano, Tomokazu Shimizu, Hideki Ishida and Kazunari Tanabe
Department of Urology, Tokyo Women's Medical University, 8-1 Kawada-cho, Shinjuku-ku, Tokyo 162-8666, Japan

Gao Hongjun, Luo Xiangdong, Liang Taisheng, Lu Shangguang, Liang FangFang, Dong Yu, Tan Zhen and Wu Zhen
RuiKang Hospital, Affiliated to GuangXi Chinese Traditional Medicine College, Nanning 530011, China

Christine Chmielewski
Department of Medicine, Thomas Jefferson University, 2228 South Broad Street, Philadelphia, PA 19145, USA

Edward J. Filippone, Rakesh Gulati and Eric Newman
Department of Medicine, Thomas Jefferson University, 2228 South Broad Street, Philadelphia, PA 19145, USA
Division of Nephrology, Thomas Jefferson University, Philadelphia, PA 19107, USA

John L. Farber
Department of Pathology, Thomas Jefferson University, Philadelphia, PA 19107, USA

Gabriele Piffaretti
Vascular Surgery, Department of Surgery and Morphological Sciences, Insubria University School of Medicine, Circolo University Teaching Hospital, Via Guicciardini 9, 21100 Varese, Italy

Marco Franchin and Matteo Tozzi
Vascular Surgery, Department of Surgery and Morphological Sciences, Insubria University School of Medicine, Circolo University Teaching Hospital, Via Guicciardini 9, 21100 Varese, Italy

Center for Research on Organ Transplantation, Insubria University School of Medicine, Circolo University Teaching Hospital, 21100 Varese, Italy

Gabriele Soldini
Center for Research on Organ Transplantation, Insubria University School of Medicine, Circolo University Teaching Hospital, 21100 Varese, Italy
General Surgery 1, Department of Surgery and Morphological Sciences, Insubria University School of Medicine, Circolo University Teaching Hospital, 21100 Varese, Italy

Alexander Bullen and Mita M. Shah
Division of Nephrology-Hypertension, University of California San Diego, San Diego, CA, USA

Saúl Pampa-Saico, Sara Jiménez-Alvaro, Fernando Caravaca-Fontán, Ana Fernández-Rodríguez and Roberto Marcén
Department of Nephrology, Hospital Universitario Ramón y Cajal, Carretera de Colmenar Viejo Km. 9.100, 28034 Madrid, Spain

Maite Rivera-Gorrín
Department of Nephrology, Hospital Universitario Ramón y Cajal, Carretera de Colmenar Viejo Km. 9.100, 28034 Madrid, Spain
Department of Medicine, Universidad de Alcalá, 28805 Madrid, Spain

Juan Sánchez
Department of Radiology, Hospital Universitario Ramón y Cajal, 28034 Madrid, Spain

Antonio Chinchilla
Department of Vascular Surgery, Hospital Universitario Ramón y Cajal, 28034 Madrid, Spain

Ryan J. Hendrix, Paulo N. Martins, Aaron Ahearn, Adel Bozorgzadeh and Babak Movahedi
University of Massachusetts Medical School, Department of Surgery, Division of Organ Transplantation, USA

Jeffrey S. Stoff
University of Massachusetts Medical School, Department of Medicine, Division of Nephrology, USA

Judith Desoutter, Marie-Joëlle Apithy, Ségolène Bartczak and Nicolas Guillaume
Department of Histocompatibility, Amiens University Medical Center, 80000 Amiens, France

Akihito Sannomiya, Ichiro Nakajima, Yuichi Ogawa, Kotaro Kai, Ichiro Koyama and Shohei Fuchinoue
Department of Surgery, Kidney Center, Tokyo Women's Medical University, Tokyo, Japan

Luca Lanfranco, Arnaud Del Bello and Laure Esposito
Department of Nephrology and Organ Transplantation, CHU Rangueil, Toulouse, France

Melanie Joly, Noelle Cognard, Peggy Perrin, Bruno Moulin and Sophie Caillard
Department of Nephrology and Transplantation, University Hospital of Strasbourg, Strasbourg, France

Nassim Kamar
Department of Nephrology and Organ Transplantation, CHU Rangueil, Toulouse, France
Université Paul Sabatier, Toulouse, France
INSERM U1043, IFR-BMT, CHU Purpan, Toulouse, France

Tamara Wanigasekera, Donal J. Sexton and Colm Magee
Transplant, Urology and Nephrology Directorate, Beaumont Hospital, Dublin 9, Ireland

Rachel J. Grainger
Department of Clinical Microbiology, Beaumont Hospital, Dublin 9, Ireland

Felix Cheung, MerritMarion Debartolo and April Adams Szafran
Department of Urology, Stony Brook University Medical Center, Stony Brook, NY 11794, USA

Leonard Michael Copertino
Department of Surgery, Stony Brook University Medical Center, Stony Brook, NY 11794, USA

Chelsea Caron Estrada
Department of Transplant, Stony Brook University Medical Center, Stony Brook, NY 11794, USA

Patrick Gerard Lynch
Division of Nephrology, Stony Brook University Medical Center, Stony Brook, NY 11794, USA

Frank Sam Darras
Department of Urology, Stony Brook University Medical Center, Stony Brook, NY 11794, USA
Department of Transplant, Stony Brook University Medical Center, Stony Brook, NY 11794, USA

Hannelore Sprenger-Mähr, Emanuel Zitt and Karl Lhotta
Department of Nephrology and Dialysis, Academic Teaching Hospital Feldkirch, 6800 Feldkirch, Austria
Vorarlberg Institute for Vascular Investigation and Treatment, Academic Teaching Hospital Feldkirch, 6800 Feldkirch, Austria

Afschin Soleiman
Clinical Pathology and Cytodiagnostics, 6060 Hall in Tirol, Austria

Noura Aloudah and Khaled O. Alsaad
Department of Pathology and Laboratory Medicine, King Abdulaziz Medical City, Riyadh, Saudi Arabia
College of Medicine, King Saud bin Abdulaziz University for Health Sciences, Riyadh, Saudi Arabia

Abdullah Alharbi
Department of Pathology and Laboratory Medicine, King Abdulaziz Medical City, Riyadh, Saudi Arabia

Maram S. Al Turki
College of Medicine, King Saud bin Abdulaziz University for Health Sciences, Riyadh, Saudi Arabia

Tracey Salter, Hannah Burton and Rachel Hilton
Departments of Nephrology and Transplantation, Guy's and St Thomas' NHS Foundation Trust, London, UK

Sam Douthwaite
Department of Virology, Guy's and St Thomas' NHS Foundation Trust, London, UK

William Newsholme
Department of Infectious Diseases, Guy's and St Thomas' NHS Foundation Trust, London, UK

Catherine Horsfield
Department of Histopathology, Guy's and St Thomas' NHS Foundation Trust, London, UK

Yuta Takezawa, Yoshifumi Kadono, Takahiro Nohara and Atsushi Mizokami
Department of Urology, Kanazawa University Hospital, 13-1 Takara-machi, Kanazawa, Japan

Ian Zheng, Mahmoud Alameddine, Joshua S. Jue, Ali Yusufali and Gaetano Ciancio
Department of Surgery, Division of Transplantation, Miami Transplant Institute, University of Miami Miller School of Medicine, Miami, FL 33136, USA

Yaohong Tan
Department of Pathology, University of Miami Miller School of Medicine, Miami, FL 33136, USA

Zhobin Moghadamyeghaneh
Department of Surgery, Division of Transplantation, Miami Transplant Institute, University of Miami Miller School of Medicine, Miami, FL 33136, USA
Department of Surgery, University of California, San Francisco, CA 94143, USA

Ahmed Farag
Department of Surgery, Division of Transplantation, Miami Transplant Institute, University of Miami Miller School of Medicine, Miami, FL 33136, USA
Department of Surgery, Zagazig University School of Medicine, Zagazig, Egypt

A. J. Vicéns-Morton, C. Callaghan and J. Olsburgh
Guy's and StThomas NHS Foundation Trust, Renal Department, London, UK

Jose Iglesias
Department of Nephrology, Jersey Shore University Medical Center, Neptune, NJ 07753, USA
Rowan University School of Osteopathic Medicine, Stratford, NJ 08084, USA

Kandria Jumil Ledesma and Paul J. Couto
American University of Antigua College of Medicine, Coolidge, Antigua and Barbuda

Jessie Liu
Ocean Renal Associates, 210 Jack Martin Boulevard, Brick, NJ 08724, USA

Raj Purgus and Tristan Legris
Centre de Néphrologie et Transplantation Rénale, Hôpital Conception, Assistance Publique-Hôpitaux de Marseille, Marseille, France

Romain Vial, Alexandre Decourt, Noémie Jourde-Chiche and Valérie Moal
Centre de Néphrologie et Transplantation Rénale, Hôpital Conception, Assistance Publique-Hôpitaux de Marseille, Marseille, France
Aix-Marseille University, Marseille, France

Christine Zandotti
Fédération de Bactériologie-Virologie-Hygiène, Hôpital Timone, Assistance Publique-Hôpitaux de Marseille, Marseille, France

Sophie Alain
Laboratoire de Bactériologie-Virologie-Hygiène, Centre Hospitalier Universitaire, Limoges, France

Charleric Bornet
Pharmacie Hospitalière, Hôpital Conception, Assistance Publique-Hôpitaux de Marseille, Marseille, France

Laurent Daniel
Aix-Marseille University, Marseille, France
Laboratoire d'Anatomie Pathologique, Hôpital Timone, Assistance Publique-Hôpitaux de Marseille, Marseille, France

Shohei Kawaguchi, Takashi Shima and Chikashi Seto
Department of Urology, Toyama Prefectural Central Hospital, Toyama, Japan

Takahiro Nohara, SatokoMatsuyama, Yoshifumi Kadono and Atsushi Mizokami
Department of Integrative CancerTherapy and Urology, Kanazawa University Graduate School of Medical Science, Kanazawa, Japan

Chikako Nose, Junya Yamahana and Masahiko Kawabata
Department of Internal Medicine, Toyama Prefectural Central Hospital, Toyama, Japan

R. C. Minnee, H. J. A. N. Kimenai and J. N. M. Ijzermans
Department of Surgery, Division of HPB and Transplant Surgery, Erasmus University Medical Center (Erasmus MC), Rotterdam, Netherlands

J. van de Wetering
Department of Nephrology, Erasmus University Medical Center (Erasmus MC), Rotterdam, Netherlands

Deepak Shankar Ray and Sharmila Thukral
Rabindranath Tagore International Institute of Cardiac Sciences, Narayana Health Hospitals, 124 EM Bypass, Mukundapur, Kolkata, India

Massini Merzkani, Ezra Israel and Mala Sachdeva
Division of Kidney Diseases and Hypertension, North Shore University Hospital and Long Island Jewish Medical Center, Hofstra Northwell School of Medicine, Great Neck, NY, USA

Go Anan, Masaki Shimbo, Fumiyasu Endo and Kazunori Hattori
Department of Urology, St. Luke's International Hospital, Tokyo, Japan

Koji Nanmoku, Takaaki Kimura, Yasunaru Sakuma and Takashi Yagisawa
Surgical Branch, Institute of Kidney Diseases, Jichi Medical University Hospital, Shimotsuke, Japan

Masahiko Nagahama and Yasuhiro Komatsu
Division of Nephrology, Department of Medicine, St. Luke's International Hospital, Tokyo, Japan

Giovanni Varotti, Alessia Terulla, Massimo Bertocchi and Iris Fontana
Kidney Transplant Unit, IRCCS San Martino University Hospital, IST National Institute for Cancer Research, Genoa, Italy

Ferdinando Dodi
Department of Infectious Disease, IRCCS San Martino University Hospital, IST National Institute for Cancer Research, Genoa, Italy

Anna Marchese
Department of Microbiology, IRCCS San Martino University Hospital, IST National Institute for Cancer Research, Genoa, Italy

Idris Yakubu and Tracy Sparkes
Pharmacy, University of Maryland Medical Center, Baltimore, MD, USA

Abdolreza Haririan and Stephen Bartlett
University of Maryland School of Medicine, Baltimore, MD, USA

Index

P

R

S

T

U

V